Adversity, Stress, and Psychopathology

ADVERSITY, STRESS, AND PSYCHOPATHOLOGY

Edited by
BRUCE P. DOHRENWEND

New York   Oxford
OXFORD UNIVERSITY PRESS
1998

Oxford University Press

Oxford   New York
Athens   Auckland   Bangkok   Bogota
Bombay   Buenos Aires   Calcutta   Cape Town
Dar es Salaam   Delhi   Florence   Hong Kong   Istanbul
Karachi   Kuala Lumpur   Madras   Madrid
Melbourne   Mexico City   Nairobi   Paris
Singapore   Taipei   Tokyo   Toronto   Warsaw

and associated companies in
Berlin   Ibadan

Library of Congress Cataloging-in-Publication Data
Adversity, stress, and psychopathology /
edited by Bruce P. Dohrenwend.
p.   cm.
Includes bibliographical references and index.
ISBN 0-19-512192-9
1. Mental illness — Etiology.   2. Suffering — Psychological aspects.
3. Stress (Psychology).   4. Stress (Physiology).
5. Psychology, Pathological — Etiology.
I. Dohrenwend, Bruce Philip, 1927 – .
RC455.4.S87A39   1998   616.89′071 — dc21   97-41525

9   8   7   6   5   4   3   2   1

Printed in the United States of America
on acid-free paper

To Barbara

Preface

When I began research on adversity, stress and psychopathology 40 years ago, environmental factors were generally thought to be the main causes of all the major types of psychiatric disorder with no known organic basis. This assumption about environmental primacy has been giving way over the past 25–30 years to a *Zeitgeist* favoring biological factors that trace mainly to genetic inheritance.

Such shifts have happened before, with the result that important work gets neglected and important lines of research go under- or unexplored. As it has done in the past in the other direction, I believe that the pendulum of ideas about causation has swung too far—this time away from environmental factors rather than biological factors. I have organized this book in an attempt to put things in better balance by demonstrating that environmental adversity and stress play major roles in the development of psychopathology, and by suggesting how much more can be learned about their contribution.

The starting point for this volume was a conference on the title theme at the 1994 Annual Meeting of the American Psychopathological Association (APPA) where most of the contributors gave presentations. Since then these presentations have been expanded into chapters and supplemented by additional contributions to increase coverage. Many of the chapters were revised and updated even in the month before the manuscript was submitted to Oxford University Press.

To be asked to set the theme and then to organize the APPA program was both an opportunity and a challenge. The opportunity was to bring together the work of an extraordinary group of researchers who have made major contributions to our knowledge of adversity, stress and psychopathology. The challenge was to assess the evidence from this work on the role of adversity and to integrate the leads from the various lines of work into a coherent framework that will facilitate understanding and provide a basis for further research.

I received a great deal of help in recruiting the investigators whose work appears in this volume. This assistance came from the scholars whose terms as APPA Officers and Council members overlapped with my terms as Vice President, President Elect and, then, President, of APPA. The other Officers and Council members were James Barrett, Magda Campbell, C. Robert Cloninger, Patricia Cohen, Ellen Frank, John E. Helzer, Leonard L. Heston, David S. Janowsky, Sheppard Kellam, Elizabeth Squires-Wheeler, and Myrna M. Weissman. The Officers and Council members also helped me to choose the winners of the Hoch and Zubin Awards, George W. Brown and Alexander H. Leighton, respectively, whose presentations are included in this volume.

The Chairperson of each the sessions, now expanded into Parts I–V of this book, was much more than a timekeeper. Each Chairperson formally commented on the papers in his or her session, and these commentaries were the bases for the Introductions to Parts I–V. When additional papers were added to a section following the meeting, I co-authored the introduction with the session chair and added comments on the additional papers. In addition, each session Chair shared with me the job of editorial review of the papers in his/her section as they were transformed into chapters. The Chairpersons were Morton Beiser, Evelyn J. Bromet, William W. Eaton, David Mechanic, and Robert M. Rose. I am most grateful to them.

I would also like to express my appreciation to Marian Reiff for assistance in getting this manuscript together that went well beyond the usual organizational tasks and could only have been provided by someone who is herself a research scientist. And my thanks go as well to my wife, Catherine J. Douglass. She is a lawyer, not a research scientist, and her critical readings of my Introduction to the volume as a whole and the two concluding chapters in Part VI were often a spur to greater clarity.

Finally, I would like to note that this book is dedicated to Barbara Snell Dohrenwend who died in 1982. Her influence has remained pervasive. I hope she would have liked what we have done.

B.P.D.

New York, N.Y.
August 1997

Contents

Contributors

PATRICIA ANDRESKI
Department of Psychiatry
Henry Ford Hospital
Detroit, Michigan 48202

JAMES C. ANTHONY
Prevention Research Center
Johns Hopkins University
School of Hygiene and Public Health
Baltimore, Maryland 21224

JOCELYNE BACHEVALIER
Department of Neurobiology
University of Texas Medical School
Houston, Texas 77030

MORTON BEISER
Culture Community & Health Study
Clarke Institute of Psychiatry
Toronto, Ontario MST IR8 Canada

CONNIE L. BEST
Medical University of South Carolina
Crime Victim Research and Treatment
   Center
Charleston, South Carolina 29425

NAOMI BRESLAU
Department of Psychiatry
Henry Ford Hospital
Detroit, Michigan 48202

EVELYN J. BROMET
Department of Psychiatry
State University of New York at Stony
   Brook
Stony Brook, New York 11794

GEORGE W. BROWN
Social Policy/Social Science
Bedford/Royal Holloway College
London WC1B 3RA England

MARTHA L. BRUCE
The New York Hospital—Cornell Medical
   Center
Westchester Division
Department of Psychiatry
White Plains, New York 10605

PAULA J. CLAYTON
Department of Psychiatry
University of Minnesota
Minneapolis, Minnesota 55455

GLENN DAVIS
Department of Psychiatry
Henry Ford Hospital
Detroit, Michigan 48202

MARY AMANDA DEW
University of Pittsburgh
Medical Center
Western Psychiatric Institute & Clinic
Pittsburgh, Pennsylvania 15213

BRUCE P. DOHRENWEND
Columbia University
New York State Psychiatric Institute
New York, New York 10032

WILLIAM W. EATON
Department of Mental Hygiene
School of Hygiene and Public Health
Johns Hopkins University
Baltimore, Maryland 21205

BELLE FEDERMAN
School of Hygiene and Public Health
Johns Hopkins University
Baltimore, Maryland 21224

ELLEN FRANK
University of Pittsburgh Medical Center
Western Psychiatric Institute
Pittsburgh, Pennsylvania 15213

ROBERT GIEL
WHO Collaborating Center
Academisch Ziekenhuis
9700 RB Groningen, The Netherlands

WESLEY E. HAWKINS
Prevention Research Center
Johns Hopkins University
School of Hygiene and Public Health
Baltimore, Maryland 21224

A. SCOTT HENDERSON
Psychiatric Epidemiology Research Center
The Australian National University
Canberra, ACT 2600 Australia

DANIEL B. HERMAN
Columbia University
New York State Psychiatric Institute
New York, New York 10032

JORDAN KARP
University of Pittsburgh Medical Center
Western Psychiatric Institute
Pittsburgh, Pennsylvania 15213

STANISLAV V. KASL
Department of Epidemiology and Public
    Health
Yale University School of Medicine
New Haven, Connecticut 06510

TERENCE M. KEANE
National Center for PTSD
VA Medical Center
Boston, Massachusetts 02130

KENNETH S. KENDLER
Department of Psychiatry
Medical College of Virginia
Virginia Commonwealth University
Richmond, Virginia 23298

SHEPPARD G. KELLAM
Prevention Research Center
Johns Hopkins University
School of Hygiene and Public Health
Baltimore, Maryland 21224

DEAN G. KILPATRICK
Medical University of South Carolina
Crime Victim Research and Treatment
    Center
Charleston, South Carolina 29425

ROBERT KOHN
Department of Psychiatry
Brown University
Butler Hospital
Providence, Rhode Island 02906

GARY W. KRAEMER
Department of Psychiatry
University of Wisconsin-Madison
Harlow Primate Laboratory
Madison, Wisconsin 53715

KATHRYN E. LASCH
The Health Institute
New England Medical Center
Boston, Massachusetts 02111

ALEXANDER H. LEIGHTON
Department of Community Health/
    Epidemiology
Faculty of Medicine, Dalhousie University
Halifax, Nova Scotia B3H 4H7 Canada

MARY CLARE LENNON
SMS School of Public Health
Columbia University
New York, New York 10032

ITZHAK LEVAV
Mental Health Program
Pan American Health Organization
World Health Organization
Washington, DC 20037

BRUCE G. LINK
New York State Psychiatric Institute
Columbia University
New York, New York 10032

LAWRENCE S. MAYER
Prevention Research Center
Johns Hopkins University
School of Hygiene and Public Health
Baltimore, Maryland 21224

DAVID MECHANIC
Institute for Health, Health Care Policy
    and Aging Research
Rutgers University
New Brunswick, New Jersey 08903

JERROLD MIROTZNIK
Brooklyn College
City University of New York
Brooklyn, New York 11210

RICHARD F. MOLLICA
Program in Refugee Trauma
Harvard University
Cambridge, Massachusetts 02138

GUEDALIA NAVEH
Department of Psychiatry
Columbia University
New York, New York 10032

SUZANNE C. OUELLETTE
Graduate School and University Center
The City University of New York
Department of Psychology
New York, New York 10036

CHARLES POOLE
Program in Refugee Trauma
Harvard University
Cambridge, Massachusetts 02138

GEORGE W. REBOK
Prevention Research Center
Johns Hopkins University
School of Hygiene and Public Health
Baltimore, Maryland 21224

HEIDI S. RESNICK
Medical University of South Carolina
Crime Victim Research and Treatment
    Center
Charleston, South Carolina 29425

JUDITH ROBERTSON
Department of Psychiatry
Washington University
St. Louis, Missouri 63110

LEE N. ROBINS
Department of Psychiatry
Washington University
St. Louis, Missouri 63110

EUNICE RODRIQUEZ
Department of Human Service Studies
Cornell University
Ithaca, New York 14853

ROBERT M. ROSE
McArthur Foundation
Health Program
Chicago, Illinois 60603

BENJAMIN E. SAUNDERS
Medical University of South Carolina
Crime Victim Research and Treatment
    Center
Charleston, South Carolina 29425

SHARON SCHWARTZ
School of Public Health
Columbia University
New York, New York 10032

PATRICK E. SHROUT
Department of Psychology
New York University
New York, New York 10003

ANDREW E. SKODOL
Columbia University
New York State Psychiatric Institute
New York, New York 10032

ANN STUEVE
School of Public Health
Columbia University
New York, New York 10032

EZRA S. SUSSER
Columbia University
New York State Psychiatric Institute
New York, New York 10032

ELMER L. STRUENING
Columbia University
New York State Psychiatric Institute
New York, New York 10032

SVANG TOR
Program in Refugee Trauma
Harvard University
Cambridge, Massachusetts 02138

CATHY SPATZ WIDOM
School of Criminal Justice
State University of New York at Albany
Albany, New York 12222

Adversity, Stress, and Psychopathology

Introduction

Bruce P. Dohrenwend

Over the years, assumptions about the causes of most of the behaviors that we now describe as "psychiatric disorders" have tended to change more with the Zeitgeist than with scientific evidence (see Dohrenwend & Dohrenwend, 1981a, pp. 131–133). In 1855, for example, when Edward Jarvis published his groundbreaking epidemiological research on the unusually high rates of "insanity" in the "pauper" class compared to rates in the "independent" class in Massachusetts, his assumption and that of other experts was that factors resulting from genetic inheritance were more important than social environmental factors in causing both the psychological problems and the poverty. Jarvis took particular note of the fact that disproportionately large numbers of the poor and insane were new Irish immigrants. As Grob (1971) pointed out in his historical introduction to the re-publication of Jarvis's study:

Like others coming from the same background, Jarvis saw the genteel New England society that he loved being eroded. . . . In a very real sense, therefore, some of the points that he attempted to make . . . were a reflection of his own ideology. . . . What Jarvis did was to take a series of statistics and read them in the light of his own moral assumptions. (p. 56)

Especially in the United States, this belief in the paramount role of genetic inheritance began to change under the impact of two major events: the stock market crash in 1929 followed by the Great Depression and the U.S. experience with World War II beginning in 1941 (see Leighton, Chapter 28, this volume). The Great Depression made it clear that a person could become poor for reasons other than inherited disabilities (e.g., Elder, 1974), and research during World War II showed that situations of extreme environmental stress arising out of combat and imprisonment could produce severe psychopathology in previously normal persons (see Dohrenwend & Dohrenwend, 1969; Dohrenwend, 1979), some of it long lasting (Beebe, 1975; Eitinger, 1964). In the United States especially, it became almost a given that environmental adversity was of paramount importance in the etiology of all of the major types of psychiatric disorder, including schizophrenia. The most sweeping statement of this position took the form of the proposition that sick and disorganized societies produced sick and disorganized citizens (e.g., Dunham, 1955; Faris & Dunham, 1939; Frank, 1936; Leighton, 1959). Similar ideas were put forward specifically about the putative causal role of lower "social class" or socioeconomic status (SES) (e.g., Hollingshead & Redlich, 1958; Srole et al., 1962).

The assumption about the primacy of environment has tended to give way since the 1960s as a Zeitgeist favoring biological factors, especially those that trace to genetic inheritance, has become dominant. This change has been coincident with the advent of new drug treatments and the strong research results from the family, twin, and adoption studies conducted by behavioral geneticists, especially with schizophrenia (e.g., Gottesman & Shields, 1976; Heston, 1966; Kety, 1965; Kety et al., 1976; Rosenthal & Kety, 1968). Moreover, the evidence from these three strategies is becoming compelling for other important types of disorders, including depression (Torgersen, 1986), alcoholism (Cloninger et al., 1981; Goodwin, 1979), drug abuse (Cadoret et al., 1986), and antisocial personality (Crowe, 1974; Hutchings & Mednick, 1975).

While these studies show that genetic factors contribute to these disorders, they also show that genetic factors alone cannot account for them (see Dohrenwend, 1976; Gottesman & Shields, 1976; Merikangas, 1990; Plomin, 1990). For example, even with schizophrenia, where the evidence for genetic factors is strongest, the concordance rate in monozygotic twins is far from 100%. For the environmentally oriented researcher, however, this argument by subtraction is not very satisfactory. He or she is faced with an inchoate pile of leftovers and the challenge to provide a similar demonstration that environmental factors are important in the etiology of any of these disorders. As Gottesman and Shields (1976) noted with regard to schizophrenia, "the burden of proof has shifted from showing that genes are important to showing that environment is important" (p. 367).

In the context of today's Zeitgeist and the persuasiveness of the behavioral genetics research, this challenge is more general than the one posed by Gottesman and Shields in relation to schizophrenia. In a paper titled "What About Environment?", for example, Heston (1988) starts with schizophrenia but goes much further:

Perhaps more effort has gone into defining environmental factors contributing to this disease than any other medical or surgical condition. Yet we cannot specify a single environmental contributor to etiology. Given a pair of newborn [monozygotic] twins and told that one of the pair will become schizophrenic, we could not specify environmental conditions that would produce schizophrenia in that twin. (p. 208)

Heston continues:

The same is true of affective illness, the anxiety states, and so on through our classification until at last we come to chemical dependency. Here are exceptions because we can specify environmental factors, for example, alcohol. If alcohol is not introduced, then alcoholism is not manifest. (p. 208)

Shortly after the appearance of Heston's paper, Guze (1989) published an article with a similarly challenging title, "Biological Psychiatry: Is There Any Other Kind?" In it, he wrote:

No one has presented convincing evidence that most individuals exposed to a particular psychologically meaningful experience develop a particular disorder. . . .

The point I am making is not that psychologically meaningful experiences are irrelevant to the development of psychiatric disorders. I remain agnostic about their ultimate importance because, in the great majority of instances, these putative causes of psychiatric disorders reflect only the usual range of human troubles that most people experience without becoming ill. (p. 317)

This text was organized in part as a response to this challenge. One of its purposes, therefore, is to examine evidence on the question of whether adverse environmental conditions are important in the etiology of psychiatric disorders. A second purpose is to develop a framework of concepts, ideas, and suggestions that will stimulate further research.

A START ON DEFINING ADVERSITY

Webster's Ninth New Collegiate Dictionary (1987) defines the adjective *adverse* as "acting against or in a contrary direction" and, more personally, as "opposed to one's interests" (p. 59). The noun *adversity* refers correspondingly to a "calamitous or disastrous experience" and "a condition of suffering, destitution, or affliction" (p. 59). A more inclusive synonym for adversity is *misfortune*, which, like adversity, "may apply to either the incident or conjunction of events that is the cause of an unhappy change of fortune or to the ensuing state of distress" (p. 759). "Adversity" itself "applies to a state of grave or persistent misfortune," as distinguished from *mishap*, which applies to a trivial instance of bad luck" (p. 759).

ADVERSE LIFE EVENTS

Life events can be important representations of adversity. Within the framework of the dictionary distinctions made above, we will restrict the definition of an adverse event to the actual incident regardless of the distressed reaction to it. We will also pay special attention to events that, as the dictionary definitions imply, represent "bad luck" in the sense that their occurrence is not influenced by the actions or behavior of the individual who experiences them. "Adversity" in this sense of ominous inevitability, regardless of the exposed person's prior behavior, defines the purest form of fateful environmental influence. It consists of a set of "unpropitious or calamitous" circumstances implying previous well-being (*Webster's*, 1961, p. 14). Near approximations of these fateful events, or combinations of such events, occur in natural and human-made disasters, including combat during wartime. These extreme situations are the subjects of Part I of this volume, with chapters by Levav on the Holocaust; Mollica, Poole, and Tor on the experiences of refugees from oppression in Cambodia; Keane on posttraumatic stress disorder (PTSD) in relation to exposure of U.S. soldiers to combat in Vietnam; and Giel on nonmilitary disasters.

Natural and human-made disasters that target whole communities or groups are, fortunately, rare at most times in most societies. Yet, as the review of epidemiological studies in Part III by Kohn, Dohrenwend,

and Mirotznik shows, psychopathology is not rare. Moreover, the various types of psychiatric disorders and symptoms of distress subsumed under the term *psychopathology* are not randomly distributed within societies. Rather, rates of various types of disorders and symptoms of distress vary with such factors as gender and SES. These differences in rates of psychopathology raise major questions about the possible impact of different exposure to adversity experienced by members of different groups; for example, the social causation–social selection issue posed by contrasting attempts to explain inverse relations between SES and various types of psychopathology that is investigated by Dohrenwend, Levav, Shrout, and their colleagues in Part III.

If we are to assess the role of event-related adversity in the occurrence of psychopathology in the general population, we must consider possibly stressful events that occur more frequently in the lives of individuals than the events in the extreme situations of human-made and natural disasters described in Part I. Individual examples of such major, stressful events in more usual situations are the topics of Part II of this volume. These include experiencing the death of a loved one (Clayton), undergoing a marital separation or divorce (Bruce), losing a job (Kasl, Rodriguez, and Lasch), becoming homeless (Herman, Susser, and Struening), suffering a serious physical illness or injury of various types (Dew), contracting HIV infection (Ouellette), or being a victim of child abuse (Widom) or rape (Kilpatrick, Resnick, Saunders, and Best). In assessing the impact of such experiences as representations of adversity, we must face the fact that the individual's behavior plays a large part in the occurrence of many of these events and that, to the extent that it does, individuals can create the "calamitous circumstances" to which they are exposed (see especially Stueve et al. and Robins and Robertson in Part III and Kendler in Part V). Their infidelity, for example, can lead to the institution of a divorce action by their spouses; their poor performance can precipitate loss of a job; their poor health habits can contribute to a serious physical illness; their carelessness, to an injury; and so on. Fatefulness, and hence the role of adverse environment in the sense of misfortune, is thus a matter of degree. The distinction, however, is of central importance in research on life events (Dohrenwend, 1979; Rutter, 1986, especially p. 1084). An analysis of the complexity of dealing with this question can be found in the concluding segment of this monograph (Part VI).

MODIFYING AND AMPLIFYING FACTORS

Returning again to the dictionary definition of adversity as exposure to unpropitious or calamitous circumstances implying previous well-being, we must recognize that not only fatefulness but also "previous well-being" is a relative matter. Whereas fatefulness varies with the degree to which the occurrence of an event is influenced by environmental factors compared to the personal predispositions and behavior of the individual, the degree of previous well-being is likely to vary with both antecedent personal characteristics and dispositions, and with prior and still ongoing situations that are the subject matter of Part IV. Moreover, as the title of Part IV suggests, differences in personal predispositions and in factors in the ongoing situation can function to increase or decrease the impact of both fateful and nonfateful events.

For these reasons, we conceive of life stress processes as consisting of three main components (Dohrenwend & Dohrenwend, 1981b). The first is the stimulus component of *proximal life events* introduced above. As was noted, these can range from extreme events, such as human-made or natural disasters, to more usual events, such as deaths of significant others, physical illnesses or injuries, marital separation, or loss of job (see Parts I and II).

The second component is the *ongoing social situation*, as discussed in Part IV, consisting of the activities of the individual in such settings as the domestic arrangement (Lennon), occupation (Link, Lennon, and Dohrenwend), and social network in which the individual was involved prior to the occurrence of the life event(s) (Henderson). The ongoing situation is likely to both affect and be affected by the occurrence of the life event(s). Characteristics of the ongoing situation can prove assets (e.g., supportive social networks) or liabilities (occupations with noisome characteristics).

The third component consists of the *personal predispositions* of the individual exposed to the life event. These characteristics involve such factors as the individual's genetic vulnerabilities in relation to health outcomes; intelligence; physical strength and stamina; past history of experiences with episodes of psychiatric disorders, physical illnesses and injuries, and other distal life events that are likely to have influenced the individual's personality, beliefs, values, and goals; those same beliefs, values, and goals (see especially Brown in Part III); and personality characteristics that are likely to be related to the individual's ability to cope with the events and changing situation (see Skodol in Part IV).

PSYCHOPATHOLOGY

By "psychopathology," I mean the kinds of signs, symptoms, and behaviors described in psychiatric nomenclatures, especially the third and fourth editions of the *Diagnostic and Statistical Manual of Mental Disorders* of the American Psychiatric Association (1980, 1987, 1994). The focus is on the types of diagnostic groupings and scales that are related to differences in gender and SES. These include schizophrenia, major depression, antisocial personality, alcoholism, substance use disorders, PTSD, and nonspecific distress or demoralization (see Kohn, Dohrenwend, and Mirotznik in Part III).

Advances have been made in the measurement and classification of psychopathology since the 1970s, and many of these are utilized in the work reported in this volume. (A variety of reliable research diagnostic interviews and psychometric scales are now available.) In the absence of satisfactory laboratory tests, however, all of these are based on personal interviews or self-report questionnaires, and there is controversy both about the merits of the differing procedures for measuring the individual signs, symptoms, and behaviors (e.g., Dohrenwend, 1990; Kendler et al., 1996; Robins, 1985) and about how to classify them into diagnoses. Controversies about PTSD provide particularly vivid examples (e.g., Kinzie & Goetz, 1995; Young, 1995). The classification issues will be best resolved when more is learned about etiology. Meanwhile, the multimethod procedure that I personally favor for present measurement and classification purposes that rely on interviews is described by Dohrenwend, Levav, Shrout, and co-workers in Part III.

COMPLEMENTARY PERSPECTIVES AND RESEARCH STRATEGIES

None of the studies and approaches described in Parts I–IV of this volume is experimental. None deals centrally with genetic factors or physiological correlates of disorders other than PTSD. Part V addresses these matters by including complementary experimental approaches illustrated by chapters on computer simulations (Shrout and Link), studies of primates (Kraemer and Bachevalier), and the implementation of preventive strategies (Kellam, Mayer, Rebok, and Hawkins); a chapter describing a behavioral genetic approach to studying life events (Kendler); a chapter on the physiological correlates of depression (Frank and Karp); and, in historical context, a chapter describing something of the complexity of the challenge of integrating lines of research operating on different levels, from molecules to social organizations (Leighton).

OVERVIEW AND INTEGRATION

The last part of this volume (Part VI) contains my overview and integration of what has gone before. I start with what I think has been shown about the importance of adversity and stress. I then take up the challenge of integrating the leads from each line of research represented in the preceding parts of this volume and set forth my suggestions for future research.

REFERENCES

American Psychiatric Association. (1980). *Diagnostic and statistical manual of mental disorders* (3rd ed.) Washington, DC: American Psychiatric Press.

American Psychiatric Association. (1987). *Diagnostic and statistical manual of mental disorders* (3rd ed., rev.). Washington, DC: American Psychiatric Press.

American Psychiatric Association. (1994). *Diagnostic and statistical manual of mental disorders* (4th ed.). Washington, DC: American Psychiatric Press.

Beebe, G. W. (1975). Follow-up studies of World War II and Korean War prisoners. II: Morbidity, disability, and maladjustments. *American Journal of Epidemiology*, 20, 400–422.

Cadoret, R., Troughton, E., O'Gorman, E. H., et al. (1986). An adoption study of genetic and environmental factors in drug abuse. *Archives of General Psychiatry*, 43, 1131–1136.

Cloninger, R. C., Bohman, M., & Sigvardsson, S. (1981). Inheritance of alcohol abuse: Cross fostering analysis of adopted men. *Archives of General Psychiatry*, 38, 861–868.

Crowe, R. R. (1974). An adoption study of antisocial personality. *Archives of General Psychiatry*, 31, 785–791.

Dohrenwend, B. P. (1976). Clues to the role of socioenvironmental factors. *Schizophrenia Bulletin*, 2, 440–444.

Dohrenwend, B. P. (1979). Stressful life events and psychopathology: some issues of theory and method. In J. F. Barrett, R. M. Rose, & G. L. Klerman (Eds.), *Stress and mental disorder* (pp. 1–15). New York: Raven Press.

Dohrenwend, B. P. (1990). The problem of validity in field studies of psychological disorders revisited. *Psychological Medicine*, 20, 195–208.

Dohrenwend, B. P., & Dohrenwend, B. S. (1969). *Social status and psychological disorder: A causal inquiry*. New York: John Wiley & Sons.

Dohrenwend, B. P., & Dohrenwend, B. S. (1981a). Socioenvironmental factors, stress, and psychopathology—Part 1: Quasi-experimental evidence on the social causation-social selection issue posed by class differences. *American Journal of Community Psychology*, 9, 129–146.

Dohrenwend, B. S., & Dohrenwend, B. P. (1981b). Socioenvironmental factors, stress, and psychopathology—Part 2: Hypotheses about stress processes linking social class to various types of psychopathology. *American Journal of Community Psychology*, 9, 146–159.

Dunham, H. W. (1955). Mental disorder in the community. In A. M. Rose (Ed.), *Mental health and mental disorder: A sociological approach* (pp. 168–179). New York: W. W. Norton.

Eitinger, L. (1964). *Concentration camp survivors in Norway and Israel*. London: Allen & Unwin.

Elder, G. H. (1974). *Children of the Great Depression*. Chicago: University of Chicago Press.

Faris, R. E. L., & Dunham, H. W. (1939). *Mental disorders in urban areas: An ecological study of schizophrenia and other psychoses*. Chicago: University of Chicago Press.

Frank, L. K. (1936). Society as the patient. *American Journal of Sociology*, 42, 335–344.

Goodwin, D. W. (1979). Alcoholism and heredity: A review and hypothesis. *Archives of General Psychiatry*, 36, 57–61.

Gottesman, I., & Shields, J. (1976). A critical review of recent adoption, twin, and family studies of schizophrenia: Behavioral genetics perspectives. *Schizophrenia Bulletin*, 2, 360–401.

Grob, G. N. (1971). Introduction. In E. Jarvis: *Insanity and idiocy in Massachusetts: Report of the Commission on Lunacy, 1855* (pp. 1–73). Cambridge, MA: Harvard University Press.

Guze, S. B. (1989). Biological psychiatry: Is there any other kind? *Psychological Medicine*, 19, 315–323.

Heston, L. L. (1966). Psychiatric disorders in foster home reared children of schizophrenic mothers. *British Journal of Psychiatry*, 112, 819–925.

Heston, L. L. (1988). What about environment? In D. L. Dunner, E. S. Gershon, & J. E. Barrett (Eds.), *Relatives at risk for mental disorder* (pp. 205–213). New York: Raven Press.

Hollingshead, A. B., & Redlich, F. C. (1958). *Social class and mental illness*. New York: John Wiley & Sons.

Hutchings, B., & Mednick, S. (1975). Registered criminality in the adoptive and biological parents of registered male criminal adoptees. In R. R. Fieve, H. Brill, & D. Rosenthal (Eds.), *Genetic research in psychiatry* (pp. 105–116). Baltimore: Johns Hopkins Press.

Jarvis, E. (1855). *Insanity and idiocy in Massachusetts: Report of the Commission of Lunacy*. Cambridge, MA: Harvard University Press.

Kendler, K. S., Gallagher, T. J., Abelson, J. M., et al. (1996). Lifetime prevalence, demographic risk factors, and diagnostic validity of nonaffective psychoses as assessed in a U.S. community sample. *Archives of General Psychiatry*, 53, 1022–31.

Kety, S. S. (1965). Biochemical theories of schizophrenia. *International Journal of Psychiatry*, 1, 255–269.

Kety, S. S., Rosenthal, D., & Wender, P. H. (1976). Studies based on a total sample of adopted individuals and their relatives: Why they were necessary, what they demonstrated and failed to demonstrate. *Schizophrenia Bulletin*, 2, 413–428.

Kinzie, J. D., & Goetz, R. R. (1995). A century of controversy surrounding posttraumatic stress-spectrum syndromes: The impact on DSM-III and DSM-IV. *Journal of Traumatic Stress*, 9, 159–179.

Leighton, A. H. (1959). *My name is Legion: Stirling County Study* (Vol. I.) New York: Basic Books.

Merikangas, K. (1990). The genetic epidemiology of alcoholism. *Psychological Medicine*, 20, 11–22.

Plomin, R. (1990). The role of inheritance in behavior. *Science*, 248, 183–188.

Robins, L. N. (1985). Epidemiology: Reflections on testing the validity of psychiatric interviews. *Archives of General Psychiatry*, 38, 381–9.

Rosenthal, D., & Kety, S. S. (Eds.). (1968). *Transmission of schizophrenia*. London: Pergamon.

Rutter, M. (1986). Meyerian psychobiology, personality development, and the role of life experiences. *American Journal of Psychiatry*, 143, 1077–1087.

Srole, L., Langner, T. S., Michael, S. T., et al. (1962). *Mental health in the metropolis: The Midtown Manhattan Study* (Vol. I). New York: McGraw-Hill.

Torgensen, S. (1986). Genetic factors in moderately severe and mild affective disorders. *Archives of General Psychiatry*, 43, 222–226, 1986

Webster's new collegiate dictionary. (1961). Springfield, MA: C. & C. Merriam Co.

Webster's ninth new collegiate dictionary. (1987). Springfield, MA: Merriam-Webster, Inc.

Young, A. (1995). Reasons and causes for posttraumatic stress disorder. *Transcultural Psychiatric Research Review*, 32, 287–298.

I

EXTREME SITUATIONS

Morton Beiser

There are reasons why investigators such as Keane and Giel study the horrible; Mollica and Levav, the unthinkable. First and foremost, we know too little about how to help people who become the psychiatric casualties of exposure to military combat, to natural and civilian disasters, and, perhaps worst of all, to inhuman cruelty. Research can provide frameworks for intervention and can make important contributions to theory about stress and coping. Ultimately, the two goals are linked: the better our theory about cause, effect, and mitigating circumstances, the more effective intervention is likely to be.

Leitmotifs in the form of recurring questions unite the four chapters in this section. Does extreme adversity have long-term psychological and psychophysiological effects? Is there evidence for a dose–response relationship that would lend credence to an etiological link between experience and hypothesized outcome? Do personal vulnerabilities existing prior to exposure contribute to ensuing psychopathology? Does exposure to severe adversity sensitize survivors to future traumas? Are particular types of adversity associated with specific patterns of distress?

DOES EXPOSURE TO EXTREME ADVERSITY HAVE LONG-TERM EFFECTS?

The chapters in this section are grounded in different types of scientific discourse—epidemiology, clinical observation, participant–observation studies, and quasi experiments. Despite their paradigmatic and methodological differences, the authors clearly agree that extreme adversity gives rise to psychopathological consequences, and that these consequences may outlive the stressor itself. None of the chapters refers to recent twin studies. However, research within this framework demonstrating increased risk for post-traumatic stress disorder (PTSD) among combat-exposed versus non-combat-exposed twins (Goldberg et al., 1990) provides additional evidence supporting the assertion that external stress of extreme proportion creates longstanding emotional distress. Evidence for a dose–response relationship supplied by Keane, Levav, and Mollica and colleagues provides additional support for the posited etiological link between adversity and psychopathology.

The mental health field has struggled for a long time to define the role of trauma in precipitating longstanding distress. The various incarnations of the American Psychiatric Association's (APA's) *Diagnostic and Statistical Manual of Mental Disorders* (*DSM*) over the past 40 years chronicle what Levav refers to as the nature–nurture struggle. In 1952, the APA issued the *DSM-I*. The Foreword, describing how the manual benefitted from "the experiences of psychiatrists of World War II, (and) the results of several years' usage by the military and Veterans Administration of a revised army nomenclature," reveals the impact that war and its aftermath exerted on nosological formulation. The *DSM-I* explicitly acknowledged that extraordinary external stress, which it classified as combat related or civilian catastrophe, could result in what it called "Gross Stress Reaction." This version of the psychiatric nomenclature was unequivocal in asserting that symptoms caused by Gross Stress Reaction were transient and reversible.

Gross Stress Reaction no longer appears in the 1968 revision, issued as the *DSM-II*. Although combat-related disorders were listed as an example of "Adjustment Reactions of Adult Life," they were still understood as distress that was presumably relieved by removal from the battlefield. The decision to include nontransient symptoms under "Anxiety Neurosis" implicitly assigns etiological primacy to predisposition over trauma.

Another of the century's "great" battles, the Vietnam war, influenced the creation of a new category, "Post-Traumatic Stress Disorder," which appeared for the first time in the *DSM-III* of 1980. The category has been retained, more or less in its original form, in 1994's *DSM-IV*. In a look backward to the *DSM-I* and Gross Stress Reaction, the PTSD concept assigns etiological significance to external stress.

PERSONAL VULNERABILITY AS A PREDISPOSING FACTOR VERSUS EXPOSURE AS A SENSITIZER TO SUBSEQUENT EXPOSURE

Even though only 6 of the 17 symptoms that define PTSD are physiological (the remainder, dealing with intrusive thoughts and avoidant behavior are psychological), Keane's elegant studies suggest that psychophysiological reactivity predicts diagnosis two times out of three. Other research (Solomon & Mikulincer, 1988) has suggested that the occurrence of stress reaction during combat constitutes a risk factor for the later appearance of PTSD. The fact that physiological reactivity predicts membership in a category largely defined by behaviors such as intrusive recollections of past events and feelings of detachment suggests that physiology plays a role, as either an etiological or a mediating agent, in the creation of PTSD. As Keane points out, the alternative hypotheses, that pre-existing psychophysiological vulnerability may be a risk factor for PTSD, or that the development of a stress reaction under conditions of adversity sensitizes people to subsequent aversive stimuli, demand further study.

TYPES OF ADVERSITY AND PATTERNS OF DISTRESS

The chapters in this section suggest the need to develop a typology of adversity that might be related to differences in the patterning or intensity of subsequent distress. After explicitly posing this question, Mollica and colleagues go on to question whether traumas such as starvation and head injury during torture may be particularly pathogenic. In a similar vein, Giel suggests the importance of distinguishing between natural and human-made disasters. A consideration of the range of disasters described in these chapters suggests that human-made adversities might be usefully subdivided into those resulting from accident or human error, a category that would include Chernobyl, and those inflicted by design, for example, torture and concentration camps. It seems plausible to hypothesize that a situation in which there is clearly someone to blame may evoke a psychological response different from one in which the locus of responsibility is unclear. Part of the cathartic power of the Nuremberg trials derives from their serving to establish the concept that individuals are responsible for heinous acts, whether or not these are sanctioned by authority. By contrast, the responsibility for events like Chernobyl tends to be more diffuse. It is even more difficult—although, as Giel points out, not impossible—to find someone to blame for an event like an earthquake.

The possibility that different types of adversity give rise to different forms of distress is related to a question raised by Levav: Does the current nosology do justice to the effects of extreme adversity? Levav's response would probably be a resounding "no." The criteria for PTSD do not, for example, include the complaints most frequently associated with the KZ, or concentration camp, syndrome. According to Levav's chapter, these include irritability, fatigability, and dysphoria. Consistent with these observations, Mollica and co-workers comment that the survivors of Pol Pot's brutality frequently report depression as well as somatic symptoms. Perhaps the *DSM* system's goal of specifying inclusion and exclusion criteria sufficiently specific to produce nonoverlapping categories compromises its ability to do complete justice to the full range of postadversity phenomena. Alternatively, perhaps a concentration camp experience evokes a different set of reactions than the combat-related experiences that seem to supply most of the underpinning for the PTSD description.

In response to extreme adversity, people do more than develop symptom complexes. As Giel points out, other effects include changing one's threshold for defining illness, changing one's attributional framework regarding illness and health, and changing one's attitudes toward and demands for service.

WHERE NEXT?

After experiencing adversity, many people react with longstanding emotional distress. "Many" means something less than 100%, an observation suggesting that exposure does not constitute a complete explanation for subsequent disorder. Future investigations should include a focus on risk and protective factors that help explain early reactions to adversity as well those contributing to the perpetuation of distress.

The dose–response data suggest that the greater the intensity of exposure, the greater the vulnerability to disorder. The level of pre-exposure physiological reactivity may supply another piece of the vulnerability puzzle. Understanding the role that protective factors might play in moderating the early effects of adversity would contribute to theory as well to the conceptualization of possible preventive strategies for high-risk conditions. Unfortunately, existing literature offers few guides to such understanding. Based on the demonstration that current social support buffers the aftereffects of adversity, Levav posits that social resources may play a similar role during the original traumatic experience. Although this is a reasonable suggestion, establishing a link between social support and emotional experience in the aftermath of adversity does not ensure that the same process affects reactions during the experience of trauma.

The fact that most disasters can be neither predicted nor prevented places limits on what can be done to help ease their early effects. However, the elucidation of factors that contribute to the perpetuation as well as the resolution of long-term reactions holds out promise for the development of intervention strategies. What combination of personal and social resources has, for example, made it possible for people such as Eli Weisel and Aaron Appelfeld, witnesses to the worst of the Holocaust, to continue to tell their stories 50 years after liberation, while another survivor, the renowned Primo Levi, chose death over the continuation of his chronicles?

To date, most research about the aftereffects of exposure to adversity has been cross sectional. The literature provides hints that reactions may change as a function of length of time since exposure. Furthermore, the changes may not be linear, that is, gradually decreasing or increasing with distance from the event. Instead, life period transitions or changes in circumstance may affect the ability of the past to influence current emotional status (Beiser, 1987, 1988).

To master disastrous experience, according to Giel, survivors have a need to search for, or even to create, meaning. Behavioral scientists and mental health workers also sift the ashes of tragedy in the hope of finding meaning. Levav, Keane, Giel, and Mollica and co-workers have addressed this formidable task with rigor and humanity.

REFERENCES

American Psychiatric Association. (1952). *Diagnostic and statistical manual of mental disorders*. Washington, DC: American Psychiatric Press.

American Psychiatric Association. (1968). *Diagnostic and statistical manual of mental disorders* (2nd ed.). Washington, DC: American Psychiatric Press.

American Psychiatric Association. (1980). *Diagnostic and statistical manual of mental disorders* (3rd ed.). Washington, DC: American Psychiatric Press.

American Psychiatric Association. (1994). *Diagnostic and statistical manual of mental disorders* (4th ed.). Washington, DC: American Psychiatric Press.

Beiser, M. (1987). Changing time perspective and mental health among Southeast Asian refugees. *Culture, Medicine and Psychiatry, 11,* 437–464.

Beiser, M. (1988). Influences of time, ethnicity, and attachment on depression in Southeast Asian refugees. *American Journal of Psychiatry, 145,* 46–51.

Beiser, M., & Hyman, I. (1997). Refugees' time perspective and mental health. *American Journal of Psychiatry, 154,* 996–1002.

Goldberg, J., True, W. R., Eisen, S. A., & Henderson, W. G. (1990). A twin study of the effects of the Vietnam War on post-traumatic stress disorder. *JAMA, 263,* 1227–1232.

Solomon, Z., & Mikulincer, M. (1988). Psychological sequelae of war. A 2-year follow-up study of Israeli combat stress reaction casualties. *Journal of Nervous and Mental Disease, 176,* 264–269.

1

Individuals Under Conditions of Maximum Adversity: The Holocaust

Itzhak Levav

To our sorrow, human-made situations of extreme adversity have not been erased from the globe since the world discovered the atrocities perpetrated by the Nazi regime in Europe. Indeed, contemporary history has been dotted by frequent loathsome events; witness to this are the persecutions and tortures committed by oppressive military governments wherever they take root or by the atrocities committed of late by warring factions on each other and on civilians in such places as Rwanda and the former Yugoslavia (Basoglu, 1993).

It is fitting to ask whether these events leave psychopathological scars on the victims. If the answer is positive, are these scars short or long lived? Is there a dose effect, so that the greater the traumatization the more severe the effect? Does the posttraumatic stress syndrome, as currently defined, encompass all the psychopathological wounds typically shown by survivors? Is there a premorbid personality constellation that renders an individual specially vulnerable to the effects of massive assaults? Are the survivors particularly vulnerable to renewed stressful situations? Finally, is there any evidence that the effects of a severe en-

vironmental trauma are transmitted to a nonexposed second generation, perpetuating the psychological damage? To answer these questions, there is no more appropriate population to study than those who survived the Nazi persecution, whether in ghettos, hiding, disguise, forced labor, or extermination camps.

Many of the above questions have already been answered in full or in part by the available literature (see Eitinger and Krell's bibliography prepared in 1985). The chief aims of this chapter are to provide a summary of the epidemiological evidence published in English that appears most robust to me, to identify gaps in knowledge, and to establish the case for additional research—if warranted.

THE PSYCHOPATHOLOGICAL EFFECTS OF NAZI PERSECUTION

Jews as well as non-Jews were victims of the Nazis. All groups were persecuted, incarcerated, and tortured, either for who they were (Chodoff, 1963; Eitinger, 1972) or for what

13

they did or may have done. The Jewish population is the main focus of this chapter because the assault on them was greater than on other groups, as evidenced by their considerably higher mortality rates (Bauer, 1982), and because the results are better documented. Furthermore, the persecution of the Jews lasted longer; it began before the establishment of the camps with the enactment of the racial laws in 1933 and the confinement into ghettos where families were torn apart, atrocities witnessed, and hunger and other material deprivations suffered. The fear for one's life and those of beloved others was thus instilled early. If the individual was sent to a camp in the infamous cattle railway cars, additional assaults that were endured shattered any remaining personal sense of coherence (Antonovsky, 1979). Succinctly, these assaults may be grouped as follows:

–Physical (e.g., beatings, hunger, exposure to extreme temperatures, forced labor)

–Psychological (e.g., fear of death, insult to self-worth)

–Psychosocial (e.g., disruption of one's closest social support group)

–Cultural–religious (e.g., anti-Semitism)

Survivors who escaped death had to endure at least two subsequent stressful events: the liberation, with the feared discovery of being alone or almost alone in the world as a result of the murder of family members and friends, and resettlement in new surroundings after additional hardships, such as active rejection by neighbors in some of their countries of origin (e.g., Poland) and immigration difficulties to pre-statehood Israel under the British Mandate or to America. Each of these implied additional coping challenges at a time when the individual's resistance resources (Antonovsky, 1979) were undermined by physical and mental disease and by little or no social supports. Therefore, in assessing the stressors undergone by the survivors, it should be noted that there were a multiplicity of them

rather than a discrete one and that they were present for protracted periods rather than at a single point in time. These characteristics led authors to refer to such aggregate of stressors as "massive psychic trauma" (Krystal, 1968) or "massive cumulative trauma" (Keilson, 1992).

Clinical observations on the effects of the Nazi persecution started before the war ended. Psychiatrists and psychologists (e.g., Bettelheim, 1943; Frankl, 1961; Kral, 1951; and others) later documented observations they themselves made while interned in ghettos or concentration camps during the war. Immediately after the war ended, mental health professionals assigned to the liberating units and to displaced persons camps recorded their first impressions. The number of these observations escalated as countries and international organizations had to deal with compensation claims and establish rehabilitation programs.

As indicated earlier, the clinical literature on the Holocaust victims is now abundant. Without exception, clinical psychiatrists and psychoanalysts from countries of markedly different political persuasion and organization [e.g., Krystal (1968), in the United States; Eitinger (1964) in Israel and Norway; and Ryn (1990) in former communist Poland] repeatedly observed that survivors suffered from many disabling symptoms constituting syndromes that necessitated special labeling (see "The Concentration Camp Syndrome," below).

Of this type of studies, Eitinger's report (1964) is most informative because it covers a heterogeneous group of survivors derived from in- and outpatient psychiatric populations (subgroups I, IV, and V); claimants (subgroup II); and individuals in active work in contrasting societal organizations, kibbutz, and urban settings (subgroups III and VI). These groups (total $n = 590$) had been subjected to differing degrees of persecution, from mild to most severe (Table 1.1). Eitinger found that a cluster of symptoms, the "concentration camp syndrome" (see below), was conspicuously present, although with different frequencies according to the subgroup. Among the Norwegian survivors,

Table 1.1. Frequency of symptoms in selected samples of individuals who underwent Nazi persecution (%)

Symptoms	Norwegian samples[°]			Israeli samples[†]		
	I (n = 96)	II (n = 152)	III (n = 80)	IV (n = 396)	V (n = 92)	VI (n = 66)
Increased fatigability	37.5	80.2	23.7	15.3	60.8	50.0
Disturbances in memory/ Difficulty in concentration	33.3	79.6	10.0	23.1	49.9	27.3
Dysphoria, bitterness	40.6	63.1	—	10.5	40.2	16.6
Emotional instability	26.0	65.7	33.7	28.9	67.3	38.4
Sleep disturbances	40.6	55.2	8.7	35.5	65.2	28.7
Feelings of insufficiency	29.1	48.6	3.7	?	36.9	18.1
Reduced initiative	26.0	44.7	7.5	?	46.7	27.3
Nervousness, irritability	60.4	76.9	36.2	27.6	66.7	74.2
Vertigo	28.1	40.1	5.0	18.2	31.5	28.7
Vegetative lability	11.4	42.1	6.2	12.5	52.1	36.4
Headaches	36.4	55.9	8.7	25.9	65.2	43.9
Marked symptoms of anxiety	31.2	51.3	12.5	35.5	59.7	28.7
Nightmares	20.8	37.5	3.7	6.7	56.5	57.5
Periods of depression	31.2	51.3	6.2	24.9	59.7	28.7

From Eitinger, L. *Concentration camp survivors in Norway and Israel*. The Hague: Martinus Nijhoff. 1972.

[°]I, patients hospitalized, Oslo, 1945–1961. II, patients specially referred, Oslo, 1957–1961. III, former prisoners, controls.

[†]IV, inmates in mental hospitals, October 1, 1961. V, clinic patients. VI, kibbutz members.

the percentage of "concentration camp syndrome" ranged from 6.2% for fully active individuals (subgroup III) to 80.9% for the claimant subgroup (subgroup II). Among the Israeli survivors, the percentages ranged from 26.8% for the subgroup of psychotic inpatients (subgroup IV) to 55.4% for the ambulatory neurotic patients (subgroup V). Even among the fully working kibbutz members (subgroup VI), the syndrome was identified in 34.9%.

However enlightening the clinical literature is, it does suffer from serious biases, as acknowledged by Eitinger (1964) himself. These biases result from, for example, selectivity, limited diagnostic reliability, and possible self-serving interest on the part of the patient in the case of examinations conducted during compensation claims.

In view of the above problems, epidemiological community studies offer a better framework to truly assess the psychopatho-logical effect of persecution. Curiously enough, these studies are few in number and were late in being conducted, most likely because treatment and legal demands were more pressing. Several of these community surveys had other goals than to investigate psychiatric conditions of survivors and included relevant questions almost incidentally (Sigal & Weinfeld, 1989). Seven studies provide epidemiological data (Table 1.2): four of them (Antonovsky et al., 1971; Eaton et al., 1982; Fennig & Levav, 1991; Levav & Abramson, 1984) were household surveys that included Jewish respondents who had been in Europe during World War II and respondents of similar origin who were not in Europe at the time, the latter serving as a comparison or control group. A fifth study was based on comprehensive health examinations conducted for screening purposes in a large medical center (Carmil & Carel, 1986). Finally, two studies (Ei-

Table 1.2. Epidemiological studies on the traumatic effects of Nazi persecution

Authors	Year	Place	Measures[a]	World War II experience	Findings	n[b]
Household surveys of Holocaust survivors						
Antonovsky et al.	1971	City-wide, Israel	Health status, well-being, role satisfaction	Varied	Affected	77 women
Eaton et al.	1982	Montreal	Langner Scale	Varied	Affected	135 both sexes
Levav and Abramson	1984	Jerusalem	CMI Scale	Varied	Affected	380 both sexes
Fenig and Levav	1991	Tel Aviv	PERI Demoralization Scale	Forced labor camps/ghetto/hiding	Affected	76 women
Other studies of Holocaust survivors						
Carmil and Carel	1986	Israel	Battery of several items on emotional stress	Varied	Affected	2159 both sexes
Other studies of concentration camp inmates						
Helweg-Larsen et al.	1952	Copenhagen	Questionnaires, clinical examination	Police force, resistance movement	Affected	710 men 562 men and 10 women
Eitinger and Strom	1966	Norway	Clinical examination	Prisoners of war	Affected	498 both sexes

[a]CMI, Cornell Medical Index; PERI = Psychiatric Epidemiology Research Interview.

[b]n refers to victims only.

tinger & Strom, 1973; Helweg-Larsen et al., 1952), were based on special population groups, largely of non-Jewish civilians of Danish and Norwegian nationalities, who had been interned in German concentration camps.

Household Surveys

In three of the four studies of this type, populations were investigated with the use of scales measuring nonspecific psychological distress (Link & Dohrenwend, 1980): the 22-item Langner Scale (Eaton et al., 1982), an abbreviated measure of the Cornell Medical Index (CMI) (Levav & Abramson, 1984), and the Demoralization Scale of the Psychiatric Epidemiology Research Interview (PERI) (Fennig & Levav, 1991). In the fourth study, Antonovsky et al. (1971) used a battery of items measuring different dimensions of health in women, including

mental health. [The measure of health status included (1) overall menopausal symptoms, "psychic menopausal symptoms," "psychosomatic and somatic menopausal symptoms"; (2) overall ratings by physicians, comprising physical and emotional symptoms and functioning; (3) well-being, self-evaluation of overall life situation and coping, and mood tone and worries scales; and (4) role satisfaction.] None of these four studies, however, used a standard method of psychiatric diagnosis.

Three of them (Antonovsky et al., 1971; Fennig & Levav, 1991; Levav & Abramson, 1984) were conducted in Israel, and one in Montreal, Canada (Eaton et al., 1982), between 25 and 40 years after liberation. The sample populations ranged from 76 to 380. Two were limited to women (Antonovsky et al., 1971; Fennig & Levav, 1991), while the other two included both genders. The results uniformly showed that the survivors' health status was adversely affected regardless of the measures utilized (see Table 1.1).

Although psychiatric diagnoses were not made, it is worth noting for later discussion the results obtained in two of the studies with measures of anxiety and mood states. Antonovsky et al. (1971) found that general practitioners, when asked about their survivor patients who were randomly included in the survey, reported that 33% were in a worse health status as compared with 10% of the controls. Lower moods were reported by 61% and 46% among the index and the comparison groups, respectively; for the worries scale—a proxy for anxiety—the respective proportions were 56% and 30%. All these differences reached statistical significance. In Eaton et al.'s 1982 Canadian survey, the depression subscale of the 22-item Langner Scale differed little between the index and comparison groups: 48% in survivors versus 40% in controls. The respective figures for the anxiety subscale were 33% and 8%.

Levav and Abramson (1984) used an abbreviated CMI scale of accepted validity and reliability. Survivor mean scores were significantly higher than the scores of controls, even after adjustments were made for age, educational level, and respondent's appraisal that he or she had endured a hard life. The most recent survey, by Fennig and Levav (1991), using the Demoralization Scale of the PERI, found again that survivors had a higher rate of demoralization: 70% for former concentration inmates in contrast to 16% among the comparison group. The cutoff point used to establish the rate of demoralization had been determined in a previous methodological study conducted in Israel comparing psychiatric cases and community controls (Shrout et al., 1986).

Community Surveys

The research design in Carmil and Carel's study (1986) differed from that in previous surveys, yet it is of considerable interest to us because it included large numbers of individuals of both sexes (those living in Europe during World War II, $n = 2159$; comparison group, $n = 1150$) under conditions of full employment save for a tiny proportion of retired workers. Subjects had been screened for reasons totally unrelated to the issue under discussion. Of further interest is the fact that, in the aggregate, subjects in the index group were slightly younger, and most measures of physical health (cholesterol, glucose in blood, and systolic blood pressure) did not differ between groups. The only statistically significant differences recorded for physical health were found among the men; index cases were slightly lower in height and lighter in weight and had a lower diastolic blood pressure. In assessing the results, it should be noted that the index group was composed of individuals with different types and degrees of exposure to Nazi persecution.

The dimension "emotional distress" was measured with a set of items extracted from the large battery of questions routinely presented to the screened individuals (e.g., Are you frequently anxious, depressed, or crying? Have you seriously considered committing suicide in the last year? Have you lately been seen regularly by a psychologist or a psychiatrist? Do you suffer from serious psychological problems? Do you have unrealistic fears? Are you often so angry that you lose control? Do you suffer from sleep disturbances?). Results showed that there were statistically significant differences among women for all items except sleep disturbances and suicidal thoughts; in all cases the index group scored higher. No statistically significant differences were found among men, although index cases consistently reported more frequent positive responses.

Two additional observations emerged from these five epidemiological studies. First, the effects of traumatization were evident long after the war. Of note, respondents in these surveys were examined in contexts totally unrelated to secondary gain; in three surveys, relevant questions about World War II experiences followed items on the respondent's emotional status to avoid leading cues. These results are consistent with findings from epidemiological studies conducted

Table 1.3. Psychological community-based studies on the traumatic effects of Nazi persecution

Authors	Year	Place	Measures	World War II experience	Findings	$n°$
Nadler and Ben-Shushan	1989	Urban & kibbutz, Israel	Clinical analysis questionnaire; Tennessee self-concept scale	Concentration camp	Affected	34, both sexes
Dor-Shav	1978	Tel Aviv, Israel	Multiple tests (embedded figures; human figure drawing; block design/WAIS[†]; Rorschach inkblot; Bender Gestalt; Catell's personality factor questionnaire)	Concentration camp	Affected	42, both sexes

°n refers to victims only.

[†]WAIS, Wechsler Adult Intelligence Scale.

long after World War II on severely mal-treated Australian (Venn & Guest, 1991) and U.S. prisoners of war in the Pacific theater (e.g., Goldstein et al., 1987; Sutker et al., 1993). In this latter group of inquiries, however, the conscious or unconscious search for personal benefits cannot be completely ruled out.

Additional evidence on the mental status of the Holocaust survivors come from two small Israel-based psychological studies carried out in the community [Table 1.3; (Dor-Shav, 1978; Nadler & Ben-Shushan, 1989)]. The latter investigation consisted of a study of dimensions of well-being and self-esteem among survivors 40 years after the end of the war. The findings showed that their responses were less favorable than those among controls. The earlier study (Dor-Shav, 1978), which explored different personality dimensions using tests commonly applied in clinical practice, found that survivors appeared more impaired than controls.

The second conclusion that emerges from a closer look at the findings reported in the community surveys is that their results should be regarded as conservative indicators of psychological impact, because most studies inquired in very general terms about the nature of exposure to Nazi persecution

("Were you in Europe during World War II?"). Conceivably, the differences would have been greater if the comparison between index cases and controls had singled out those who formerly had been in extermination camps, where the stress had been more severe, from those who had experienced other types of persecution. Indeed, the surveys that inquired into these experiences more specifically (Fennig & Levav, 1991; Sigal & Weinfeld, 1989), clearly showed that the more severely traumatizing the condition (in the latter study, from confinement in a ghetto, to hiding, to forced labor camp, to extermination camp), the more marked the damage as reflected in the measure used, thus constituting a true dose–response effect. In this study, the mean demoralization scores, adjusted for education, social class, and a measure of social supports, climbed from 1.7 for those who had been in ghetto or in hiding, to 2.0 for those who had been in concentration camps. This finding is further buttressed by special population studies such as those related to compensation claims of Jewish Nazi victims (see Hafner, 1968), other Holocaust survivors (Robinson et al., 1994), and Danish members of the resistance movement who were in German concentration camps (Helweg-Larssen et al., 1952).

Other Studies of Concentration Camp Inmates

Two studies were conducted with former German prisoners of war (POWs) (largely non-Jewish civilians), one in Norway (Eitinger & Strom, 1973), and one in Denmark (Helweg-Larsen et al., 1952). They each offer distinct methodological advantages, such as careful enumeration procedures, relatively large sample sizes, and high completion rates (see Table 1.2). Internment in this case included prisons or camps in Germany as well as in the occupied countries of Central Europe. Life conditions, on the whole, were less brutal than for the Jews, but these prisoners were not spared from death, either during internment or after liberation, or from a high degree of suffering. Unlike the Jews, however, their repatriation, if not totally uneventful, was to a family and a caring country.

Eitinger and Strom (1973), with the aid of multiple sources, painstakingly built a register of the Norwegian World War II POWs. This register, considered complete except for approximately 500 POWs presumed missing, constituted a considerable improvement over methods used in a previous report (Strom et al., 1962). Of the 4768 former POWs who were alive at liberation, less those who died before the field work was conducted ($n = 763$), emigrated ($n = 123$), or were not traced ($n = 71$), Eitinger and Strom selected a representative sample of 498, including 18 women. They identified an equal number of carefully matched controls from the local health insurance offices. In this study, morbidity was evaluated using clinical means: sick leave periods, hospital admissions, and the recorded diagnosis (as customary at the time, no standard method of diagnosis was used). The period of follow-up varied, ranging from 6 to 21.6 years, according to the availability of the information.

Sick leave periods were more frequent and extended among ex-POWs. An identical finding was made regarding number and length of hospitalization periods of any kind. As for psychiatric morbidity, ex-POWs had more frequently been diagnosed than controls as suffering from "neurosis, nervousness" (24.2%–9.4%); "abuse of alcohol and drugs" (7.0%–1.6%); and "psychosis" (3.0%–1.0%). For all three diagnostic categories, ex-POWs had more frequent measures of severity of the disorder (e.g., number of sick periods per sick person, number of sick days per sick period, number of hospitalized patients per group, total number of days in hospital, etc.).

The study conducted in Denmark (Helweg-Larsen et al., 1952) included two selected populations: 710 members of the police force deported "en bloc" to Germany on September 19, 1944, who were serving in Copenhagen at the time of the field work (September 1948), and 572 members of the resistance movement who had been deported to German concentration camps and/or prisons during the war and were living in Copenhagen at the time of the investigation (May–September 1947).

Members of the resistance were asked to fill out questionnaires regarding their deportation, specific symptoms of disease at different points in the study periods, and their social conditions. This information was supplemented and revised on the basis of personal interviews; additional information was obtained from different sources. A group of subjects ($n = 52$), selected partly on the basis of their answer to the questionnaires and partly at random, were subjected to a thorough psychiatric investigation. A somewhat similar procedure, although briefer, was followed with the policemen. Findings showed that 2½ years after repatriation, 78% of the 566 members of the resistance and 63% of the 710 members of the police force who filled out the questionnaires "stated that they had, or still have, neurotic symptoms of varying degree of severity . . . ," whereas only 30% and 43%, respectively, had a "normal working capacity" after liberation. By 1947 the following were the complaints of the members of the resistance in descending order of frequency: restlessness, 63%; excessive fatigue, 58%; irritability, 47%; headache/muscular pain, 47%; emotional instability, 46%; increased sleep requirement, 40%; insomnia, 40%; defective memory, 39%; depression, 36%; increased consumption of alcohol, 20%; and sexual difficulties, 19%. In 61% of these ex-POWs, symptoms of "repatriation neurosis" had persisted at the time of examination in 1947.

As noted in the earlier set of household surveys, the authors demonstrated that the various conditions of deportation and the intensity of the symptoms of starvation (a measure of victimization) correlated positively with the difficulties in social readaptation during the first 2–3 years after liberation. An additional important contribution made by these studies was that subjects were judged by the authors, based on relevant items included in the questionnaires, as having been adequately adjusted regarding both work and psychiatric status before internment. This would obviously point to the greater importance of the traumatic events, compared to previous personality vulnerabilities, to the observed psychopathology. This matter is considered further below (see "Premorbid Factors and Extreme Conditions").

Other groups of POWs subjected to prolonged and extremely harsh conditions during their confinement during World War II (e.g., Beebe, 1975), the Korean conflict (e.g., Sutker et al., 1991), and the Vietnam war (e.g., Ursano, 1981) have also been studied epidemiologically years after repatriation. Some of the U.S. studies, however, are problematic because of the selectivity of the samples, the small sample sizes, the occasional absence of a control group, the diagnostician's knowledge of the identity of the subject, and the relatively low response rates. In contrast, with rare exception these problems were present in the Scandinavian surveys.

More recent studies have improved their methods over earlier ones, among them the use of standard instruments for psychiatric diagnoses. As an illustration of such POW-based studies published in the last decade, consider Tennant et al.'s investigation in Australia (1986). One hundred seventy POWs from Sidney who were badly mal-treated during their prolonged captivity under the Japanese, and 172 nonimprisoned former combatants from the same city, of whom almost every one also fought in the Pacific, responded to several self-report instruments (e.g., Zung's depression inventory) and an abbreviated version of the Diagnostic Interview Schedule. The participation rates were 88% for the POWs and 86% for the other former combatants. Former POWs were found to have more psychiatric disorders (71%,) than the comparison group (46%); the differences were highly statistically significant. POWs scored higher in Zung's depression inventory (34.4 compared with 29.6 in the other group, p <.01). Interestingly, no differences were found for state and trait anxiety as measured by the Spielberger's Scale. Because the authors did not state whether the single diagnostician who conducted the interviews was blind to the respondent's status (POW or other), the results from the self-administered instruments are probably less open to bias.

Conclusions

Taken together, the two set of studies reviewed in this section, community surveys of Holocaust survivors and special population groups composed of German POWs and resistance members, have conclusively shown that highly traumatized individuals (on the aggregate, the former group more than the latter both during and after the war) suffer from long-lasting psychopathology whatever the measures used. Research conducted on other POWs further reinforces these conclusions.

THE CONCENTRATION CAMP SYNDROME

The diagnosis of post-traumatic stress disorder (PTSD) as we know it today and the clinical literature based on World War II observations, were obviously not available at the end of the war when Holocaust survivors were examined clinically by psychiatrists. At the time, psychiatrists who examined survivors had to face a mental condition with which they were unfamiliar as diagnosticians; neither did they clearly understand its etiology. Initially, the concomitant presence of physical disorders, the effect of hunger, and the knowledge that survivors suffered head traumas as a result of beatings led examiners to believe that the condition was organic in its basis, rather than psychological or mixed. Eitinger (1961, 1964), a leading researcher on the mental status of the survivors, was so inclined and argued his case most persuasively.

The fact that survivors presented a constellation of different symptoms that did not fit any known category following a situation in which they all had suffered persecution led psychiatrists to label the syndrome by its origin, "KZ-syndrom," "survivor syndrome," and the like. Would contemporary classifications accommodate such a category? Apparently not, because this type of syndrome does not appear in the *Diagnostic and Statistical Manual of Mental Disorders* (third edition, revised) (*DSM-III-R*; American Psychiatric Association, 1987). A contemporary American clinician would probably settle for a PTSD diagnosis, especially because of the recurrent nightmares and the persistent sleep problems so frequently observed in veterans. In contrast, the tenth International Classification of Diseases (ICD-10) does refer to conditions resulting from concentration camp experiences in the F.62.0 category under "enduring personality change after catastrophic experience" (World Health Organization, 1992).

Does the diagnosis of PTSD, however, cover all manifestations of the concentration camp syndrome as we know it today based on the available Holocaust literature? Eitinger (1961, 1964) identified 11 symptoms as pathognomonic of the concentration camp syndrome (see Table 1.1). For this author, the number of symptoms present in any combination was correlated with his degree of certainty that the syndrome was indeed present. Thus, if there were seven to ten symptoms he would have high certainty; if

six, moderate certainty; if five, limited certainty; and if there were less than five symptoms, he considered the syndrome as absent. Of Eitinger's 11 symptoms, only four are to be found in the PTSD disorder as it appears in the *DSM-III-R* (see Table 1.4). Matussek (1975), in a separate well-studied group of concentration camp survivors, attempted to describe the frequency of their complaints. Of note, 6 of the 12 complaints he characteristically found in 10% or more of the cases are included in the PTSD description of the disorder (Table 1.5). Eitinger and Matussek agreed that items on dysphoric mood or its equivalent are included in the syndrome; similar findings were made by Hafner (1968) in a review of the psychiatric status of 324 compensation cases. However, these types of symptoms (e.g., dysphoric mood) have been omitted in the PTSD description.

A study that reclassified symptoms recorded in a large number of compensation files was able to establish the presence of PTSD disorder in survivors. The investigators also found that the frequency of symptoms was greater for those survivors who had been in extermination camps (Kuch & Cox, 1992) (Table 1.6). This study, however, is not fully contributory to our discussion because it does not tell us whether symptoms currently classified in other disorders were simply left out when they did not fit the purpose of the exercise. It would thus appear that, among concentration camp survivors, there were co-morbid manifestations of at least two syndromes, in a proportion that we are not able to establish reliably: PTSD and a likely residual state of a pathological grief reaction (Jacobs, 1993). Indeed, some of the symptoms not included in the PTSD coincide with those in the cluster described by Clayton and Darvish (1979) in their study of bereavement. The losses that the survivors endured (from 80% to 90% of the survivors interviewed by Eitinger in 1964 in Israel had lost most of their closest relatives), with little or no possibilities for adequate mourning, would make this hypothesis rather plausible. Parenthetically, Tennant et al. (1986), based on their

Table 1.4. Comparison between *DSM-III-R* PTSD and the concentration camp syndrome

PTSD according to *DSM-III-R*	Concentration camp syndrome according to Eitinger°
A. Event outside the range of usual experience	

B. At least one:
    Recurrent and extensive distressing recollection
    Recurrent distressing dreams
    Sudden acting/feeling as if events were returning
    Distress at exposure to symbols/resemblance of event	

C. Persistent avoidance of stimuli, at least three:
    Efforts to avoid thoughts/feelings
    Efforts to avoid activities/situations
    Psychogenic amnesia
    Diminished interest in significant activities
    Feelings of detachment
    Restricted range of affect
    Sense of a foreshortened future	

D. Persistent symptoms of increased arousal, at least two:
    Difficulty falling/staying asleep
    Irritability/outburst of anger
 	
    Difficulty concentrating
    Hypervigilance
    Exaggerated startle response
    Physiologic reactivity symbolizing/resembling an aspect of traumatic events
	Sleep disturbances
	Nervousness, irritability, restlessness
	Emotional instability
	Failing memory and difficulty in concentration

E. Duration of symptoms in B, C, and D of at least 1 month	Fatigue Headaches Dysphoric moodiness Vertigo Loss of initiative Vegetative lability Feeling of insufficiency

From Eitinger, L. *Concentration camp survivors in Norway and Israel*. The Hague: Martinus Nijhoff, 1972.

°If 7 or more items, high certainty (+++); if 6 items, moderate certainty (++); if 5 items, minimum certainty (+); if 4 or less items, absent.

experience with POWs, stated: "depending on the nature of the stress (e.g., multiple losses of comrades) . . . other conditions such as depressive disorders may also result; post traumatic stress disorder may *not* [italics added] be the only outcome of severe stress." As noted above, the clinical literature on the Holocaust survivors often refers to an anxious and depressed condition with

PTSD components wherein sleep disturbances are salient and may be objectively recorded (Hefez et al., 1987).

At least three additional issues have occupied the interest of those who studied the direct effects of the Holocaust among the victims. These are the role played by the premorbid personality in the emergence of the KZ syndrome, social bonding as a pro-

Table 1.5. Frequency of complaints in selected concentration camp survivors (%)

Complaints	One diagnosis[°] (n = 50)	Multiple diagnoses[†] (n = 14)	Total (n = 64)
Anxiety dreams[‡]	69	86	72
Anxiety states	37	71	45
Paranoid ideation	16	7	14
Feelings of hatred	18	29	20
Agitation/irritability/nervousness[‡,°°]	67	64	66
Memory/concentration difficulties[‡,°°]	47	64	51
Mistrust/shyness/poor social contact[‡]	37	43	38
Feelings of isolation[‡]	33	29	32
Depression/compulsive brooding[°°]	73	64	71
Sleep problems[‡,°°]	63	71	65
Disturbed vitality[°°]	20	29	22
Tiredness/apathy[°°]	59	43	55

From Matussek, P. *Internment in concentration camps and its consequences*. New York: Springer-Verlag, 1975.

[°]One diagnosis: either chronic reactive depression, neurotic reaction, neurasthenia, or organic brain damage.

[†]Multiple diagnosis; any combination of the above.

[‡]Items in *DSM-III-R* PTSD syndrome.

[°°]Items in Eitinger's "concentration camp syndrome."

tective factor, and the possible vulnerability of the survivor facing renewed stressors. These three issues are discussed in turn.

Premorbid Factors and Extreme Conditions

The discussion of whether each individual has a psychological "breaking point" was a matter of clinical and legal interest after the war. If a KZ syndrome was entirely dependent on the individual's *Anlage*, no material compensation should be forthcoming to the victim. Orthodox psychoanalytical theory, by postulating the importance of early infantile conflicts, would therefore undermine the role played by current stressors. (This issue seemed to have disconcerted psychoanalysts; see Rapaport, 1968). In contrast, those who upheld the independent effect of victimization gave full justification to the medico-legal basis for the current claimant's predicament.

The role of famine in the impairment of mental functions was less under dispute; compensations based on brain changes resulting from starvation were granted with greater ease (see Helweg-Larssen et al., 1952), but psychologically based trauma was questioned. Eitinger and Major (1993) wrote "The official school of German psychiatry strictly kept to the Jaspers' criteria on psychogenesis, which accepted that substantial psychological trauma could produce serious psychological reactions [I would add, regardless of the premorbid personality]. However, it was argued, with the cessation of the cause, the reaction should disappear too, like the so-called jail psychosis" (p. 626). Evidence in the psychiatric literature on the Holocaust emerging from solid research rather than from mere doctrine is rather meager. To buttress that evidence we may turn to related literature, that on highly traumatized prisoners, such as veterans of World War II and the Vietnam war.

Table 1.6. Frequency of reclassified *DSM-III-R* PTSD symptoms in a selected sample of Holocaust survivors (%)

Symptom	Total sample (n = 124)	Concentration camp survivors (n = 78)	Tattooed concentration camp survivors (n = 20)
B(1) Intrusive recollections	55.6	65.4	80.0
B(2) Recurrent nightmares	83.1	87.2	90.0
B(3) Feelings of recurrence	2.4	1.3	5.0
B(4) Intense distress over reminders	75.0	79.5	75.0
C(1) Avoidance of thoughts and feelings	38.7	48.7	45.0
C(2) Avoidance of activities and situations	50.0	64.1	70.0
C(3) Psychogenic amnesia	3.2	3.8	10.0
C(4) Diminished interest	64.5	66.7	65.0
C(5) Detachment	31.5	37.2	35.0
C(6) Restricted affect	28.2	33.3	35.0
C(7) Sense of foreshortened future	26.6	28.2	35.0
D(1) Sleep disturbance	96.0	98.7	100.0
D(2) Irritability/anger	51.6	51.3	50.0
D(3) Difficulty concentrating	66.9	67.9	75.0
D(4) Hypervigilance	53.2	61.5	70.0
D(5) Exaggerated startle response	13.7	14.1	25.0
D(6) Physiologic reactivity	60.5	69.2	75.0

From Kuch, K., and Cox, B. J. Symptoms of PTSD in 124 survivors of the Holocaust. *American Journal of Psychiatry*, 149, 337–340, 1992.

In Eitinger and Strom's study (1973), as mentioned above, appropriate controls matched by sex, occupation, and age bracket were used. The authors found no reason to suspect that the higher frequency of nervousness or alcohol abuse in the POW group was not related to the war effect, assuming that prior personality vulnerabilities were equally frequent in both groups and that the only major distinguishing factor between them was past imprisonment.

Strom et al. (1962), in a paper on 100 prisoners of war referred by the Norwegian authorities for investigation of their disability, report that "in 10 of them slight deviations in childhood existed, 11 described themselves as sensitive, . . . 6 had to be described as un-harmonious, unstable individuals prior to arrest. More important still is the fact that all of them, with the exception of 3, had been in comparatively long-term

and regular employment before the war" (p. 46). These latter findings, however biased the overall study was by the nature of the sampled cases, are nevertheless of interest because they are based on a disabled population judged to deserve compensation.

Eitinger (1964), in his study in Norway and Israel, inquired about premorbid factors and concluded that personality characteristics did not play a role in the aftereffects of the trauma. Regrettably, we do not have the operational definitions used by the author for each category, nor was the investigator blind to the group to which the ex-inmate belonged. Earlier, Helweg-Larssen et al. (1952) had arrived at an identical conclusion in their Danish study, stating that "the main impression is that the repatriates, with regard to both occupation and social position, form a representative section of the population, so that there is no reason for assuming that a greater or smaller degree of pre-dispositions to difficulties in psychological and social readjustment [had been] present" (p. 415).

More recently, Sutker et al. (1993) compared a group of 36 POWs from World War II and 29 combat veterans 40 years after the Pacific war on a number of psychiatric disorders. Current PTSD diagnoses were more frequently made in the former group (70% met criteria) than among the latter (18%, a statistically significant difference) despite similar "personal background characteristics" in which "both had stable emotional and behavioral adjustment during the developmental years, school suspensions or truancy were reported with low frequency, and none of the men admitted substance abuse, arrests as adults, employment difficulties, psychiatric care, or suicide attempts prior to military service" (p. 242). (These measures were obtained using a structured questionnaire.) The major reservation regarding this study is that the researchers did not indicate whether subjects were assessed blindly as to their group affiliation (POW or veteran). Closure on this subject is still to be reached given the above-reported study limitations.

Ursano's clinical study (1981) on six Vietnam POWs is an interesting addition to this literature because his observations were based on intensive psychiatric evaluations that were conducted at both precaptivity and postliberation stages. Based on his findings, Ursano concluded that "neurotic illness can develop under unusually stressful conditions in individuals with no predisposition to psychiatric illness" (p. 318). The small sample size, however, limits the potential contribution of the study. In a companion paper, Ursano et al. (1981) reported findings on 332 Air Force Vietnam POWs made at repatriation. Psychiatric disorders (methods of diagnosis unreported), were found in 23% of them. Five years later an evaluation of 253 of these POWs showed a slight increase in this percentage. These results, although not based on a random sample derived from the total population of POWs, nevertheless are worth considering

because, as the authors noted, "the repatriated POWs [had been] highly screened for flying. They [had been] free of psychiatric disease, were educated, intelligent, successful, motivated" (p. 313).

In summary, the evidence in the literature assigns greater pathogenic weight to massive and cumulative trauma (nurture) than to previous personality (nature). A study on World War II veterans (Lee et al., 1995) supports such a conclusion, at least insofar as war-related PTSD is concerned. The dose–effect, measured by the type of persecution endured, found both in clinical and epidemiological studies, further strengthens the above conclusion.

Role of Social Bonds in Protection from the Aftereffects of Trauma

Antonovsky et al. (1971), reporting on the aftereffects of trauma (see above), noted that not all survivors were found to have an adversely affected health condition. Indeed, "40% of the camp survivors were rated by their physicians as being in excellent or quite good health for women of their age" (p. 40). The authors, led by a focus on health rather than on disease, posed the intriguing question of why, despite repeated traumas, their health condition was no different from that of controls. Survivors, responding to different researchers, stated that a number of factors protected them in the camps against the unbearable stressors, among these were luck, faith in God, and the presence of a relative or friend or the support of a fellow inmate.

Davidson (1979) and others, based on clinical observations, hypothesized that social supports had a buffering effect. Empirical findings on the former inmates that would confirm these reports are not available, except for the study by Fennig and Levav (1991) that investigated the effects of contemporary social support on the mean scores of demoralization in a group of female survivors and in community counterparts after controls (e.g., social class) were introduced in the multivariate analysis. As expected, the higher the scores on the measure they used to elicit the presence of contemporary social supports, the lower the values on the scale of demoralization, ranging from an adjusted mean score of 1.44 for the lowest quartile of support to 1.02 for the highest. The study was not able to explore, however, whether the effect obtained may in turn derive from the protected capacity of the subject's personality to establish, sustain, and enjoy these supports.

Vulnerability of Survivors to Renewed Stress

Shuval (1957-58), in a study conducted in Israel 5 years after the end of the war, argued for the "hardening effect" of previous trauma, a feature that would protect individuals facing renewed life challenges. However, other authors conducting more recent research have been troubled by its possible undermining role. Three studies have been published on this subject, one that refers to possible social threats (anti-Semitism) and two that involve life-threatening stressors: cancer and war under passive conditions.

The first study (Weinfeld et al., 1981) focused on a set of political science questions that were included in the survey of psychiatric symptoms cited above (Eaton et al., 1982). Holocaust survivors (n = 135) residing in Montreal were compared with 120 Jewish city residents born somewhere other than in Canada and 196 Canada-born respondents on two items purported to measure perceived anti-Semitism and other related issues. Contrary to the authors' hypothesis, the results showed that no differences were recorded in the perception of a possible threat arising from the unsettling political changes that the province of Quebec was undergoing at the time.

Two complementary studies conducted in Israel were reported on Holocaust survivors facing the threat of cancer. The authors had posited that several defense mechanisms, mainly denial, that must be adequately mobilized when facing cancer may no longer effectively operate in the survivors. In the first study, Baider and Sarell (1984) compared a group of Holocaust survivors (n =

26) with another group of Europe-born patients who were not survivors (n = 24). The former group scored significantly higher on items measuring low moods and anxiety. In part one of the second study, Baider et al. (1992) compared two groups of rather well-matched cancer patients, survivors and nonsurvivors (both n = 53), on the Brief Symptom Inventory (BSI) and on the Psychosocial Adjustment to Physical Illness Scale, a measure of functioning. The uncontrolled BSI scores were consistently elevated among survivors, indicating higher emotional distress; in their functioning, however, they did not differ from that of the comparison group. In part two of their report, Baider et al. (1993) compared two groups of Holocaust survivors, cancer patients (n = 57) and healthy controls (n = 50), on the BSI. As was expected, the results showed that the former group had statistically significantly higher scores than the comparison group on almost all subscales, even after relevant variables known to affect the results (age and education) were controlled. Both studies, regrettably, suffer from methodological problems (e.g., sample design and a cross-sectional design that does not allow for baseline measures) that are worth overcoming in future research because such studies may identify a population group with emotional vulnerabilities when facing a life-threatening stressor.

Finally, a study was reported by Solomon and Prager (1992), consisting of an assessment of the distress scores measured by a questionnaire that included the state–trait anxiety inventory and a modified scale based on relevant items from the *DSM-III-R* criteria for PTSD administered to elderly Holocaust survivors (n = 61) and nonsurvivors (n = 131). Both groups had been exposed to the Iraqi Scud attacks on Israeli cities during the Gulf war. The results showed that survivors scored marginally higher on both instruments. However, the gap in information resulting from the unavailability of before-the-event measures, as in the preceding cancer studies, and the lack of adequate specifications on the sampling procedures and the continent of origin of the comparison group, renders this inquiry a tentative, although suggestive, exploration.

The issue of heightened vulnerability among survivors to renewed stressors, as it emerges from the studies reviewed here, awaits definitive investigation; its theoretical and practical importance fully justifies further research efforts.

THE QUESTION OF THE INDIRECT EFFECTS OF NAZI PERSECUTION ON THE SECOND GENERATION

Numerous clinic-based observations have suggested that some of the effects of the persecution of parents were transmitted to their offspring (Sigal & Weinfeld, 1989; Solkoff, 1981, 1992). The traumatization suffered by the survivors—with its prolonged psychopathological and psychosocial after-effects, including familial losses, often of spouse and children; the frequent hastily contracted marriages upon liberation; and problems arising from resettlement— among other factors, were thought to impair parenting abilities. Several mediating mechanisms that affected the survivor's family as a functioning unit were postulated, such as overinvolvement, withdrawal, inability to exert control, parental affective unavailability, and undue degree of preoccupation with past experiences (see Levine, 1982; Sigal & Weinfeld, 1989; among others). Other imputed mechanisms referred to psychological processes during child development, such as difficulties in the individuation–separation phase (Freyberg, 1980).

These clinical studies, although methodologically inadequate because of selectivity, small sample sizes, absence of adequate controls, and a host of other factors (Solkoff, 1981, 1992), nevertheless served to raise the interest of researchers. Indeed, there are four implications arising from these observations if taken at face value: clinical, legal, ethical, and sociopsychiatric. As for the latter, demonstrating that the second generation may show higher rates of the types of disorders affecting the parents would pro-

vide persuasive grounds to conclude that the transmission of environmentally induced psychopathology (whether learned or due to other mechanisms) does exist and it is measurable, just as genetics-oriented researchers were successful in proving familial transmission resulting from genetic factors (Kety et al., 1978). An additional scientific advantage of examining this type of traumatized population is the possibility of screening out the effect of a common environment, a problem affecting research where children and parents live together (Kety, 1976).

The clinical studies alluded to earlier focused on families that sought psychiatric assistance (e.g., Rakoff et al., 1966, among many others) following a disorder or complaint (e.g., depressive mood, conduct disorder) of a child. It is noteworthy that, with only a single exception where psychiatric instruments were applied for diagnosis (Schwartz et al., 1994), all studies conducted in the community on the mental status of the second generation, including control populations, involved scales that measured psychological symptoms and personality characteristics rather than psychiatric diagnosis made by trained clinicians. Furthermore, almost all of the controlled studies investigated adolescents or young adults (Solkoff, 1981, 1992; Eitinger & Major, 1993) but not children, who would be in a period of the life cycle when contact with the parents is more intense and continuous.

Most community-based studies were handicapped by problems of sample design and low response rates. Studies originating in Australia (Halik et al., 1990), Canada (e.g., Russell, 1980) (with the exception of Sigal and Weinfeld's inquiry in 1987, which used an acceptable population base), and the United States (e.g., Weiss et al., 1986) for the most part relied on population lists provided by Jewish organizations that do not include all potential respondents; research that was conducted in Israel shared only in part such shortcomings. Additionally, the limited completion rates in both the index and control groups threatened the robustness of the findings, because there is an obvious potential risk of modification of the findings as a result of the effect of nonrespondents.

Solkoff (1981, 1992), Ryn (1990), and Eitinger and Major (1993) have provided detailed reviews of studies on the second generation. Suffice it to mention here that, in stark contrast to the clinical observations, the studies conducted in the community did not show evidence that the offspring of concentration camp survivors have more psychopathology than controls. To be more precise, there are studies that show dissimilar findings in the index subjects and the controls, for example, in reference to family behaviors and attitudes (Last & Klein, 1984; Podietz et al., 1984) and capacity to externalize aggression (cf., Nadler et al., 1985, later criticized by Silverman, 1987). None of these characteristics, however, was found to have clinical significance. Lichtman's study (1984) did find that children of survivors scored higher on the Minnesota Multiphasic Personality Inventory anxiety scales, but methodological problems related to sample selection seriously undermined the results.

In contrast, Schwartz et al. (1994) have conducted the only study that yielded standard psychiatric diagnoses in a two-stage procedure for case identification and diagnosis (Levav et al., 1993). In addition, this investigation relied on an unbiased population source to extract its sample, had a high response rate, and used adequate statistical methods for analysis. Their cohort study comprised young Israel-born adults (ages 25–35) that included 291 second-generation survivors in the screening stage and 147 in the diagnostic stage. The respondents reported the main parental exposure to the different types of Nazi persecution (concentration camp, confinement to a ghetto, or in hiding). The investigation included a suitable group of controls, children whose Europe-born parents had not been in World War II (n = 957 for the screening stage and 476 for the diagnostic). The findings showed that 1 year prevalence rates for the group of disorders studied by the Schedule for Affective Disorders and Schizophrenia/Research Diagnostic Criteria (SADS/RDC) in the diagnostic stage (Levav et al., 1993), including

depressive and anxiety categories, did not reveal differences between both group of respondents, thus confirming the above-noted results. Furthermore, they did not find higher rates of PTSD (measured by two different scales in the screening stage) among the index respondents who had been in combat after the age of 18 in the different Israel–Arab wars than among the controls with similar exposure. Of interest, however, is the fact that lifetime RDC rates were higher in the index group, tentatively suggesting that disorders may have been present earlier in life when the respondents were living in the parental home.

An interesting investigation, by Major (1996) in Norway reinforces the above hypothesis. Major's study, although unavoidably limited by the tiny number (n = 7) of parent survivors included (they represented all those Jews who returned alive from Germany and had children), showed that, when the offspring (n = 19) were young, they exhibited more disorders than the controls (n = 37) (children of Norwegian Jews who fled to Sweden in a rescue operation). No such differences were elicited during adulthood.

With the last two cited studies it is possible to conclude that the methodological issues that marred previous research and that prompted Solkoff (1992) to state that "the [current] findings on the transgenerational effects of the Holocaust-related trauma [are] at best problematic" (p. 342) may now be approaching resolution. Granted, results based on both studies have some limitations: Schwartz et al. (1994) do not report on the possible diagnoses of childhood disorders among the second generation of survivors because the psychiatric instruments used in their study were not designed to make such diagnosis. Major (1996) based her information on the respondents' retrospective report without conducting additional checks; this type of report risks reliability flaws (Bromet et al., 1986). Yet the concurrent evidences of these studies as to the present psychiatric status of the second generation, coupled with the consistent negative findings of almost all other studies done in young adults (Sigal & Weinfeld, 1989; Solkoff, 1992), should now lead researchers to ask what protective factors both enabled the children, if indeed they were affected, to subsequently free themselves from additional psychopathology, and enable the psychologically impaired individuals to fulfill their parenting functions, rather than to investigate whether transmission of the after-effects of the trauma and its sequelae is present (Levav et al., 1998).

CONCLUSION

The abundant clinical literature and the more limited number of epidemiological studies regarding the late effects of the Holocaust leave no doubts that the psychological wounds of the war left evident scars long after the ordeal ended. These findings would provide ample confirmation to the logic of the victimization model as posited by Dohrenwend and Dohrenwend (1981).

From a research vantage point, however, this issue is complex and requires some further discussion. Dohrenwend and Dohrenwend (1969) established the exclusion criteria that research data should meet to enable the determination that "concentration camp experiences produced persistent psychological disorder" (p. 120). These conditions consist of ruling out the existence of premorbid components, the role of physical injury or defects, the presence of current stresses, and the role of secondary gains. Based on their analysis of Eitinger's (1964) work in Norway and Israel, reviewed above, Dohrenwend and Dohrenwend argued that those criteria were met only in part; thus "the existence of environmentally produced persistent psychological disorders in human beings is not proved . . . but [it] could also [be] conclude[d] that because of the nature of the problem it may never be better proved" (1969, pp. 120–121).

Has 25 years of additional research successfully met those four conditions? Admittedly, no study by itself met all criteria. As in a mosaic, the figure emerges, with varied degrees of completeness, from the apposition of multiple components, including the community-based studies on the Holocaust survivors, the examinations of Norwegian and Danish POWs interned in Germany during World War II, and the studies of the Australian and U.S. POWs from the Pacific, Korean and Vietnam theaters.

The community studies conducted in Israel and Canada, taken singly or collectively, conclusively showed that demoralization was higher among Holocaust survivors than among suitable controls. The fact that such a condition was identifiable over three decades after the war may be surprising, yet these findings are consistent with those made on POWs who also underwent life situations of maximum adversity. Thus the research issue no longer is whether demoralization, as an indicator of psychopathology, is present in past victims (recall that psychiatric disorders were not investigated), but rather what contributes to symptom maintenance. The role of secondary gain as a sustaining factor of stress-induced psychopathology has been well documented in psychiatric combat reactions and may be imputed in the maintenance of the concentration camp syndrome in those survivors examined in clinics. However, secondary gain may be an overplayed factor when respondents are investigated in their own households during unrelated health examinations. Note that Thygesen et al. (1970) identified a cluster of marked psychological symptoms in a group of nonclaimant Danish former concentration camp inmates ($n = 52$), and yet no secondary gains could be thought to be at stake in this group. Further studies are thus in place to ascertain the possible sensitization of formerly severely traumatized individuals to stressful life events and daily hassles to explain one possible set of factors that may contribute to symptom maintenance.

The degree of interaction between nature and nurture in the case of individuals under maximum adversity is a matter often contaminated by doctrine rather than explained by solid facts; the accumulated combined information on Holocaust survivors and POWs would suggest that the more stressful the circumstances, the lesser the role played by premorbid factors.

Physical factors obviously cannot be ruled out completely in the study populations because subjects endured prolonged undernutrition and brain trauma that could have resulted in irreversible brain changes (modern methods of neuroimaging may be contributory). Yet this issue may not be theoretically relevant to establishing the causal association between "unfavourable environments and psychological disorder" (Dohrenwend & Dohrenwend, 1969), because the latter could be the final clinically identifiable common path for the effects of all stressors. (If this exclusion condition is deemed necessary by some, the composite research mosaic alluded to earlier could include psychiatric observations made during combat, where most of these physical factors are not present.)

In conclusion, it is safe to admit that the field of social psychiatry has gained considerable knowledge since Dohrenwend and Dohrenwend (1969) reviewed Eitinger's study (1964) regarding the aftereffects of trauma in individuals who have faced maximum adversity. However, it also must be admitted that these gains are somewhat tempered by the methodological limitations of the research conducted so far, as mentioned also in this review.

The epidemiological research agenda on the different topics related to the survivors of maximum adversity (the Holocaust and other origins, since the number of the former are dwindling) remains widely open; the matter of resilience is a mere illustration of one of the scarcely researched issues. The clarification of the protective mechanisms of individuals facing maximum adversity is of theoretical and practical importance and potentially extensive to those individuals subjected to more common types of adverse situations, such as extreme poverty or repeated maltreatment. Studies addressed to health- rather than disease-related topics may also consider the issue of parenting by severely traumatized individuals; as noted earlier, the research findings on the second generation of survivors makes this subject an intriguing area of inquiry (Garland, 1993; Levav et al., in press).

Lindemann (1969), in his discussion of a paper describing the effects of Nazi persecution, pointed out that its documentation is merited by the ethical issues involved and by its relevance to social psychiatry. As long as the wolf and the lamb have not learned to live in peace together, as prophesied in the Bible, the subject of the Holocaust and its aftermath and of other similar persecutions will sadly remain with us, and continue to occupy the attention of mental health researchers and clinicians and of the civilized community of humankind.

Acknowledgments: Drs. B. P. Dohrenwend, J. J. Sigal, and H. Dasberg reviewed earlier drafts of this paper. Drs. M. Levav and R. Kohn provided bibliographical assistance. Mrs. S. della Grota typed the tables. Their help is gratefully acknowledged.

REFERENCES

American Psychiatric Association. (1987). *Diagnostic and statistical manual of mental disorders* (3rd ed., rev.). Washington, DC: American Psychiatric Press.

Antonovsky, A. (1979). *Health, stress and coping.* San Francisco: Jossey-Bass.

Antonovsky, A., Maoz, B., Dowty, N., et al. (1971). Twenty-five years later: A limited study of the sequelae of the concentration camp experience. *Social Psychiatry, 6,* 186–193.

Baider, L., Peretz, T., & Kaplan De-Nour, A. (1992). Effect of the Holocaust on coping with cancer. *Social Science and Medicine, 34,* 11–15.

Baider, L., Peretz, T., & Kaplan De-Nour, A. (1993). Holocaust cancer patients: A comparative study. *Psychiatry, 56,* 349–355.

Baider, L., & Sarell, M. (1984, Fall). Coping with cancer among Holocaust survivors in Israel: An exploratory study. *Journal of Human Stress,* pp. 121–127.

Basoglu, M. (1993). Prevention of torture and care of survivors: An integrated approach. *JAMA, 270,* 606–611.

Bauer, Y. (1982). *A history of the Holocaust.* New York: Franklin Watts.

Bebbe, G. W. (1975). Follow-up studies of World War II and Korean War prisoners. II: morbidity, disability, and maladjustments. *American Journal of Epidemiology, 101,* 400–422.

Bettelheim, B. (1943). Individual and mass behavior in extreme situations. *Journal of Abnormal and Social Psychology, 38*, 417–452.

Bromet, E. J., Dunn, L. O., Connell, M. M., Dew, M. A., & Schulberg, H. C. (1986). Longterm reliability of diagnosis lifetime major depression in a community sample. *Archives of General Psychiatry, 43*, 435–440.

Carmil, D., & Carel, R. S. (1986). Emotional distress and satisfaction in life among Holocaust survivors—a community study of survivors and controls. *Psychological Medicine, 16*, 141–149.

Chodoff, P. (1963). Late effects of the concentration camp syndrome. *Archives of General Psychiatry, 8*, 323–333.

Clayton, P. J., & Darvish, H. S. (1979). Course of depressive symptoms following the stress of bereavement. In J. Barrett, R. M. Rose, & G. L. Klerman (Eds.), *Stress and mental disorder* (pp. 121–136). New York: Raven Press.

Davidson, S. (1979). Massive psychic traumatization and social support. *Journal of Psychosomatic Research, 23*, 395–402.

Dohrenwend, B. P., & Dohrenwend, B. S. (1969). *Social status and psychological disorder: A causal inquiry.* New York: John Wiley & Sons.

Dohrenwend, B. P., & Dohrenwend, B. S. (1981). Socioenvironmental factors, stress, and psychopathology—Part 2: Hypotheses about stress processes linking social class to various types of psychopathology. *American Journal of Community Psychology, 9*, 146–159.

Dor-Shav, N. K. (1978). On the long range effects of concentration camp internment on Nazi victims: 25 years later. *Journal of Consulting and Clinical Psychology, 46*, 1–11.

Eaton, W. W. (1981). Long-term effects of the Holocaust on selected social attitudes and behaviors of survivors: A cautionary note. *Social Forces, 60*, 1–19.

Eaton, W. W., Sigal, J. J., & Weinfeld, M. (1982). Impairment in Holocaust survivors after 33 years: Data from an unbiased community sample. *American Journal of Psychiatry, 139*, 773–777.

Eitinger, L. (1961). Pathology of the concentration camp syndrome. *Archives of General Psychiatry, 5*, 371–379.

Eitinger, L. (1964). *Concentration camp survivors in Norway and Israel.* London: Allen & Unwin.

Eitinger, L. (1972). *Concentration camp survivors in Norway and Israel.* The Hague: Martinus Nijhoff.

Eitinger, L., & Krell, R. (1985). *The psychological and medical effects of concentration camps and related persecutions on survivors of the Holocaust.* Vancouver: University of British Columbia Press.

Eitinger, L., & Major, E. F. (1993). Stress of the Holocaust. In L. Glodberger & S. Breznitz (Eds.), *Handbook of stress: Theoretical and clinical aspects* (2nd. ed.) (pp. 617–637). New York: The Free Press.

Eitinger, L., & Strom, A. (1973). *Mortality and morbidity after excessive stress: A follow-up investigation of Norwegian concentration camp survivors.* New York: Humanities Press.

Fennig, S., & Levav, I. (1991). Demoralization and social supports among Holocaust survivors. *Journal of Nervous and Mental Disease, 179*, 167–172.

Frankl, V. E. (1954). Group therapeutic experiences in a concentration camp. *Group Psychotherapy, 7*, 81–90.

Freyberg, J. T. (1980). Difficulties in separation-individuation as experienced by offspring of Nazi Holocaust survivors. *American Journal of Orthopsychiatry, 50*, 87–95.

Garland, C. (1993). The lasting trauma of the concentration camps. *BMJ, 307*, 77–78.

Goldstein, G., van Kammen, W., Shelly, C., Miller, D. J., & van Kammen, D. P. (1987). Survivors of imprisonment in the Pacific theater during World War II. *American Journal of Psychiatry, 144*, 1210–1213.

Hafner, H. (1968). Psychological disturbances following prolonged persecution. *Social Psychiatry, 3*, 79–88.

Halik, V., Rosenthal, D. A., & Pattison, P. E. (1990). Intergenerational effects of the Holocaust: Patterns of engagement in the mother-daughter relationship. *Family Process, 29*, 325–339.

Hefez, A., Metz, L., & Lavie, P. (1987). Longterm effects of extreme situational stress on sleep and dreaming. *American Journal of Psychiatry, 144*, 344–347.

Helweg-Larson, P., Hoffmeyer, H., Kieler, J., et al. (1952). Famine disease in German concentration camps. Complications and sequelae. *Acta Psychiatrica et Neurologica Scandinavica, Supplementum, 83*.

Jacobs, S. (1993). *Pathologic Grief.* Washington, DC: American Psychiatric Press.

Keilson, H. (1992). *Sequential traumatization in children.* Jerusalem: Magness Press.

Kety, S. S. (1976). Studies designed to disentangle genetic and environmental variables in schizophrenia: Some epistemological questions and answers. *American Journal of Psychiatry, 133,* 1134–1137.

Kety, S. S., Wender, P. H., & Rosenthal, D. (1978). Genetic relationships within the schizophrenia spectrum: Evidence from adoption studies. In R. L. Spitzer & D. F. Klein (Eds.), *Critical issues in psychiatric diagnosis* (pp. 213–223). New York: Raven Press.

Kral, A. V. (1951). Psychiatric observations under severe chronic stress. *American Journal of Psychiatry, 108,* 185–192.

Krystal, H. (1968). *Massive Psychic Trauma.* New York: International University Press.

Kuch, K., & Cox, B. J. Symptoms of PTSD in 124 survivors of the Holocaust. *American Journal of Psychiatry, 49,* 337–340.

Last, U., & Klein, H. (1984). Impact of parental Holocaust traumatization on offsprings' reports of parental child-rearing practices. *Journal of Youth and Adolescence, 13,* 267–283.

Lee, K. A., Vaillant, G. E., Torrey, W. C., & Elder, G. H. (1995). A 50-year prospective study of the psychological sequelae of World War II combat. *American Journal of Psychiatry, 152, 4,* 516–522.

Levav, I. & Abramson, J. H. (1984). Emotional distress among concentration camp survivors: A community study in Jerusalem. *Psychological Medicine, 14,* 215–218.

Levav, I., Kohn, R., Dohrenwend, B. P., Shrout, P. E., Skodol, A. E., Schwartz, S., Link, B. G., & Naveh, G. (1993). An epidemiologic study of mental disorders in a 10 year cohort of young adults in Israel. *Psychological Medicine, 23,* 691–707.

Levav, I., Kohn, R., & Schwartz, S. (in press). The psychiatric after-effects of the holocaust on the second generation. *Psychological Medicine.*

Levine, H. R. (1982). Toward a psychoanalytic understanding of children of survivors of the Holocaust. *Psychiatric Quarterly,* 70–92.

Lichtman, H. (1984). Parental communication of Holocaust experience and personality characteristics among second-generation survivors. *Journal of Clinical Psychology, 40,* 914–924.

Lindemann, E. (1969). Discussion of Haefner, H. Psychosocial changes following racial and political persecution. *Association for Research in Nervous and Mental Disease–Research Publications, 47,* 101–117.

Link, B., & Dohrenwend, B. P. (1980). Formulation of hypotheses about the true prevalence of demoralization in the United States. In B.

P. Dohrenwend, B. S. Dohrenwend, S. Schwartz, M. Gould, et al. (Eds.), *Mental illness in the United States. Epidemiological estimates.* New York: Praeger.

Link, B., & Dohrenwend, B. P. (1980). Formulation of hypotheses about the true prevalence of demoralization in the United States. In B. S. Dohrenwend, B. S. Dohrenwend, M. Schwartz-Gould, B. Link, R. Neugebauer, & R. Wunsch-Hitz (Eds.), *Epidemiologic estimates* (pp. 114–132). New York: Praeger.

Major, M. F. (1996). The impact of the Holocaust on the second generation: Norwegian Jewish Holocaust survivors and their children. *Journal of Traumatic Stress, 9,* 441–452.

Matussek, P. (1975). *Internment in concentration camps and its consequences.* New York: Springer-Verlag.

Nadler, A., Kav-Venaki, S., & Gleitman, B. (1985). Transgenerational effects of the Holocaust: Externalization of aggression in second generation Holocaust survivors. *Journal of Consulting and Clinical Psychology, 53,* 365–369.

Nadler, A., & Ben-Shushan, D. (1989). Forty years later: Long-term consequences of massive traumatization as manifested by Holocaust survivors from the city and the kibbutz. *Journal of Consulting and Clinical Psychology, 57,* 287–293.

Podietz, L., Zwerling, I., Ficher, I., et al. (1984). Engagement in families of Holocaust survivors. *Journal of Marital and Family Therapy, 10,* 43–51.

Rakoff, V., Sigal, J. J., & Epstein, N. B. (1966). Children and families of concentration camp survivors. *Canada's Mental Health, 14,* 24–26.

Rappaport, E. A. Beyond traumatic neurosis: A psychoanalytic study of late reactions to concentration camp trauma (1968). *International Journal of Psychoanalysis, 49,* 719–731.

Robinson, S., Rapaport-Bar-Sever, M., & Rapaport, J. (1994). The present state of people who survived the Holocaust as children. *Acta Psychiatric Scandinavica, 89,* 242–245.

Russell, A. (1980). Late effects: Influence on the children of the concentration camp survivor. In J. E. Dimsdale (Ed.), *Survivors, victims and perpetrators* (pp. 175–203). Washington, DC: Hemisphere.

Ryn, Z. (1990). The evolution of mental disturbances in the concentration camp syndrome (KZ-Syndrom). *Genetic, Social and General Psychology Monographs, 116,* 21–36.

Schwartz, S., Dohrenwend, B. P., & Levav, I. (1994). Non-genetic familial transmission of psychiatric disorders? Evidence from the children of the Holocaust. *Journal of Health and Social Behavior, 354,* 385–402.

Shrout, P. E., Dohrenwend, B. P., & Levav, I. (1986). Screening scales from the Psychiatric Epidemiology Research Interview PEP. In M. M. Weissman, J. K. Meyers, & C. E. Ross (Eds.), *Community surveys of psychiatric disorders* (pp. 249–275. New Brunswick, NJ: Rutgers University Press.

Shuval, J. T. (1957-58). Some persistent effects of trauma: Five years after the Nazi concentration camps. *Social Problems, 5,* 230–243.

Sigal, J. J., & Weinfeld, M. (1987). Mutual involvement and alienation in families of Holocaust survivors. *Psychiatry, 50,* 280–288.

Sigal, J. J., & Weinfeld, M. (1989). *Trauma and rebirth. Intergenerational effects of the Holocaust.* New York: Praeger.

Silverman, W. K. (1987). Methodological issues in the study of transgenerational effects of the Holocaust: Comment on Nadler, Kav-Venaki, and Gleitman. *Journal of Consulting and Clinical Psychology, 55,* 125–126.

Solkoff, N. (1981). Children of survivors of the Nazi Holocaust: A critical review of the literature. *American Journal of Orthopsychiatry, 51,* 29–42.

Solkoff, N. (1992). Children of survivors of the Nazi Holocaust. A critical review of the literature. *American Journal of Orthopsychiatry, 62,* 342–358.

Solomon, Z., & Prager, E. (1992). Elderly Israeli Holocaust survivors during the Persian Gulf War: A study of psychological distress. *American Journal of Psychiatry, 149,* 1707–1710.

Strom, A. (1968). *Norwegian concentration camp survivors.* Oslo: Universitesforlaget.

Strom, A., Refsum, S. B., Eitinger, L., Gronvik, O., Lonnum, A., Engeset, A., Osvik, K., & Rogan, B. (1962). Examination of Norwegian ex-concentration camp prisoners. *Journal of Neuropsychiatry, 4,* 43–62.

Sutker, P. B., Allain, A. N., & Winstead, D. K. (1993). Psychopathology and psychiatric diagnoses of World War II Pacific theatre prisoner of war survivors and combat veterans. *American Journal of Psychiatry, 150,* 240–245.

Tennant, C. C., Goulston, K. J., & Dent, O. F. (1986). The psychological effects of being a prisoner of war: Forty years after release. *American Journal of Psychiatry, 143,* 618–621.

Thygesen, P., Hermann, K., & Willanger, R. (1970). Concentration camp survivors in Denmark. Persecution, disease, disability, compensation. *Danish Medical Bulletin, 17,* 65–108.

Ursano, R. J. (1981). The Vietnam era prisoner of war: Precaptivity personality and the development of psychiatric illness. *American Journal of Psychiatry, 138,* 315–318.

Ursano, R. J., Boydstun, J. A., & Wheatley, R. D. (1981). Psychiatric illness in U.S. Air Force Viet Nam prisoners of war: A five-year follow-up. *American Journal of Psychiatry, 138,* 310–314.

Venn, A. J., & Guest, C. S. (1991). Chronic morbidity of former prisoners of war and other Australian veterans. *Medical Journal of Australia, 155,* 705–712.

Weiss, E., O'Connell, A. N., & Siiter, R. (1986). Comparison of second-generation Holocaust survivors, immigrants, and non-immigrants on measures of mental health. *Journal of Personality and Social Psychology, 4,* 828–831.

World Health Organization. (1992). *The ICD-10 classification of mental and behavioural disorders, clinical descriptions and diagnostic guidelines.* Geneva: World Health Organization.

2

Symptoms, Functioning, and Health Problems in a Massively Traumatized Population: The Legacy of the Cambodian Tragedy

Richard F. Mollica
Charles Poole
Svang Tor

In 1990, a team of researchers from the Harvard Program in Refugee Trauma (HPRT), with the co-sponsorship of the World Federation for Mental Health (WFMH) and the Ford Foundation (Bangkok), conducted a population-based survey of Cambodians living in the refugee camp known as Site 2. Containing more than 150,000 displaced persons, Site 2 was for over a decade the largest camp for displaced Cambodians along the Thai border (Fig. 2.1) [World Health Organization (WHO), 1986].

From as early as 1988, the Thai government, the United Nations, and numerous voluntary agencies had acknowledged that immediate action was needed to remedy the deteriorating social and psychological conditions in Site 2 and the other border camps [Committee for the Coordination of Services to Displaced Persons Thailand (CCSDPT), 1988]. Preliminary reports by the WHO (Diekstra, 1988) and the WFMH

(Mollica & Jalbert, 1989; Mollica et al., 1989) suggested a great impact of trauma and confinement on this population. To obtain detailed, population-based information for improving the psychosocial environment of the Thai camps, the HPRT conducted a household survey to measure the extent of trauma, the physical and mental health symptoms, and the relative disability of the adult community living in the camps. Preliminary scientific findings and policy recommendations have been reported previously (Mollica et al., 1993).

This chapter presents additional findings to continue the evaluation of the psychosocial impact of mass violence on this civilian refugee population. The principal aim is to identify differences by gender in traumatic experiences, psychiatric and physical symptoms, and social and economic limitations. In addition, preliminary results are presented on "dose–response" relationships

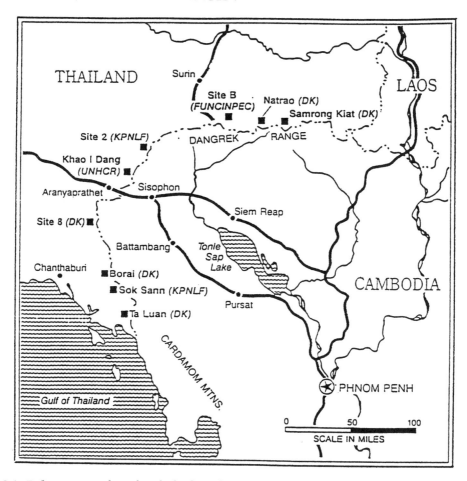

Figure 2.1. Refugee camps along the Thailand-Cambodia border. Abbreviations: DK, Democratic Kampuchea; FUNCINPEC, National United Front for an Independent, Neutral, Peaceful and Cooperative Cambodia; KPNLF, Khmer People's National Liberation Front; UNHCR, United Nations High Commissioner for Refugees. [From Lawyers Committee for Human Rights, 1987, with permission.]

between cumulative trauma and symptoms of depression and post-traumatic stress disorder.

BACKGROUND

It is estimated that 1.5 million to 3.0 million Cambodians, or 20%–40% of the total population, died between 1975 and 1979 under the communist Khmer Rouge regime led by Pol Pot (Hannum, 1989; Kiljunen, 1985). In 1979 and 1980, with the regime's collapse, hundreds of thousands of malnourished and diseased Cambodians fled to safety in Thai-

land (Centers for Disease Control, 1979, 1980; Glass et al., 1980). Initially, under the auspices of the United Nations High Commissioner for Refugees, many of the refugees were resettled to the United States and other Western nations. However, this early resettlement program was stopped by the Thai government, leaving more than 300,000 Cambodian refugees, who were assembled into enclosed camps along the Thai-Cambodian border (Rogge, 1992).

Site 2 was a long, oval perimeter (Fig. 2.2) bounded by a barbed wire fence and policed by the Thai military, who strictly controlled entry and egress. Within Site 2,

THE PLAN OF SITE 2 CAMP
SCALE 1:10,000

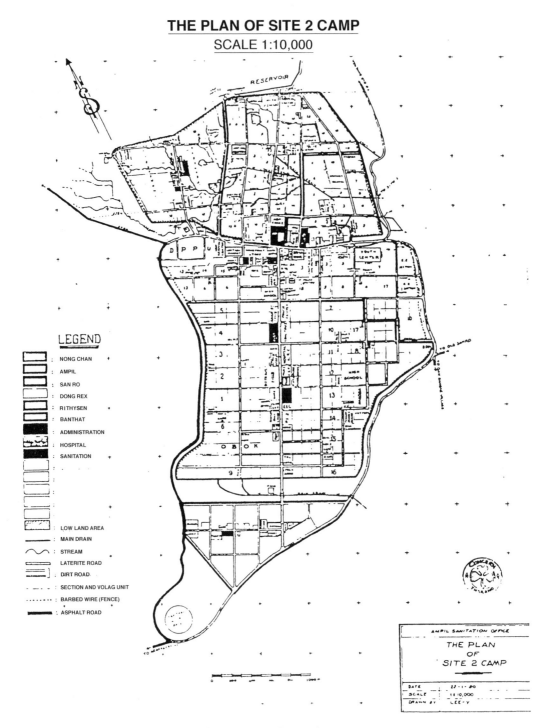

Figure 2.2. Grid map of Site 2.

the Cambodian population was housed in small bamboo structures, with families of six allocated housing units 4 × 6 m in size. A mean of 16 families shared each common latrine (WHO, 1986). The camp population was totally dependent upon the United Nations for all subsistence (Reynell, 1989). The camp had no electricity, and water was scarce because it had to be trucked in daily. Primary schools provided limited education to grade 6, adult education and vocational training were minimal, farming was prohibited, and only limited employment for additional food rations was legally allowed. Food consisted of a monotonous daily diet of fish and rice donated by the international community. Western medical services, in contrast to the extreme poverty and material deprivation of the camp, were extensive and effective.

Like the other Thai border camps for Cambodians, Site 2 was unsafe. During the time of the survey, for instance, Vietnamese troops occupied Cambodia and were routinely shelling the camps. Because of the changing military and political situation in Cambodia, the population of Site 2 had to be relocated on numerous occasions. In addition to shelling and military attacks, the residents feared violence from bandits, the Cambodian guerrillas fighting the Vietnamese, and the Thai security officers. At the time of the survey, United Nations reports revealed a dramatic increase in violence between camp residents [United Nations Border Relief Operation (UNBRO), 1985]. Lack of effective justice and police systems seemed to contribute to greater violence among neighbors and family members, permitting outsiders to prey violently upon the community (Lawyers Committee for Human Rights, 1987, 1989).

METHODS

The study consisted of a cross-sectional survey of demographic information, trauma experiences, psychiatric symptoms, health status, and physical and social functioning in a random sample of Site 2 residents. The project, which included informed consent from all participants, was approved by the Medical Ethics Committee of UNBRO and by the Human Subjects Committee of the Harvard School of Public Health.

Participants were selected by multistage, area probability sampling. Site 2 was divided into five camps (Nong Chan, San Ro, and Ampil in Site 2 North and Rithysen and Dong Rek in Site 2 South), with each camp laid out in a gridlike pattern (Fig. 2.2). One hundred sampling points were distributed among the camps in proportion to the number of households in each camp, using census estimates from UNBRO (Rithysen received 39%; Ampil, 22%; Nong Chan, 18%; Dong Rek, 14%; and San Ro, 7%). Using the grid map (Fig. 2.2), the assigned sampling points were distributed randomly throughout each camp's geographic area. The order of points within camps and the starting place within points were randomly assigned. A sampling point was considered complete when interviews were completed for ten households within that point. A household was considered complete if interviews were conducted with persons in each of the three phases of the study: (1) one adult age 18 years or older, randomly selected from the household roster (the phase forming the subject of the present report); (2) all teenagers in the household age 16 or 17 years; and (3) all children in the household age 12 or 13 years plus one parent of each child.

Because details of the development and testing of the interview schedule and of the recruitment and training of the interviewers are described fully elsewhere (Mollica et al., 1993), a brief synopsis is provided here. The interview schedule consisted of sections previously translated and used in Khmer populations and sections newly adapted and translated for this study. The section on demographic items was adapted from a previous survey of Site 2 residents (Lynch, 1989). The sections on health status and on physical and social functioning were adapted from the short form of the Medical Outcomes Study (Steward et al., 1988). The sections on trauma history and symptoms of post-traumatic stress disorder were drawn from the 15-item section on depressive symptoms from the Cambodian version of the Hopkins Symptom Checklist–25 (Mollica et al., 1987a) and from the Cambodian version of the Harvard Trauma Questionnaire (Mollica et al., 1992), which consisted in this study of 16 criterion symptoms for post-traumatic stress disorder and an additional 15 culturally dependent symptoms derived from clinical experience with Cambodian refugees. Both sets of symptom questions referred to the week prior to the interview and were scored on a four-point scale (1, not at all; 2, a little; 3, quite a bit; 4, extremely). In keeping with previous work (Mollica & Caspi-Yavin, 1991; Mollica et al., 1987a, 1992, 1993), the symptom scores for individual participants were computed as the arithmetic means of the item-specific scores, thus retaining the three-point range (1.00 to 4.00). Criteria ranges of greater than 1.75 on the depressive symptom scale and greater than 2.50 on the scale of post-traumatic stress symptoms have been validated against clinical diagnoses and found to have high sensitivity among Southeast Asian refugees in a clinic setting in the United States (Mollica et al., 1987a, 1992).

The interviews were conducted in Khmer by volunteer residents of Site 2, equally distributed by gender, who received 4 days of training. Their first two interviews were observed by Cambodian supervisors. The interviewers were randomly assigned to the primary sampling units after exclusion of the units in which they resided. The interviews averaged approximately 90 minutes in length.

Aside from cross-tabulated descriptive statistics, the analyses in the present report include the use of scatterplot smoothing to examine the relationship of cumulative trauma to educational level and year of arrival in refugee camps (SAS System, Release 6.08 for Microsoft Windows, Cary, NC) and logistic regression modeling to quantify the relationship of psychiatric symptoms to cumulative trauma (LogXact-Turbo, Version 1.0, Cytel Software Corporation, Cambridge, MA).

RESULTS

Demographics

Of the 1000 adults randomly selected for participation, 998 were interviewed and 5 were eliminated from the analysis for being under age (Table 2.1). The preponderance of women reflects the gender distribution of the camp population, because men were more likely to be involved in military activities outside the camp. The majority of respondents were young to middle-aged adults, married, poorly educated, and from Battambang province. Ninety-eight percent described themselves as Buddhist. The men were more highly educated than the women, and proportionately more of the men were married. Most of the participants had been in Thai border camps for at least 10 years and at Site 2 for 5 years.

Trauma

The mean numbers of trauma events reported under Pol Pot and the Khmer Rouge (1975–1979) were 14 among the men and 12 among the women (Table 2.2). Cumulative trauma under the Khmer Rouge was strongly related to early arrival in Site 2 and to level of education (Table 2.2). The relationships of year of arrival and education to cumulative trauma in the Pol Pot era are described in further detail in Figure 2.3. Trauma in this time period shows little association with year of arrival in Thai border camps in general, with the exception of a slight increase among those arriving in 1986 and 1987 and a slight decrease among those arriving in 1989 (see Fig. 2.3). Year of arrival in the Site 2 camp, however, is strongly related to trauma under the Khmer Rouge. The 26 participants who arrived in the Site 2 camp prior to 1984 reported substantially more trauma events than those who arrived contemporaneously in other camps or who arrived subsequently at any camp (Fig. 2.3A). Those who joined the Site 2 camp in 1984 and 1985, when the camp grew vastly in size as a consolidation of several other

Table 2.1. Demographic characteristics of 993 adult residents of Site 2, Thailand, 1990, by gender

Characteristic	Category	Men (n = 383)		Women (n = 610)		Total (n = 993)	
		n	Percent	n	Percent	n	Percent
Age (years)	18–24	42	11.0	95	15.6	137	13.8
	25–34	146	38.1	243	39.8	389	39.2
	35–44	106	27.7	167	27.4	273	27.5
	45–90	89	23.2	105	17.2	194	19.5
Marital status	Never married	35	9.1	24	3.9	59	5.9
	Married	328	85.6	386	63.3	714	71.9
	Widowed	12	3.1	99	16.2	111	11.2
	Separated	5	1.3	89	14.6	94	9.5
	Divorced	3	0.8	12	2.0	15	1.5
Education (years)	0	55	14.4	231	37.9	286	28.8
	1–5	171	44.6	279	45.7	450	45.3
	6–10	114	29.8	74	12.1	188	18.9
	11–20	34	8.9	9	1.5	43	4.3
	Unknown	9	2.4	17	2.8	26	2.6
Province of origin	Battambang	178	46.5	323	53.0	501	50.5
	Kandal	29	7.6	35	5.7	64	6.4
	Phnom Penh	24	6.3	59	9.7	83	8.4
	Siem Reap	23	6.0	39	6.4	62	6.2
	Other	105	24.4	121	19.8	226	22.8
	Unknown	24	6.3	33	5.4	57	5.7
Year of arrival in any border camp	1979–1983	279	72.8	469	76.9	748	75.3
	1984–1990	101	26.4	135	22.1	236	23.8
	Unknown	3	0.8	6	1.0	9	0.9
Year of arrival in Site 2	1979–1983	14	3.7	12	2.0	26	2.6
	1984–1990	365	95.3	587	96.2	952	95.9
	Unknown	4	1.0	11	1.8	15	1.5

camps, and those who arrived in the 2 years prior to the survey, reported relatively little Pol Pot era trauma. Participants arriving in Site 2 in the intervening years reported an intermediate level of trauma under the Khmer Rouge.

There has been considerable anecdotal reporting in newspapers and biographies (Ngor, 1987) that highly educated persons were singled out by the Khmer Rouge for special abuse. In particular, Cambodian survivors of the Pol Pot era have indicated that the wearing of eyeglasses was interpreted by the Khmer Rouge as a sign of higher education, elevated social class, and Western corruption. It has been said that, if the Khmer Rouge found a pair of eyeglasses in the possession of an incarcerated person, it could lead to immediate maltreatment, torture, or even execution. Therefore, in addition to the trend among all participants, separate trends are shown for those who reported a need to wear eyeglasses and for those who did not (Fig. 2.3B). Among persons who did not wear eyeglasses, trauma did not begin to rise sharply with education

Table 2.2. Cumulative trauma in the Pol Pot era (1975–1979) and in the year prior to interview and prevalence of elevated scores for symptoms of depression and post-traumatic stress among 993 adult residents of Site 2, Thailand, 1990, by demographic characteristics

| Characteristic | Category | n | Mean number of trauma events | | Percent with elevated symptom scores | |
			1975–1979	Past year	Depressive[°]	Posttraumatic stress[†]
Total	All	993	12.6	0.9	67.9	37.2
Gender	Male	383	14.0	1.0	63.7	34.2
	Female	610	11.8	0.7	70.5	39.0
Age (years)	18–24	137	11.4	1.0	59.8	31.4
	25–34	389	12.8	0.8	64.0	30.1
	35–44	273	13.4	0.9	69.6	41.4
	45–90	194	12.2	0.8	78.9	4.95
Marital status	Never married	59	12.2	0.9	55.9	23.7
	Married	709	13.1	0.8	64.7	34.3
	Disrupted	225	11.4	1.1	81.4	49.8
Education (years)	0	286	11.9	0.8	72.7	41.3
	1–5	450	11.8	0.8	66.4	35.6
	6–10	188	14.3	0.9	62.2	30.9
	11–20	43	17.7	1.1	67.4	48.8
	Unknown	26	14.8	1.2	80.8	46.2
Province of origin	Battambang	501	11.8	0.7	65.1	34.3
	Kandal	62	13.8	1.2	68.8	43.8
	Phnom Penh	83	14.2	1.1	77.1	37.4
	Siem Reap	62	14.8	0.8	75.8	50.0
	Other	226	12.9	0.7	67.7	37.2
	Unknown	57	12.6	1.9	70.2	40.4
Year of arrival in any border camp	1979–1983	748	12.1	0.9	66.0	36.4
	1984–1990	236	14.4	0.7	75.0	41.1
	Unknown	9	12.0	0.4	33.3	0.0
Year of arrival in Site 2	1979–1983	26	21.0	0.6	84.6	80.8
	1984–1990	952	12.3	0.9	67.5	35.9
	Unknown	15	17.4	0.3	60.0	40.0

[°]Depressive symptom score greater than 1.75 (see text).

[†]Post-traumatic stress symptom score peater than 2.50 (see text).

until they had achieved approximately 12 years of schooling. Among those who wore eyeglasses, the increase in trauma began much earlier, at about 5 years of schooling. These results suggest that wearing eyeglasses did in fact cause individuals to receive more trauma than those who did not wear eyeglasses, above the independent effect of education. The 41 respondents who needed eyeglasses and who had more than 10 years of education reported by far the greatest degrees of cumulative trauma during that time period.

In Site 2 during the year immediately prior to the survey, cumulative trauma was greatly reduced. Respondents reported ex-

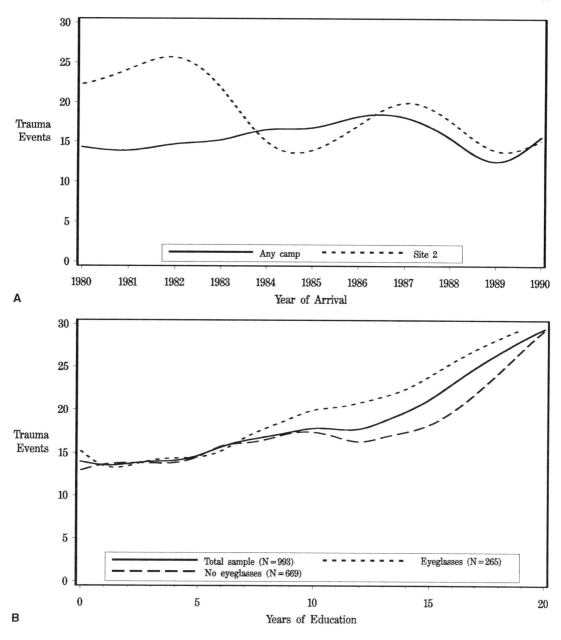

Figure 2.3. Cumulative trauma in the Pol Pot era (1975–1979) reported by 993 adult residents of Site 2, Thailand, 1990. *A*: Trauma events in relation to year of arrival in Thai border camps. *B*: Trauma events in relation to years of education, by need for eyeglasses.

periencing a mean of approximately one trauma event in this period (Table 2.2). These distributions were skewed in the opposite direction of the distributions of Pol Pot era trauma, however, because 45% of men and 53% of women reported zero trauma events in the past year (Fig. 2.4B).

As under the Khmer Rouge, men reported more trauma than women in the camp. However, the early arrivals in Site 2, who had experienced high levels of cumulative trauma in the Pol Pot era, reported relatively little trauma in the camp (Table 2.2). Participants from Kandal and Phnom Penh

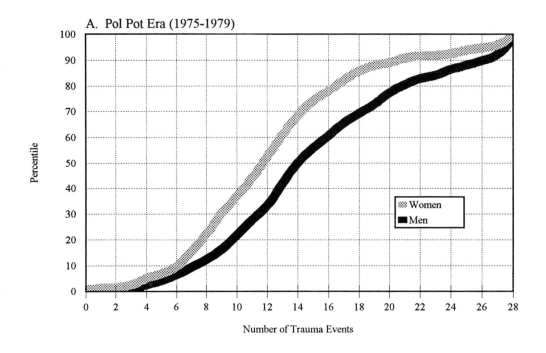

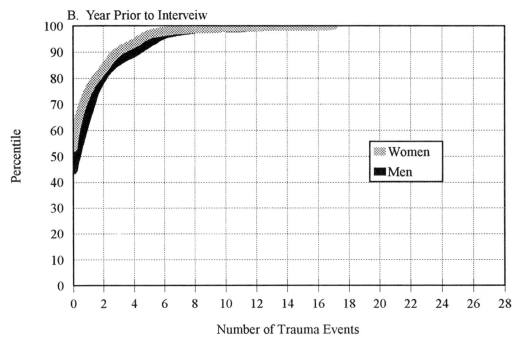

Figure 2.4. Distribution of cumulative trauma in the Pol Pot era (1975–1979) (A) and in the year prior to interview (B) reported by 993 adult residents of Site 2, Thailand, 1990.

reported relatively more trauma in the camp and those from Battambang, Siem Reap, and other provinces relatively little.

Of the 28 specific trauma events, 13 were reported by a majority of the men and 10 by a majority of the women in the Pol Pot era (Fig. 2.5A). The excess among men was apparent to varying degrees for all events. Lack of food, water, and shelter; murder of a family member or friend; forced labor; ill health with no medical care; and brainwashing and witnessing of brainwashing, beatings, and torture were essentially ubiquitous under the Khmer Rouge. Trauma in the past year consisted primarily of experiences related to the quality of camp life, such as lack of food, water, and shelter; witnessing of knifing and axing was the most frequently reported event involving violence (Fig. 2.5B). None of the trauma events, including unspecified forms of torture and specific forms such as near-suffocation with a plastic bag, reached absolute zero frequency in the camp.

Psychiatric Symptoms

Approximately two-thirds of the respondents had depressive symptom scores and about one-third had post-traumatic stress symptom scores in the clinical ranges (Table 2.2). Elevated depressive and post-traumatic stress symptom scores were particularly prevalent among women, the elderly, persons of disrupted marital status (widowed, divorced, or separated), participants from Siem Reap, and those who said they had joined the Site 2 camp prior to 1984. Participants from Phnom Penh had relatively high levels of depressive symptoms, but not of post-traumatic stress symptoms. Respondents who lacked any formal education reported the most depressive symptoms, but post-traumatic stress symptoms were most common among the most highly educated.

Health Status and Social Functioning

About one-third of the Site 2 residents interviewed described their health status as "poor," and a majority responded affirmatively to the question, "Does your health keep you from working at a job, doing work around the house, or going to school?" (Table 2.3). Relatively long-term disability (> 3 months) was much less common, being reported by only one-fifth of the respondents. Self-perceptions of poor health and of impaired functioning were most common among women, the elderly, persons who had ever been married, those with the least formal education, those from Phnom Penh and Siem Reap, and those who had arrived in any border camp prior to 1984.

Despite the widespread self-perceptions of poor health and functional impairment, nearly half of the respondents were engaged in income-generating activity in Site 2 (Table 2.3). The highest proportions of persons doing something to earn a living were among men, persons in the intermediate age groups (25–44), ever-married persons, the more highly educated, those who came from Kandal and Phnom Penh, and those who said they had joined the Site 2 camp before 1984.

A majority of respondents reported short-term and long-term health-related limitations of physical activity (Fig. 2.6). Limitations of any duration in engaging in the most vigorous activities were reported more commonly by women (Fig. 2.6A), but the female excess was not present for relatively long-term limitation (Fig. 2.6B). Men reported a much higher prevalence than women of long-term limitation in the least vigorous activities [eating, dressing, bathing, or using the toilet (Fig. 2.6B)].

The most common specific health problems reported by Site 2 respondents were frequent headaches, dizziness, weakness, and poor appetite, all of which were reported by more than 50% of men and women (Fig. 2.7). The women reported higher prevalences of all health-specific problems except for head injury and paralysis in an extremity.

Cumulative Trauma and Psychiatric Symptoms

Table 2.4 shows associations between elevated psychiatric symptoms and cumulative

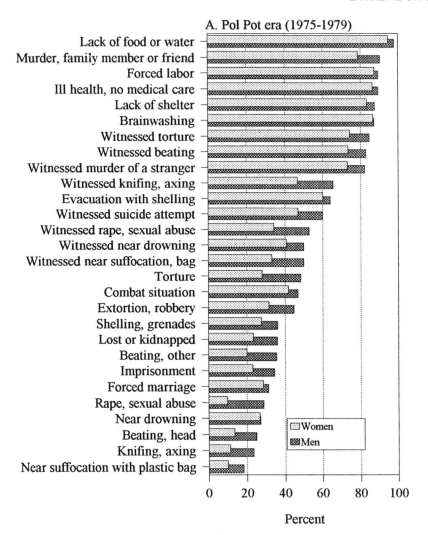

Figure 2.5. Specific trauma events in the Pol Pot era (1975–1979) (*A*) and in the year prior to interview (*B*) reported by 993 adult residents of Site 2, Thailand, 1990. *Illustration continues on opposite page.*

trauma in the Pol Pot era (1975–1979). Pronounced upward trends, in the nature of "dose–response" relationships, are apparent. At the very highest levels of cumulative trauma, scores in the clinical ranges were nearly ubiquitous for symptoms of depression and post-traumatic stress. The associations shown were computed after controlling for age, gender, education level, marital status, and cumulative trauma in Site 2 during the year prior to interview.

DISCUSSION

This survey quantifies the massive trauma experienced by Site 2 residents during the Pol Pot era (1975–1979) and the dramatic reduction, but not elimination, of trauma in the refugee camp environment. In spite of the improvement of camp life over the Khmer Rouge work camps, respondents indicated that Site 2 had problems of safety and protection, material assistance, and vulnerability to shelling and bombing. These

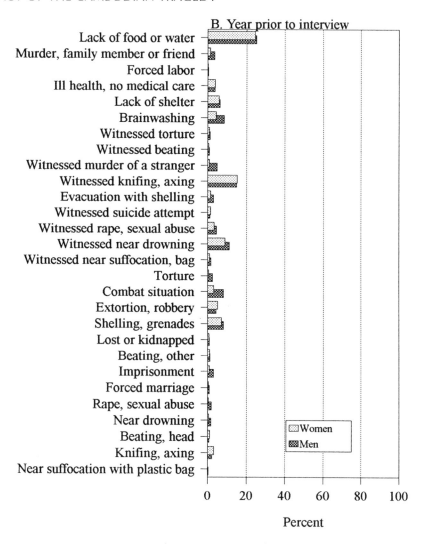

Figure 2.5. *Continued*

findings are consistent with the reports of the United Nations (UNBRO, 1985) and the international community (Amnesty International, 1986; CCSDPT, 1988; Crossette, 1988; Lawyers Committee for Human Rights, 1987, 1989) serving the Cambodian refugees on the Thai border.

Interestingly, the survey data confirm two widely held historical beliefs regarding the Thai border camps. The first consists of previously anecdotal claims that educated Cambodians were targets of the Khmer Rouge's worst aggression (Ngor, 1987). Familiar refugee tales that even eyeglasses would be taken as a sign of education and of association with corrupt Western society, and thus would cause the wearer to be singled out for particularly violent abuse (as depicted, for example, in the motion picture *The Killing Fields*), are substantiated by our data.

Second, the data seem to bear out stories that early arrivals in the camps that were forerunners to Site 2 were severely traumatized by the Khmer Rouge. Although Site 2 was officially founded in 1985, it was an amalgamation of many smaller camps previously established on the Thai border by the Khmer People's National Liberation

Table 2.3. Self-reported poor health, health-related inability to work, and employment status reported by 993 adult residents of Site 2, Thailand, 1990, by demographic characteristics

Characteristic	Category[a]	Self-reported poor health (%)	Health prevents working at a job, etc. (%)		Working to earn a living in Site 2 (%)
			Any duration	> 3 months	
Total	All	36.3	58.5	19.3	46.1
Gender	Male	30.3	50.9	19.1	65.0
	Female	40.0	63.3	19.5	34.3
Age (years)	18–24	16.1	45.3	16.8	30.7
	25–34	33.4	54.8	20.6	45.5
	35–44	37.0	56.8	20.2	58.6
	45–90	55.2	77.8	17.5	40.7
Marital status	Never married	11.9	35.6	20.3	30.5
	Married	34.6	58.8	20.4	51.8
	Disrupted	48.2	63.6	15.4	31.8
Education (years)	0	41.6	66.8	19.6	31.5
	1–5	36.7	57.1	17.8	45.8
	6–10	26.6	48.4	19.2	64.9
	11–20	30.2	53.5	27.9	67.4
	Unknown	50.0	73.1	30.8	42.3
Province of origin	Battambang	36.5	55.9	18.0	45.3
	Kandal	31.2	60.9	26.6	57.8
	Phnom Penh	38.6	69.9	18.1	56.6
	Siem Reap	41.9	62.9	19.4	32.3
	Other	35.0	58.8	26.8	45.6
	Unknown	35.1	56.1	19.3	42.1
Year of arrival in any border camp	1979–1983	38.6	60.4	20.9	45.6
	1984–1990	29.2	53.0	14.0	48.3
	Unknown	22.2	34.4	33.3	33.3
Year of arrival in Site 2	1979–1983	34.6	61.5	34.6	76.9
	1984–1990	36.3	58.3	18.7	45.3
	Unknown	33.3	66.7	33.3	46.7

[a]Numbers of participants are given in Tables 2.1 and 2.2.

Front (KPNLF). Thus, the small number of respondents who said they had joined the camp at Site 2 in earlier years undoubtedly were referring not to the formal designation of "Site 2" or even to a particular geographic location, but to one of the highly mobile camps of refugees that the KPNLF had established early on and that ultimately were incorporated into Site 2. One of these forerunner camps, Nong Chan, moved six times between 1983 and 1985 (Lawyers Committee for Human Rights, 1987). Cambodians who have resettled in the United States recall that Nong Chan included politicians and government officials who had been ousted by the Khmer Rouge (S. Tor & M. Oeur-

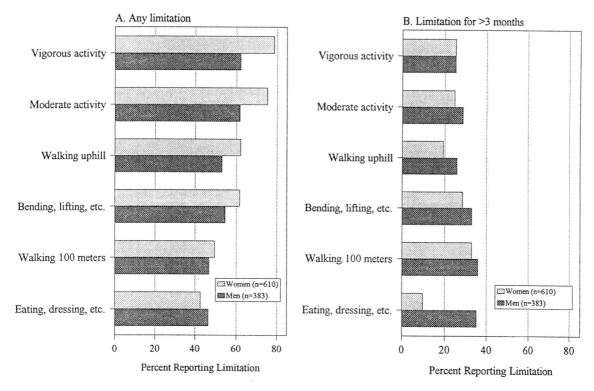

Figure 2.6. Health-related physical limitations of any duration (A) and for more than 3 months (B) reported by 993 adult residents of Site 2, Thailand, 1990, by gender.

Chum, personal communication). Such persons would have been expected to receive especially harsh treatment.

These confirmations of international reports and refugee stories support the survey responses as generally accurate. It would be difficult to imagine that biased respondents would be sophisticated enough to create associations between trauma in the Pol Pot era and such characteristics as the need for eyeglasses or joining the camp at Site 2 before it was formally given that name.

It not surprising that men reported more traumatization than women, both under the Khmer Rouge and in the camp environment. These results are consistent with reports of the dramatic killing of men by the Khmer Rouge and the subsequent enlistment of Cambodian men in the fight to liberate their country from occupation by the Khmer Rouge and Vietnamese communists (Kiljunen, 1984). Although Site 2 was a civilian camp, it provided manpower to Cam-

bodian resistance fighters, who were politically associated with the camp. Neither is it surprising that more than one in four men reported rape or sexual abuse during the Pol Pot era, because anecdotal reports are plentiful of male prisoners being sexually humiliated by their Khmer Rouge captors. In the Cambodian culture, men are not as ashamed or inhibited as women in reporting this form of abuse (Mollica & Son, 1989).

The greater degree of cumulative trauma among the male respondents, however, was not sufficient to create a higher prevalence among men of many psychosocial outcomes, including depressive and post-traumatic stress symptoms, than among women. Differences in baseline prevalence may be partially accountable [e.g., the well-known and consistently reported elevation of depressive symptoms among women (Weissman & Klerman, 1977)] in populations not selected for experiencing high levels of extreme trauma. Also potentially explanatory are hy-

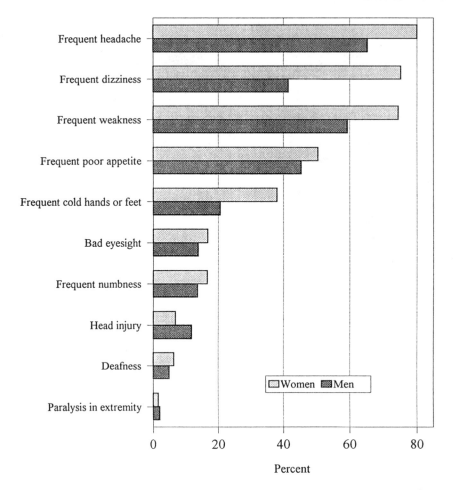

Figure 2.7. Specific health problems reported by 993 adult residents of Site 2, Thailand, 1990.

pothetical gender differences in susceptibility and in the kinds of trauma experienced, which a crude measure of cumulative trauma (number of reported trauma events in a specific time period) would not be expected to capture. As an obvious example, the frequency of widowed persons was much greater among women (16%) than among men (3%) in this study. Policy analyses concerning repatriation of Site 2 residents (Thorn, 1988) and numerous United Nations reports on refugees world-wide (United Nations Economic and Social Council, 1990; United Nations Security Council, 1992) have highlighted refugee women, especially those who are uneducated, widowed, and responsible for the care of large households. Additional analyses

of the data from the present investigation will be devoted to disentangling the complex interrelationships among specific kinds and degrees of trauma, psychiatric symptoms, impaired physical condition, and demographic characteristics such as gender.

By combining culturally valid measures for psychiatric symptoms, self-perceptions of health status, and an assessment of social and physical limitations, this survey was able to quantify associations between these elements for the first time in a refugee camp population. For example, it is known qualitatively from clinical studies that refugees (including Cambodian refugees) suffer from major depressive disorder and post-traumatic stress disorder (Mollica et al., 1987b), that Holocaust survivors and survi-

Table 2.4. Associations between cumulative trauma in the Pol Pot era (1975–1979) and elevated scores[*,†] for symptoms of depression and post-traumatic stress among 993 adult residents of Site 2, Thailand, 1990

Number of trauma events	Number of persons	Depressive symptoms[*]			Post-traumatic stress symptoms[†]		
		Prevalence (%)	Relative odds[‡]	95% confidence interval	Prevalence (%)	Relative odds[‡]	95% confidence interval
0–4	41	36.6	1.		17.1	1.	
5–8	141	57.4	2.4	1.1–5.1	22.7	1.3	0.5–3.5
9–12	267	67.8	3.5	1.7–7.2	28.8	1.6	0.7–4.0
13–16	259	69.1	4.0	1.9–8.3	37.5	2.7	1.1–6.7
17–20	131	67.2	3.8	1.7–8.4	37.4	2.8	1.1–7.2
21–24	56	67.9	3.5	1.4–8.8	51.8	5.2	1.8–14.8
25–28	98	93.9	41.6	13.8–125.6	79.6	27.7	10.0–76.7

[*]Depressive symptom score greater than 1.75 (see text).

[†]Post-traumatic stress symptom score greater than 2.50 (see text).

[‡]The estimated odds ratios are from logistic regression models controlling age, gender, education, marital status, and cumulative trauma in the year prior to interview.

vors of war trauma suffer from somatic complaints (Chodoff, 1963; Katon et al., 1982; Levav, 1994; Shalev et al., 1990) and poor perceived health status (Solomon & Mikulincer, 1987), and that functional disability coexists in individual patients with depressive disorders and symptoms across cultures (Ormel et al., 1994). The present study, given its size and design as an epidemiological investigation, permits expression of these phenomena in numerical terms.

This survey reveals, that for a civilian population with excellent medical care and few chronic illnesses, the adult residents of Site 2 in high numbers felt generally sick and depressed, and that their health was negatively affecting their ability to work and function. The cross-sectional data are limited in their ability to shed light on how and why these associations occur. Nevertheless, it can be concluded from the high overall prevalence of adverse status on measures of psychiatric symptoms, physical health, and social function, and from the strong "dose–response" relations between symptoms and cumulative trauma, that the level of negative health and mental health impact is high.

At the time of the survey, in 1990, were the majority of Site 2 residents suffering from a clinically diagnosable major depressive disorder? The answer to this question is unknown, because psychiatric interviews by clinicians of survey respondents were not feasible (Dohrenwend, 1990; Dohrenwend et al. 1980). The adult residents of Site 2 appeared comparable in their level of symptoms and disability to the patient populations diagnosed with major depression in a cross-national study by the WHO (i.e., those persons experiencing a depressive episode as diagnosed by the tenth edition of the International Classification of Diseases) (Ormel et al., 1994). Yet it is fascinating that, in spite of this picture of profound and widespread depressive affect, more than half of the men and one-third of the women were working to earn a living. Despite strict camp restrictions against employment, the black market economy of the Site 2 community was reminiscent of those created by prisoners of war, whose resourcefulness at survival is legendary even under the most oppressive conditions (Radford, 1945). Although the high level of daily activity of Site 2 residents seems to argue against the inference that most camp residents had clinical depression, it is possible that the unremitting stress of camp life did little to alleviate the negative psychosocial processes that were begun during the mass violence of the Pol Pot era. The dose–response-like effects strongly indicate that the Pol Pot era trauma continued, 10 years after it was sustained, to exert a prominent impact on the psychosocial well-being of Site 2 residents, an impact differentially distinct from the effects of the harsh life in the camp. We thus raise the hypothesis that the original psychiatric symptoms were initiated during the Pol Pot era, that the general feelings of poor health and physical complaints ensued subsequently, and that a mutual re-enforcement occurred between symptoms and disability during the refugee camp period. Additional analyses of the Site 2 data, as well as future ethnographic studies and longitudinal follow-up, will help clarify the association of work with psychiatric symptoms and the relative ability of income generating and socially productive activities to protect and ameliorate the psychosocial suffering of mass violence.

Acknowledgements: This research was supported in part by the Ford Foundation, the Pew Charitable Trusts, and an anonymous donor.

We gratefully acknowledge the contributions of the following people to the design and conduct of this study: Douglas Bennett, M.D., Maudsley Hospital, London, England; Ronald Bass and Martin Frankel, Ph.D., Louis Harris & Associate; James Lavelle, LICSW, and Savuth Sath, Harvard Program in Refugee Trauma; and Karen Donelan, Ed.M. and Robert J. Blendon, Sc.D., Health Policy and Management, Harvard School of Public Health. Special appreciation is expressed to the Khmer refugees who participated as interviewers and respondents in this survey.

REFERENCES

Amnesty International. (1986). *Thailand: Torture of three Kampuchean nationals.* London: Amnesty International (AI Index: ASA 39/05/86).

Centers for Disease Control. (1979). Health status of Kampuchean refugees—Sakaeo, Thailand. MMWR. *Morbidity and Mortality Weekly Report, 28,* 545–546.

Centers for Disease Control. (1980). Follow-up on health status of Kampuchean refugees—Thailand November 1979—February 1980. MMWR. *Morbidity and Mortality Weekly Report, 29,* 218–225.

Chodoff, P. (1963). Late effects of the concentration camp syndrome. *Archives of General Psychiatry, 8,* 323–333.

Committee for the Coordination of Services to Displaced Persons Thailand. (1988). *Marking time: The human cost of confinement.* (Annual conference proceedings, 1988). Bangkok.

Crossette, B. (1988, June 26). After the killing fields: Cambodia's forgotten refugees. *The New York Times.*

Diekstra, R. F. W. (1988). *Psychosocial and mental health problems of the Khmer refugees in Site 2 and Site 8 of the Thai-Kampuchean border.* Geneva: World Health Organization, Division of Mental Health.

Dohrenwend, B. P. (1990). The problem of validity in field studies of psychological disorders revisited. *Psychological Medicine, 20,* 195–208.

Dohrenwend, B. P., Dohrenwend, B. S., Gould, M. S., et al. (Eds.). (1980). *Mental illness in the United States.* New York: Praeger.

Glass, R. I., Cates, W., Jr., Nieburg. P., et al. (1980). Rapid assessment of health status and preventive-medicine needs of newly arrived Kampuchean refugees, Sakaeo, Thailand. *Lancet. 1,* 868–872

Hannum, H. (1989). International law and Cambodian genocide: The sounds of silence. *Human Rights Quarterly, 11,* 82–138.

Katon, W., Kleinman, A., & Rosen, G. (1982). Depression and somatization: A review. *American Journal of Medicine, 72,* 127–135.

Kiljunen, K. (Ed). (1984). *Kampuchea: A decade of genocide.* London: Zed Press.

Kiljunen, K. (1985). Power politics and the tragedy of Kampuchea during the seventies. *Bulletin of Concerned Asian Scholars, 17,* 49–64.

Lawyers Committee for Human Rights. (1987). *Seeking shelter: Cambodians in Thailand: A report on human rights.* New York.

Lawyers Committee for Human Rights. (1989). *Problems in the protection of Vietnamese and Cambodians in Thailand and the admission of Indochinese refugees into the United States.* New York.

Levav, I. (1994, March). *Individuals under conditions of maximum adversity: The Holocaust.* Paper presented at the meeting of the American Psychopathological Association. New York.

Lynch, J. (1989). *Border Khmer: A demographic study of the residents of Site 2, Site B, and Site 8.* Bangkok: The Ford Foundation.

Mollica, R. F., & Caspi-Yavin, Y. (1991). Measuring torture and torture-related symptoms. Psychological Assessment. *Journal of Consulting and Clinical Psychology, 3,* 1–7

Mollica, R. F., Caspi-Yavin, Y., Bollini, P., et al. (1992). The Harvard Trauma Questionnaire: Validating a cross-cultural instrument for measuring torture, trauma, and posttraumatic stress disorder in Indochinese refugees. *Journal of Nervous and Mental Disease, 180,* 111–116.

Mollica, R. F., Donelan, K., Tor, S., et al. (1993). The effect of trauma and confinement on functional health and mental health status of Cambodians living in Thailand-Cambodia border camps. *JAMA, 270,* 581–586.

Mollica, R. F., & Jalbert, R. R. (1989). *Community of confinement: The mental health crisis in Site Two (displaced persons camps on the Thai-Kampuchean border).* Alexandria, VA: World Federation for Mental Health.

Mollica, R. F., Lavelle, J., Tor, S., et al. (1989). *Turning point in Khmer mental health: Immediate steps to resolve the mental health crisis in the Khmer border camps.* Alexandria, VA: World Federation for Mental Health.

Mollica, R. F., & Son, L. (1989). Cultural dimensions in the evaluation and treatment of sexual trauma: An overview. *Psychiatric Clinics of North America, 12,* 363–379.

Mollica, R. F., Wyshak, G., deMarneffe, D., et al. (1987a). Indochinese versions of the Hopkins Symptom Checklist-25: A screening instrument for the psychiatric care of refugees. *American Journal of Psychiatry, 144,* 497–500.

Mollica, R. F., Wyshak, G., & Lavelle, J. (1987b). The psychosocial impact of war trauma and torture on Southeast Asian refugees. *American Journal of Psychiatry, 144,* 1567–1572.

Ngor, H. (1987). *A Cambodian odyssey.* New York: Macmillan.

Ormel, J., VonKorff, M., Bedirhan, T., et al. (1994). Common mental disorders and disability across cultures: Results from the WHO collaborative study on psychological problems in general health care. *JAMA, 272,* 1741–1748.

Radford, R. A. (1945). The economic organization of a P.O.W. camp. *Economica*, new series V, 12, 189–201.

Reynell, J. (1989). Political pawns: Refugees on the Thai-Kampuchean border. Oxford: Refugees Studies Program.

Rogge, J. R. (1992). Return to Cambodia: The significance and implications of past, present, and future spontaneous repatriations. In F. C. Cuny, B. Stein, & P. Reed (Eds.), *Repatriation during conflict in Africa and Asia.* Dallas: Center for the Study of Societies in Crisis.

Shalev, A., Bleich, A., & Ursano, R. J. (1990). Posttraumatic stress disorder: Somatic comorbidity and effort tolerance. *Psychosomatics, 31,* 197–203.

Solomon, A., & Mikulincer, M. (1987). Combat stress reactions, post traumatic stress disorder, and somatic complaints among Israeli soldiers. *Journal of Psychosomatic Research, 31,* 131–137.

Steward, A. L., Hays, R. D., & Ware, J., Jr. (1988). Communication: The MOS short-form general health survey. *Medical Care, 26,* 724–734.

Thorn, L. (1988). *From rice truck to paddy field.* Bangkok: Innomedia Co. Ltd.

United Nations Border Relief Operation (UMBRO). (1985). *Monthly protection reports.* Bangkok, Thailand.

United Nations Economic and Social Council. (1990). *Peace: Refugee and displaced women* (Document E/CN.6/1991/4). New York.

United Nations Security Council. (1992). *Report of the Secretary General on Cambodia* (Document S23613). New York.

Weissman, M. M., & Klerman, G. L. (1977). Sex differences and the epidemiology of depression. *Archives of General Psychiatry, 34,* 98.

World Health Organization. (1986). Report on the WHO/UN Health Mission to the Thai-Kampuchean border: Health conditions in the Kampuchea–Thailand border encampments, January–February 1986.

3

Psychological Effects of Military Combat

Terence M. Keane

Until the 20th century, chronicling the psychological effects of exposure to war on soldiers was the domain of poets such as Homer (*The Iliad*, *The Odyssey*), playwrights such as Shakespeare (*Henry IV*), and novelists such as Stephen Crane (*The Red Badge of Courage*). Beginning with Freud and continuing into the early part of this century, the psychological and physiological effects of war were seen as sequelae of exposure to massive deprivation and rigorous physical conditions as well as explosives (e.g., the term "shell shock" was used to describe a psychological condition that was thought to have developed as a function of proximity to explosions). This work clearly placed the psychological effects of war in the medical arena, and both neurologists and psychiatrists began to study more closely the effects of exposure to overwhelming and life-threatening stressors (see Weathers et al., 1995).

During World War II, consistent descriptions of the effects of military experiences on soldiers began to emerge. Classic texts by Kardiner (1947) and Grinker and Spiegel (1945) provided compelling descriptions of the phenomenology, nosology, assessment, and treatment of war-related stress disorders. These works clearly set the stage for contemporary research on post-traumatic

stress disorder (PTSD) in general, and on combat stress disorders specifically. In the 1970s, as a function of the Vietnam war, a series of scientific studies addressed the effects of this war on U.S. soldiers. Although clearly a distinctive war from a sociopolitical perspective, the scope and the nature of the Vietnam war's psychological aftereffects shared many characteristics with those of other wars. Veterans reported a wide range of disabling psychological problems that included anxiety and depression, nightmares, sleep disturbance, dissociative-like flashback experiences, and psychophysiological reactivity to cues of traumatic events (Figley, 1978; Wilson, 1978). This psychophysiological reactivity was seen by some researchers as central to PTSD and its adverse psychosocial consequences.

This chapter presents information from two key studies that contribute to our understanding of the effects of exposure to combat. The first is the National Vietnam Veterans Readjustment Study (NVVRS), a major epidemiological effort to estimate the prevalence of PTSD in the Vietnam veteran population. The second is a multisite study of the psychophysiological parameters of PTSD and the extent to which psychophysiological reactivity, long viewed as a major feature of PTSD, was indeed a fundamental component that could be reliably observed in laboratory settings. This is known as the PTSD in Vietnam Veterans (PIVVET) study.

NATIONAL VIETNAM VETERANS READJUSTMENT STUDY

In addition to the psychological and psychophysiological symptoms reported by Vietnam veterans in earlier studies, data indicated that the war had profound social, marital, and interpersonal effects on its participants. Interestingly, other studies conducted concurrently concluded that the adverse effects of exposure to war were a function of pre-existing psychopathology, substance abuse, behavioral problems, and other known risk factors that predisposed these individuals to develop combat-related disorders (Helzer, 1984; Helzer et al., 1987; Worthington, 1977). These studies placed greater emphasis on these pre-existing characteristics than on levels of combat exposure in the ultimate development of psychopathology.

All these studies suffered from serious, and perhaps even fatal, methodological flaws influencing the validity of conclusions drawn from them. Their primary value was in alerting society to the large number of individuals who served in Vietnam who were having adjustment problems, and to the fact that many people sent to Vietnam possessed characteristics that placed them at some risk for the development of disorder when exposed to stress. None of the studies could accurately inform the public about the number of veterans with psychological problems or the variables that would predict disorder or adjustment. For example, virtually all of the studies conducted in the 1970s and early 1980s suffered from difficulties in sampling. No study included a representative sample of veterans who had served in the war, and most samples either were drawn by convenience or were clinical samples of patients seeking services at different institutions. Some samples of veterans were so small that it was impossible for them to yield reliable findings of the current status of Vietnam

veterans (Helzer et al., 1987). Moreover, the typical study either did not measure PTSD at all or did so using instruments that had questionable reliability and validity. Because of these limitations, it was virtually impossible to comprehensively understand the psychological and social effects of service in Vietnam. What we needed was a study that would permit policy makers to understand as specifically as possible the psychological effects of exposure to combat in Vietnam. Such a study would serve to elucidate the psychosocial problems of Vietnam veterans and guide policy makers in constructing a social policy that would be optimally beneficial to veterans and their families.

To accomplish this, in 1984 the U.S. Congress mandated an epidemiological study of the psychological and social effects of the Vietnam War on its veterans. This study was to address many of the methodological and measurement flaws noted in previous studies and provide information to resolve some of the discrepancies in the scientific literature regarding the long-term effects of the war on its participants. To this end, a study designed to measure premilitary, military, and postmilitary factors to determine the contribution of each to the overall functioning of Vietnam veterans was proposed.

The NVVRS was funded by the U.S. Department of Veterans Affairs (DVA) and conducted under contract with the Research Triangle Institute (RTI) of North Carolina. The study (Kulka et al., 1988) had three primary objectives: (1) to determine the prevalence of PTSD and other psychological disorders that might have occurred as a result of participation in the Vietnam War; (2) to examine the current life adjustment of individuals who participated in the war; and (3) to study factors related to the development of PTSD.

The design of this research study incorporated a number of significant features that would permit conclusions to be drawn regarding the extent to which any problems found would be specific to service in the Vietnam war zone. The design featured the following three comparison groups: (1) a representative sample of Vietnam-theater veterans, (2) a sample of Vietnam-era veterans who did not serve directly in the war zone but who did serve in the military during the same time period, and (3) a civilian sample that was comparable on variables such as age, sex, race, and education. In drawing the Vietnam-theater veteran sample, all U.S. veterans from 1964 to 1975 who served in the Vietnam theater or in the airspace above or the seas surrounding the theater had known probabilities of being included in the study. In addition, the sampling strategy employed in this project oversampled certain subgroups of the population in order to draw conclusions specifically about each group. The groups oversampled were (1) African-Americans, (2) Hispanic-Americans, (3) women, and (4) those who received physical injuries as a result of the war.

Pretest Validation Study

At the time the NVVRS was initiated, few measures of PTSD possessed acceptable psychometric properties. Given the scope and the importance of this project for public policy, there was considerable interest in ensuring that any measures used had demonstrated reliability and validity, as well as acceptable levels of sensitivity and specificity. To assure the use of appropriate measures, the RTI research group conducted a pretest validational study examining the performance of numerous candidate measures.

In this pretest validational study, multiple sites using very experienced clinicians examined more than 200 veteran patients with known diagnoses (some with PTSD, some without PTSD, and some with disorders other than PTSD). From this pretest validational study, several measures of PTSD were selected, including a PTSD module of the Diagnostic Interview Schedule (Robins et al., 1981) to be used by lay interviewers in conducting the survey portion of the study; the Mississippi Scale for Combat-Related PTSD, a self-report measure for combat-related PTSD and related symptomatology (Keane et al., 1988a); and the Structured Clinical Interview for *DSM-*

III-R (SCID) PTSD module to be used by clinicians in a second stage of the study when examining a portion of the sample derived from the initial screening by lay interviewers. At this second stage the Keane PTSD (PK) Scale of the Minnesota Multiphasic Personality Inventory–2 (MMPI-2) (Keane et al., 1984) and the Stress Response Rating Scale (Weiss et al., 1984) were also employed in the context of examining the "clinical subsample."

The procedures designed for use in this study stem from Dohrenwend's two-stage approach to assessment of psychopathology in field settings (Dohrenwend & Shrout, 1981). Stage one included a survey conducted by lay interviewers who were well trained in the administration of the specific assessment instruments to be used. The second stage of this design included a clinician's assessment conducted by clinical psychologists, psychiatrists, and doctoral-level nurses and social workers. The clinician's assessment was reserved for all cases deemed positive on the lay survey (Mississippi Scale score $\geq$ 89), but also included all cases that were seen as high risk for disorder (e.g., high combat exposure) and a randomly selected subsample of all negative cases. This two-stage strategy permitted an examination of the reliability and accuracy of the lay survey case identification; it also provided the opportunity to adjust information about cases on the basis of this additional, clinically derived information. Ultimately, the strategy employed by the researchers in this study was to assign a probability of PTSD "caseness" depending upon variables collected in the lay interview adjusted by information collected in the clinician's assessment.

Results of the NVVRS

Findings from the NVVRS indicated that, among male Vietnam-theater veterans, current rates of PTSD were 15.2% compared with 2.5% among Vietnam-era veterans and 1.2% among the civilians. These differences between the Vietnam-theater veterans and the two comparison groups reached statistical significance. In terms of lifetime prevalence of PTSD among male theater veterans, a prevalence rate of 30.9% was observed. Using an estimate of 3.14 million American people having served in Vietnam, the study projected approximately 479,000 cases of current combat-related PTSD in the Vietnam-theater sample. In addition, approximately twice that number had PTSD at one time or another since their return from the war.

Among women, the prevalence rate of current PTSD for the Vietnam-theater veterans was 8.5% compared to 1.1% for Vietnam-era veterans and 0.3% for the matched civilian comparisons. The majority of women who served in Vietnam were nurses; consequently, the matched civilian comparison group was not representative of the general population. Lifetime prevalence rates of PTSD among the Vietnam-theater veteran women were 26.9%.

The NVVRS also found notable differences in current prevalence of PTSD among racial and ethnic subgroups. Among the white/other veterans, there was a prevalence rate of 13.7% for current PTSD. Among African-American veterans, there was a prevalence of 20.6% of current PTSD, and among Hispanic-American veterans, the prevalence of current PTSD was 27.8%. These differences were striking in terms of the magnitude of differential effects of the war and also for their policy implications. Subsequent analyses of these findings revealed that, controlling for levels of combat and war-zone stress exposure, the differences between African-Americans and whites were no longer statistically significant, while the differences between Hispanic-Americans and these two groups remained statistically significant, although at a substantially reduced level. These findings indicated that resulting differences in prevalence rates were largely a function of differences in reported levels of combat and war-zone stress exposure: this was particularly true for the African-American cohort.

Data in this study were also analyzed by examining differences in current PTSD rates among those exposed to high rates of war-zone stress. Among male veterans, those exposed to low or moderate stress during the course of their service had a prevalence rate of PTSD of 8.5%; those exposed to high amounts of war-zone stress had a current prevalence rate of 35.8%. Similarly, women veterans who were exposed to low or moderate war-zone stress during their service in Vietnam had a current prevalence rate of 2.5%, whereas those exposed to high war-zone stress had a current prevalence rate of 17.5%. (In interpreting these results, it is essential to know that war-zone stress was defined differently for men and women because of the different roles in which men and women served during the Vietnam War.)

Importantly, the high rates of PTSD among the Vietnam-theater veteran subjects still exceeded the rates of this disorder in the comparison groups even when numerous predisposing risk factors or personal characteristics were controlled statistically. Specifically, a wide range of demographic variables (including age, sex, race, and education), socioeconomic status variables, quantitative measures of the subject's childhood and adolescent social environment, the presence of delinquent or antisocial behavior, the presence of psychological and psychiatric disorders, and a wide range of biopsychosocial factors previously found to be related to the development of psychopathology were examined. Even with all of these variables controlled statistically, there were still differences between the Vietnam-theater veterans and both Vietnam-era veterans and civilian controls in terms of prevalence of current PTSD. These findings strongly indicate that the source of the difference in current psychological problems among the Vietnam-theater veteran group and the other comparison groups was service in the war zone. Furthermore, the strong relationship between war-zone stress exposure variables and PTSD pointed to specific experiences (i.e., life threat from traumatic events) that occurred in Vietnam as the pathogenic variables leading to disorder. Studies examining the nature of

PTSD using the NVVRS data confirm these factors as important variables (e.g., King et al., 1995), thus further contributing to the knowledge base on the issue of causation.

What does it mean to have PTSD? An examination of the many psychosocial variables measured in this study provided important insights to factors associated with PTSD. Individuals who have PTSD or who have ever had it seem more likely to develop at least one other psychological disorder during the course of their lives. Typically, this is a substance abuse or depressive disorder. One-half of individuals with PTSD currently have another psychological disorder. Moreover, PTSD veterans were 5 times more likely to be unemployed at the time of the survey than theater veterans without PTSD. Seventy percent of PTSD veterans have been divorced; 35% have been divorced two or more times. Fifty percent reported high levels of marital problems and 55% reported high levels of parenting problems associated with their children. Twenty-five percent of Vietnam-theater veterans with PTSD report being very dissatisfied with their lives.

Other important social variables were also associated with a diagnosis of PTSD. Forty-seven percent of PTSD veterans reported being isolated; 35% reported being homeless at one time since their separation from the military. Moreover, 37% of PTSD veterans reported being involved in six or more acts of violence in the past year, with a mean of 13.3 acts of aggression. Relatedly, 50% of PTSD veterans reported being arrested or jailed once, and 34% reported being arrested or jailed more than once. Among these individuals, 12% were arrested for a felony. In addition, 40% of PTSD veterans scored highest on ratings of hostility, anger, and aggression. For all of these problems, the rates among PTSD veterans were at least twice those of Vietnam-theater veterans without PTSD.

In conclusion, the prevalence of PTSD among Vietnam-theater veterans appeared to be high for lifetime and current rates of disorder. These high rates of disorder were accompanied by a wide range of psycholog-ical and social problems that place these individuals at great risk in contemporary society. In addition, the problems observed in the NVVRS appeared to be a function of war-zone stress exposure, rather than of pre-existing conditions or circumstances that led individuals into the military or into Vietnam specifically. The problem of PTSD among Vietnam-theater veterans is significant to public health in the United States. With 3.14 million veterans of Vietnam, plus their spouses and children, many of whom have related psychological and social problems, this disorder represents a major concern for the United States in terms of delivery of appropriate social and mental health services.

As the first comprehensive study conducted by any nation to examine the psychosocial consequences for soldiers of participating in a war, the NVVRS demonstrated convincingly that the environment to which we expose military personnel in war and peacekeeping efforts can place them at considerable risk for the development of longstanding, serious, and in some cases debilitating psychological problems. These findings may be useful in identifying who is at greatest risk for the development of psychological disorders as well as for encouraging the development of programs and procedures that may prevent disorder among combatants. In particular, efforts to train soldiers in a variety of adaptive and self-help skills prior to exposure to massive stressors may prove to be a worthwhile enterprise. Second, providing the opportunity for psychological debriefing following exposure to massive stressors may also prevent development of untoward expectations, provide an opportunity to normalize an individual's psychological reactions, and provide requisite social support to assist people in their own psychological recovery from this exposure. Identifying methods for implementing these interventions are matters for further research. The remainder of this chapter is devoted to a description of some of the main work underway to expand knowledge about the nature of PTSD—knowledge on which preventative and remedial efforts must be based.

PSYCHOPATHOLOGY AND PSYCHOPHYSIOLOGY OF CHRONIC PTSD

Problems of Vietnam veterans, particularly PTSD, have been major concerns of the DVA and the Department of Defense for an extended time. The DVA has been especially interested in the development of contemporary methods for assessing PTSD in order to assist clinicians in the provision of appropriate treatment and to assist adjudicators in determining disability compensation claims. In addition to issues of psychological assessment, studies of the psychopathology associated with the disorder are lacking and are sorely needed. The diagnostic criteria and description of PTSD contained in the *Diagnostic and Statistic Manual of Mental Disorders* (third edition, revised) (*DSM-III-R*) of the American Psychiatric Association (1987) derive from numerous clinical studies of veterans and the observations of clinicians who work with them. Further work on the phenomenology of PTSD is warranted.

Psychophysiological reactivity in PTSD has been observed clinically for many years. Kardiner (1941), in his studies of World War I veterans, referred to the disorder as a "physio-neurosis" because of the many somatic complaints and problems he noted among war veterans. Gillespie's (1942) study of veterans' complaints also specified generalized muscle tension, including headache and backache, as well as heart palpitations and panic reactions, as central features of the disorder. Also noticing this same pattern of psychophysiological reactions among trauma-exposed veterans were Grinker and Spiegel (1945), who observed excessive muscle tension, startle reactions, and a wide range of psychophysiological and psychosomatic symptoms among combatants.

One question that arose from these observations was the extent to which the psychophysiological reactions that were apparent among war trauma survivors were predominantly tonic phenomena as well as phasic reactions. A second and related issue was the extent to which the phasic reactions occurred specifically in response to trauma-related cues or, rather, were a more generalized reaction to any stimulation. Evidence supporting the trauma specificity of the physiological reactions would provide support for the role of the traumatic events in the development of the disorder.

The early observations by clinicians led to a number of experimental studies that examined psychophysiological parameters among combat veterans. Wenger (1948) examined three groups of subjects: (*1*) 225 subjects with "operational fatigue," (*2*) 98 subjects with neurotic disorder, and (*3*) 448 subjects who were normal Air Force students. This comparative study measured baseline differences in psychophysiological functioning. Wenger found differences in the operational fatigue group (predecessor of PTSD) when compared to the neurotics and the Air Force students on the following measures: salivary output, systolic and diastolic blood pressure, heart rate, respiration rate, palmar conductance, sinus arrhythmia, finger temperature, and mean tidal air values. In all cases the operational fatigue subjects demonstrated higher levels of arousal than did either of the two comparison groups. This study did not involve any experimental manipulation, nor did it involve exposure to neutral or relevant stressors, but it did demonstrate clearly that, even at baseline, subjects with war stress–related problems performed differently on psychophysiological variables than did comparison groups of subjects.

Dobbs and Wilson (1960) examined 8 decompensated veterans (probable PTSD) and compared them to 13 compensated combat veterans and 10 nonveteran student controls. This study presented combat cues, including flashing lights and sounds of weapons firing, to the participants. At baseline, the researchers found that the decompensated veterans had higher heart rates than did either of the two comparison groups. Perhaps more striking was their inability to measure any psychophysiological variables during the presentation of combat cues because of the high levels of arousal exhibited by the decompensated veterans and their inability to remain in the experimental situation.

Using more contemporary methods for psychophysiological measurement and cue presentation, Blanchard et al. (1982) examined 11 Vietnam veterans with a diagnosis of PTSD and compared them with nonveteran normal controls. They presented auditory combat cues, alternating with neutral cues, while measuring heart rate, blood pressure, electromyogram (EMG), and skin conductance. Psychophysiological reactivity, and in particular elevation in heart rate, was demonstrably different among the PTSD veterans. Using simply heart rate reactivity, this study correctly classified 95.5% of the subjects in either the PTSD or the no-PTSD groups. The sole subject who was incorrectly classified was a PTSD subject taking a major tranquilizer.

Malloy et al. (1983) examined a group of PTSD veterans and compared them with two distinct groups, veterans with psychiatric diagnoses and well-adjusted combat veterans. Using visual and auditory cues of combat, these researchers measured heart rate and skin conductance as well as subjective measures of distress. Employing all measures of arousal (physiological and subjective), they were able to successfully classify 100% of the subjects of the study into PTSD and no-PTSD groups. Relying exclusively on the physiological measures, the correct classification rate of PTSD and no-PTSD subjects was 80%.

Utilizing the experimental model for the study of emotion developed by Lang (1977), Pitman et al. (1987) examined psychophysiological reactivity in 15 PTSD veterans and 18 combat veteran controls. They employed combat and noncombat imagery that contained relevant traumatic and nontraumatic life experiences for each of the subjects. Measures of heart rate, skin conductance, and EMG led to 100% correct classification of PTSD subjects and 61% classification of no-PTSD subjects in this study (i.e., high sensitivity and moderate specificity).

These contemporary studies of psychophysiological reactivity to combat cues resulted in impressive overall classification rates with particularly strong sensitivity and good specificity. These studies occurred in three separate research laboratories over approximately 6 years. Replications of these findings within these same laboratories and in additional laboratories led to concrete evidence that veterans with PTSD suffered from strong physiological reactions to relevant cues, and that this reactivity might be helpful in our understanding of the disorder and in the development of non-self-report assessment methods. Baseline differences in physiological measures appeared in some studies but not in all, leaving open the possibility that veterans with PTSD might suffer from both tonic and phasic physiological arousal problems.

Despite the strengths of these cross-laboratory findings, however, numerous methodological problems limited the extent to which firm conclusions could be drawn regarding the utility of psychophysiological reactivity in assessing PTSD. These limitations included (1) the small sample sizes contained in virtually all of the studies conducted, (2) PTSD base rates in the studies that exceeded expected base rates of PTSD in the help-seeking population, (3) the inclusion of non-treatment-seeking controls, (4) the absence of any cross-validation information on the classification rates, (5) limited test–retest reliability particularly among the physiological variables, and (6) the absence of a complete utility analysis (i.e., sensitivity rates, specificity rates, predictive power of a positive test, and predictive power of a negative test). The presence of these limitations led to the development of a multisite clinical trial that could address the question of whether physiological parameters could be useful in the diagnosis and classification of patients with PTSD; this trial would contain sufficient subjects and power to address this question in a thorough manner.

THE PIVVET COOPERATIVE STUDY

Funded by the DVA Cooperative Study Program, the PIVVET study attempted to address each of the methodological limitations identified in the psychophysiological literature to date. It had as its objective the development of a physiological indicator for the presence of PTSD when compared to a comprehensive examination and diagnosis by a trained clinical psychologist.

This study employed as subjects male Vietnam-theater veterans who enrolled in the study via a consecutive cohort admission procedure across the various sites involved. All subjects were drug and alcohol free at the time of the research, and urinalyses confirmed the absence of illicit drugs in subjects included in the analyses. Exclusion criteria for the study included the presence of cardiovascular disease, organic mental disease, and any of the spectrum psychotic disorders. The primary hypothesis was that variables from the psychophysiological protocol would predict the clinicians' diagnosis of PTSD obtained from the SCID PTSD module.

Methods

Subjects

Included in this study were 1240 male Vietnam veterans recruited from 15 Veterans Affairs (VA) Medical Centers across the United States. All subjects were seeking services and were therefore comparable in nature to VA patients for whom the diagnostic test was intended (Kraemer, 1992).

Subjects in the study averaged 41 years of age. Among those diagnosed with PTSD, there was a mean of 13.6 years of education; for those without PTSD, the average education was 14.6 years. Annual income for the PTSD subjects was $12,560; for those with no PTSD annual income was $25,270. Percent disability for the PTSD group was 31; for the no-PTSD group, it was 21.7. The number of jobs per subject in the PTSD group was 27.6; for the no-PTSD group the mean was 11.5.

In the PTSD group 8.3% had at least one criminal arrest since discharge, compared with 2.6% in the no-PTSD group. With respect to marital histories, 40.8% of the

Table 3.1. Psychometric data on PIVVET participants

	PTSD	No-PTSD
Combat Exposure Scale score	28.8 (high)	17.9 (moderate)
Vietnam trauma (yes)	99%	81.4%
Mississippi Scale score (mean)	123.0	78.1
MMPI PK scale (mean)	30.4	13.9

PTSD group had been married more than once; among the no-PTSD group, 26.6% had been married more than once. PTSD subjects reported an average of 5.0 hours of sleep per night, while the no-PTSD subjects averaged 6.5 hours per night. Table 3.1 presents psychometric data for participants.

Diagnostic Co-morbidity

For subjects who met diagnostic criteria for PTSD, 24.6% reached criteria for a current diagnosis of alcohol abuse, compared to 13.9% of those without PTSD. Fourteen percent of PTSD subjects met criteria for drug abuse, while only 6.3% of those without PTSD met these criteria. Similarly, subjects with PTSD met criteria for panic disorder more frequently, with 13.4% in the PTSD group reaching criteria and none without PTSD receiving this diagnosis. Major depression, a frequently co-occurring diagnosis with PTSD, was found in 34.5% of the PTSD subjects, while only 5.9% of those without PTSD met criteria for a current diagnosis of major depressive disorder.

With regard to *DSM-III-R* Axis II disorders, 18% of PTSD subjects also met criteria for borderline personality disorder, compared to only 3.4% without PTSD. The figures for antisocial personality disorder were 10.6% for those with PTSD and 3.0% for those without PTSD.

Assessment Measures

Clinicians employed the SCID (Spitzer & Williams, 1985) to examine patients for the

Table 3.2. Psychophysiological assessment
protocol

Condition	Length of presentation (min)
Baseline 1	10
Mental arithmetic	1–2
Baseline 2	5
Neutral slides	9.5
Baseline 3	5
Combat slides	7
Baseline 4	5
Neutral script 1	2
Combat script 1	2
Neutral script 2	2
Combat script 2	2
Baseline 5	5
Debriefing	

presence of PTSD and a wide range of Axis
I and Axis II disorders. In addition to this
diagnostic instrument, all subjects completed the War Stress Inventory I and II,
developed by Rosenheck and Fontana
(1989) to assess broad-spectrum psychological and social problems in VA patients. Self-
report scales included in the assessment battery were the Mississippi Scale for
Combat-Related PTSD (Keane et al.,
1988a), the Combat Exposure Scale (Keane
et al. 1989b), and the MMPI-2 and the
Keane PTSD scale contained within it
(Keane et al. 1984).

Psychophysiological Assessment Procedure

Table 3.2 summarizes the psychophysiologic
assessment procedure for each subject in
the study. It combines exposure to a neutral
stressor consisting of a mental arithmetic
task (serial 7s), exposure to neutral slides
(i.e., snow-covered mountains) and an accompanying sound track of classical music,
combat stressor slides and sounds (i.e., a
military unit landing in a heavy combat area
in Vietnam), and the script-driven imagery
that compared neutral (i.e., relaxing in a favored area) and combat (i.e., the most dis-

tressing event from their Vietnam experience) scripts developed for each person
individually (see Lang, 1977; Pitman et al.,
1987). Measures obtained during the course
of the assessment procedure were heart
rate, systolic and diastolic blood pressure,
EMG, and skin conductance.

RESULTS

Analytic Plan

We divided the subjects into a training sample and a cross-validation sample representing approximately 60% and 40% of the total
sample, respectively. Data presented here
are from the analyses completed to date and
are taken from the training sample only.
Keane et al. (1988b) present a more thorough description of the data-analytic approach planned for use in the study, including the methods employed in data reduction
for the psychophysiological measures.

Figure 3.1 presents the mean heart rate
in beats per minute (bpm) for these subjects
(n = 672) during baseline and experimental
test conditions. In general, PTSD veterans
demonstrated greater heart rate at baseline
when compared to no-PTSD veterans. Differential elevations were also observed for
the mental arithmetic condition, the combat
slide condition, and the combat script condition on this measure. Comparisons of
mean heart rate in response to the combat
versus neutral conditions also revealed a statistically significant difference for the combat slides (PTSD mean = 2.1 bpm; no-
PTSD mean = 0.5 bpm) and the combat
scripts (PTSD mean = 2.9 bpm; no-PTSD
mean = 1.9 bpm).

Figure 3.2 presents the mean skin conductance data for both conditions. In comparisons of the combat with the neutral conditions, the PTSD group exhibited a greater
increase in skin conductance (mean = 0.75
mS) compared to the no-PTSD group
(mean = 0.33 mS). Similarly, the PTSD subjects demonstrated greater change in skin
conductance as a function of the combat
scripts when compared with the neutral
scripts. Subjects with PTSD exhibited a
mean change of 0.73 mS, while those in the

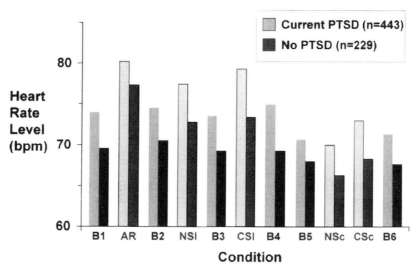

Figure 3.1. Mean heart rate levels at various baseline and test conditions. (Conditions: B1, baseline 1; AR, mental arithmetic; B2, baseline 2; NSl, neutral slides; B3, baseline 3; CSl, combat slides; B4, baseline 4; B5, baseline 5; NSc, neutral script; CSc, combat script; B6, baseline 6.)

no-PTSD group exhibited a mean change of 0.44 mS.

Lateral frontalis EMG data provided similar effects for the PTSD and no-PTSD subjects. Figure 3.3 presents the data across the experimental protocol for EMG. Statistically significant differences were observed in the means of combat minus neutral change scores on this variable as well. For the com-bat slides minus the neutral slides, the mean differences were 0.92 mV for the PTSD group and 0.28 mV for the no-PTSD group. For the scripts a similar pattern emerged. The PTSD group's mean difference was 1.20 mV, while the no-PTSD group's mean difference was 0.42 mV. Comparable findings were obtained for the systolic and diastolic blood pressure recordings.

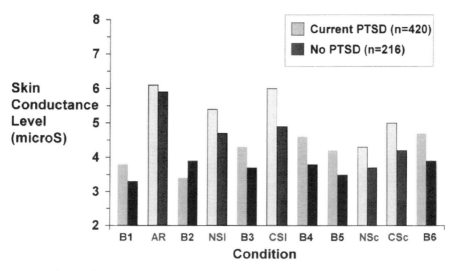

Figure 3.2. Mean skin conductance levels at various baseline and test conditions. (For explanation of conditions, see Figure 3.1.)

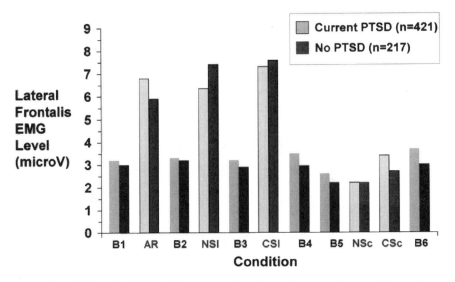

Figure 3.3. Mean lateral frontalis EMG levels at various baseline and test conditions. (For explanation of conditions, see Figure 3.1.)

We submitted all data from the psychophysiological protocol (reduced into change scores) to a logistic regression procedure to determine accuracy of classification by diagnostic grouping. Using the mean differences from neutral to combat stimulus presentation for each of the measures (heart rate, skin conductance, EMG, systolic and diastolic blood pressure, and subjective units of distress), the procedure correctly classified 65% of the subjects in the training sample.

DISCUSSION

Preliminary findings from the PIVVET study indicate that, for a substantial number of combat veterans with PTSD, there remain measurable increments in psychophysiological reactivity to cues of combat experiences some 20 or more years following the life experiences. The analyses conducted to date indicate that this reactivity may be a useful adjunct to more traditional approaches to assessment, such as the clinical interview and psychometric tests. Estimates of diagnostic accuracy in the cross-validation sample will contribute further to our understanding of the reliability of these findings of psychophysiological reactivity.

Psychophysiological reactivity in PTSD is also being replicated across populations. Orr et al. (1993) found similar elevations across measures in both World War II and Korean veterans with PTSD. Shalev et al. (1993) found that a group of male and female Israeli citizens traumatized by a variety of noncombat life experiences also exhibited this reactivity. Moreover, Blanchard et al. (1994) found evidence for psychophysiological reactivity in PTSD resulting from motor vehicle accidents.

Thus the findings of psychophysiological reactivity to cues of the original trauma appear to occur in different wars, cultures, genders, and types of traumas. Possibly most important from an understanding of the etiology of this disorder is the finding that the reactivity is most clearly observed in response to the cues that are relevant to the traumatic events themselves. Other stressful cues, sounds, or stimuli do not appear to evoke the same level of physiological reactivity as do the cues of the traumatic events.

These findings also raise other questions of central importance in our growing understanding of this disorder. Specifically, future studies are now needed to address the underlying biological mechanisms that are responsible for the development and the maintenance of this reactivity. Delineation of these factors might spur the recognition and implementation of effective treatment interventions. A related question is whether successful treatment of this physiological reactivity through behavioral or psychopharmacological methods would yield an improved clinical outcome in terms of symptomatology and psychosocial functioning.

Left unanswered in this study is the extent to which the observed autonomic elevations are a function of a predisposition to develop PTSD or a consequence of the disorder. Future studies of the genetic predisposition to developing PTSD will shed light on this issue. Either interpretation is consistent with the findings of this study. Clearly a person-by-event interaction offers the most appealing interpretation of the findings, with personal characteristics encompassing genetic, physiological, and psychological factors.

The findings also replicate previous studies demonstrating hyperreactivity in PTSD and support the inclusion of arousal reduction methods in the treatment of PTSD (Keane et al., 1989a). Techniques that involve the repeated presentation of trauma-related cues in careful and systematic ways (i.e., the exposure therapies) would seem to be particularly warranted. Given the clinical complexity of PTSD cases, it is likely that the most effective interventions will be multiphasic in nature and will require numerous interventions in addition to exposure therapy. This would be especially true for chronic cases of PTSD with high rates of comorbid psychological problems such as those seen in combat-related PTSD.

CONCLUSION

The NVVRS and the PIVVET study are two of the largest studies conducted to date on the effects of war. Both studies provide information on the adverse long-term effects of exposure to life threat and terror. The NVVRS findings indicate that psychological and social problems plague veterans of war for at least 20 years following participation.

At least as tragic is the apparent effects of the war on PTSD veterans' spouses and children, both of whom seem to have more problems of a clinically significant nature than the families of survivors who did not develop PTSD.

The PIVVET study provided important information on the physiological representation of PTSD and the stimulus characteristics that seem to elicit pathological elevations in heart rate, blood pressure, muscle tension, and skin conductance. It is clear from these data that parameters of reactivity constitute a significant part of the PTSD clinical picture and that, even in laboratory based protocols, cues reminiscent of traumatic life experiences are able to evoke measurable physiological reactions.

Taken collectively, these studies provide important new information on the role of life stressors in inducing psychopathology. Even controlling for a host of pre-existing and demographic variables, the NVVRS demonstrated that war-zone stress exposure was strongly associated with the ultimate development of PTSD. The PIVVET study indicated that psychophysiological reactivity to cues of the traumatic events identified PTSD veterans seeking services while not identifying those combat veterans without PTSD. Although it is always difficult to draw inferences about causal agents in the absence of experimental paradigms, these studies add further support to our understanding of the relationship between exposure to war and the subsequent development of serious problems in long-term psychological and social adjustment.

REFERENCES

American Psychiatric Association. (1987). *Diagnostic and statistical manual of mental disorders*, (3rd ed. rev.). Washington, DC: American Psychiatric Association.

Blanchard, E. B., Hickling, E. J., Taylor, A. E., Loos, N. R., & Gerardi, R. J. (1994). The psychophysiology of motor vehicle accident related posttraumatic stress disorder. *Behavior Therapy*, 25, 453–467.

Blanchard, E. B., Kolb, L. C., Pallmeyer, T. P., & Gerardi, R. (1982). A psychophysiological study of post traumatic stress disorder in Vietnam veterans. *Psychiatric Quarterly, 534,* 220–229.

Dobbs, D., & Wilson, W. P. (1960). Observations on the persistence of traumatic war neurosis. *Journal of Nervous and Mental Disease, 21,* 686–691.

Dohrenwend, B. P., & Shrout, P. E. (1981). Toward the development of a two-stage procedure for case identification and classification in psychiatric epidemiology. *Research in Community and Mental Health, 2,* 295–323.

Figley, C. R. (Ed.). (1978). *Stress disorders among Vietnam veterans: Theory, research, and treatment.* New York: Brunner/Mazel.

Gillespie, R. D. (1942). *Psychological effects of war on citizen and soldier.* New York: W. W. Norton.

Grinker, R., & Spiegel, J. P. (1945). *Men under stress.* Philadelphia: Blakiston.

Helzer, J. (1984). The impact of combat on alcohol use by Vietnam veterans. *Journal of Psychoactive Drugs, 16,* 183–191.

Helzer, J. E., Robins, L. N., & McEvoy, L. (1987). Post-traumatic stress disorder in the general population: Findings of the Epidemiologic Catchment Area survey. *New England Journal of Medicine, 317,* 1630–1634.

Kardiner, A. (1941). *The traumatic neuroses of war.* New York: Hoeber.

Keane, T. M., Caddell, J. M., & Taylor, K. A. (1988a). The Mississippi Scale for Combat-Related PTSD: Three studies in reliability and validity. *Journal of Consulting and Clinical Psychology, 56,* 85–90.

Keane, T. M., Fairbank, J. F., Caddell, J. M., & Zimering, R. T. (1989a). Implosive (flooding) therapy reduces symptoms of PTSD in Vietnam veterans. *Behavior Therapy, 20,* 245–260.

Keane, T. M., Fairbank, J. A., Caddell, J. M., Zimering, R. T., Taylor, K. L., & Mora, C. A. (1989b). Clinical evaluation of a measure to assess combat exposure. *Psychological Assessment: A Journal of Consulting and Clinical Psychology, 1,* 53–55.

Keane, T. M., Kolb, L., & Thomas, R. T. (1988b). *A psychophysiological study of chronic PTSD* (Vol. 1) (Department of Veterans Affairs Cooperative Study #334). Washington, DC: Department of Veterans Affairs.

Keane, T. M., Malloy, P. F., & Fairbank, J. A. (1984). Empirical development of an MMPI subscale for the assessment of combat-related posttraumatic stress disorder. *Journal of Consulting and Clinical Psychology, 52,* 888–891.

King, D. W., King, L. A., Gudanowski, D. M., & Vreven, D. L. (1995). Alternative representations of war zone stressors: Relationships to posttraumatic stress disorder in male and female Vietnam veterans. *Journal of Abnormal Psychology, 104,* 184–196.

Kraemer, H. C. (1992). *Evaluating medical tests: Objective and quantitative guidelines.* Newbury Park, CA: Sage Publications.

Kulka, R. A., Schlenger, W. E., Fairbank, J. A., Hough, R. L., Jordan, B. K., Marmar, C. R., & Weiss, D. S. (1988). *National Vietnam Veterans Readjustment Study (NVVRS): Description, current status, and initial PTSD prevalence estimates.* Research Triangle Park, NC: Research Triangle Institute.

Lang, P. J. (1977). Imagery in therapy: An information processing analysis of fear. *Behavior Therapy, 8,* 862–886.

Malloy, P. F., Fairbank, J. A., & Keane, T. M. (1983). Validation of a multimethod assessment of post-traumatic stress disorders in Vietnam veterans. *Journal of Consulting and Clinical Psychology, 51,* 488–494.

Orr, S. P., Pitman, R. K., Lasko, N. B., & Herz, L. R. (1993). Psychophysiological assessment of posttraumatic stress disorder imagery in World War II and Korean combat veterans. *Journal of Abnormal Psychology, 102,* 152–159.

Pitman, R. K., Orr, S. P., Forgue, D. F., de Jong, J. B., & Claiborn, J. M. (1987). Psychophysiologic assessment of posttraumatic stress disorder in Vietnam combat veterans. *Archives of General Psychiatry, 44,* 970–975.

Robins, L. N., Helzer, J. E., Croughan, J., & Ratcliff, K. (1981). National Institute of Mental Health Diagnostic Interview Schedule. *Archives of General Psychiatry, 38,* 381–38.

Rosenheck, R., & Fontana, A. (1989). *War Stress Inventory I and II.* (Available from the authors at West Haven VA Medical Center, Northeast Program Evaluation Center, West Haven, CT).

Shalev, A. Y., Orr, S. P., & Pitman, R. K. (1993). Psychophysiologic assessment of traumatic imagery in Israeli civilian patients with posttraumatic stress disorder. *American Journal of Psychiatry, 150,* 620–624.

Spitzer, R., & Williams, J. (1985). *Structured Clinical Interview for DSM-III-R, patient version*. New York: New York State Psychiatric Institute, Biometrics Research Department.

Weathers, F. W., Litz, B. T., & Keane, T. M. (1995). Military trauma. In J. R. Freedy & S. F. Hobfoll (Eds.), *Traumatic stress: From theory to practice* (pp. 103–128). New York: Plenum.

Weiss, D., Horowitz, M. J., & Wilner, N. (1984). The Stress Response Rating Scale: A clinician's measure for rating the response to serious life-events. *British Journal of Clinical Psychology*, 23, 202–215.

Wenger, M. A. (1948). Studies of autonomic balance in army and air forces personnel. *Comparative Psychology Monographs*, 19, No. 4.

Wilson, J. P. (1978). *Identity, ideology, and crisis: the Vietnam veteran in transition* (Vols. 1 and 2). Cincinnati, OH: Disabled American Veterans.

Worthington, E. R. (1977). Post-service adjustment and Vietnam era veterans. *Military Medicine*, 142, 865–866.

4

Natural and Human-Made Disasters

Robert Giel

Reflecting on her experience some seven months after the earthquake of December 1988, an Armenian psychiatrist in the town of Leninakan summed it up in a few terse sentences: "At the time I did not even know what I was doing, looking down and seeing that I was running barefooted on broken glass. I felt nothing, we were totally unprepared." Next, she started to cry, explaining:

When I talk again about what happened that day, I see once more that young man holding desperately onto something while the house around him collapsed. I still see the fires, the vacant eyes, the staring faces. You could not reach them. Of course, people did what you required them to do, but you could not get through to them. Since that day we have worked continuously to forget, but now we are simply exhausted.

Of her four colleagues in the psychiatric dispensary of Leninakan, one died in the disaster and two had left the town because they were burnt out. She herself had lost her daughter. Recounting her flashback, this doctor describes her personal, deeply imprinted experience of the impact of a disaster that destroyed about 80% of the buildings of Leninakan and killed from 20,000 to 30,000 of its 270,000 inhabitants. Nobody knows the exact figure because by no means have all bodies been recovered, and at the

time the town was full of unregistered refugees from Nagorno–Karabach, a contested Armenian enclave across the border with Azerbaijan.

This earthquake is a classic example of a major natural disaster, an "act of God," although, in their retrospective search for meaning, people were inclined to connect the earthquake with Soviet nuclear testing, giving it a human-made perspective and establishing blame.

Quarantelli (1985) identified two opposing views with regard to the mental health aftermath of major disasters affecting communities. One view holds that disasters are traumatic life events, producing "very pervasive, deeply internalized, and essentially negative psychological effects. Disaster victims are viewed primarily as attempting to cope with the meaning of the trauma and disaster impact" (p. 191). The second view is "that community disasters have differential rather than across-the-board effects. Some of the effects are positive as well as negative; many of the latter are relatively short in duration. The varying problems of victims are more closely related to the postimpact organized response than they are to the disaster impact itself." Quarantelli's review indicates that the matter may never be decided, because no two disasters are com-

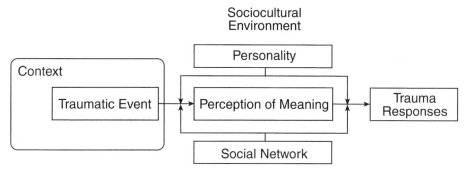

Figure 4.1. Relationship between traumatic events and sociopsychological reactions. [Adapted from Kleber & Brom, 1992.].

pletely similar with regard to their conditions or the manner in which they are researched. In all probability, the two positions are not really oppositional but additional.

This chapter deals with two disasters not only in terms of individual loss and trauma but also as a basic disruption of the social context (Fritz, 1961) within which individuals and groups function, and therefore as a radical departure from the pattern of normal social expectation (Wallace, 1957). In comparing the Armenian earthquake of 1988 with the human-made nuclear disaster of Chernobyl in 1986, I discuss some of the mechanisms involved in the process of restoring social identity—in other words, the transformation of a disorganized society of victims into a community of survivors. To Figley (1985) the basic issue is this "transformation from being a victim to being a survivor. The survivor draws on the experiences of coping with the catastrophe as a source of strength, while the victim remains immobilized" (p. 399). In his opinion the fundamental questions the victim has to answer in order to become a survivor are: (*1*) What happened? (*2*) Why did it happen? (*3*) Why did I act as I did then? (*4*) Why did I act as I have since then? and (*5*) What if it happens again? (p. 404).

Figley considers the cognitive processing of the traumatic event during and following a catastrophe of prime importance. In his conceptual model the level of traumatic stress is considered to be a function of two major sets of variables: the individual's coping ability (including his or her utilization of social support), and the individual's situation within the catastrophe, which may be either passive (immobile and helpless) or active (able to modulate the stressor). My basic assumption, therefore, is that the relationship between the traumatic events and the sociopsychological reactions is not a direct one (see Figure 4.1) (Kleber & Brom, 1992). It is mediated, among other variables, by the context of the traumatic event and by the way in which this is perceived by the public, including the victims. Important contextual features of a disaster are its cause, its scale, and whether it was anticipated, and therefore the degree of preparedness of the population.

Green (1982) proposed an additional contextual dimension, refining the notion of scope: whether a disaster is central or peripheral with respect to a community. After a train disaster happens to people who have come together by chance, survivors return to their respective geographic communities, where the physical setting and the social support networks are still intact. The disaster is peripheral to the community, and, although the survivors' support networks may require guidance and, particularly, information, no substitute needs to be provided. An intermediate type of disaster, according to Green, would be one that occurs to a group of people within a community and hence affects the whole community in some sense (e.g., a coal mine cave-in), but in which there are still many unaffected members of the community and the physical settings remain unchanged. The most central type of disaster is one in which the whole physical and organizational structure of the community is changed (flood, landslide, tornado), because homes are destroyed and survivors are relocated in different surroundings with strangers.

The sociocultural environment exerts its influence on a community's response to disaster through people's attitudes toward loss and death, their ways of coming to terms with loss, and the attribution of personal and public control over events in general (e.g., locus of control; Rotter, 1966). Therefore, important notions regarding a disaster are its perceived predictability, probability, and controllability as a hazard.

The findings presented in this chapter are based not on systematic research but on observations and numerous interviews, both arranged and spontaneous, with villagers, townspeople, authorities, health workers, and the general public through formal and more often informal interpreters (League of the Red Cross and Red Crescent Societies, 1990). These organizations and interviews occurred at the sites of two large-scale disasters. Three fact-finding visits of approximately 10 days each were made to the Leninakan earthquake disaster area on behalf of the World Health Organization; the third visit to Leninakan included a seminar in post-traumatic stress for Armenian health workers. A traveling mission of 2 weeks' duration was made on behalf of the League of Red Cross and Red Crescent Societies to areas in Belorussia and the Great Russian Federation affected by the Chernobyl nuclear incident, during 1989 and 1990. In addition, I was rapporteur to a WHO Workshop on the psychosocial aspects of the Chernobyl incident, which was held in Kiev in May 1990. Also during the latter visit, a day of discussions was organized with the general public, health workers, and local authorities in an affected area in the Ukraine. Because no clear and unambiguous local statistics were available, all figures mentioned should be taken as provisional only.

People interviewed did not appear to feel restricted in what they could say; on the contrary, many accounts were openly critical of the authorities.

AFTERMATH OF THE CHERNOBYL NUCLEAR ACCIDENT

In the early morning of April 26, 1986, one of the reactors at Chernobyl, in the Ukraine, exploded during an experiment. Two employees died immediately; 29 others, employees and firefighters, died later of radiation sickness. Between 250 and 300 people were admitted to the hospital because of radiation sickness but have since been discharged alive (Mould, 1988; Pohl, 1987). It took about 13 days to extinguish the fire in the graphite of the reactor, during which time large quantities of different radionuclides were emitted. The largest contamination occurred within the 30 km zone around the reactor; the immediate area was evacuated within days and the remainder of the area within weeks after the accident. This involved evacuation of approximately 100,000 people. Outside the 30 km zone, the contamination occurred in irregular patterns depending on meteorological conditions, which had a major influence on the levels of deposition from the radioactive plume.

Initially, the main concern was with the short-lived radioisotopes of iodine. Uncertainty remains about the distribution of these isotopes, as well as the effectiveness of the countermeasure of distributing iodine tablets, particularly to children. However, the main problem is contamination of the soil with radioactive cesium (the half-life of the more dominant cesium isotope, cesium 137, is approximately 31 years). Strontium 90 plays a less important role; it poses problems because of the difficulties in measuring the levels present in the environment.

Three zones of contamination are now distinguished:

1. Regions with cesium 137 contamination between 1 and 15 Ci/sq km: zone of occasional control

2. Regions with contamination between 15 and 40 Ci/sq km: zone of permanent control

3. Regions with contamination in excess of 40 Ci/sq km: zone of strict control

Although any radioactive contamination is in principle undesirable, there is general agreement among scientists that life in zone 1 should pose very few problems. The major problems occur in zones 2 and 3. Approximately 10,000 sq km are considered to be contaminated with more than 15 Ci/sq km cesium 137, of which 7000 sq km are in Belorussia, 2000 in the Great Russian Federation, and 1000 in the Ukraine. In Belorussia alone, more than 100,000 persons with roughly 30,000 children live in these two zones.

The necessity of relocating people from contaminated zones is not a decision that can be based purely on clearly defined dose levels. With ionizing radiation, one cannot distinguish a safe dose range from that which implies some level of increased risk. In none of the contaminated regions outside the 30 km zone is there a danger of acute radiation effects with observable symptoms. The danger is from late effects, which occur with small probabilities after several years (mainly leukemias) or after decades (generally other cancers). A small increase of hereditary damage resulting from mutations of germ cells is also possible. According to present knowledge, a lifetime radiation dose of 35 rem (0.35 Sv), may increase the contribution of cancer deaths to total mortality from approximately 20% to perhaps 22%. However, such small increases are difficult to observe statistically. The average "normal" lifetime doses of radiation from all sources is from 0.2 to 1 Sv (Kellerer, 1989).

As far as we could ascertain in our discussions with the public and the authorities in the area, it took several years for the above picture to emerge. Therefore, the context of the Chernobyl accident is that of a central disaster with a delayed but extensive ripple effect of a growing awareness of risk. The radioactive threat was unmistakable to the workers in the power station, and

was immediately acknowledged by the authorities in Moscow, who took over management of the crisis in the grandest possible way. At the same time, the public were kept ignorant. On the first day following the accident, people in Pripyat, Chernobyl, and Kiev were still out in the streets enjoying the sun in a cloudless sky. The first public ripple appeared late on April 28, with a subdued announcement in the Radio Moscow news bulletin, later followed by a brief and reassuring message from the U.S.S.R. Council of Ministers in *Pravda*, stating that the radiation situation at the power station and the adjoining areas had been stabilized (Voznesenskaya, 1987).

In the meantime, the first wave of evacuations from within a radius of 15 km of the power station had already taken place, and people from all over the Soviet Union were engaged in a massive cleanup operation. According to the authorities in Minsk, 600,000 people became involved in this enormous cleanup of parts of the Ukraine, Belorussia, and the Great Russian Federation. Their presence caused the ripples of the original disaster to deepen and to spread wider, carrying an invisible and ill-understood impact. This situation lingered on until March 1988, at which time the authorities could no longer withhold information from the public. From that time on, they started a campaign to regain credibility with the public, and all newspapers now carry the latest readings on radioactivity in the various areas.

In the Belorussian and Great Russian Federation villages I visited, the disaster was perceived as having been caused by the residents of another republic. The Army was considered to have worsened the situation because of its rumored attempts to use rockets to make the radioactive cloud shed its radionuclides before they could contaminate the major population centers in the republics.

People always mentioned, almost in the same breath, another man-made disaster, the Great Patriotic War (World War II), describing the devastation these republics suffered during that period and how they recovered. Minsk, for example, was almost completely destroyed, and in Belorussia alone, 1.5 million people are said to have died during the war (by comparison, the present population is 10.5 million). People in these republics take pride in their nationality and their national language. This is probably an additional reason for the disagreement about the tolerable level of radiation. In Belorussia, the radiation exposure in the the zone of occasional control was taken as sufficiently unsafe to justify relocation, and a lifetime dose of 0.35 Sv was considered as too high, and more a political than a biological issue. Opinion polls appeared to indicate that many people, particularly young parents with children, want to move out.

Individually, people tended to worry about three questions:

1. *What does the already received dose of radiation mean for my present health? How many of my present problems can be ascribed to radioactivity in the environment?* A Red Cross center I visited, which during an average week was attended by 60 elderly people for physical checkups of various kinds, was referring about 20% of its patients for radiological investigations for complaints such as dizziness, headache, or hypertension, to which the relationship of irradiation is tenuous. The impression of clinic workers was that illness behavior had doubled or tripled. Incidences of hypertension, diabetes, chronic bronchitis, ischemic heart disease, cholecystitis, diseases of the nervous system, neurasthenic syndromes, and other health problems were listed as having increased since the accident.

2. *What will become of my children? In what way is their health threatened?* Typical of such concerns were the worried questions of a mother with two asthmatic children, who could not quite believe that this condition may have little to do with radioactivity. In one of the villages I found that, for fear of irradiation, children were kept in school for 12 hours a day and fed

canned food that is supposed to be uncontaminated. The teachers complained that the children were apathetic. In Minsk, three mothers with children with various cancers were in a state of desperation, accusing the authorities of indifference. Again, the relationship of these cases to the accident was not quite straightforward.

3. *What kind of life do I have to live if I am not free to roam the woods and collect mushrooms like I used to do or to cultivate my land, or if I must be very cautious about the food I buy in the market?* In this respect, the situation appeared quite complex. In some villages the land was safe but not the houses; in others, the reverse applied. Sometimes one village and its land were safe, but not another village where the children used to go to school or where the market and post office used to be. People also were aware that the risks are not the same for all ages, which may result in the breaking up of three-generation families. Rumor had it that even the "zero ground" within a radius of 30 km around the reactor was being repopulated with several hundred people, most of them elderly.

Little was known by the public of the morbidity risks of radioactive contamination. Predisaster patterns of morbidity were not always available, and, even if they were, the attribution of differences between those and present patterns can pose problems. For example, the area is known to be naturally deficient in iodine, which has resulted in thyroid malfunction in approximately 25% of the population in some locations. During my visit, thyroid problems were being found in as many as 47% of people in some locations. Do such differences reflect increased morbidity caused by irradiation, more intensive and wider screening of the populace, or changes in the criteria for thyroid malfunction? In some places an increase in the number of cases of tuberculosis had been reported. Can this be attributed to irradiation-induced deterioration of the immune system or to lower rates of presymptomatic diagnosis resulting from people's refusal to have any more medical X-rays for fear of adding to their lifetime dose of radiation? What is the contribution of the symptoms of stress resulting from the indeterminate radioactive threat to the perception of sickness?

The figures obtained locally suggested increased health awareness and illness behavior on the part of the population and increased diagnostic sensitivity on the part of the medical profession; real changes in the pattern of morbidity, however, were unclear. The medical authorities spoke of "generalized radiophobia." This psychiatric labeling was unjustified, because people's fears were not "irrational"; the morbidity risk was quite real, if not immediate. Time has shown that radioactive contamination is widespread and occurs in irregular patterns, justifying careful monitoring. Illness behavior as well as migration appeared to be ways of coping with a hazard perceived as unpredictable and uncontrollable, its probability still a matter of controversy for scientists and its impact different among the generations affected. What other ways than radiophobia exist to become a survivor, except indifference to the risks?

THE AFTERMATH OF THE ARMENIAN EARTHQUAKE

The Armenian earthquake took the country by surprise in terms of its magnitude, but it occurred in a geologically unstable area. Therefore, although it was uncontrollable, it was a predictable and probable event. Attempting to comprehend what happened, many people I interviewed explained how this catastrophe confirmed the tragic fate of the Armenian people: earlier earthquakes; the "forgotten genocide" (Dadrian, 1989) by the Turks in 1894–1896 and in 1909 and 1915; the incorporation into the Soviet Union; and the struggle with Azerbaijan over Nagorno-Karabakh and the perceived lack of support from Moscow in that struggle. The traumatic reality of the disaster was re-

peatedly linked to the historical plight of the Armenian people, emphasizing their unhappy identity and a spirit that was nevertheless indestructible.

The lasting state of arousal of the populace was evident in my interpreter, a young teacher. In the middle of a conversation she suddenly got restless, wanting to leave the prefab building in which we were sitting. I had not observed, as she had, that the ground had trembled and the lamp had started swinging as a heavy truck passed by in the street. A few months earlier she had been in school teaching when laborers used explosives to demolish a neighborhood building that had become unsafe. Teachers and students started screaming and ran from the school. Fearing collapse, nobody wanted to enter the building again, and the school had to be closed. Since then, she has been out of work.

Many people feared heights or high ceilings. Sudden noise startled people. Children had nightmares and did not want to be left alone. Pregnant women were afraid their babies would die born with a malformation. Even though a year had passed since the earthquake, people were still depressed, anxious, and exhausted. An aid and research program, initiated by the Armenian Relief Society of the Western United States subsequently confirmed the lasting nature of these symptoms, particularly in children and young adults (Goenjian et al., 1994; Pynoos et al., 1993). The program also established a relationship between people's closeness to the epicenter and the severity of psychological symptoms, and they concluded that the earthquake was a psychiatric calamity, especially for the children in the region.

The social consequences of the disaster were considerable, because people lacked social resources. The role of the Communist Party was limited because it has no deep roots in society. The central Komsomol office in Yerevan had the difficult task of tracing missing people during the chaotic postimpact phase. On the whole, however, people had little respect for the party's leaders, who discussed models of behavior but did not themselves set the proper example.

The Armenian Orthodox Church oversaw the rites at life's turning points, but its priests otherwise had very little interaction with the people, although religious interest was returning (Goenjian, 1993). Labor unions were important because they were the guardians of material social security, and they were in close contact with the survivors and their families, offering the means for obtaining material support. The social stronghold, however, was still the family, under the leadership of the eldest male or any other member who emerged spontaneously as the main resource person.

The contribution of the medical profession was a much debated issue. They saw themselves as hard-working and poorly paid servants of the public. Nevertheless, there were the persistent stories of doctors requiring a fee before they would render treatment, even to those under duress of the disaster. The medical profession has been severely criticized by the media and the political leadership. Psychiatrists in particular had a poor reputation. The clinics and hospitals in which they work were repugnant to the public, and they themselves were seen as agents of social control, with their frightening diagnostic labels, psychotropic drugs, and electroconvulsive therapy (ECT). To have been sent to a psychiatric clinic or hospital was itself seen as an induction into madness.

With regard to organizing rehabilitation, the public perception of more or less total dependence on Moscow led the community to see itself as caught in a bureaucratic vicious circle. Because the bureaucrats in Moscow were seen as always having to "push the button" to initiate relief activities, and because it would take ages for them to do so, it made little sense to the local residents to even initiate administrative procedures. In this way, local helplessness was again and again confirmed.

More than 1 year after the disaster, the cemetery still was the focal point where people tried to come to terms with their traumatic experiences, and where much of the grieving was being done. Much money was spent on large tombstones with photographs of those who perished. There were always people busy with flowers around the graves, and the sick joke most often repeated was that more time and money were being spent on the dead than were ever during their lifetimes. The town itself was still very much in ruins, with few new buildings and many people still living in prefab housing and some kind of containers. Electricity and water were available but the supply was not entirely reliable. There were almost no shops. The surviving children should have returned several months ago from the holiday camps where they were taken immediately after the disaster, but they had not yet come back because the town was still lacking in infrastructure. This meant that the both painful and joyful reunion of what was left of many families had been postponed.

Grieving had not been completed, and women were taking a leading role in the mourning. One group of women met every week while their husbands waited outside. The women, some of them teachers, spoke of the vivid dreams in which the children they lost beckoned them from beyond the grave. They cried and wished to be with their dead children, so much so that their living children begged to be with their deceased brothers or sisters. The teachers among them could not tolerate the laughter of their students. Photographs of dead children in their coffins were passed around. These women were inconsolable and rejected the suggestion that life was worth living for the sake of those still alive. They felt guilty and were not yet able to let the past rest.

In some respects, traditional social patterns were changing. Parents who lost their partners had to fulfill a double role. Women with professional careers as teachers or doctors could no longer afford to stay away from home, because there was no one else to look after the children; some even had to look after the remnants of other incomplete families. The assistant mayor for social affairs of Leninakan underlined the burden women in particular have to carry. He had to give counsel to hundreds of them every week; they were lost in this bureaucracy dominated by males. Pamphlets and posters with information served no purpose because people wanted to unburden themselves from their personal misery, and they did not bother to read such material. The media were no help either because they mentioned only what went wrong.

There was jealousy of neighbors who survived without a scratch. Other couples who had barely escaped with their lives attributed a deeper meaning to their marriage. One year after the disaster, many still struggled with the burning question, "Why me? To what purpose?"—as if there can be a rational answer to this question in the face of such a major natural disaster.

COMPARING THE TWO DISASTER SITUATIONS

These two traumatic situations, both totally unforeseen by their victims, differed immensely with regard to Figley's (1985) first fundamental question, "What happened?" The impact of the earthquake in Armenia was overwhelmingly and tangibly evident to everyone because of the tremor itself, the immense death toll, and the vast material destruction. The threat itself passed as suddenly as it had occurred. Every survivor had his or her ordinary expectations of reality violently shaken and replaced by a horrifying imprint of an incomprehensible new reality, to be experienced again and again in the form of nightmares and flashbacks. However, the two worlds could to some extent be integrated on historical grounds, in a sense reinforcing Armenian national identity. The difficult and tiresome processes of mourning, restoration, and rehabilitation could at least begin. The stream of aid from abroad widened the crack made in the Iron Curtain by *perestroika*, gradually shifting the public locus of control from external to more internal. One can speculate that the earthquake also shook public attitudes in the capital and other less affected areas, and was a factor in preparing the ground for self-determination and the war being waged

on Azerbaijan, after the breakup of the U.S.S.R.

Outside the 30 km zone around Chernobyl, however, there was no real impact other than a growing awareness of something being terribly wrong, of some intangible threat. People's strong desire, even today, for repeated measurements of radioactivity in the environment and for medical examination of every ailment shows that they are still striving to find out what has happened.

This technological disaster brings out the issue of risk or hazard *perception*. The context in which the two disasters centrally affected complete communities is different, not only in terms of speed, extent, and death toll, but particularly in the perception of risk and in the signal potential of the two disasters (Slovic, 1986, 1987, 1990). When experts judge risk, their responses correlate highly with technical estimates of annual fatalities. Concerning the Chernobyl disaster, these estimates were low and almost indistinguishable from predisaster statistical probabilities of dying of cancer (Ilyin et al., 1990), but they are also changing and increasing with time because of growing insight (Kellerer, 1989).

The judgments of lay people are related more to other hazard characteristics, for example, whether the hazard has catastrophic potential, is a threat to future generations, is involuntary, is known to those exposed, is known to science, is controllable, or has an equal distribution of risks and benefits. In these respects, everything related to nuclear energy scores very poorly, is greatly feared, and causes a strong sense of uncertainty, much more so than an earthquake. People tend to adopt particular strategies when dealing with uncertainty. Anxiety, incomprehension of what is meant by probability, orientation toward opinions communicated by the media, and personal experience regularly result in over- or underestimation of risk and in unshakably biased perceptions of "reality." New evidence is accepted only if it supports existing opinions. Otherwise, it is rejected out of hand as unreliable, erroneous, or unrepresentative. The strength with which this happens depends on the firmness of the original conviction, with, in the extreme, the victim being completely at the mercy of the conceptualizations of the authorities. Such a coping strategy is revealed in the change in the individual's perception of the same risk when it is presented in terms of survival instead of mortality.

The signal potential of both disasters concerns the new information they provide about the likely occurrence of similar or more destructive mishaps. The informativeness or signal value of an event, and thus its potential social impact, appears to be systematically related to the previously mentioned characteristics of a hazard (Slovic, 1987). An accident that takes many lives may produce little social disturbance if it occurs as part of a familiar and well-understood system (earthquake). However, a smaller accident (in terms of its death toll) involving an unfamiliar, poorly understood system (nuclear energy) may have immense social consequences if it is perceived as a harbinger of further possibly catastrophic mishaps. Compared with the much-discussed Chernobyl accident of 1986, the Armenian earthquake of 1988, with its much heavier death toll, is already a forgotten event.

Coping strategies depend very much on people's perception of meaning. In this respect, the two disasters show some similarity but also tremendous differences. In both cases, the disasters are put in the general perspective of affecting populations with a history of being victims but also tenacious survivors. There the similarity ends because, from an individual point of view, the Armenians are coping by mourning their lost ones. They continue to do so by searching for the remains of the deceased and by keeping their memories alive at the cemetery. They also have firm objectives, (i.e., rebuilding their towns and reconstructing their communities).

In contrast, people in the contaminated areas of Chernobyl, rather than having to deal with actual losses, continue to live with the threat of losing their health. One aspect of their increased "illness behavior" is that their access to readings of radioactivity and their knowledge of its consequences, and of the meaning and background of their complaints, will assist them in coping with the stressful situation of permanent uncertainty. Therefore, it appears irrational not to have informed people for fear of causing panic. The combination of unconfirmed rumor and ignorance, on the contrary, must have promoted apprehension rather than prevented it.

Since there was no observable impact in either Belorussia or the Great Russian Federation, but rather more of a ripple effect, one would not expect post-traumatic stress reactions with flashbacks and triggering events, such as were in evidence in Leninakan (e.g., the flight reaction caused by the tremor from a truck passing in the street). The emergency situation caused by radioactive contamination appears more enduring.

The answer to Figley's second question, "Why did it happen?", is straightforward. In the case of Chernobyl, people (managers of the plant) were culpable and have been punished. In addition, the authorities are accused of allowing dependency on nuclear energy. In Leninakan, there are no such easy answers to this question, nor such resolutions as punishment or the closure of plants. Accusations that Soviet nuclear testing was responsible for the earthquake did not convince many people and should be seen not as rational but as unconvincing attempts to explain the inexplicable.

Figley's third and fourth questions, "Why did I act as I did then?" and "Why did I act as I have since then?", do not seem pertinent in the contaminated areas in Belorussia and the Great Russian Federation. In a sense, there are "no survivors" in those areas because on the whole there have been few visible victims yet, in terms of death or destruction, except for those whose farming or selling of food has been affected or who otherwise had to change their way of life. The questions and solutions of mothers and their young children, who want to move away, are obviously quite different from those of the elderly, who are not inclined to leave.

In Leninakan, several years after the disaster, these are still burning questions. Particularly, mothers were accusing themselves of not having been able to prevent the deaths of their children, although they were in no position to do so. Many admitted that since the disaster they have sought refuge in hyperactivity, which tended to numb awareness of their real situation. The grief groups and the activities at the cemetery appear to have an aspect of healing recapitulation, but at the same time they incorporate an element of self-victimization in the entertaining of wounds and in the resulting economic burden.

The role of the social network also differs in the two disasters. Whereas in Armenia it is important for the remaining family members to be together and support one another, in the contaminated areas near Chernobyl the presence of the youngest generation poses a threat because of the long-term consequences of radiation for their health. Mothers with young children want to move out, while the elderly want to stay. Age strongly affects the perception of meaning of the event.

CONCLUSION

The effects of the two disasters appear different but not in a positive way. At the moment, at least, it is difficult to discern any positive effects. Psychosocial rehabilitation appears difficult in both cases, for different reasons. In Armenia, for political and historical reasons it will not be easy for people to overcome their passive-dependent role, although the war with Azerbaijan may be evidence that this has indeed happened. In the areas contaminated with radionuclides in and around Chernobyl, the disastrous threat lingers on and will do so for many years. Whereas in Armenia, post-traumatic stress disorder and outright depression can be expected, in the contaminated areas the health care system will have to cope with increased illness behavior in general. This can only become clear against a background of solid epidemiological data.

REFERENCES

Dadrian, V. N. (1989). Genocide as a problem of national and international law: The World War I Armenian case and its contemporary legal ramifications. *Yale Journal of International Law, 14*, 221–334.

Figley, C. R. (1985). From Victim to Survivor: Social Responsibility in the Wake of Catastrophe. In C. R. Figley (Ed.), *Trauma and its wake. The study and treatment of post-traumatic stress disorder. Vol. I.* (pp. 398–415). New York: Brunner/Mazel.

Fritz, C. E. (1961). Disaster. In R. K. Merton & R. A. Nisbet (Eds.), *Contemporary social problems* (pp. 148–171). New York: Harcourt, Brace and World.

Goenjian, A. (1993). A mental health relief programme in Armenia after the 1988 earthquake: Implementation and clinical observations. *British Journal of Psychiatry, 163*, 230–239.

Goenjian, A. K., Najarian, L. M., Pynoos, R. S., Steinberg, A. M., Manoukian, G., Tavosian, A., & Fairbanks, L. A. (1994). Post-traumatic stress disorder in elderly and younger adults after the 1988 earthquake in Armenia. *American Journal of Psychiatry, 151*, 895–901.

Green, B. L. (1982). Assessing levels of psychological impairment following disaster: Consideration of actual and methodological dimensions. *Journal of Nervous and Mental Disease, 70*, 544.

Ilyin, L. A., Balonov, M. I., Buldakov, L. A., et al. (1990). Radiocontamination patterns and possible health consequences of the accident at the Chernobyl nuclear power station. *Journal of Radiologic Protocol, 10*, 13.

Kellerer, A. M. (1989). Die neue Bewerung der Strahlenrisiken: Folgerungen aus der Revision der Dosiemetrie in Hiroshima und Nagasaki. In W. Koehnlein, et al. (Eds.), *Die Wirkung niedriger Strahlendosen* (pp. 37–55). Berlin: Springer.

Kleber, R. J., & Brom, D. (1992). *Coping with trauma: Theory, prevention, and treatment.* Lisse: Swets en Zeitlinger.

League of Red Cross and Red Crescent Societies. (1990). *Report on assessment mission to the areas affected by the Chernobyl disaster, U.S.S.R.* Geneva: International Red Cross.

Mould, R. F. (1988). *Chernobyl: The real story.* New York: Pergamon.

Pohl, F. (1987). *Chernobyl: A novel.* New York: Bantam Books.

Pynoos, R. S., Goenjian, A., Tashjian, M., Karakashian, M., Manjikian, R., Manoukian, G.,

Steinberg, A. M., & Fairbanks, L. A. (1993). Post-traumatic stress reactions in children after the 1988 Armenian earthquake. *British Journal of Psychiatry, 163,* 239–247.

Quarantelli, E. L. (1985). An assessment of conflicting views on mental health: The consequences of traumatic events. In C. R. Figley (Ed.), *Trauma and its Wake. The study and treatment of post-traumatic stress disorder. Vol. I* (pp. 173–215). New York: Brunner/Mazel.

Rotter, J. B. (1966). Generalized expectancies for internal versus external control of reinforcement. *Psychological Mongraphs,* No. 80.

Slovic, P. (1986). Informing and educating the public about risk. *Risk Analysis, 6,* 403.

Slovic, P. (1987). Perception of risk. *Science, 236,* 280–285.

Slovic, P. (1990). Perception of risk from radiation. In W. K. Sinclair (Ed.), *Radiation protection today—the NCRP at sixty years* (pp. 73–97). Bethesda, MD.

Voznesenskaya, J. (1987). *The star Chernobyl.* London: Methuen

Wallace, A. F. C. (1957). Mazeway disintegration: The individual's perception of sociocultural disorganization. *Human Organization, 16,* 23.

II

INDIVIDUAL EVENTS

William W. Eaton
Bruce P. Dohrenwend

Major individual events that are negative generally occur in more usual situations than the extreme situations of human-made and natural disasters described in the previous section. In Part II we turn to an examination of eight such adverse events: child abuse, unemployment, bereavement, homelessness, human immunodeficiency virus (HIV) infection, victimization (especially rape), divorce, and physical illness. On the basis of reviews of previous research and presentation of original analyses of data from prospective and longitudinal studies, important information is provided about the nature of these events as likely risk factors for various types of disorder.

The focus on individual events contrasts with the influential work of Holmes and Rahe (1967), which had as its underlying theory the notion that an accidental confluence of events and circumstances caused distress, mental disorder, and physical illness by upsetting a homeostatic equilibrium. The model of Holmes and Rahe grouped together all events and circumstances that required adjustment into a single, overall score. However, the underlying notion of accidental confluence—essentially a Poisson process—hindered the development of the-

ory and preventive action. Soon further theoretical developments specified categories or dimensions of events, such as desirable versus undesirable, predictable versus unpredictable, controllable versus uncontrollable, and exits versus entrances. These categories increased the potential of the type of approach used by Holmes and Rahe to contribute to etiological understanding of mental disorders. Here we consider the effects of specific events, one by one, without necessarily trying to link them into categories.

The dominant strategy at the time of Holmes and Rahe's publication in 1967 was retrospective and often involved use of case–control designs. Methodological criticisms led to emphasis on the need for prospective and longitudinal strategies such as those described in this section. Increasing appreciation of the epidemiological approach in psychiatry, and of the issue of statistical power, also led to larger sample sizes in many studies, despite the large costs involved. The chapters in this section contain examples of specific adverse events defining cohorts for longitudinal studies that compare exposed to unexposed populations. These cohort studies have the potential to contribute good answers to etiological questions, at substantially less cost than large longitudinal studies of general populations, but they will necessarily have difficulty contributing to a general theory of adverse events and circumstances, because comparisons across different types of events will not be feasible when the specific type of event defines the cohort for follow-up. However, research on specific events can evolve into preventive intervention research trials, and full-scale prevention efforts, much more feasibly than strategies focused on multiple categories of events.

There is an interesting parallel between the development of theories about the nature and role of events over the last quarter-century or so and the development of concepts of mental disorder. At the time Holmes and Rahe published their unidimensional approach to measuring life events in terms of the cumulative amount of change they were likely to introduce, the definition of mental disorder, especially in the United States, was oriented toward unitary or global concepts such as "caseness" and "impairment" (Leighton et al., 1963; Srole et al., 1962). Now we are studying specific mental disorders with precise operational criteria. Against this background, a number of important theoretical questions can be raised. How do specific events fit into theoretically meaningful categories? Is it necessary to categorize events in order to develop a useful theory? Will the usefulness of the theory depend on the specific disorder, or can it apply to a range of disorders? Is the development of a theory based on categories of events necessary for prevention efforts to take place? Can we develop a theory general enough to cover the range of adverse situations and events that the human organism experiences on its journey through life? These are questions to keep in mind while reading the chapters in this section.

It seems clear from the chapters by Widom and by Clayton that child abuse and spousal bereavement are causally related to major depression. The relation of the other types of negative events to various types of psychopathology appears more complicated.

The chapters by Kasl and his colleagues on unemployment, Bruce on divorce, Kilpatrick et al. on victimization, and Herman and co-workers on homelessness show that each of these types of events includes highly varied subtypes. Instances of any one type can differ in source (e.g., unemployment resulting from being fired in contrast to unemployment caused by a plant shutdown) and severity (e.g., rapes that involve life threat and injury in contrast to those that do not), depending, for example, on the circumstances under which they occurred. The complexities of relations of physical illnesses to psychiatric disorders make this a challenging and important field unto itself, as is evident in the chapter by Dew.

It is difficult, and probably not very useful, to consider positive aspects of stress when the events are as all-encompassing and life threatening as those considered in the previous section on extreme situations. In the present section, with its focus on events that are stressful but more nearly within the range of usual experience, the "dosage" of adversity, on the average, is probably lower. At some point in the range of severity, the possibility arises that stress will have positive effects instead of, or in addition to, negative effects. This possibility is raised in the discussion of "psychological growth" by Ouellette in her chapter on AIDS and by Kasl and colleagues in relation to the apparent absence of negative effects of the stress of retirement.

Ouellette notes that social support often contributes to lower demoralization—feeling better—among those experiencing HIV-related stress. She also points out that, as time passes, there apparently is increasingly less negative psychological effect of loss of friends and partners in HIV-positive men. This decrease in the effect of bereavement over time suggests that the individuals are learning to adapt to stress. Such evidence of adaptation is also found in the wider literature on stressful life events. For example, Eaton (1978) found in an analysis of longitudinal data that, when life event stressors at the follow-up wave are adjusted, life event stressors at the prior wave can be seen to have a protective effect on level of distress or demoralization experienced. This analysis suggests that something like inoculation may have occurred. In more general terms, confronting adversity may contribute in some way to the search for meaningful existence in which all humans engage. The stress itself, or the act of overcoming it, may contribute to that search.

Overall, however, the more usual results presented in this section have to do with negative effects. It would seem that we have, or are close to having, undeniable evidence of the etiological effects of adverse life events and circumstances on various types of psychopathology, ranging from diagnosable disorder to symptoms of psychological distress. This evidence takes us closer to the possibility of developing preventive interventions. We need to learn, for example, how much it costs to reduce, by a quantifiable amount, exposure to such adverse circumstances as child abuse, victimization, and homelessness. Combining information on the malleability of the circumstances leading to the occurrence of such events with epidemiological knowledge of the attributable risks (Kleinbaum et al., 1982) they represent would make it possible to plan rational programs directed at reducing their most serious psychopathological consequences (Mrazek & Haggerty, 1994).

REFERENCES

Eaton, W. W. (1978). Life events, social supports, and psychiatric symptoms: A reanalysis of the New Haven data. *Journal of Health and Social Behavior, 19,* 230–234.

Holmes, T. H., & Rahe, R. H. (1967). The Social Readjustment Rating Scale. *Journal of Psychosomatic Research, 11,* 213–218.

Kleinbaum, D. G., Kupper, L. L., & Morgenstern, H. (Eds.). (1982). *Epidemiologic research: Principles and quantitative methods.* London: Lifetime Learning Publications.

Leighton, D. C., Harding, J. S., Macklin, D. B., et al. (1963). *The character of danger.* New York: Basic Books.

Mrazek, P. J., & Haggerty, R. J. (Eds.). (1994). *Reducing risks for mental disorders: Frontiers for preventive intervention research.* Washington, DC: National Academy Press.

Srole, L., Langner, T. S., Michael, S. T., et al. (1962). *Mental health in the metropolis.* New York: McGraw-Hill.

5

Childhood Victimization: Early Adversity and Subsequent Psychopathology

Cathy Spatz Widom

Adversity: "exposure to a set of unpropitious or calamitous circumstances implying previous well-being."
—*Webster's*, 1961:14

Childhood experiences such as physical and sexual abuse and neglect are adverse events with immediate and long-term consequences. However, in considering child abuse and neglect as examples of adverse life events that have the potential to affect development and subsequent psychopathology, the assumption of "well-being" in the child's life *prior* to the victimization experience may not be a reasonable one. Although certain forms of childhood victimization may indeed be viewed as acute stressors, child abuse and neglect often occur against a background of more chronic adversity in multiproblem homes. Child abuse or neglect may be only one of a family's problems. Thus the general effects of other family characteristics, such as poverty, unemployment, parental alcoholism or drug problems, or other inadequate social and family functioning, must be recognized and disentangled from the specific effects of childhood abuse or neglect.

Often, outcomes attributable to childhood abuse and/or neglect may not be distinguishable from outcomes associated with co-occurring family problems. For example, in a review of the child sexual abuse literature, Beitchman et al. (1991) concluded that most of that literature has "been vague in separating effects directly attributable to sexual abuse from effects that may be due to pre-existing psychopathology in the child, family

dysfunction, or to the stress associated with disclosure"(p.538).

The purpose of this chapter is fourfold. First, drawing on past literature, I illustrate the range of outcomes associated with child abuse and neglect. Second, I describe some of my own research from a prospective cohort design study, documenting the long-term consequences of early childhood victimization across a number of domains of functioning. Third, I call attention to potential differences in consequences as a function of the gender of the child and the context in which the abuse or neglect occurs. Fourth, the last part of this chapter speculates on a number of ways in which childhood victimization may influence the development of these outcomes and raises some issues for future research.

CONSEQUENCES OF CHILDHOOD VICTIMIZATION

A number of reviews have described the impact of different types of child maltreatment (Augoustinos, 1987; Beitchman et al., 1991; Browne & Finkelhor, 1986; Kendall-Tackett et al., 1993; Milner, 1991; National Research Council, 1993; Urquiza & Capra, 1990; Widom, 1989c; Wolfe, 1987). Physical consequences may range from minor injuries to severe brain damage and even death. Cognitive effects may be manifest in attentional problems, learning disorders, or poor school performance. Psychological consequences range from chronic low self-esteem, anxiety, and depression (Allen & Tarnowski, 1989; Kaufman, 1991; Kazdin et al., 1985; Lipovsky et al., 1989; Peters, 1988; Stein et al., 1988) to alcohol and other substance abuse (Ladwig & Anderson, 1989; Root, 1989), and other self-destructive behaviors and suicide attempts (DeWilde et al., 1992; Green, 1978; Walsh & Rosen, 1988). Behaviorally, the consequences range from poor peer relations to physical aggression and antisocial behavior (Kolko et al., 1990) and to extraordinarily violent behaviors (Lewis et al., 1979, 1982; Maxfield & Widom, 1996; Widom, 1989b). Thus not only is the behavior of abused and neglected children potentially damaging to them, but it also appears to be damaging to others.

Gender Differences

Gender differences in the consequences of childhood victimization have not received major scholarly attention, although some writers have discussed gender differences in the manifestations of distress and have suggested a certain conformity to gender roles, (Dohrenwend & Dohrenwend, 1976; Downey et al., 1994; Horwitz & White, 1987; Widom, 1984). For example, Downey et al. (1994) have suggested that gender differences in the consequences of abuse may parallel gender differences in expressions of psychopathology and that aggression and depression may be different expressions of the same underlying distress, perhaps reflecting different strategies for maintaining self-esteem in the face of perceived rejection.

A few studies have reported differences in the reaction of boys and girls to abuse. One study found boys to have more externalizing and girls to have more internalizing symptoms (Friedrich et al., 1986). Livingston (1987) examined depression and conduct disorders in sexually abused children and found that girls were overrepresented among abuse victims with depressive disor-

ders and underrepresented among abuse victims with conduct disorders. Dodge et al. (1990) found a much larger increase over base rates in depression among physically harmed girls, compared to a lesser increase among physically harmed boys.

However, at least three factors introduce complexity into the study of gender differences in the consequences of childhood victimization. First, some of the lack of attention to gender differences in consequences may result from the small number of male victims of sexual abuse in most studies and lower rates of reporting childhood sexual abuse in boys (Finkelhor, 1990). Second, certain forms of psychopathology and psychiatric diagnoses are more prevalent in one sex than the other (Robins & Regier, 1991; Widom, 1984). On that basis alone, it would be expected that certain outcome patterns will interact with the sex of the respondent. Third, it is also possible that different outcomes reflect gender differences in response to different types of abuse. That is, if boys and girls experience different types of childhood victimization, then the consequences might also be expected to differ. Thus type of childhood abuse or neglect might be the critical variable in determining a person's risk for subsequent problem behaviors.

Contextual Variables

Understanding the impact of childhood abuse and neglect also requires consideration of contextual variables (Widom, in press). There is emerging evidence that the long-term impact of childhood trauma may depend on the larger context, that is, the family's or community's reaction to it (Briere & Runtz, 1988; Harris et al., 1990; Terr, 1983). Some ways of handling or responding to incidents of abuse or neglect may act to buffer the child and in turn lead to better outcomes for that child, whereas other responses may act to exacerbate these already vulnerable children.

Premature babies generally do relatively poorly in school (Drillen, 1964). However, the long-term disadvantage for the premature infant is especially marked if the child is raised in an unstable, disturbed family setting. Premature children raised in stable homes showed no or minimal disadvantage. Terr (1983) found that pre-existing family pathology contributed to individual differences in the long-term adjustment of children kidnapped and held for 48 hours in an underground hideout. Four years after the kidnapping, the children from troubled families were more maladjusted than children from healthier families. Gibbin et al. (1984) suggest that abuse or neglect will not necessarily predict the developmental outcome of the child. They found that the provision of appropriate play materials and maternal involvement were more discriminating in predicting outcome than abuse/control status alone. Thus the presence or absence of abuse may interact with other aspects of the child's environment to determine outcome.

Similarly, the long-term consequences of childhood victimization may be affected by practices of the community and justice and social service systems in which the child lived. For example, some have suggested that the relationship between early childhood victimization and problem behaviors in adolescence may be in part a function of juvenile justice system practices that disproportionately label and adjudicate maltreatment victims as juvenile offenders (Smith et al., 1980). Wyatt (1990) has called attention to the ways in which racial and ethnic minority children can encounter discrimination, affecting their self-esteem and exacerbating initial or lasting effects of earlier childhood victimization. Finally, other research suggests a link between parental alcoholism and child abuse (Famularo et al., 1986; Reider et al., 1989) and parental alcoholism and subsequent alcoholism in offspring (Cloninger et al., 1985; Goodwin et al., 1973, 1977). If parents with alcohol problems are more likely to abuse or neglect their children, then there are multiple reasons for expecting that their offspring will be at increased risk for the development of alcohol problems. This complexity is illustrated by research by Kroll et al. (1985),

who found that the abusive parent for a sample of abused male alcoholic Veterans Administration patients was almost always the natural father, who was an alcoholic. The effects of this familial influence must be disentangled from the effects of an abusive or neglectful home environment. Taken together, these studies suggest the importance of specifying the context in which traumatic events occur and incorporating contextual variables into analyses of consequences.

A PROSPECTIVE COHORT STUDY: DESIGN AND METHODOLOGY

Phase I

In 1986 I began research to document the long-term consequences of early child abuse and neglect. The initial focus was on delinquency, criminality, and violent criminal behavior (Widom, 1989b). This research involved a prospective cohort design, in which children who were abused and neglected approximately 20 years earlier were compared with a matched control group of children of the same age, sex, race, and approximate family social class. In the first phase of the research, official criminal histories were compiled for these individuals from three levels of law enforcement (local, state, and federal) and comparisons between abused and neglected individuals and controls were made. [For complete details of the study design and subject selection criteria, see Widom (1989a)].

The prospective nature of this design permits some issues of causality to be examined and helps to disentangle the effects of childhood victimization from other potentially confounding effects. Because of the matching procedure, the subjects are assumed to differ in the risk factor (having experienced childhood sexual or physical abuse or neglect). Because it is not possible to randomly assign subjects to groups (and obviously this could not be done), the assumption of equivalency for the groups is an approximation.

The abused/neglected group (n = 908) was composed of substantiated cases of childhood physical and sexual abuse or neglect processed during the years 1967–1971 in the county juvenile or adult criminal court (situated in a metropolitan area in the Midwest). These are cases of early child abuse and neglect, restricted to children who were 11 years of age or less at the time of the abuse or neglect incident.

Physical abuse cases included injuries such as bruises, welts, burns, abrasions, lacerations, wounds, cuts, bone and skull fractures, and other evidence of physical injury. *Sexual abuse* cases varied from those involving relatively nonspecific charges of "assault and battery with intent to gratify sexual desires" to more specific ones of "fondling or touching in an obscene manner," sodomy, incest, and so forth. *Neglect* cases reflected a judgment that the parents' deficiencies in child care were beyond those found acceptable by community and professional standards at the time. These neglect cases represented extreme failure to provide adequate food, clothing, shelter, and medical attention to children.

A matched control group (n = 667) was established. Children who were under school age at the time of the abuse/neglect incident were matched with children of the same, sex, race, date of birth (± 1 week), and hospital of birth through the use of county birth records. For children of school age, records of more than 100 elementary schools for the same time period were used to find matches with children of the same sex, race, date of birth (± 6 months), class in same elementary school during the years 1967–1971, and home address. Overall, there were matches for 74% of the abused and neglected children.

Phase II

In 1989, I began the second phase of this research to trace, locate, and interview these abused/neglected individuals (more than 20 years after their childhood victimization) and controls. Two-hour follow-up interviews were conducted during 1989 and 1995. The interviews consisted of a series of structured and semistructured questions and rating scales, measures of IQ and reading ability, and a psychiatric assessment—the National Institute of Mental Health Diagnostic Interview Schedule (Version III, Revised) (DIS-III-R; Robins et al., 1989).

Interviewers were blind to the purpose of the study, to the inclusion of an abuse and neglect group, and to the participants' group membership. Similarly, the subjects were blind to the purpose of the study. Subjects were told that they had been asked to participate as part of a large group of individuals who grew up in that area during the late 1960s and early 1970s. After the study was described, subjects who agreed to participate signed a consent form indicating their willingness to participate.

The findings described here are based on interviews with 1196 individuals. Of the original sample of 1575 participants, 82% were located and 76% interviewed. Of the people not interviewed, 39 were deceased, 9 were incapable of being interviewed, 284 were not found, and 47 refused to participate (a refusal rate of 3%). Comparison of the current follow-up sample with the original sample indicated no significant differences in terms of percent male, white, abused/neglected, poverty in childhood census tract, or mean current age. The interviewed group (follow-up sample) was significantly more likely to have an official criminal arrest record than the original sample of 1575 (50% of the current sample versus 45% of the original sample). However, this is not surprising because people with a criminal history are generally easier to find, in part because they have more "institutional footprints" to assist in locating them.

Approximately half the sample was female (48.7%) and about two-thirds were white (62.9%). The mean age of the sample at the time of the interview was 28.7 [standard deviation (SD) = 3.84]. There were no differences between the abused and neglected group and controls in terms of gender, race/ethnicity, or age.

The interview was designed with particular awareness of the potential difficulty of

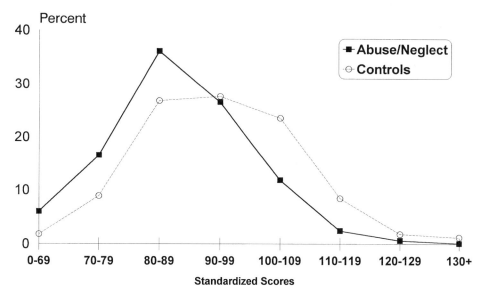

Figure 5.1. Distribution of IQ scores in follow-up sample ($n = 1185$).

obtaining information from subjects about sensitive topics. With clinical research, there is always a trade-off between being sensitive to the needs and experiences of the person interviewed and eliciting sufficient information by adequate probing without becoming leading or overly intrusive.

RESEARCH FINDINGS

Intellectual Outcomes

Figure 5.1 presents the distribution of IQ scores (Quick Test, Ammons & Ammons, 1962) assessed at approximately age 29. This figure reveals that the sample as a whole is functioning at the lower end of intellectual performance and that the majority of both the abused/neglected and control groups score below the mean standardized score of 100. Furthermore, despite the overall low level of performance, abused/neglected individuals scored significantly lower on IQ than controls. These lower levels of IQ in the abused/neglected group, in comparison with the controls, persist in multivariate regression equations with controls for age, sex, race, and criminal history (see Perez & Widom, 1994).

The average highest grade of school completed for the follow-up sample as a whole was 11.47 years (SD = 2.19), although abused/neglected individuals had completed significantly less school (mean = 10.99, SD = 1.99) than controls (mean = 12.09, SD = 2.29) ($t_{1,193} = 8.88$, $p < .001$). Whereas two-thirds of the control group had completed high school, less than half (48%) of the abused/neglected children at follow-up had done so.

Behavioral and Social Outcomes

The interview asked about employment status both at the time of the interview and over the last 5 years. Occupational status of the sample was coded according to the Hollingshead Occupational Coding Index (Hollingshead, 1975). Occupational levels of the subjects ranged from 1 (laborer) to 9 (professional). The median occupational level of the sample was semiskilled workers, and less than 7% of the overall sample was in levels 7–9 (managers through professionals). In terms of occupational status at the time of the interview (Fig. 5.2), significantly more of the abused/neglected individuals were in menial and semiskilled occupations than controls (62% vs. 45%, $p < .001$). Con-

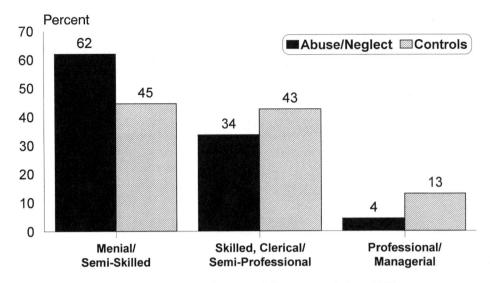

Figure 5.2. Occupational status in follow-up sample ($n = 1167$).

versely, more of the controls were work-ing in higher occupational levels, from skilled ($p < .01$) to professional ($p < .001$) occupations.

Employment history findings (Fig. 5.3) are based on a measure used by Robins and Regier (1991, p. 103). Individuals who are currently *unemployed* may be temporarily out of work or not working for a number of reasons, such as being a student, a house-wife, retired, or incapacitated. Furthermore, a person's current work status may be long or short term. *Underemployment* is defined as a "total of six months or more out of the five years prior to the interview when ex-pected to work—that is, excluding periods when one was not in the work force for the reasons listed above" (Robins & Regier, 1991, p. 103). In the Epidemiological Catchment Areas study, about 13% of the total sample met the definition of under-employment (Robins & Regier, 1991). Here, significantly more of the abused/neglected individuals were underemployed over the

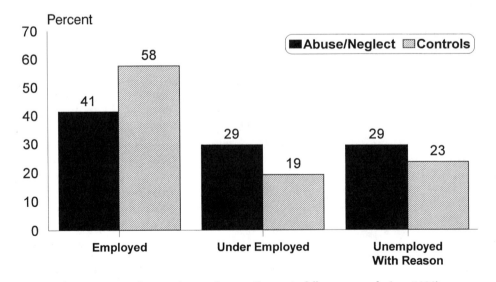

Figure 5.3. Employment history for past 5 years in follow-up sample ($n = 1196$).

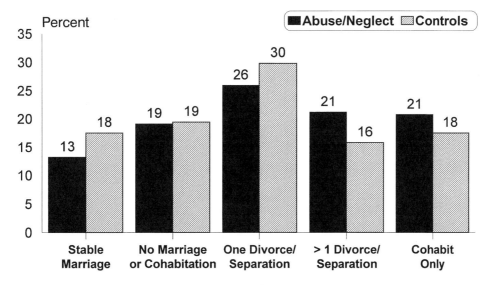

Figure 5.4. Marital history in follow-up sample (n = 1196).

past 5 years than controls (29% versus 19%, respectively; p < .001). Not surprisingly, controls were more often employed (58% versus 41%, respectively, p < .001). At the same time, more than a fifth of both groups (29% of the abuse/neglect group and 23% of the controls) were unemployed during that 5 year time period.

Childhood victimization is associated with consequences for interpersonal relationships as well (Fig. 5.4). Whereas almost a fifth of the controls in the sample reported a stable marriage, only 13% of the abused/neglected group reported that kind of relationship. More abused/neglected individuals reported a history of multiple divorces and separations than controls (p < .05).

As reported previously, early childhood victimization is also associated with in-

creases in risk for official criminal behavior—arrests for delinquency, adult criminality, and violence. Table 5.1 summarizes these results *for the follow-up sample* (i.e., 1196 of the original 1575 subjects) to provide a more complete picture of these individuals and the extent to which childhood victimization has influenced their subsequent lives. [These findings should not be confused with those published previously (Widom, 1989b; Maxfield & Widom, 1996), which report rates of arrest for the original entire sample of 1575.] The odds of an arrest for a juvenile crime in these abused/neglected individuals are 1.9 times higher than that for the controls, and those for an adult arrest 1.6 times higher. Being abused or neglected as a child also has an impact on a person's risk of an arrest for a violent

Table 5.1. Childhood victimization and criminality in follow-up sample (n = 1196)

	Abuse/neglect (%) (n = 676)	Control (%) (n = 520)	Odds ratio	Confidence interval
Juvenile arrest	31.2°°°	19.0	1.9	1.5–2.5
Adult arrest	48.4°°°	36.2	1.6	1.3–2.1
Any arrest	56.5°°°	42.5	1.8	1.4–2.2
Violent arrest	21.0°	15.6	1.4	1.1–1.9

°p ≤ .05; °°p ≤ .01; °°°p ≤ .001.

Table 5.2. Childhood victimization and psychopathology in follow-up sample (n = 1196)

	Abuse/neglect (%) (n = 676)	Control (%) (n = 520)	Odds ratio	Confidence interval
Suicide attempt	18.8°°°	7.7	2.8	1.9–4.0
Antisocial personality disorder diagnosis	18.4°°°	11.2	1.8	1.3–2.5
Alcohol abuse/dependence diagnosis	54.5	51.0	1.2	0.9–1.4

°p ≤ .05; °°p ≤ .01; °°°p ≤ .001.

crime [odds ratio (OR) = 1.4]. Abused/neglected individuals are clearly at increased risk for arrest in adolescence (before age 18) and adulthood, but a substantial group of abused/neglected children did *not* become delinquents, adult criminals, or violent offenders.

Psychological and Emotional Consequences

Psychological and emotional consequences are illustrated here by three indices of psychopathology—suicide attempts and diagnoses of antisocial personality disorder (ASPD) and alcohol abuse and/or dependence according to criteria in the *Diagnostic and Statistical Manual of Mental Disorders (Third Edition, Revised)* (*DSM-III-R*; American Psychiatric Association, 1987). Table 5.2 presents these psychiatric sequelae for abused/neglected individuals and controls.

Overall, abused/neglected individuals in this sample are significantly more likely to report having made suicide attempts (OR = 2.8) and to meet *DSM-III-R* criteria for ASPD (OR = 1.8) than controls, findings that persist despite controls for age, sex, race, and criminal history. [Further discussion of the findings with regard to antisocial personality disorder can be found in Luntz and Widom (1994)]. Despite high rates of alcohol abuse in this sample, the abused/neglected children as a group were not at increased risk for lifetime diagnoses of alcohol abuse and/or dependence compared to controls. Although this finding differs from other research reporting a connection between child abuse and alcohol problems, methodological differences between this study and most others might account for this discrepancy (see Widom et al., 1995).

Table 5.3 presents psychopathology associated with childhood abuse/neglect by gen-

Table 5.3. Childhood victimization and psychopathology in follow-up sample, by Gender

	Abuse/neglect (%)	Control (%)	Odds ratio	Confidence interval
Women				
Suicide attempt	24.3°°°	8.6	3.4	2.0–5.7
Antisocial personality disorder diagnosis	9.8°	4.9	2.1	1.1–4.1
Alcohol abuse/dependence diagnosis	43.8°°	32.8	1.6	1.1–2.2
Number of cases	338	224		
Men				
Suicide attempt	13.4°°	6.9	2.1	1.2–3.7
Antisocial personality disorder diagnosis	27.0°°	16.7	1.8	1.2–2.8
Alcohol abuse/dependence diagnosis	65.4	67.0	0.9	0.7–1.3
Number of cases	338	276		

°p ≤ .05; °°p ≤ .01; °°°p ≤ .001.

Note: Number of cases varies slightly because of missing data.

Table 5.4. *DSM-III-R* diagnosis of ASPD in offspring as a function of criminality in parents

	Abuse/neglect (%)	Controls (%)	Row significance
Either parent arrested	21.9 (365)	18.8 (170)	n.s.
Neither parent arrested	14.2 (310)	7.4 (350)	°°°
Column significance	°	°°°	

°$p \leq .05$; °°$p \leq .01$; °°°$p \leq .001$.

Note: Number of cases indicated in parentheses.

der. For women, abuse and neglect were associated with increased risk for all three forms of psychopatholgy presented here: suicide attempts (OR = 3.4) and lifetime *DSM-III-R* diagnoses of alcohol abuse and/or dependence (OR = 1.6) and ASPD (OR = 2.1). For men, abuse and neglect were associated with increased risk for suicide attempts (OR = 2.1) and ASPD (OR = 1.8) but not for alcohol problems. Interestingly, it is primarily the neglected women who were at greatest risk for subsequent alcohol problems, not the physically or sexually abused women (Widom et al., 1995).

Contextual Factors

Tables 5.4 and 5.5 illustrate the importance of the context in which the abuse and neglect occurs and the influence of contextual variables on subsequent outcomes. Table 5.4 shows the relationships among childhood victimization, having a parent with an arrest,

and the likelihood that the offspring will have a diagnosis of ASPD in this sample of abused/neglected individuals and controls. Among individuals whose parents were arrested, abuse and neglect did *not* lead to increased risk of ASPD in the offspring. However, among those who reported that their parents were not arrested, being abused or neglected in childhood was associated with significantly increased risk of ASPD diagnosis ($\chi^2 = 7.12$, df = 379, $p < .01$).

Table 5.5 presents the relationships among childhood victimization, having a parent with an alcohol and/or drug problem, and the likelihood of being diagnosed with alcohol abuse and/or dependence in adulthood. Having a parent with an alcohol and/or drug problem was associated with a significant increase in risk in the offspring's having a diagnosis of alcohol abuse and/or dependence ($p < .001$), regardless of whether the person was abused or neglected

Table 5.5. *DSM-III-R* diagnosis of alcohol abuse/dependence in offspring as a function of alcohol/drug problems in parents

	Abuse/neglect (%)	Controls (%)	Row significance
Either parent with alcohol/drug problem	63.2 (389)	56.5 (196)	n.s.
Neither parent with alcohol/drug problem	42.6 (284)	47.5 (324)	n.s.
Column significance	°°°	°	

°$p \leq .05$; °°$p \leq .01$; °°°$p \leq .001$.

Note: Number of cases indicated in parentheses.

in childhood or not. For this sample overall, being abused or neglected in childhood was *not* associated with increased risk for alcohol problems.

Thus the consequences of childhood victimization depend in part on the context in which the abuse or neglect experiences occur. The relationship between parental characteristics and the likelihood of psychopathology in offspring varies by type of parental characteristics and type of outcome. For ASPD, childhood victimization is associated with increased risk regardless of parental characteristics. That is, even among children whose parents are not criminal, abuse and neglect is associated with increased risk of antisocial behavior in the offspring. For alcohol abuse, having a parent who has alcohol problems is more important in determining a person's own alcohol problems than whether abuse or neglect occurred.

CONCLUSIONS

Clearly, the consequences of childhood victimization extend well beyond childhood and adolescence and persist into young adulthood. Childhood abuse and neglect affect a wide range of domains of later functioning, including intellectual and academic performance, as well as behavioral, social, psychological, and emotional outcomes. Furthermore, these sequelae most likely represent only the tip of the iceberg. However, some of the expected outcomes (such as the increased risk for alcohol problems) did not emerge, raising questions about at least one presumed consequence.

These findings also illustrate the importance of gender and contextual variables in understanding the consequences of early childhood victimization. On the one hand, the increased risk for ASPD in men clearly conforms to gender roles and with the notion that men are more likely to direct their pain and suffering outwardly. Similarly, the increased risk for alcohol problems in women is consistent with a gender role ex-

pectation and with the notion that women are more likely to manifest their distress in more inward directions. On the other hand, we found that abused and neglected women are also at risk for ASPD and for criminal behavior (findings not shown here; see Maxfield & Widom, 1996). Thus we may need to reconsider the two pathways—internalizing and externalizing—that have formed the basis for expectations about the ways in which men and women manifest their responses to distress.

Characteristics of parents influenced the likelihood of subsequent psychopathology in their offspring in two different ways. First, consistent with previous literature, having a parent who was arrested increased the likelihood of the offspring's being diagnosed as having ASPD, regardless of abuse or neglect versus control group status. However, in the absence of parental criminality, being abused or neglected was also associated with increased risk of ASPD. Therefore, in addition to complicating attempts to understand the consequences of childhood victimization, these findings suggest multiple factors in the development of ASPD.

Second, a different picture and set of relationships was found for alcohol abuse. The interrelationships among parental characteristics, childhood victimization, and subsequent alcohol problems in offspring revealed that the critical variable associated with increased risk for subsequent alcohol problems in this sample was parents' alcohol and/or drug problems. This strong influence of parental characteristics on the offspring's subsequent alcohol problems (regardless of abuse/neglect status) warrants more careful consideration but is consistent with earlier literature on the genetic transmission of alcoholism (Cloninger et al., 1985; Goodwin et al., 1973, 1977).

One of the difficulties in assessing risk of negative consequences for abused and neglected children is the co-occurrence of other problems (or co-morbidity) in the children and their parents. Other research has found that adverse effects interact with one another, so that their combined effects may be greater than their sums considered separately (Rutter, 1979). Whether this interaction effect applies to childhood victimization is not known, although it is likely. The question arises as to whether the presence or absence of certain characteristics or other adverse events influence a child's response to the experiences of childhood victimization. Because childhood victims may be at risk for the development of multiple problem behaviors, an examination of the co-occurrence of problems may be a useful direction for future research. For example, the co-occurrence of alcoholism, ASPD, and substance use has been noted among male jail detainees (Abram, 1990). Alcoholics often attempt destructive behaviors, including suicide (Schuckit, 1986), and the diagnosis of alcoholism is complicated by the presence of ASPD, which in turn includes components of criminal behavior and sexual promiscuity. Engaging in any one of these behaviors, then, might increase the likelihood of involvement in other at-risk behaviors.

Substantially less is known than one would wish about the long-term consequences of childhood victimization and the processes linking child abuse and neglect with later outcomes. Considering the areas of functioning potentially linked to childhood victimization, it is likely that there are multiple pathways by which these early stressful and abusive life experiences influence behavior.

This work has not yet tried to distinguish among the possible mechanisms by which early childhood victimization affects subsequent development and particular forms of psychopathology. A number of potential mechanisms may be at work. Although it is possible that children are simply modeling their parents' behaviors, it is also possible that child abuse or neglect may lead to immediate sequelae that then have an irremediable effect on the subsequent development of the child, and this, in turn, may be related to later outcomes. For example, some forms of physical abuse (battering) or severe neglect (malnutrition, dehydration,

or failure to thrive) may lead to developmental retardation (low IQ), which in turn may affect school performance, the likelihood of truancy, delinquency, and so on.

Some of the pathways from abuse and neglect in childhood to adult outcomes may be direct—persisting through adolescence, young adulthood, and into adulthood. Abused and neglected children have shown aggressiveness and behavior problems in childhood and have manifested higher rates of delinquency in adolescence and antisocial and criminal behavior in adulthood. It is also likely that this pathway leads to abusive behavior in the home, as in spouse or child abuse (Campbell & Humphries, 1984; Fagan & Browne, 1990). However, for many abused and neglected children, the consequences of childhood victimization do *not* follow a direct pathway to delinquency or aggressive behaviors. A substantial group appears to manifest the consequences of their earlier childhood victimization in other ways, such as in self-destructive behaviors or suicide attempts.

Early child abuse and neglect may lead directly to altered patterns of behavior, the results of which might become manifest only some years later, although the behavior is in place during early childhood. A child's sensitivity or vulnerability to stress may be modified. Thus some consequences of childhood victimization may be manifest immediately, whereas others may be temporally delayed and appear less directly related.

Abuse or neglect may encourage the development of certain styles of coping that might be less than adaptive. For example, these early experiences might lead to the development of impulsive behavioral styles, which in turn are related to deficiencies in problem-solving skills or inadequate school performance, or to less than adequate functioning in occupational spheres and ASPD. Adaptations that might appear to be functional at one point in time in the development of the person (e.g., avoiding an abusive parent, running away, or desensitizing oneself against feelings) may later compromise the person's ability to draw upon the environment in a more adaptive and flexible way. These initial adaptations may place the child at subsequent risk for further negative situations or subsequent victimizations that may trigger the development of various forms of psychopathology.

Some outcomes may be an indirect by-product of these early adverse life experiences. Abuse and/or neglect may lead to changed environments or family conditions that, in turn, may later predispose a person to problem behaviors. These early adverse experiences may lead to the child's exposure to further harmful life experiences, which in turn lead to the development of psychopathology. In this way, psychopathology may result not so much from the abuse or neglect experience itself but as a result of the chain of events subsequent to the abuse or neglect. For example, being taken away from one's biological parents subsequent to the abuse and neglect incident(s) and placed in foster care may be associated with deleterious effects, or being placed outside the home may be associated with negative outcomes for *some* abused and neglected children (Widom, 1991).

No doubt there are many other possible mechanisms as well. Hopefully, future explanatory models developed to explain the long-term consequences of childhood victimization will examine the role of a number of these possible mechanisms, because it is unlikely that one mechanism will "fit" all cases of abuse and neglect.

A few caveats are needed. These findings are based on substantiated court cases of childhood physical and sexual abuse and neglect and most likely represent the most extreme cases processed through the system (Groeneveld & Giovannoni, 1977). Furthermore, these cases were processed during the years 1967–1971, before the child abuse laws were passed. Many cases were not reported and never came to the attention of the authorities. These findings, then, are not generalizable to unreported or unsubstantiated cases of abuse and neglect, or to cases of childhood adoption, because these were excluded (Widom, 1989a). Cases that came to the attention of the courts were skewed toward the lower end of the socioeconomic spectrum; thus cases and controls in this study are predominantly from the lower social classes. Given the importance of contextual factors, it would be inappropriate to generalize from these findings to cases of abuse and neglect in middle class individuals. The consequences of abuse and neglect for children living in middle- or upper-class families may be dramatically different from those studied here. Further research is needed with abused and neglected middle-class children followed prospectively into adulthood.

Research in the field of child abuse and neglect is relatively young. Although there are characteristics of childhood victimization experiences that may distinguish them from other adverse and traumatic life events, theory and methods in the field of child maltreatment research will ultimately benefit from cross-fertilization with the broader literature on adversity, stress, and psychopathology.

Acknowledgments: This research was supported by grants from the National Institute of Justice (86-IJ-CX-0033, 89-IJ-CX-0007, and 94-IJ-CX-0031), National Institute on Alcohol Abuse and Alcoholism (AA09238), and National Institute of Mental Health (MH49467). Points of view are those of the author and do not necessarily represent the position of the U.S. Department of Justice or the other federal agencies supporting this research. The author is grateful to Patricia J. Glynn and Suzanne Luu for help in the preparation of this chapter.

REFERENCES

Abram, K. (1990). The problem of co-occurring disorders among jail detainees: Antisocial disorder, alcoholism, drug abuse, and depression. *Law and Human Behavior, 14*, 333–345.

Allen, D., & Tarnowski, K. (1989). Depressive characteristics of physically abused children. *Journal of Abnormal Child Psychology, 17*, 1–11.

American Psychiatric Association. (1987). *Diagnostic and statistical manual of mental disorders* (3rd ed., rev.). Washington, DC: American Psychiatric Press.

associated with childhood sexual victimization in a nonclinical adult sample. *Child Abuse and Neglect, 12,* 51–60.

Browne, A., & Finkelhor, D. (1986). Impact of sexual abuse: A review of the research. *Psychological Bulletin, 99,* 66–77.

Campbell, J., & Humphreys, J. (1984). *Nursing care of victims of family violence.* Reston, VA: Reston Publishing Co.

Cloninger, C. R., Bohman, M., Sigvardsson, S., & VonKnorring, A. L. (1985). Psychopathology in adopted-out children of alcoholics: The Stockholm adoption study. In M. Galanter (Ed.), *Recent developments in alcoholism* (Vol. 3) (pp. 37–51). New York: Plenum.

DeWilde, E. J., Kienhorst, I. C., Diekstra, R. F., & Wolters, W. H. (1992). The relationship between adolescent suicidal behavior and life events in childhood and adolescence. *American Journal of Psychiatry, 149,* 45–51.

Dodge, K. A., Bates, J. E., & Pettit, G. S. (1990). Mechanisms in the cycle of violence. *Science, 250,* 1678–1683.

Dohrenwend, B. P., & Dohrenwend, B. S. (1976). Sex differences in psychiatric disorders. *American Journal of Sociology, 81,* 1447–1154.

Downey, G., Feldman, S., Khuri, J., & Friedman, S. (1994). Maltreatment and childhood depression. In W. M. Reynolds & H. F. Johnson (Eds.), *Handbook of depression in children* (pp. 481–508). New York: Plenum.

Drillen, C. M. (1964). *The growth and development of the prematurely born infant.* Baltimore: Williams & Wilkins.

Fagan, J., & Browne, A. (1990). *Marital violence: Physical aggression between men and women in intimate relationships* (Background paper for the Panel on the Understanding and Control of Violent Behavior). Washington, DC: National Research Council.

Famularo, R., Stone, K., Barnum, R., & Wharton, R. (1986). Alcoholism and severe child maltreatment. *American Journal of Orthopsychiatry, 56,* 481–485.

Finkelhor, D. (1990). Early and long-term effects of child sexual abuse: An update. *Professional Psychology: Research and Practice, 21,* 325–330.

Friedrich, W. H., Urquiza, A. J., & Beilke, R. L. (1986). Behavior problems in sexually abused young children. *Journal of Pediatric Psychology, 11,* 47–57.

Gibbin, P. T., Starr, R. H., & Agronow, S. W. (1984). Affective behavior of abused and control children: Comparison of parent-child interactions and the influence of home environment variables. *Journal of Genetic Psychology, 144,* 69–82.

Goodwin, D. W., Schulsinger, F., Hermansen, L., Guze, S. B., & Winokur, G. (1973). Alcohol problems in adoptees raised apart from alcoholic biological parents. *Archives of General Psychiatry, 28,* 238–243.

Goodwin, D. W., Schulsinger, F., Knop, F., Mednick, S., & Guze, S. B. (1977). Alcoholism and depression in adopted-out daughters of alcoholics. *Archives of General Psychiatry, 34,* 751–755.

Green, A. H. (1978). Self-destructive behavior in battered children. *American Journal of Psychiatry, 135,* 579–582.

Groeneveld, L. P., & Giovannoni, J. M. (1977). Disposition of child abuse and neglect cases. *Social Work Research and Abstracts, 13,* 24–30.

Harris, T., Brown, G. W., & Bifulco, A. (1990). Loss of parent in childhood and adult psychiatric disorder: A tentative overall model. *Development and Psychopathology, 2,* 311–328.

Hollingshead, A. B. (1975). *Four factor index of social class* (working paper). New Haven, CT: Yale University.

Horwitz, A. V., & White, H. R. (1987). Gender role orientations and styles of pathology among adolescents. *Journal of Health and Social Behavior, 28,* 158–170.

Kaufman, J. (1991). Depressive disorders in maltreated children. *Journal of the American Academy of Child and Adolescent Psychiatry, 30,* 257–265.

Kazdin, A., Moser, J., Colbus, D., & Bell, R. (1985). Depressive symptoms among physically abused and psychiatrically disturbed children. *Journal of Abnormal Psychology, 94,* 298–307.

Kendall-Tackett, K. A., Williams, L. M., & Finkelhor, D. J. (1993). The impact of sexual abuse on children: A review and synthesis of recent empirical studies. *Psychological Bulletin, 113,* 164–180.

Kolko, D., Moser, J., & Weldy, S. (1990). Medical/health histories and physical evaluation of physically and sexually abused child psychiatric patients: A controlled study. *Journal of Family Violence, 5,* 249–266.

Kroll, P. D., Stock, D. F., & James, M. E. (1985). The behavior of adult alcoholic men abused as children. *Journal of Nervous and Mental Disease, 173,* 689–693.

Ladwig, G. B., & Anderson, M. D. (1989). Substance abuse in women: Relationship between chemical dependency of women and past reports of physical abuse and/or sexual abuse. *International Journal of the Addictions, 24,* 739–754.

Lewis, D. O., Pincus, J. H., Shanok, S. S., & Glaser, G. (1982). Psychomotor epilepsy and violence in a group of incarcerated adolescent boys. *American Journal of Psychiatry, 139,* 882–887.

Lewis, D. O., Shanok, S. S., Pincus, J. H., & Glaser, G. H. (1979). Violent juvenile delinquents: Psychiatric, neurological, psychological, and abuse factors. *Journal of the American Academy of Child Psychiatry, 10,* 1161–1167.

Lipovsky, J. A., Saunders, B. E., & Murphy, S. M. (1989). Depression, anxiety, and behavior problems among victims of father-child sexual assault and nonabused siblings. *Journal of Interpersonal Violence, 4,* 452–468.

Livingston, R. (1987). Sexually and physically abused children. *Journal of the American Academy of Child and Adolescent Psychiatry, 26,* 413–415.

Luntz, B. K., & Widom, C. S. (1994). Antisocial personality disorder in abused and neglected children grown-up. *American Journal of Psychiatry, 151,* 670–674.

Maxfield, M. G., & Widom, C. S. (1996). The cycle of violence: Revisited six years later. *Archives of Pediatrics and Adolescent Medicine, 150,* 390–395.

Milner, J. S. (Ed.). (1991). Special issue: Physical child abuse. *Criminal Justice and Behavior, 18,* 1–112.

National Research Council. (1993). *Understanding child abuse and neglect.* Washington, DC: National Academy Press.

Perez, C., & Widom, C. S. (1994). Childhood victimization and longterm intellectual and academic outcomes. *Child Abuse and Neglect, 18,* 617–633.

Peters, S. D. (1988). Child sexual abuse and later psychological problems. In G. E. Wyatt & G. J. Powell (Eds.), *Lasting effects of child sexual abuse.* Newbury Park, CA: Sage.

Reider, E. E., Zucker, R. A., Maguin, E. T., Noll, R. B., & Fitzgerald, E. E. (1989, August). *Alcohol involvement and violence toward children among high risk families.* Paper presented at the annual meeting of the American Psychological Association. New Orleans.

Robins, L. N., Helzer, J. E., Cottler, L., & Goldring, E. (1989). *National Institute of Mental Health Diagnostic Interview Schedule (DIS-III-R).* St. Louis: Washington University.

Robins, L. N., & Regier, D. A. (Eds.). (1991). *Psychiatric disorders in America: The Epidemiological Catchment Area Surveys.* New York: The Free Press.

Root, M. P. (1989). Treatment failures: The role of sexual victimization in women's addictive behavior. *American Journal of Orthopsychiatry, 59,* 542–549.

Rutter, M. (1979). Protective factors in children's response to stress and disadvantage. In M. V. Kent & J. E. Rolf (Eds.), *Primary Prevention of Psychopathology: Social Competence in Children* (Vol. 3, pp. 49–74). Hanover, NH: New England Press.

Schuckit, M. A. (1986). Primary men alcoholics with a history of suicide attempts. *Journal of Studies on Alcohol, 47,* 78–81.

Smith, C. P., Berkman, D. J., & Fraser, W. M. (1980). *A preliminary national assessment of child abuse and neglect and the juvenile justice system: The shadows of distress.* Washington, DC: Office of Juvenile Justice and Delinquency Prevention.

Stein, J. A., Golding, J. M., Siegel, J. M., Burnam, M. A., & Sorenson, S. B. (1988). Long-term psychological sequelae of child sexual abuse: The Los Angeles Epidemiologic Catchment Area Study. In G. E. Wyatt & G. J. Powell (Eds.), *Lasting effects of child sexual abuse* (pp. 135–154). Newbury, Park, CA: Sage Publications.

Terr, L. A. (1983). Chowchilla revisited: The effects of psychiatric trauma four years after a school-bus kidnapping. *American Journal of Psychiatry, 140,* 1543–1550.

Urquiza, A. M., & Capra, M. (1990). Impact of sexual abuse: Initial and long-term effects. In M. Hunter (Ed.), *Sexually abused male: Prevalence, impact, and treatment* (Vol. 1, pp. 105–135). Lexington, MA: Lexington Books.

Walsh, B. W., & Rosen, P. (1988). *Self-mutilation: Theory, research, and treatment.* New York: The Guilford Press.

Widom, C. S. (1984). Sex roles, criminality, and psychopathology. In C. S. Widom (Ed.), *Sex roles and psychopathology* (pp. 187–213). New York: Plenum.

Widom, C. S. (1989a). Child abuse, neglect, and adult behavior: Research design and findings on criminality, violence, and child abuse. *American Journal of Orthopsychiatry,* 59, 355–367.

Widom, C. S. (1989b). The cycle of violence. *Science,* 244, 160–166.

Widom, C. S. (1989c). Does violence breed violence? A critical examination of the literature. *Psychological Bulletin,* 106, 3–28.

Widom, C. S. (1991). The role of placement experiences in mediating the criminal consequences of early childhood victimization. *American Journal of Orthopsychiatry,* 6, 195–209.

Widom, C. S. (in press). Understanding the consequences of childhood victimization. In R. M. Reece (Ed.), *The treatment of child abuse.* Baltimore: The Johns Hopkins University Press.

Widom, C. S., Ireland, T., & Glynn P. J. (1995). Alcohol abuse in abused and neglected children followed-up: Are they at increased risk? *Journal of Studies on Alcohol,* 56, 207–217.

Wolfe, D. A. (1987). *Child abuse: Implications for child development and psychopathology.* Newbury Park, CA: Sage Publications.

Wyatt, G. E. (1990). Sexual abuse of ethnic minority children: Identifying dimensions of victimization. *Professional Psychology: Research and Practice,* 21, 338–343.

In their 1993 *Handbook of Stress*, Gold-berger and Breznitz define *stressors* as external events or conditions that affect the organism. They then comment that the description of stressors and their impact on behavior is evolving, with more and more events being defined as stressors and more and more behaviors being related to them. This reminds me of Parkes's summary of the stress literature in his 1972 book, *Bereavement*. He stated

For many years researchers have studied and written about stress. The term has been used to characterize the effect of virtually any novel or unpleasant experience—from doing mental arithmetic to being involved in trench warfare, from being in an unfamiliar environment to having a limb crushed. Human beings and animals of all shapes and sizes have been tricked, confined, terrified, mutilated, shocked, puzzled, embarrassed, challenged, stumped, overwhelmed, confused, or poisoned in the widest variety of experimental conditions in attempts to track down the consequences of this ubiquitous phenomenon. Numerous books and articles describe the results of these experiments. The outcome of all this work has not been negligible but it has been disappointing. Generalizations made in one setting fail to hold up in another. Results ob-

tained with one individual are quite different with another and chemical changes in the blood which seem in one experiment to indicate the amount of stress a person is undergoing bear no relation to what is found in another.

No one would argue that the death of someone close should not be considered a stressor, and that the experience that follows should not be identified as a response to stress. In Holmes and Rahe's (1967) Social Readjustment Rating Scale, loss of a spouse is considered the most stressful life event. From other research, the loss of a child is at least as stressful, if not more so (Clayton et al., 1968; Sanders, 1979–80). *Bereavement* by definition is the reaction to a loss by death. In life, it is an unavoidable experience. Other terms that are sometimes, but should not be, used interchangeably with bereavement are *grief*, which is the emotional and psychological reaction to any loss but not limited to death, and *mourning*, which is the social expression of bereavement or grief, sometimes formalized by custom or religion. The study of bereavement impinges on many disciplines: epidemiology for base rates and risk factors; sociology and anthropology for cultural similarities and differences; neurobiology for the correlates

96

of the reaction; and psychology and psychiatry for the comparison of symptoms in bereavement to anxiety and depressive disorders and comparison of its pathological qualities to post-traumatic stress disorder and chronic depression. Bereavement can serve as an ideal model for a reaction to stress because the stress is definitive. It is *real* (not imagined, devised), *dateable* (by death certificate), current (not retrospective), and significant by anybody's standards; and the reaction can be studied immediately and in an enormous variety of ways. In many cases, it can even be studied prospectively. In addition, bereavement is not species specific, so that, like almost no other stress, it can be defined identically across species and generations of species.

STAGES

As a first step in understanding the reaction, the stages of bereavement are reviewed (Clayton, 1982). Numerous authors have studied widows and widowers and other recently bereaved individuals and have followed them prospectively. Just as with the response to stress itself, most agree that there are three stages to bereavement. Although they are labeled differently by different investigators (Clayton, 1973; Parkes, 1972; Silverman, 1966; Zisook, 1992), all agree that these stages sometimes overlap.

The first stage is *numbness*. This is precisely the term used by the majority of widows and widowers. It lasts from a few hours to a few days to a few weeks. During this stage the bereaved is dazed and in disbelief, and his or her functions are automatic, as if going through the motions. Most of what is communicated is poorly remembered, so any important information should be given verbally and in writing. Anxiety and depressive symptoms begin during this time.

Numbness flows imperceptively into the second stage, termed *depression*. Others have called it recoil, yearning, protest, and disorganization or simply acute mourning. Depressive symptoms dominate the picture, although generalized anxiety and hypervigilance are also present (Jacobs et al., 1989). Retardation as a symptom is uncommon. Hostility is also uncommon and, if present, is usually directed at the deceased. Many people begin to recover by 4 months, although they continue to have symptoms for up to 1 year and experience a mild recurrence of symptoms on holidays, birthdays, and other special events.

The third stage, *recovery* or *restitution*, is the acceptance of the death and the return of the survivor to the level of functioning established before the death.

The same reaction has also been described with other losses, such as divorce and separation, where the term "grief reaction" would be appropriate. Any significant loss, if followed immediately or within a short time by depressive symptoms, could precipitate symptoms similar to those seen in the bereavement reaction. This is why bereavement is an excellent model for a stress reaction. The important element in the reaction is timing. The universal reaction to a physical stress or insult is an immediate injury with gradual resolution. The same should apply to a psychological injury, and this very accurately describes the depression associated with bereavement (Clayton, 1990).

PSYCHOLOGICAL AND SOMATIC SYMPTOMS AND COURSE

Just as awakening to find an unknown person in your bedroom would provoke fear, so the loss of someone close provokes sadness. All authors studying bereavement have found that depressive symptoms dominate the clinical picture (Clayton, 1982), and our three separate studies of recently bereaved people concur (Clayton et al., 1968, 1971, 1980a, 1980b).

In a previous report (Clayton & Darvish, 1979), samples from two similar but separate studies (of 109 and 62 widows and widowers) were combined to yield a group of 171 white men and women. Each surviving spouse was seen at home within the first month after the death and was interviewed in a 3 hour structured and semistructured interview. The interview format had been used in an earlier study of bereaved (Clayton et al., 1968) and consisted of 47 depressive symptoms listed as significantly different in depressives than in controls (Cassidy et al., 1957), as well as quantifiable bereavement and relationship issues that were later incorporated into the Personal Resources Inventory (O'Connell et al., 1991). The survivor was asked about symptoms and feelings for three different time periods after the presence or absence of a terminal illness had been determined: "ever before" (lifetime), "during the terminal illness," and "since the death." Other symptoms of psychiatric disorder and family history were also recorded, as the interview was modeled on a forerunner of the Renard Diagnostic Interview (Helzer et al., 1991). Of the combined samples, 141 people were re-interviewed 1 year later. The average age of the combined group was 51 years.

The first sample was a random sample of 109 people (96 women and 53 men) with an average age of 61 who were chosed by a random numbers table from available death certificates. They were contacted by telephone and seen in their homes by one of three psychiatrists. (All three psychiatrists attended the first few interviews.) The acceptance rate in this sample was 58%. There were no differences in age, sex, and type of spousal death between the acceptors and the refusers. Four of the sample (4%) died during the first year of bereavement. Of the remaining 105, 92 (88%) were re-interviewed (by a different one of the three interviewers) 1 year after the first interview. Every effort was made to contact the refusers, and all indications from these efforts revealed there were no differences between those who were seen and those who were lost to follow-up. The measure of poor health in the bereaved that is easiest to measure is death within the first year. Of this group, most of the refusers were located by telephone; a search of local death certificates did not reveal the names of any who could not be traced. If all had moved out of town and died, the death rate still would not

have been significantly higher in the refusers than the acceptors.

Because of the low number of young widows and widowers in the first sample, a second study was undertaken of a consecutive sample of subjects widowed at age 45 or younger. Sixty-two people (34 women and 28 men) with an average age of 36 years were interviewed by one of three psychiatrists, two of whom were different from those participating in the first widowed study. The acceptance rate was 66%. There were no deaths during the following year, and 57 people, (92%) were re-interviewed in the same way. In the second sample, widowed persons with children answered systematic questions about the physical and mental health of three of their randomly chosen children (Van Eerdewegh et al., 1982).

In the same year the longitudinal study was undertaken, each bereaved subject was matched with three married subjects of the same sex in the same voting district and, when possible, on the same street. One year later, the first of the three controls was contacted and interviewed in regard to physical and mental health in the previous year. All controls who had lost a spouse or a first-degree relative were excluded, and the next control was chosen. In the first control sample, there were five deaths (5%), which is very similar to the death rate among the widowed sample. There were no deaths in the second control sample. In the second sample, data were also gathered in the same way about the children of the controls. Tables 6.1–6.3 summarize the responses of two groups of bereaved men and women randomly or consecutively selected and followed over 1 year, matched with two longitudinally followed groups of married controls.

Table 6.1 shows the depressive symptoms that were endorsed at 1 and 13 months. The three most common symptoms in the first month were crying, sleep disturbance, and low mood. The sleep disturbance was characterized as trouble falling asleep, trouble staying asleep, and early morning awakening, problems identical to those reported in major depressives (Pasternak et al., 1994). Most respondents reported no dreaming, some reported pleasant dreams, and a few had nightmares. This is similar to the sleep and dreaming patterns reported after extreme situational stress (Hefez et al., 1987). Other common depressive symptoms were also present. Restlessness rather than retardation characterized the motor symptoms. The weight loss of the bereaved could be profound, with some losing up to 18 kg. The guilt reported referred almost exclusively to the events surrounding the terminal illness or the death.

By the end of the first year, the somatic symptoms had improved remarkably, although restlessness remained unimproved and sleep was still a problem. Death wishes were expressed, but suicidal thoughts were rare. If they did occur, they occurred in young males. Other psychological symptoms of depression were far less common and less likely to improve. Feelings of worthlessness actually increased in frequency by the end of the first year. This is consistent with what Parkes (1972) concluded was the most typical psychophysiological response of animals to stress. Referring to sympathetic stimulation and parasympathetic inhibition, he noted three distinct components of the overall response: level of arousal, autonomic disturbance, and emotional reaction. It seems that the level of arousal and the autonomic disturbance are prominent early in bereavement and that the emotional reaction surfaces later.

Symptoms were examined by age, sex, and length of the deceased spouse's terminal illness (Clayton & Darvish, 1979). Young widowed people had significantly more symptoms at 1 month but by 13 months were similar to older bereaved people. Men reported more alcohol consumption at 1 month and the percentage "using" alcohol increased by 13 months. Length of terminal illness (and its corollary, anticipation of death) had very little effect on outcome. A full depressive syndrome as defined by Feighner et al.(1972) was present in 42% of the bereaved at 1 month and 16% at 1 year. The best predictor of depression at 1 month

was the presence of poor physical or mental health prior to the death of the spouse. The best predictor of depression at 1 year was depression at 1 month. There were very few new cases of depression.

Table 6.1. Frequency of depressive symptoms at 1 and 13 months

Symptom	1 Month % reporting (n = 149°)	13 Months % reporting (n = 149°)
Crying	89	33°°
Sleep disturbance	76	48°°
Low mood	75	42°°
Loss of appetite	51	16°°
Fatigue	44	30[†]
Poor memory	41	23°°
Loss of interest	40	23°°
Difficulty concentrating	36	16°°
Weight loss of 2.25 kg or more	36	20[†]
Feeling guilty	31	12°°
Restlessness (n = 89)	48	45
Reverse diurnal variation	26	22
Irritability	24	20
Feels someone to blame	22	22
Diurnal variation	17	10
Death wishes	16	12
Feeling hopeless	14	13
Hallucinations	12	9
Suicidal thoughts	5	3
Fear of losing mind	3	4
Suicide attempts	0	0
Feeling worthless	6	11
Feels angry about death	13	22[†]
Depressive syndrome	42	16°°

° Sample size varies from symptom to symptom; n mostly 148

[†] Significant by McNemar's chi-square; df = 1, $p \leq .02$.

[‡] Significant by McNemar's chi-square; df = 1, $p \leq .01$.

°° Significant by McNemar's chi-square; df = 1, $p \leq .001$.

From Clayton, P. J. (1982). Bereavement. In E. S. Paykel (Ed.), *Handbook of affective disorders*. London: Churchill Livingstone.

As Table 6.2 shows, when the frequency of depressive symptoms occurring at any time during the first year was compared between the bereaved and the community controls, all symptoms were more common among the bereaved. Hallucinations were reported by the bereaved, a finding also noted by Rees (1971) and Grimby (1993). Delusions were rarely reported, although they were inquired about. Grimby's longi-

Table 6.2. Frequency of depressive symptoms at any time in the first year of bereavement and in controls

Symptom	Probands % reporting (n = 149°)	Controls % reporting (n = 131°)
Crying	90	14[††]
Sleep disturbance	79	35[††]
Low mood	80	18[††]
Loss of appetite	53	4[††]
Fatigue	55	23[††]
Poor memory	50	22[††]
Loss of interest	48	11[††]
Difficulty concentrating	40	13[††]
Weight loss of 2.25 kg or more	47	24[††]
Feeling guilty	38	11[††]
Restlessness	63	27[††]
Irritability	35	21[†]
Diurnal variation	22	14
Death wishes	22	5[††]
Feeling hopeless	19	4[°°]
Hallucinations	17	2[††]
Suicidal thoughts	8	1[†]
Fear of losing mind	7	5
Suicide attempts	0	0
Worthlessness	14	15
Depressive syndrome	47	8[°°]

° Sample size varies from symptom to symptom.

[†] Significant by chi-square, df = 1, $p < .05$.

[†] Significant by chi-square, df = 1, $p < .01$.

[°°] Significant by chi-square, df = 1, $p < .0005$.

[††] Significant by chi-square, df = 1, $p < .0001$.

From Clayton, P. J. (1982) Bereavement. In E. S. Paykel (Ed.), *Handbook of affective disorders*. London: Churchill Livingstone.

tudinal study, although with an older group, nicely replicated the findings reported here, indicating that low mood, loneliness, and crying were the cardinal symptoms of bereavement, with loneliness persisting the longest. He did not include sleep disturbance as a possible symptom. Anxiety, identified as feelings of restlessness and nervousness but not anxiety attacks, was also common. Grimby felt that restlessness represented a search for the lost object.

Table 6.3 shows the frequency of depressive symptoms at 13 months according to whether the symptoms were present at 1 month. As stated previously, those who had symptoms or the depressive syndrome at 1 month were more likely to have the same symptoms or syndrome at 1 year than those who had no symptoms at 1 month. The percentage of subjects reporting new symptoms or the depressive syndrome is very similar to that found in the controls (Table 6.2). This emphasizes the very important point that delayed grief was not reported more frequently in those who had experienced bereavement than in control groups who had no such loss. The longer the time between the event and the onset of depression, the more questionable the association becomes.

Finally, a subset of the bereaved were matched by age and sex to inpatients who were depressed, and their symptoms were compared (Clayton et al., 1974). The most significant differences between the depressed patients and the bereaved subjects were in in the psychological symptoms. Approximately half the depressed patients admitted to feelings that they would rather be dead, having suicidal thoughts, showing retardation, and feeling themselves to be a burden, hopeless, or worthless, with none of the matched bereaved patients reporting those symptoms. The only symptom more common in the bereaved was crying easily. The average number of symptoms in the depressed patients was 15, compared with 7 in the bereaved. Patients with depression experienced their condition as a change (not their usual selves), which led them to seek help and to define themselves as patients,

Table 6.3. Frequency of depressive symptoms at 13 months

Symptom	Those with symptoms at 1 month		Those without symptoms at 1 month (new symptom)	
	% Reporting	n	% Reporting	n
Crying	36	132	6	16
Sleep disturbance	59	113	11	35
Low mood	49	111	22	37
Loss of appetite	28	76	4	72
Fatigue	45	65	19	83
Poor memory	34	61	15	88
Loss of interest	40	57	12	84
Difficulty concentrating	33	52	6	94
Weight loss of 2.25 kg or more	22	51	17	92
Feeling guilty	25	49	6	97
Restlessness	63	43	28	46
Reverse diurnal variation	39	38	17	109
Irritability	37	35	15	113
Feels someone to blame	63	32	11	111
Diurnal variation	24	25	7	122
Death wishes	33	24	7	124
Feeling hopeless	55	20	6	128
Hallucinations	29	17	6	131
Suicidal thoughts	0	8	3	139
Fear of losing mind	0	5	4	143
Suicide attempts	0	0	0	147
Feeling worthless	56	9	8	139
Feel angry about death	63	19	16	128
Depressive syndrome	27	63	8	86

From Clayton, P. J. (1982). Bereavement. In E. S. Paykel (Ed.), *Handbook of affective disorders*. London: Churchill Livingstone.

whereas the bereaved considered their responses normal and understandable.

This reinforces several points about the usual response to a death and perhaps to other natural stresses. As Freud (1917/1957) indicated, in the bereaved, disturbance of self-regard is absent. This was confirmed by Breckenridge et al. (1986), who reported that in 196 elderly recently (within 2 months) bereaved and 145 comparison individuals, self-deprecatory cognitions occurred with similar frequency. The ruminative guilt of the depressed patient is rare, as is morbid cultivation or mummification of the deceased, as practiced by Queen Victoria (Longford, 1964). Suicidal thoughts are uncommon. Retardation is rare. We never observed a retarded depression in a bereaved person, a finding similar to those of Lindemann (1944) and Parkes (1970). The occurrence of these symptoms may indicate true psychiatric morbidity. By 1 year, most bereaved subjects could discuss the dead person with equanimity. A severe reaction to the first anniversary of the death (Bornstein & Clayton, 1972; Jacobs et al., 1987b) is rare and indicates a poor outcome. Asking about it is a good way for a clinician to assess the survivor's clinical state 1 year after the death.

THE SYNDROMES OF DEPRESSION AND GENERALIZED ANXIETY

As the *Diagnostic and Statistical Manual of Mental Disorders (Fourth Edition)* (*DSM-IV*; American Psychiatric Association, 1994) indicates, bereaved individuals commonly experience symptoms and the syndrome of major depression. There are characteristic symptoms that are abnormal, and the persistence of depression is also considered pathological. In our first study of widowhood, 35% of the subjects had a depressive syndrome at 1 month, 25% at 4 months, and 17% at 1 year (Bornstein et al., 1973). Forty-five percent were depressed at some point during the year, and 11% were depressed for the entire year. Adding the second younger sample, 42% were depressed at 1 month and 16% met the criteria at 1 year (Clayton, 1982). Forty-seven percent were depressed at some time during the year, and 11% for the entire year. As this indicates, when the younger sample was added, the percentage depressed in the immediate postbereavement period increased but was essentially the same at 13 months and among those who were chronically depressed. This is consistent with the literature (Hays et al., 1994) that indicates younger people have more severe immediate reactions, probably because all deaths at this age are untimely; they recover quickly, however, probably because they have more pathways, options, and demands for recovery. These figures are remarkably similar to those of a study extensively reported by Zisook and Shuchter (1991). They identified 2466 widows and widowers from death certificates. After soliciting volunteers by mail, they personally interviewed 350 at 2 months and re-interviewed the vast majority at 7, 13, and 24 months. The average age of their respondents was 61, and 71% were women. The majority were married for a long time. The sample, then, is almost identical to the first widowed sample reported here. They reported that 24% of the sample were depressed at 2 months, 23% at 7 months, 16% at 13 months, and 14% at 25 months (Zisook & Shuchter, 1991, 1993a, 1993b). Seven percent were chronically depressed, very similar to the 8.8% reported by Byrne and Raphael (1994). The Zisook et al. studies also found that the best predictor of depression at 13 months was depression at 2 months. Depression also correlated with a past history of poor physical health and a past history of depression. Surtees (1995), prospectively studying women whose husbands had either recently died or had a myocardial infarction, found that 48% of the bereaved developed a new episode of depression in the 27–30 weeks after the event. Very few developed new episodes of anxiety disorder. Using a broader definition of depression, in a prospective longitudinal study, Harlow et al. (1991b) reported that, in an even more elderly group, 58% were depressed at 1 month, 23% at 6 months, and 17% at 12 months. The best predictors of depression at 12 months were poor health and limitations of physical activity at baseline before widowhood (Harlow et al., 1991a). Nuss and Zubenko (1992) did telephone interviews with 50 widows about 1 year after their spouses' deaths and found

that premorbid psychiatric history predicted depression at 1 year. Only Mendes de Leon et al. (1994), who studied elderly subjects prospectively, did not report an association between increases in 1 year depression scores and prebereavement health status. They also reported a higher level of depressive symptoms persisting beyond 1 year in widows ages 65–74. Similar correlations with outcome have been shown after other stressors such as firefighting (McFarlane, 1989) and surviving an airplane crash (Smith et al., 1990). These data confirm that depression is extremely common in the first months of bereavement. Whether the defining period of time as indicated in the *DSM-IV* should be 2 months still remains questionable; probably 4–6 months is better. The symptoms dissipate slowly, with some, such as appetite, weight gain, and sexual interest, returning early and sleep disturbance being more entrenched.

New episodes of anxiety are rare (Surtees, 1995). Anxiety disorders are seen in approximately 25% of respondents in the first year of bereavement, with more than half of the cases being generalized anxiety disorder (Jacobs et al., 1990), which correlated with severe grief and depression. Because according to the *DSM-IV* a generalized anxiety disorder diagnosis cannot be made if the disorder exists only during the presence of major depression, it may be best to consider these anxiety symptoms part of depression. In another study (Hays et al., 1994), because anxiety scores did not vary by circumstance or timing of bereavement, authors concluded that it may be that anxiety is encompassed in the concept of grief.

PHYSICAL SYMPTOMS AND HOSPITALIZATION

In our studies, physical symptoms were systematically recorded (Clayton, 1974; Clayton & Darvish, 1979; Clayton, 1982). There were minimal differences between symptoms at 1 month and 13 months, indicating that physical symptoms could develop at any time during the year.

Table 6.4. Frequency of physical symptoms in 1 year in bereaved and controls

Symptom	Probands % reporting (n = 149°)	Controls % reporting (n = 131°)
Headaches	36	27
Dysmenorrhea	38	20
Other pains	44	18[†]
Urinary frequency	30	23
Constipation	27	24
Dyspnea	27	16[†]
Abdominal pain	26	11[°°]
Blurred vision	22	13
Anxiety attacks	15	8
Alcohol use	19	9[†]
Tranquilizers	46	8[††]
Hypnotics	32	2[††]
Physician visits		
3 or more	45	48
6 or more	27	29
Hospitalizations	22	14
General poor health	10	7

° Sample size varies slightly from symptom to symptom.

[†] Significant by chi-square, df = 1, $p < .05$.

[‡] Significant by chi-square, df = 1, $p < .005$.

[°°] Significant by chi-square, df = 1, $p < .001$.

[††] Significant by chi-square, df = 1, $p < .0001$.

From Clayton, P. J. (1986). Bereavement and its relation to clinical depression. In H. Hippius et al. (Eds.), *New results in depression*. Berlin: Springer-Verlag.

As Table 6.4 indicates, when bereaved subjects were compared to controls, they reported a significantly higher frequency of "other pains," shortness of breath, and abdominal pain. The most common "other pain" was arthritis and and was mainly reported by elderly bereaved. In general, however, the physical symptoms were not striking and the patients had no more doctor visits, hospitalizations, or feelings of general poor health than the controls. In a very large study of survivors of hospice care, Mor et al. (1986) suggested that incidences of physicians' visits were somewhat higher but hospitalization rates were lower among the recently bereaved than age- and sex-adjusted national norms. However, when the data analyses were restricted to "widowed," the rate of hospital use among both sexes was almost double that of other relatives, probably indicating that it was higher than the age- and sex-adjusted norms. The best predictor of both physicians' visits and hospitalization was the health status of the bereaved before the death, with poor health increasing the numbers of visits and hospitalizations.

As Table 6.4 illustrates, the *cardinal* response to stress is the increased use of alcohol, tranquilizers, and hypnotics. This was particularly true in subjects who had used these drugs before, but there was some new use of tranquilizers and hypnotics, especially taking drugs that had been prescribed for the deceased spouses. In the alcohol category, there were no new drinkers, but alcohol consumption increased in some who had not had problem drinking before. In other studies, increase in smoking also has been verified (Maddison & Viola, 1968). Mor et al. (1986) confirmed that increased use of alcohol among the recently bereaved. Valanis et al. (1987) also confirmed with a comparison group that recently bereaved men were much more likely to drink heavily that their nonbereaved counterparts and than bereaved females. Six percent of the men were classified as problem drinkers based on reporting more than three drinks a day and scoring one or more points on the Short Michigan Alcohol Screening Test (Selzer, 1971). There were no new cases of heavy drinking or problem drinking at 9 months.

These findings also have been confirmed by Zisook et al. (1990). Without a comparison group, they showed that 18% of bereaved subjects at 2 months, 25% at 7 months, and 30% at 13 months had increased their drinking and that men were at elevated risk to increase both the frequency and quantity of drinking. Although the authors did not show much change in cigarette smoking, if change occurred it was in the direction of increased rather than decreased use. The only controversy in these data is whether increased alcohol consumption continues or lessens as the time since death lengthens. They certainly emphasize that recent bereavement could lead to problem drinking and may explain late-onset substance abuse. Eaton et al. (1989) confirmed that the incidence rate for alcohol abuse/dependence (as diagnosed by Diagnostic Interview Schedule or DSM-III criteria) from the Epidemiological Catchment Area data was "bowl-shaped," with highest rates among the youngest but increases after 60 years of age. It was particularly high for men over 75, although the numbers were small. The increased mortality seen in bereavement could also be because of increased use of substances including cigarettes and alcohol.

In looking specifically at psychiatric hospitalization following a recent bereavement, there is no evidence that there is a correlation between bereavement and admission to a psychiatric hospital (Frost & Clayton, 1977). As Table 6.5 indicates, when a consecutively admitted group of psychiatric patients were matched with appropriate controls, both reported equal frequencies of bereavement within the previous 6 months or the contiguous 6 months.

MORTALITY

Numerous studies (Bowling, 1987; Clayton, 1982; Kaprio et al., 1987; Klerman & Clayton, 1984; Mellström et al., 1982; Mendes de Leon et al., 1993; Niemi, 1979) have reported on the mortality of bereavement, almost exclusively studying widows and widowers, probably because the change in marital status can be identified from archival data. It is almost universally accepted that there is an increased mortality in men up to the age of 75 during the first 6 months of widowhood. The data on mortality in women are inconsistent. The one study of adult Israeli bereaved parents (Levav et al., 1988) showed no increased mortality in parents who sons died either in war or in accidents, but an increased mortality if the parent was also divorced or widowed. The causes of death are not consistent. In widowed men, there is definitely an increase in death by su-

Table 6.5. Comparison of consecutively admitted psychiatric patients, matched controls, and psychiatric hospital survey group (point prevalence) for incidence of recent loss

Time of death	No. (%) of consecutively admitted patients ($n = 249$)	No. (%) of controls ($n = 249$)	No. (%) of survey group ($n = 95$)
Previous 6 months			
First-degree relative or spouse	5 (2)	6 (2)	3 (3)
Second-degree relative, close friend, or other	49 (20)	47 (19)	11 (12)
Previous 6 months to 1 year			
First-degree relative or spouse	7 (3)	10 (4)	2 (2)
Second-degree relative, close friend, or other	31 (12)	28 (11)	15 (16)

From Frost, N. R., & Clayton, P. J. (1977). Bereavement and psychiatric hospitalization. *Archives of General Psychiatry, 34,* 1172–1175.

icide in the first year and probably an increase in death by accident (Clayton, 1982; Helsing et al., 1982; Kaprio et al., 1987; Klerman & Clayton, 1984; MacMahon & Pugh, 1965; Mellström et al., 1982). Several studies reported an increased mortality from circulatory diseases (Kaprio et al., 1987; Kraus & Lilienfeld, 1959; Mellström et al., 1982). Two studies showed an increased mortality from infectious diseases (Helsing et al., 1982; Kraus & Lilienfeld, 1959). One also suggested that death from tumors may be overrepresented (Mellström et al., 1982), but there are numerous studies that reported no association between cancer and dying in the first year. These causes of death were similar in women.

The one study that did not show an increased mortality at any age in recent widows did show, however, an increase in relative risk of dying from cirrhosis (Helsing et al., 1982), a cause of death that appears in another study in excess on death certificates from widowers (Melström et al., 1982). The explanations for this increased risk are multiple, and prebereavement factors are certainly important. We have suggested that the excesses of drinking and smoking in the bereaved may be related to their excess mortality, especially because both occur in men. Kaprio et al. (1987) suggested, based on work by Partinen et al. (1982), that the induced disturbance of sleep may predispose to arrythmias leading to cardiac mortality. These investigators showed that Finnish men who slept more than 9 hours a night had a much higher prevalence of myocardial infarction, whereas men who slept 6 hours or less per night had a higher rate of symptomatic coronary artery disease. These results, associated with the variable finding of increased cardiovascular deaths, particularly in men, might be instrumental in explaining bereavement death.

In their series of papers on mortality and widowhood, (Helsing et al. 1981, 1982; Helsing & Szklo, 1981) showed that there was a substantial difference in mortality rates between the widowed men who remarried and those who did not, a factor that sometimes is not taken into account when working only with archival data. It is also not known whether remarriage itself protects against ill health and death or whether good health is what permits the remarriage.

PATHOLOGIC REACTIONS

Because there are an estimated 8 million deaths per year in the United States, any pathological outcome should be considered a serious health consequence (Osterweis & Townsend, 1988). Without question, the most common pathologic consequence of the loss of someone close is chronic grief. All studies have confirmed this. It occurs in at least 7%–11% of the recently bereaved. There may be different pathways to this chronic grief, as Parkes and Weiss (1983) have suggested, but prolonged severe grief, no matter how it was assessed or described, accounted for the poorest outcome.

Parkes (1993) has described the response of 17 patients who were referred for assessment and treatment after the homicide death of a close relative or friend. The most common psychiatric condition was post-traumatic stress disorder (PTSD), with haunting memories associated with nightmares that led to fear, hyperalertness, and avoidant behavior, as well as all the other symptoms of grief. As opposed to this highly selected sample, Vargas et al. (1989) reported on personal structured in-home interviews with 201 close relatives or intimate friends of victims of violent and sudden natural death. They showed that the survivors' responses could be defined by four factors, the most common one being depressive symptoms followed by preservation of the lost object, suicidal ideation, and decedent-directed anger. Thus, as opposed to avoidance, these survivors were cultivating the sense of the lost object. The high endorsement of suicidal ideation occurred because the authors combined symptoms into a factor that included "wishing you were dead" and "feeling hopeless" as well as suicidal ideation. They had only two items on decedent-directed anger, and they reported that 43% of subjects endorsed one of the two.

Anger, however, is not an absolute component of the bereavement response, and its presence or *absence* should not be considered pathological. In a previous study (Clayton et al., 1968), 5% of survivors expressed anger in the immediate postbereavement period. In the random sample of widowed people (Clayton et al., 1971), 6% expressed anger; when the younger sample was added (Clayton, 1982), the percentage rose to 13. In the same way, the absence of grief is not pathological. Parkes (1972) emphasized that there is a great deal written about repressing grief, which might imply that those who display the most minimal reactions have the poorest outcomes. The data contradict that and show that those who are most disturbed early in the bereavement are the most likely to be disturbed later. In our data from the first widowed study, there was only one subject (2%) who developed depression for the first time who had not been identified either at 1 or 4 months as depressed. In the second study of younger individuals, at most 8% developed depression. Zisook & Shuchter (1993b) reported that 11% of their sample developed a new depressive syndrome at 13 months. In addition, the absence of sleep disturbance (e.g., the absence of a symptom) at 1 month predicts a favorable outcome. Not a single person with no sleep difficulty either developed sleep difficulty or a depressive syndrome, or had any use of tranquilizers, hypnotics, or the like at 1 year. Reynolds et al. (1993) reported on sleep patterns in 27 elderly bereaved volunteers chosen because they had no depression or sleep complaints an average of 3.5 months after their spouses died. They were similar to a nonbereaved comparison group on all sleep parameters except for increased rapid eye movement density.

Several additional studies of stress should be mentioned. Studies of rape (Frank & Stewart, 1984) or catastrophic financial loss (Ganzini et al., 1990) have indicated that these stresses result in the onset of major depressive disorder and generalized anxiety disorder. Studies of disasters such as airplane crashes, tornadoes, and mass murders (North & Smith, 1990; Smith et al. 1993) have shown that between 0% and 9% of directly exposed survivors develop PTSD, whereas a much larger percentage develop depression and generalized anxiety disorder in the immediate postdisaster period. The best predictor of PTSD was the intensity of the exposure. In those who passively experienced the disaster, the best predictor of developing PTSD was predisaster psychiatric diagnosis. There is no follow-up yet on these reports, so possible long-term effects of more traumatic stresses are not known; even in these cases, however, the overwhelming first response is depression.

PREDICTORS OF OUTCOME

Numerous investigators have tried to predict which individuals might have a more serious long-range bereavement response, and there has been little consensus. Predictors of outcome depend in large part on which outcomes are measured. For example, in trying to predict the outcome of bereavement by using remarriage as the predictor, men would have the best outcome (Clayton, 1982; Schneider et al. 1996); using mortality, men would most likely have a less favorable outcome.

The most common poor outcome is a chronic depressive syndrome. As already indicated, a favorable outcome can be almost guaranteed in someone who has no sleep difficulty in the first month of bereavement, but, because this is rare, using sleep as a predictor is not helpful. Those who have no depressive syndrome also will probably do well. The best predictor of outcome, though, is good physical and mental health prior to the death. In the same way, the most clear-cut indicator of a poor outcome is poor physical or mental health prior to the death and the occurrence of a depressive syndrome in the first few months of bereavement.

All other variables are less clear. Age, sex, race, social supports, finances, number of other concurrent stresses, religious involvement, relationship to the deceased, and degree of closeness to the deceased do not invariably predict long-term outcome. Lack of social supports, low income, and young age do predict poorer immediate responses, and, of course immediate responses sometimes predict long-term outcome. The length of the terminal illness or suddenness or abruptness of the death does not necessarily predict poorer short- or long-term outcome for the bereaved. As mentioned earlier, the untimeliness of the death may be associated with having suicidal thoughts in the immediate bereavement period. In the same way, the absence of mourning does not predict a more serious outcome.

The question of who is vulnerable is important when considering or studying the treatment of the recently bereaved. Certainly one would expect that the proven efficacy for the treatment of depression with interpersonal psychotherapy would also apply to the bereaved, because one of the targeted areas for the therapy is loss, but as yet it has not been tested in recently bereaved people. There have been two open-trial studies using tricyclic antidepressants in recently bereaved subjects (Jacobs et al., 1987a; Pasternak et al., 1991). Both have shown efficacy. In the second, subjects had significant improvement in all areas of bereavement-related depression except the continued intensity of the grief (Pasternak et al., 1991), which means that the fear that some people have that antidepressants will mask normal grieving is not substantiated. As Osterweis and Townsend (1988) suggest, the efficacy of antidepressants for grief reactions has not been shown, but such use would be a new indication not currently approved by the Food and Drug Administration. Other specific stresses that result in depression, including adjustment disorder with depressed mood, might warrant similar pharmacological studies.

SUMMARY

The death of someone close is universally regarded as a stress. Bereavement is an excellent response model for a stress that produces a syndrome of depression or sadness (as opposed to a stress that produces anxiety or fear) that resolves slowly with time. Between 8% and 11% of survivors are left with chronic depression that probably warrants treatment. How this relates to other stress responses has yet to be identified. The lessons learned and the questions raised should be applicable to research concerning other stressors and other responses, as well as to improving the quality of life of the bereaved and impacting on the morbidity and mortality of those affected.

REFERENCES

American Psychiatric Association. (1994). *Diagnostic and statistical manual of mental disorders* (4th ed.). Washington, DC: American Psychiatric Press.

Bornstein, P. E., & Clayton, P. J. (1972). The anniversary reaction. *Diseases of the Nervous System, 33*, 470–472.

Bornstein, P. E., Clayton, P. J., Halikas, J. A., et al. (1973). The depression of widowhood at 13 months. *British Journal of Psychiatry, 122*, 561–566.

Bowling, A. (1987). Mortality after bereavement: A review of the literature on survival periods and factors affecting survival. *Social Science and Medicine, 24*, 117–124.

Breckenridge, J. N., Gallagher, D., Thompson, L. W., et al. (1986). Characteristic depressive symptoms of bereaved elders. *Journal of Gerontology, 41*, 163–168.

Byrne, G. J. A., & Raphael, B. (1994). A longitudinal study of bereavement phenomena in recently widowed elderly men. *Psychological Medicine, 24*, 411–421.

Cassidy, W. L., Flanagan, N. B., Spellman, M., et al. (1957). Clinical observations in manic-depressive disease. *Journal of the American Medical Association, 164*, 1535–1546.

Clayton, P. J. (1973). The period of numbness. *The Director*, 4–5.

Clayton, P. J. (1974). Mortality and morbidity in the first year of widowhood. *Archives of General Psychiatry, 30*, 747–750.

Clayton, P. (1982). Bereavement. In E. S. Paykel (Ed.), *Handbook of affective disorders*. London: Churchill Livingstone.

Clayton, P. J. (1990). Bereavement and depression. *Journal of Clinical Psychiatry, 51*, (7 Suppl.), 34–38.

Clayton, P. J., & Darvish, H. S. (1979). Course of depressive symptoms following the stress of bereavement. In J. E. Barrett et al. (Eds.), *Stress and mental disorder*. New York: Raven Press.

Clayton, P., Desmarais, L., & Winokur, G. (1968). A study of normal bereavement. *American Journal of Psychiatry, 125*, 168–178.

Clayton, P. J., Halikas, J. A., & Maurice, W. L. (1971). The bereavement of the widowed. *Diseases of the Nervous System, 32*, 597–604.

Clayton, P. J., Herjanic, M., Murphy, G. E., et al. (1974). Mourning and depression: Their similarities and differences. *Canadian Psychiatric Association Journal, 19*, 309–312.

Clayton, J., Parilla, R. H., Jr., & Bieri, M. D. (1980a). Methodological problems in assessing the relationship between acuteness of death and the bereavement outcome. In J. Reiffel et al. (Eds.), *Psychosocial aspects of cardiovascular disease: The patient, the family and the staff*. New York: Columbia University Press.

Clayton, J., Parilla, R. H., Jr., & Bieri, M. D. (1980b). Survivors of cardiovascular and cancer deaths. In J. Reiffel et al. (Eds.), *Psycho-

social aspects of cardiovascular disease: The patient, the family, and the staff. New York: Columbia University Press.

Eaton, W. W., Kramer, M., Anthony, J. C., et al. (1989). The incidence of specific DIS/DSM-III mental disorders: Data from the NIMH Epidemiologic Catchment Area Program. *Acta Psychiatrica Scandinavica, 79,* 163–178.

Feighner, J. P., Robins, E., Guze, S. B., et al. (1972). Diagnostic criteria for use in psychiatric research. *Archives of General Psychiatry, 26,* 57–63.

Frank E., & Stewart, B. D. (1984). Depressive symptoms in rape victims: A revisit. *Journal of Affective Disorders, 7,* 77–85.

Freud, S. (1957). Mourning and melancholia. In *The complete psychological works of Sigmund Freud* (Vol 14, pp. 243–258). London: Hogarth Press. (Original work published 1917)

Frost, N. R., & Clayton, P. J. (1977). Bereavement and psychiatric hospitalization. *Archives of General Psychiatry, 34,* 1172–1175.

Ganzini, L., McFarland, B. H., & Cutler, D. (1990). Prevalence of mental disorders after catastrophic financial loss. *Journal of Nervous and Mental Disease, 178,* 680–685.

Goldberger, L., & Breznitz, H. (Eds.). (1993). *Handbook of stress: Theoretical and clinical aspects* (2nd ed.). New York: The Free Press.

Grimby, A. (1993). Bereavement among elderly people: Grief reactions, post-bereavement hallucinations and quality of life. *Acta Psychiatrica Scandinavica, 87,* 72–80.

Harlow, S. D., Goldberg, E. L., & Comstock, G. W. (1991a). A longitudinal study of risk factors for depressive symptomatology in elderly widowed and married women. *American Journal of Epidemiology, 134,* 526–538.

Harlow, S. D., Goldberg, E. L., & Comstock, G. W. (1991b). A longitudinal study of the prevalence of depressive symptomatology in elderly widowed and married women. *Archives of General Psychiatry, 48,* 1065–1068.

Hays, J. C., Kasl, S. V., & Jacobs, S. C. (1994). The course of psychological distress following threatened and actual conjugal bereavement. *Psychological Medicine, 24,* 917–927.

Hefez, A., Metz, L., & Lavie, P. (1987). Long-term effects of extreme situational stress on sleep and dreaming. *American Journal of Psychiatry, 144,* 344–347.

Helsing, K. J., Comstock, G. W., & Szklo, M. (1982). Causes of death in a widowed population. *American Journal of Epidemiology, 116,* 524–532.

Helsing, K. J., & Szklo, M. (1981). Mortality after bereavement. *American Journal of Epidemiology, 114,* 41–52.

Helsing, K. J., Szklo, M., & Comstock, G. W. (1981). Factors associated with mortality after widowhood. *American Journal of Public Health, 71,* 802–809.

Helzer, J. E., Burnam, A., & McEvoy, L. T. (1991). In L. N. Robins & D. A. Regier (Eds.), *Psychiatric disorders in America: The Epidemiological Catchment Area Surveys.* New York:The Free Press.

Holmes, T., & Rahe, R. (1967). The Social Readjustment Rating Scale. *Journal of Psychosomatic Research, 11,* 213–216.

Jacobs, S., Hansen, F., Berkman, L., et al. (1989). Depressions of bereavement. *Comprehensive Psychiatry, 30,* 218–224.

Jacobs, S., Hansen, F., Kasl, S., et al. (1990). Anxiety disorders during acute bereavement: Risk and risk factors. *Journal of Clinical Psychiatry, 51,* 269–274.

Jacobs, S. C., Nelson, J. C., & Zisook, S. (1987a). Treating depressions of bereavement with antidepressants: A pilot study. *Psychiatric Clinics of North America, 10,* 501–510.

Jacobs, S. C., Schaefer, C. A., Ostfeld, A. M., et al. (1987b). The first anniversary of bereavement. *Israel Journal of Psychiatry and Related Sciences, 24,* 77–85.

Kaprio, J., Koskenvuo, M., & Rita, H. (1987). Mortality after bereavement: A prospective study of 95,647 widowed persons. *American Journal of Public Health, 77,* 283–287.

Klerman, G., & Clayton, P. (1984). Epidemiologic perspectives on the health consequences of bereavement. In M. Osterweis, F. Solomon, & M. Green (Eds.), *Bereavement: Reactions, consequences, and care.* Washington, DC: National Academy Press.

Kraus, A. S., & Lilienfeld, A. M. (1959). Some epidemiological aspects of the high mortality rate in the young widowed group. *Journal of Chronic Disease, 10,* 207–217.

Levav, I., Friedlander, Y., Kark, J. D., et al. (1988). An epidemiologic study of mortality among bereaved patients. *New England Journal of Medicine, 319,* 457–461.

Lindemann, E. (1944). Symptomatology and management of acute grief. *American Journal of Psychiatry, 101,* 141–148.

Longford, E. (1964). *Victoria R. I.* London: Wiedenfeld and Nicolson.

MacMahon, B. & Pugh T. F. (1965). Suicide in the widowed. *American Journal of Epidemiology, 81,* 23–31.

Maddison, D., & Viola, A. (1968). The health of widows in the year following bereavement. *Journal of Psychosomatic Research, 12,* 297–306.

McFarlane, A. C. (1989). The aetiology of post-traumatic morbidity: Predisposing, precipitating and perpetuating factors. *British Journal of Psychiatry, 154,* 221–228.

Mellström, D., Nilsson, Å., Odén, A., et al. (1982). Mortality among the widowed in Sweden. *Scandinavian Journal of Social Medicine, 10,* 33–41.

Mendes de Leon, C. F., Kasl, S. V., & Jacobs, S. (1993). Widowhood and mortality risk in a community sample of the elderly: A prospective study. *Journal of Clinical Epidemiology, 46,* 519–527.

Mendes de Leon, C. F., Kasl, V., & Jacobs, S. (1994). A prospective study of widowhood and changes in symptoms of depression in a community sample of the elderly. *Psychological Medicine, 24,* 613–624.

Mor, V., McHorney, C., & Sherwood, S. (1986). Secondary morbidity among the recently bereaved. *American Journal of Psychiatry, 143,* 158–163.

Niemi, T. (1979). The mortality of male old-age pensioners following the spouse's death. *Scandinavian Journal of Social Medicine, 7,* 115–117.

North, C. S., & Smith, E. M. (1990). Post-traumatic stress disorder in disaster survivors. *Comprehensive Therapy, 16,* 3–9.

Nuss, W. S., & Zubenko, G. S. (1992). Correlates of persistent depressive symptoms in widows. *American Journal of Psychiatry, 149,* 346–351.

O'Connell, R. A., Mayo, J. A., Flatow, L., et al. (1991). Outcome of bipolar disorder on long-term treatment with lithium. *British Journal of Psychiatry, 159,* 123–129.

Osterweis, M., & Townsend, J. (1988). *Mental health professionals and the bereaved* [DHHS Publication No. (ADM) 88-1554], Washington, DC: U.S. Department of Health and Human Services.

Parkes, C. M. (1970). The first year of bereavement: A longitudinal study of the reaction of London widows to the deaths of their husbands. *Psychiatry, 33,* 444–467.

Parkes, C. M., (1972). *Bereavement: Studies of grief in adult life.* New York: International Universities Press.

Parkes, C. M. (1993). Psychiatric problems following bereavement by murder or manslaughter. *British Journal of Psychiatry, 162,* 49–54.

Parkes, C. M., & Weiss, R. S. (1983). *Recovery from bereavement.* New York: Basic Books.

Partinen, M., Putkonen, P. T. S., Kaprio, J., et al. (1982) Sleep disorders in relation to coronary heart disease. *Acta Medica Scandinavica (Supplementum), 660,* 69–83.

Pasternak, R. E., Reynolds, C. F., Houck, P. R., et al. (1994). Sleep in bereavement-related depression during and after pharmacotherapy with nortriptyline. *Journal of Geriatric Psychiatry and Neurology, 7,* 71–75.

Pasternak, R. E., Reynolds, C. F., Schlernitzauer, M., et al. (1991). Acute open-trial nortriptyline therapy of bereavement-related depression in late life. *Journal of Clinical Psychiatry, 52,* 307–310.

Rees, W. D., (1971). The hallucinations of widowhood. *British Medical Journal, 4,* 39–41.

Reynolds, C. F., Hoch, C. C., Buysse, D. J., et al. (1993). Sleep after spousal bereavement: A study of recovery from stress. *Biological Psychiatry, 34,* 791–797.

Sanders, C. M. (1979–80). A comparison of adult bereavement in the death of a spouse, child, and parent. *Omega, 10,* 303–322.

Schneider, D. S., Sledge, P. A., Shuchter, S., et al. (1996). Dating and remarriage over the first two years of widowhood. *Annals of Clinical Psychiatry, 8,* 51–57.

Selzer, M. (1971). The Michigan Alcoholism Screening Test: The quest for a new diagnostic instrument. *American Journal of Psychiatry, 127,* 89–94.

Silverman, P. R. (1966). *Services for the widowed during the period of bereavement: Social work practice.* New York: Columbia University Press.

Smith, E. M., North, C. S., McCool, R. E., et al. (1990). Acute postdisaster psychiatric disorders: Identification of persons at risk. *American Journal of Psychiatry, 147,* 202–206.

Smith, E. M., North, C. S., & Spitznagel, E. L. (1993). Post-traumatic stress in survivors of three disasters. *Journal of Social Behavior and Personality, 8,* (Special Issue), 353–368.

Surtees, P. G. (1995). In the shadow of adversity: The evolution and resolution of anxiety and depressive disorder. *British Journal of Psychiatry, 166,* 583–594.

Valanis, B., Yeaworth, R. C., & Mullis, M. R. (1987). Alcohol use among bereaved and non-bereaved older persons. *Journal of Gerontological Nursing, 13,* 26–32.

Van Eerdewegh, M. M., Bieri, M. D., Parrilla, R. H., et al. (1982). The bereaved child. *British Journal of Psychiatry, 140,* 23–29.

Vargas, L. A., Loya, F., & Hodde-Vargas, J. (1989). Exploring the multidimensional aspects of grief reactions. *American Journal of Psychiatry, 146,* 1484–1488.

Zisook. S. (1992). *Grief responses—perspectives on the process of grieving.* Master's in psychiatry, pp. 20–24.

Zisook, S., & Shuchter, S. R. (1991). Depression through the first year after the death of a spouse. *American Journal of Psychiatry, 148,* 1346–1352.

Zisook, S., & Shuchter, S. R. (1993a). Major depressions associated with widowhood. *American Journal of Geriatric Psychiatry, 1,* 316–326.

Zisook, S., & Shuchter, S. R. (1993b). Uncomplicated bereavement. *Journal of Clinical Psychiatry, 54,* 365–372.

Zisook, S., Shuchter, S. R., & Mulvihill, M. (1990). Alcohol, cigarette, and medication use during the first year of widowhood. *Psychiatric Annals, 20,* 318–326.

7

The Impact of Unemployment on Health and Well-Being

Stanislav V. Kasl
Eunice Rodriguez
Kathryn E. Lasch

Studies addressing the impact of unemployment on health and well-being appear in a variety of disciplines, use a variety of research designs, and examine a variety of outcomes. The empirical evidence is therefore difficult to organize, evaluate, and summarize. In this chapter we employ the perspective of psychosocial epidemiology to bring this material together. This perspective views the findings of public health, medicine, and the social–behavioral sciences using the methodological framework of contemporary epidemiology. Admittedly, it is not adequately sensitive to such disciplines as economics and anthropology, nor does it accommodate easily the viewpoints of political science and public policy. Nevertheless, our orientation is broad enough to characterize the major issues and findings.

This chapter does not address the question of how the evidence regarding the impact of unemployment should be translated into public policy and planning. Rather, it focuses on the nature and extent of the evidence itself. In this connection, we note that any conclusion that "there is no credible evidence that unemployment impacts on" has one of two meanings: (1) there is

ample evidence for the conclusion of no impact, or (2) the issue has not been credibly examined. The former meaning is the informative one, while the latter is a particularly poor basis for discerning implications and deciding on policy.

SOME CONCEPTUAL CONSIDERATIONS

In classical occupational epidemiology, it is often a rather straightforward task to define the exposure variable and make it operational, to determine its dose and duration, and to plot the pathways of exposure, among other characteristics. In unemployment studies, the exposure variable is much more complex, much more difficult to conceptualize and measure. Simple, "objective" indicators (e.g., employed vs. unemployed) are unlikely to yield a rich understanding of the underlying processes and will contribute little to determining the impact of individual and subgroup differences.

One issue in unemployment studies centers on the meaning of work and the impact work can have on individuals and their families. Jahoda (1979) suggests that a job, aside from meeting economic needs, has additional "latent functions": it (1) imposes time structure on the day; (2) implies regularly shared experiences and contacts with others; (3) links an individual to goals and purposes that transcend his or her own; (4) defines aspects of personal status and indentity; and (5) enforces activity. Warr (1987) discusses a number of environmental features of work that he postulates are responsible for psychological well-being: opportunity for control, skill use, interpersonal contact, external goal and task demands, variety, environmental clarity, availability of money, physical security, and valued social position. An earlier review (Kasl, 1979a) offers additional formulations on the meaning of work and unemployment. In addition, for some individuals job loss may represent the termination of exposures, such as work stress or specific work hazards, that themselves may be adverse influences on health. The implication of such formulations is that the experience of job loss and unemployment is likely to be multifaceted and involve different intervening processes, moderating influences, and outcomes. At minimum, one should try to separate the effects of economic hardships from the other effects of being without a job (Jahoda, 1992), a distinction most previous studies unfortunately do not address.

The unemployment experience may also affect subgroups of individuals differently. For example, age (and stage of the life cycle) is an important consideration: the unemployment experience is likely to be different for (1) young persons completing their education and unable to find a job; (2) young workers with unclear career goals in their first jobs, which they find unsatisfying; (3) a middle-aged head of household, with dependents at home, losing a long-held job made obsolete by new technology; and (4) an elderly worker, in poor health and close to retirement, in a job that is physically demanding.

A labor economics perspective on unemployment introduces additional issues. For example, Burchell (1992) argues for the need to understand the broader context of the labor market when studying the psychological health of unemployed individuals. In particular, he points to the inappropriate neglect of other labor market phenomena such as job insecurity, promotions and demotions, and stagnated careers. Cahill (1983) argues from a broader macroeconomic perspective and argues for the need to attend to five characteristics of the current economic system: instability in the business cycle, unemployment, inequality in income distribution, capital mobility, and fragmentation of the work process.

In short, job loss as an acute event and unemployment as a potentially enduring exposure are both richly embedded in a social matrix involving the interdependence of the individual, the family, the network of friends and relatives, the immediate community, the regional economy, and society as a whole. This leaves ample room for variability of impact, linked to variations in the meaning of the experience and to the role of diverse moderators that can affect the process and the outcomes. All this represents a formidable challenge to investigators and their research designs in trying to meet their two major goals: (1) isolate one broad cause–effect relationship, that of unemployment to health and well-being, from a larger matrix of causal and reciprocal influences; and (2) capture the richness of the phenomenon of unemployment and the diversity of the underlying etiological dynamics.

SOME METHODOLOGICAL CONSIDERATIONS

The most dominant methodological issue in unemployment research centers on the distinction between causation and selection: Does the observation of poorer physical and mental health reflect the impact of unemployment, or does it, instead, denote the influence of prior characteristics of the individuals who later become unemployed? The latter alternative, biased selection into exposure status, could reflect either (1) the direct influence of health (i.e., persons with poorer health are more likely to become unemployed), or (2) the indirect influence of characteristics such as disadvantaged social status and unstable occupational career, which lead to greater likelihood both of unemployment and of poorer health. The interpretive dilemma (causation vs. selection) also applies to studies in which the independent (exposure) variable is either length of unemployment or the contrast between re-employed and continued unemployment; the poorer health of those with prolonged unemployment could again be either because this reflects a higher "dose" of the exposure variable, or because those with prior poorer health have a lower chance of being re-employed.

The evidence on unemployment and health supports both the causation and the selection interpretations (e.g., Bartley, 1988; Hammarstrom, 1994; Jahoda, 1992; Miles, 1987; Schwefel, 1986). The two interpretations are not incompatible, even within a single study. We note that this broad conclusion that the causation and selection dynamics are present is actually based on a variety of types of evidence: (1) ambiguous results where either or both interpretations are tenable, (2) evidence for selection but not causation, (3) evidence for causation (usually after statistical adjustments for some set of prior characteristics) but not selection, and (4) evidence for both within the same study. Studies that show no difference in health or well-being between the employed and the unemployed are relatively rare because selection reflects the broader effects of social disadvantage on health. Thus studies likely to show no difference are generally those in which the two groups (of employed and unemployed) are selected to be highly comparable on most background variables.

Many different study designs have been used to examine the impact of unemployment on health and well-being (Cook, 1985; Kasl, 1982; Stern, 1983). One primary distinction made among designs (e.g. Catalano, 1991; Cook, 1985) is whether the data are aggregated (also referred to as ecological or macroeconomic) or are based on individuals. Although there are occasional studies

in which the ecological analyses are cross-sectional and the unit of aggregation is some geopolitical entity (e.g., Charlton et al., 1987; Robinson & Pinch, 1987), most of the ecological analyses involve time series data in which annual fluctuations in some economic indicator, often the nationwide percentage of the labor force that is unemployed, are related to annual changes in some outcome, such as total mortality, cause-specific mortality, alcohol consumption, acts of domestic violence, and so on. These business cycle analyses are currently seen as problematic and controversial. Consequently, many authors believe that they do not have sufficient grounds either to dismiss the methodology or to trust it and accept the findings. The next section provides additional discussion of some of the issues surrounding the business cycle analyses.

With the exception of some controlled randomized intervention programs (e.g., Price, 1992; Vinokur et al., 1991), designed to promote job search skills and thereby prevent adverse mental health consequences of prolonged unemployment, the usual design in studies of unemployment and health is an observational (nonexperimental) study. The epidemiological designs represent the usual spectrum of longitudinal and cross-sectional studies. (Retrospective case–control designs are relatively rare in unemployment research, with the possible exception of suicide studies; see Platt, 1984). *Longitudinal* studies of unemployment and health can be classified into several distinct types; such a typology can organize the evidence but also illuminates important methodological issues.

1. *Natural experiments.* The typical study is one of a plant or factory closure in which all employees lose their jobs and are then followed for health status changes. Morris and Cook (1991) have discussed the advantages and disadvantages of such an approach. Among the former, the most important is the absence of self-selection. However, a comparison group of stably employed individuals is still generally needed,

and these may come from another plant or work setting that is insufficiently comparable to the one that shut down. These studies are difficult to carry out, and the number of subjects tends to be small and the follow-up period relatively short. Moreover, the specificity of the setting and the circumstances of the plant closing may restrict the generalizability of the findings. In addition, initial data collected before the plant closes are seldom true baseline data; because the subjects are aware of the impending event, many variables may show anticipatory effects (e.g., Kasl & Cobb, 1970; Kasl et al., 1968). Finally, when length of unemployment is examined as the independent variable, self-selection biases may reappear in the design because prior poor health may lead to greater difficulty in obtaining new employment; however, one would expect the study to have some relevant health data and to be able to carry out the appropriate statistical adjustments.

2. *Longitudinal comparisons of the employed and unemployed.* This design is rather weak when no baseline data are available on health and social characteristics of the two cohorts. This weakness is aggravated if the "exposed" cohort has been unemployed for a long time and if no retrospective data are available on the circumstances of the original job loss. Conversely, if the unemployed cohort has already experienced adverse health changes by the start of the follow-up, then adjustments for initial differences will overcorrect in analyses intended to adjust only for self-selection.

3. *Follow-up of the unemployed to detect benefits of re-employment.* This design can offer highly suggestive results if the unemployed show an improvement in health or well-being after becoming re-employed, if this improvement brings them up to par with the continuously employed, and if the continuously unemployed do not show such an improvement. The reasonable inference is that the variable showing improvement had declined earlier because of the impact of the unemployment. Two caveats are in order here. First, if the unemployment experience had already produced irreversible changes by the start of follow-up (but this cannot be detected, given the design), then the failure to show improvement after re-employment should not lead to the interpretation that this variable is not affected by unemployment. Second, the usual monitoring of a cohort may not be sufficiently frequent to identify correctly the underlying temporal sequence. For example, recovery from depression among the unemployed may precede finding a new job, while failure to recover from depression may interfere with job search. Thus self-selection is at work in the observed association with re-employment. This could be the case even if there is a true initial impact of unemployment on depression.

Cross-sectional designs showing an association between unemployment and poor health normally cannot disentangle the causation-versus-selection interpretations. Statistical adjustments can be made for the influence of stable social characteristics, such as education, but these can control, at best, for indirect selection only. However, there may be special circumstances that allow for more extensive statistical controls and thus stronger inferences. For example, retrospective information regarding original circumstances of the job loss might identify a subgroup of unemployed to whom self-selection processes are unlikely to apply. As another example, it may be that we have quite precise population norms for the prevalence of a certain outcome, such as clinical depression. If a cross-sectional study is carried out in a community that experienced a sharp rise in unemployment and only self-selection is present, then the unemployed will be "recruited" from the ranks of the previously employed but depressed community residents. The prevalence of depression in the total community will remain unchanged and the prevalence among the employed will be lower than expected. Obviously, this scenario requires great precision in estimates and precisely applicable population norms.

It is useful to come back to the earlier distinction between designs using aggregate data versus data on individuals. There is a *hybrid* design in which data on individuals are supplemented with ecological information on economic indicators for the community or the region (e.g., Dooley et al., 1988). This is a strong design, particularly when longitudinal data are collected. Specifically, it enables one to answer two additional questions: (*1*) Do changes in community level of unemployment impact on the health and well-being of those who remain employed? (*2*) Do the levels of community unemployment moderate the impact on the unemployed (e.g., the impact on the individual unemployed person could be greater when the community level of unemployment is high vs. when it is low)?

A NOTE ON BUSINESS CYCLE ANALYSES

There is no doubt that the foremost practitioner of the aggregate time series approach during the last 20 years has been M.H. Brenner (e.g., Brenner, 1983, 1987a, 1987b, 1987c; Brenner & Monney, 1983). Although his approach has become more sophisticated over the years, and his statistical models have included a longer list of potential confounders and control variables, his fundamental strategy has remained the same: to demonstrate that fluctuations in some economic indicator, such as unemployment and business failures, are causally associated with fluctuations in some adverse outcome, particularly total or cause-specific mortality. Adjustments are made for various short- and long-term trends, and time lags of varying lengths are explored. The unvarying conclusion in Brenner's reports is that, indeed, un-

employment adversely affects a nation's health.

Brenner's work has been controversial from the beginning. Some early critics (e.g., Eyer, 1977a, 1977b) did not object to the overall macroeconomic strategy as much as to the broad conclusions; that is, they saw an association of mortality rates with business booms, not economic depressions. Other critics (e.g., Cohen & Felson, 1979) were disturbed by the strong inferences for public policy drawn from such difficult-to-interpret data-analytical strategies. The last 10–15 years have produced numerous critical examinations of this methodology and of the results it has yielded (e.g., Colledge, 1982; Forbes & McGregor, 1987; Gravelle et al., 1981; Kasl, 1979b, 1982; Morris & Cook, 1991; Sogaard, 1992; Spruit, 1982; Starrin et al., 1990; Wagstaff, 1985). The net effect of such scrutiny has been to provide a basis for considerable skepticism about the data and the conclusions. At the same time, there is no consensus about what exactly is wrong with the methodology, how exactly it may bias the findings, and what are the correct analytical strategies. Dooley and Catalano (1988), themselves quite sophisticated researchers, arrive at an indeterminate conclusion that "the field is uncertain how to interpret the findings from the aggregate time series approach" (p. 6).

Briefly, some of the criticisms of Brenner's work and of the aggregate time series approach have been: (*1*) inability to understand and follow the actual methods used, based on information provided; (*2*) inability to replicate the findings using the *same* data; (*3*) inability to obtain similar results when carrying out attempted cross-validation with comparable data; (*4*) apparent arbitrariness of selected time lags; (*5*) insufficient justification for de-trending strategies, which often drastically alter the findings; (*6*) difficulty in estimating the magnitude of effects attributable to economic variables; and (*7*) inappropriateness of units of analysis (e.g., total country) when there is substantial variation in the independent and dependent variables at levels of smaller geopolitical units, suggesting the need for a finer grained analysis. It might also be noted that all analyses so far have been of past trends; no investigator seems to have attempted to develop a model from past data to forecast future trends, or to use one segment of past data to develop a model to "forecast" trends in a later segment of past data. Developing successful models that predict future trends would address the criticism that the analyses are tailor made and distorted in order to obtain the expected results.

Perhaps the most common criticism of the aggregate time series approach is that it is vulnerable to the ecological fallacy (Robinson, 1950): aggregate-level relationships do not necessarily apply to individuals and, specifically, we cannot conclude that the higher mortality applies to the unemployed individuals. However, this may not be a fully appropriate criticism, because Brenner is interested in documenting the adverse impact on all individuals, whether or not they themselves are unemployed. However, other technical issues remain: (1) individual-level relationships can be vastly magnified at the aggregate level, and thus ordinarily negligible confounders can create strong spurious associations at the aggregate level; and (2) specific variables may lose their usefulness when aggregated in a certain way, such as measuring per capita alcohol consumption in analyzing heart disease mortality (Brenner, 1987a) when one needs a different measure, percentage of moderate drinkers in the population.

THE IMPACT OF UNEMPLOYMENT ON MORTALITY

There are a number of epidemiological studies that have examined the relationship between unemployment and mortality. Three British reports are based on the follow-up of men in the Office of Population Censuses and Surveys (OPCS) longitudinal study (Moser et al., 1984, 1986, 1987). Men who were seeking work during the week before the 1971 survey had a higher age-adjusted mortality [standardized mortality ratio (SMR) = 136] during the following

decade than would be expected from the rates in the total OPCS. Adjustment for social class reduced this excess to a SMR of 121. Particularly high mortality was observed for suicide (SMR = 169). Although the authors could not control statistically for possible prior health status differences, they argued that the pattern of results (cause-specific analyses, overall mortality trends over time) did not suggest a strong effect of self-selection. Women whose husbands were seeking work had higher mortality (SMR = 120), which was only slightly diminished by controlling for social class. A shorter follow-up of men after the 1981 census confirmed the earlier findings but obtained a somewhat lower adjusted SMR of 112. Analyses by regions of the country suggested that the region with the highest mortality and unemployment rates had higher SMRs as a result of unemployment.

In a report by Morris et al. (1994) based on a prospective cohort study (British Regional Heart Study), all men (ages 40–59) had been continuously employed for at least 5 years before initial screening. On a postal questionnaire 5 years later, they indicated changes in employment during the previous 5 years. Then they were followed for 5.5 years (after the questionnaire) for mortality. Compared to the continuously employed men, those who had some unemployment (but not as a result of illness, according to self-reports) showed an elevated age-adjusted relative risk (RR) of 1.59. This was reduced only slightly to RR = 1.47 with further adjustment for social class, smoking, alcohol intake, and pre-existing disease at screening. Two additional groups are of interest: those "retired not due to illness" had an RR of 1.86, and those "unemployed or retired due to illness" had an RR of 3.14. Both values are adjusted for the full set of covariates. The RR for retirement suggests that it is a more adverse experience than unemployment—an improbable conclusion, given the uniform evidence that retirement per se does not have a negative impact on mortality (e.g., Kasl, 1980). The high value of 3.14 for those citing illness as reason for not working reveals the inadequacy of baseline health status adjustments that used data from the time when all respondents were still continuously employed. This suggests that baseline health status must be updated in such studies and/or supplemented with adjustments for reports of illness reasons for not working.

A number of additional reports are available for Sweden (Stefansson, 1991), Finland (Martikainen, 1990), Denmark (Iversen et al., 1987), and Italy (Costa & Segnan, 1987); they all use designs similar to the British OPCS analyses. Several conclusions can be derived from these studies:

1. Excess mortality associated with unemployment is observed in all studies, with the magnitude of effect generally between SMRs of 150 and 200, adjusted for age and socioeconomic status.
2. Gender differences were examined in two studies, with the Danish data showing no gender difference in magnitude of effect attributable to unemployment, while the Swedish data showed a much weaker impact on women (SMR = 114).
3. Adjustments for sociodemographics generally reduce the magnitude of effect, while additional adjustments for various (imperfect) indicators of health status make much less of a difference.
4. Younger subjects tend to show stronger effects of unemployment, but occupational status data do not show consistent differences across subgroups.
5. Cause-specific analyses suggest that suicides, accidents, violent deaths, and alcohol-related deaths tend to be especially elevated but do not explain all of the excess mortality.
6. Analyses by regional unemployment rates were possible in the Danish data. These showed that, in regions of higher unemployment, the impact attributable to the unemployed status of individuals was weaker, thus contradicting the British OPCS results (Moser et al., 1986).

These results from Europe are contradicted by a U.S. study that matched U.S. Census Bureau Current Population Surveys to the National Death Index (Sorlie & Rogot, 1990). After adjusting for age, education, and income, the SMRs related to unemployment among those 45–64 years of age were 107 for men and 81 for women; neither was significantly different from SMR of 100, which reflects the mortality of the total sample. There was some hint of an effect among younger men (35–44), but the numbers were too small to yield a reliable finding. This discrepancy with the European data is not easily explained, particularly in that the "social net" protecting the unemployed is believed to be stronger in these European countries than in the United States.

It is worth emphasizing that strong causal inferences are seldom justified from these observational studies. Even apparently good evidence, such as the unemployment–suicide association, is neither so consistent nor so compelling so as to allow the conclusion that the causal issue has been settled (Dooley et al., 1989; Platt, 1984; Platt et al., 1992). Platt (1984) points out that the prior role of psychiatric illness in both the unemployment and the (later) suicide has not been satisfactorily ruled out.

THE IMPACT OF UNEMPLOYMENT ON MORBIDITY

Studies of unemployment and physical morbidity introduce a new concern not applicable to mortality studies: the measurement of health status outcomes. There are at least two concerns. First, the influence of psychological distress on some measures could be substantial: that is, physical symptoms and complaints could be due to the distress rather than to some underlying physical condition, or distress could lower the threshold for reporting existing physical symptoms. Second, measures based on seeking and/or receiving care could indicate differences in illness behavior rather than underlying illness. Occasionally, it may be simply too difficult to determine what is being measured. Thus, in a well-designed prospective study of the effects of closure of a sardine factory in Norway (Westin, 1990a, 1990b; Westin et al., 1988, 1989), the rates of disability pensions granted observed over a 10 year follow-up period were higher, compared with rates at a nearby "sister factory" that did not close. Although these pensions are granted "for medical conditions only," it is still difficult to know what exactly is being assessed and what health status differences would have been observed with other types of measurements.

Of the ten *longitudinal* studies of factory closures reviewed by Morris and Cook (1991), most did not have direct measures of morbidity, though they obtained other related data. For example, the Westin study, in addition to data on disability pension, also obtained information on "time outside of labor force without social security coverage" and "long-term reduction in mean time spent in job." These are important indices of social impact (sensitive to the regional economy) but do not reflect morbidity. Other studies examined such outcomes as rates of medical consultation, which are difficult to interpret, particularly in the absence of a control group (Yuen & Balarajan, 1986).

There is reasonable agreement in the several available longitudinal studies that the job loss experience has a negative impact on health, although the precise nature of this impact is difficult to pinpoint. For example, in a Canadian study of factory closure (Grayson, 1989), former employees reported on a survey an average of 2.3–2.6 ailments during three occasions in a 27-month follow-up. The expected average, based on population data (adjusted for age, education, and employment status), was about 1.1. Spouses of former employees also showed elevated values (average around 3.0). What these results mean is difficult to determine. The higher prevalence was for a wide range of conditions (e.g., headaches, acute respiratory ailments, ulcers, arthritis, sight and hearing disorders, dental troubles). Only heart disease, asthma, and

endocrine diseases showed no significant differences. The authors offer the interpretation that these data indicate higher levels of stress that produce "a series of symptoms that people mistake for illness itself."

In an earlier Michigan study of two plants that shut down and several control plants (Cobb & Kasl, 1977), the number of men studied was rather small, with resultant low power to detect differences in disease conditions. However, there were two suggestive findings involving higher rates among the unemployed of (*1*) dyspepsia (ulcer activity) among those with no ulcer history, and (*2*) observed joint swellings, suggestive of rheumatoid arthritis. Measures based on administration of a 2 week health diary, including days of complaint ("did not feel as well as usual") and days of disability ("did not carry out usual activities"), showed significant fluctuations over time, but these could not be linked to employment/unemployment status changes (Kasl et al., 1975). For example, days of complaint were elevated some 6 weeks before plant closing, when all men were still working but fully aware of the coming event. Some 6 weeks after closure, when many of the men were unemployed, levels of days of complaint were significantly below average, irrespective of work status. Some 6–8 months after plant closing, the levels were elevated again, equally so for men still unemployed and for those recently re-employed or those who were stabilizing their employment.

A British study of factory closure examined the impact on general practice consultation rates (Beale & Nethercott, 1987, 1988a, 1988b). Comparisons of rates were made before and after factory closure, and changes in rates over time were assessed among cases versus controls. The factory closure was clearly associated with increased rates of consultations, referrals, and visits to the hospital. More refined analyses revealed that very common illnesses did not show the impact. Rather, the significant increase was for "chronic" illnesses, those conditions that in the past required four or more consultations per year. It is not clear if these conditions were exacerbated by the factory closure, or if there was simply a higher rate of consulting, without any underlying clinical changes. One of the reports (Beale & Nethercott, 1988b) suggests that the incidence (i.e., newly developed conditions) of chronic diseases also went up, but there is nothing in the paper describing the methodology for specifically determining incident (new) cases.

A Danish study of shipyard workers (Iversen et al., 1989) obtained somewhat different results from those noted above: The relative risk (RR) ratios of admission to hospital in the study group, compared to controls, declined from 1.29 some 4–5 years before closure to 0.74 for the 3 years thereafter. Cause-specific analyses revealed strong declines for accidents and diseases of the digestive system. Relative risk ratios increased for circulatory and cardiovascular diseases (from 0.8 to 1.6 and from 1.0 to 2.6, respectively). The authors suggest that two processes are at work: the workers are removed from workplace hazards on the one hand, and exposed to stresses of unemployment on the other.

Cross-sectional associations between unemployment and poor health status also have been reported, but these tend to be less convincing because of the incomplete way they control for selection effects. In an analysis of the Canada Health Survey data (D'Arcy, 1986; D'Arcy & Siddique, 1985), the "unemployed" respondents (those who had looked for work during the previous year) had higher rates of disability days during the previous 2 weeks, major activity limitations, health problems, hospitalizations, and physician visits. Statistical adjustments were possible only for age, sex, marital status, and socioeconomic status. The authors also noted that the impact of unemployment was stronger for women and older respondents.

A cross-sectional analysis of the British General Household Survey data (Arber, 1987) examined rates of "longstanding illness, disability, or infirmity" that limited the respondents' activities. The following SMRs were obtained: employed men, 82; unemployed men, 218; employed women, 78; un-

employed women, 136. The differences between the employed and the unemployed were maintained when respondents were stratified by levels of occupational status, ranging from professional to unskilled manual. The outcome variable in this study is somewhat awkward: It is not clear if being unemployed could have influenced the judgment that a particular condition interfered with activities.

A Dutch cross-sectional study reported on differences between long-term (at least 1 year) unemployed and employed men and women (Leeflang et al., 1992a, 1992b). Unemployed men reported higher numbers of somatic symptoms and chronic conditions (borderline significance) than employed men. No significant differences between employed and unemployed men were obtained for physician consultations, use of prescribed drugs, and percentage under treatment. For women, the results were more complicated because of the phenomenon of hidden unemployment: some unemployed women (usually those with working husbands) failed to register formally as unemployed. Still, the results were somewhat puzzling: employed women reported somewhat higher numbers of somatic symptoms and had a higher percentage under treatment, compared with either unemployed men or unemployed women; the latter groups reported higher numbers of chronic conditions, more use of prescribed drugs, and more physician consultations (registered unemployed only). This study developed a three-item measure of "health selection": changed jobs because of health, attempted and/or received disability benefits, and illness condition of at least 9 months' duration. This three-item variable had a strong influence on health status, but it is not clear from the reports how it altered the magnitude of impact of unemployment after adjusting for its influence.

Cross-sectional data on the impact of unemployment have also been reported for men in the British Regional Heart Study (Cook et al., 1982). The authors separated the unemployed into those who did and did not regard their unemployment as being due to ill health. The latter group, which is more appropriate for examining the impact of unemployment, were quite comparable to the employed men on self-reported history of chronic conditions. On four major illnesses diagnosed from the screening information, the two groups had comparable rates of bronchitis, hypertension, and obstructive lung disease; only on ischemic heart disease did the unemployed men show a significantly higher prevalence.

THE IMPACT OF UNEMPLOYMENT ON BIOLOGICAL AND BEHAVIORAL RISK FACTORS

The biological variables that have been examined in relation to unemployment include (*1*) indicators of "stress" reactivity, such as neuroendocrine changes, which do not have a well-documented relationship to specific diseases; (*2*) a very diverse set of indicators of immune functioning that are linked to possible disease outcomes theoretically rather than empirically; and (*3*) risk factors for specific diseases, typically cardiovascular disease, where the presumption is that a chronic impact on these factors as a result of unemployment translates into higher risk for clinical disease.

Studies that have examined *neuroendocrine* variables (Arnetz et al., 1987; Brenner & Levi, 1987; Brenner & Starrin, 1988; Cobb, 1974; Cobb & Kasl, 1977; Fleming et al., 1984) show a range of findings that do not allow any simple conclusion: (*1*) no effects, (*2*) large fluctuations within the continuously unemployed that are not easily linked to work status changes, (*3*) inconsistent effects of duration of unemployment, and (*4*) well-replicated strong anticipation effects. One interesting observation was that a greater magnitude of the anticipatory reaction was associated with shorter length of subsequent unemployment (Cobb & Kasl, 1977). It is likely that neuroendocrine parameters are better suited for describing acute phases of reactivity rather than chronic stress effects suggestive of increased risk of future disease.

There appears to be only one study that has examined *immune functioning* in relation to unemployment (Arnetz et al., 1987; Brenner & Levi, 1987). The results suggested that unemployment lasting more than 9 months is accompanied by a significant decrease in immune function; after 24 months of unemployment, normal reactivity was restored. There were no benefits of a psychosocial intervention administered to some of the unemployed. These findings apply to some, but by no means all, indicators of immune functioning used in the study.

The impact of employment/unemployment on *cardiovascular risk factors* has been examined in several studies. Two reports deal with threat of unemployment. Cross-sectional data on German blue-collar workers in steel and metal plants, some of which were undergoing reductions in work force (Siegerist et al., 1988), showed that "atherogenic risk" was higher among those threatened with job loss, especially those who also scored high on subjectively perceived job insecurity. Atherogenic risk was defined as the ratio of low- to high-density lipoproteins, and this was adjusted for potential confounders, such as body weight, smoking, and alcohol consumption. In another study, longitudinal data on male Swedish shipyard workers threatened with closure and on stably employed controls (Mattiasson et al., 1990) showed that serum cholesterol concentrations increased significantly among those workers threatened with job loss. The increase was greater among those with higher levels of sleep disturbance, as well as those with increases in other cardiovascular risk factors, particularly weight and blood pressure. However, no significant differential trends over time were seen for weight, blood pressure, or glucose.

Janlert et al. (1991) reported on cross-sectional results from a population survey (ages 25–64) conducted in northern Sweden. Data on lifetime history of unemployment were used to create two contrasting groups: unemployed for 1 year or more versus never unemployed or unemployed less than 1 year. Men with a history of unemployment for 1 year or more scored higher on systolic blood pressure, serum cholesterol levels, and cigarettes smoked daily, and lower on high-density lipoprotein quotient and physical activity. For women, similar differences were obtained for three of the variables (high-density lipoprotein quotient, smoking, physical activity) as well as for body mass index. The authors were unable to rule out selection as an explanation but argued that some of the variables (e.g., blood lipids) are "not directly observable" and thus are unlikely to influence employment status in any simple way.

An Irish group (Cullen et al., 1987) reported cross-sectional results from the pilot phase of a study of young men and women (16–23 years old) who were either unemployed, blue-collar trainees, or in white-collar jobs. Data on blood pressure, heart rate, height, weight, and percentage of body fat were examined. Although a few significant differences were obtained in comparisons of the three groups, none was supportive of the notion that the unemployed youth would score higher on the risk variables.

Analyses of blood pressure and serum cholesterol changes from the Michigan study of plant closure (Kasl & Cobb, 1982) revealed a substantial sensitivity of these variables to the experience of anticipating the closing of the plant, losing the job and going through a period of unemployment, and finding a new job. However, these were acute effects reflecting specific transitions. Men who continued to be unemployed did not continue to show elevated levels; levels declined even in the absence of finding a new job. Two years after the event, the men had "normal" blood pressure levels and somewhat below-normal cholesterol levels. Data on antihypertensive medications were also examined, and these revealed highly suggestive findings. Incidence of "hypertension" was significantly higher among those losing their jobs than among controls, if this incidence was indexed by new antihypertensive medication regimen of at least 3 months' duration among those without any previous history of hypertension. However, this result was determined to be due to (1)

doctors' greater readiness to initiate treatment among the unemployed and (2) the greater readiness of controls to drop out of treatment.

Several reports concern the impact of unemployment on *health habits* and *behavioral risk factors*. The typical variables examined include cigarette smoking, alcohol consumption, body weight, and physical exercise. Longitudinal data from the British Regional Heart Study (Morris et al., 1992, 1994) showed only an increase in weight attributable to unemployment; there was no evidence for such impact on cigarette or alcohol consumption. Because of the longitudinal nature of the data, the study was able to show that higher levels of smoking and heavy drinking were predictive of greater likelihood of subsequent unemployment. The Michigan data (Kasl & Cobb, 1980) showed that cigarette smoking remained quite stable and was not sensitive to the job loss experience. Data on body weight did suggest an impact; however, the effect was a decrease following reemployment rather than an increase as a result of job loss. Although subjects who lost their jobs did not show long-term trends different from controls, they did show greater temporal instability in phase-to-phase weight changes over the 2 years of observation.

Longitudinal data on alcohol consumption yield a somewhat mixed picture. In a Norwegian study of young people (ages 17–20), results showed that unemployment did not influence consumption of alcohol (Hammer, 1992); in fact, in a high-consumption subgroup, unemployment led to a decrease. These results are in agreement with the British data cited above. However, an analysis of panel data from a psychiatric epidemiological study (Catalano et al., 1993) suggested that the incidence of clinically significant alcohol abuse was greater among those who had been laid off than among those who had not been laid off. Interestingly, employed persons in communities with higher unemployment were at reduced risk of becoming alcohol abusers. This study shows the strength of the hybrid design in which both individual-level and community-level data are collected. In general, reviews of the alcohol consumption and unemployment literature (e.g., Forcier, 1988; Hammarstrom, 1994) point to many difficulties in arriving at a coherent picture regarding documented impact. For example, losing a job may increase the need for alcohol consumption but also reduce the ability of the unemployed to afford such expenditures. The conclusion that both causation and selection ("drift") dynamics are supported by the evidence is perhaps the most suitable one (Dooley et al., 1992).

National cross-sectional data on unemployment and behavioral risk factors (U.S. Department of Health and Human Services, 1988) show a mixed picture:

1. The unemployed were more likely to be current cigarette smokers, especially men ages 18–64. However, among current smokers, the unemployed men were less likely to be heavy smokers (> 25 cigarettes per day).
2. There were no notable differences on alcohol consumption.
3. The unemployed men were more likely to be physically active in leisure, but women showed no differences.
4. The unemployed were less likely to say that they had experienced "at least a moderate amount of stress" in the past 2 weeks, but they were more likely to have sought help for "personal or emotional problems" during the past year.

Clearly, in addition to whether these associations reflect selection or causation, they are also rather complicated.

THE IMPACT OF UNEMPLOYMENT ON MENTAL HEALTH AND WELL-BEING

There is little doubt that unemployment has a negative impact on mental health and well-being. However, moving beyond this broad generalization to formulate more specific conclusions becomes difficult because the evidence is less consistent and less com-

plete. Some specific questions have been proposed: Is the impact stronger for some domains of mental health and functioning and weaker for others? Are there subgroup differences in impact that point to vulnerability factors? Is there a dose–response relationship with severity (length) of unemployment? What variables moderate the impact? What processes mediate the unemployment–outcome relationship? These questions guide the review that follows but are not fully answered.

Longitudinal studies strongly support the expectation that unemployment has an adverse impact on subclinical symptomatology or symptoms of poor mental health (e.g., Brenner & Starrin, 1988; Frese & Mohr, 1987; Warr et al., 1988); it is unlikely that the impact is also on overt diagnosable clinical disorder, but only one study is available for this conclusion (Dew et al., 1987). Longitudinal studies also generally demonstrate that becoming re-employed is associated with a reduction in symptomatology (e.g., Ensminger & Celentano, 1988; Iversen & Sabroe, 1988; Kessler et al., 1987b, 1988; Warr et al., 1988). One striking exception is the report by Dooley et al., (1988), which found that the transition from unemployment to re-employment was accompanied by an increase in symptoms. The longitudinal re-employment studies also allow for an examination of selection processes that might be involved in influencing chances of re-employment. By and large, the evidence (e.g., Kessler et al., 1987a, 1988, 1989; Warr et al., 1988) suggests that levels of symptoms do not significantly predict re-employment; in such analyses, it may be necessary to control for reasons for the original unemployment and restrict the conclusions to data on those who become unemployed through no fault of their own.

In European studies, the most frequently used instrument is the General Health Questionnaire, developed by Goldberg (1978). This is best viewed as a general psychiatric screening instrument. In U.S. studies, a greater diversity of symptom checklist instruments has been in use. In general, it would appear that depressive symptoms are the most sensitive indicators of impact of unemployment. However, because symptom checklists tend to be well intercorrelated, similar findings often are obtained with other scales, such as anxiety or somatization (psychophysiological symptoms). An impact of unemployment has been described on other checklist items, such as lower self-confidence and higher externality (one's life is beyond one's control); an impact on self-esteem may be revealed only on items that reflect self-criticism (Warr et al., 1988).

Results from controlled randomized intervention programs designed to promote job search skills (Price, 1992; Vinokur et al., 1991) support the longitudinal observational studies on the reduction in symptoms of depression following re-employment. Successful intervention led to better chances of high-quality re-employment, thereby lowering levels of depressive symptoms up to 2.5 years later. The benefits of the intervention were greatest among those program participants at high risk for depression at baseline: individuals with high symptom levels, high financial hardships, and low social assertiveness.

Cross-sectional studies that address the issue of overall impact of unemployment (e.g., D'Arcy, 1986; Kessler et al., 1987a) do not extend our knowledge gained from the longitudinal studies. However, some of the studies allow for additional comparisons. For example, Hamilton et al. (1990) were able to compare the effects of actual versus anticipated unemployment: Those workers anticipating layoff scored somewhat higher (but not significantly so) on anxiety, depression, and somatization than stably employed workers. However, interaction analysis revealed that less educated blacks were especially affected by the anticipation. Additional cross-sectional studies are reviewed below as they provide insight into the role of moderating and mediating variables.

A number of studies have concerned themselves with the impact of unemployment on *young adults* (e.g., Broomhall & Winefield, 1990; Cullen et al., 1987; Graetz, 1993; Hammarstrom, 1994; Morrell et al., 1994; Schaufeli & Van Yperen, 1992; Wine-

field et al., 1993). The experience of young adults may be different than for older adults because (1) the transition is often from school to unemployment rather than from employment to unemployment, (2) the employed respondents can also experience adaptation stress because of new work role demands, and (3) other significant changes may be taking place for young adults (e.g., leaving home) that could attenuate the impact of the specific employed–unemployed contrast.

Several of the reports on young adults are based on Australian longitudinal studies. The Adelaide study (Winefield et al., 1993) showed that: (1) the difference in well-being between the employed and the unemployed was due to the fact that getting a job was associated with improved well-being rather than that becoming unemployed was associated with a decline; (2) those who were dissatisfied on their jobs (a minority) had low levels of well-being comparable to the unemployed; (3) leaving school was associated with greater impact than that due to employment status differences. A second Australian study (Graetz, 1993) obtained similar results. Specifically, symptoms of distress were highest among dissatisfied workers and lowest among satisfied workers, with the unemployed at intermediate levels. Furthermore, (1) increases in symptoms were comparable whether the transition was from employment to unemployment or from studying to unemployment, and (2) decreases in symptoms were comparable whether the transition was from unemployment to employment or from studying to employment. A third Australian study (Morrell et al., 1994) dealt only with the impact of employment–unemployment–re-employment transitions. The authors estimated that the former transition was associated with a relative risk of 1.51 of "becoming psychologically disturbed" among young people not suffering from physical ill health. Conversely, the second transition was associated with a relative risk of 1.63 of recovering from such disturbance. The authors also estimated the relative risk of becoming disturbed among those continuing to be unemployed: The estimated risks were somewhat below 1.0, suggesting an adaptation to unemployment.

A longitudinal study of Dutch technical college graduates (Schaufeli & Van Yperen, 1992) obtained somewhat different results. Specifically, unemployment was only found to be associated with psychological distress among those unemployed for more than 2 years. In addition, less psychologically distressed graduates were more likely to become re-employed, evidence for a selection effect.

Some studies have been concerned with the impact of unemployment on *women* and with possible gender differences in impact. For example, Dew et al., (1992) followed a group of women for 12 months; all were initially employed but, during follow-up, some were laid off for shorter ($\leq$ 5 months) or longer (> 5 months) periods of time. Depressive symptoms were higher only among those with longer unemployment. Anxiety-related symptoms showed no significant impact. Also, there were no differences in symptom scores as a function of whether or not the women had become re-employed. The same research team (Penkower et al., 1988) has also examined the impact of husbands' layoff on their wives' mental health. Using the Global Severity Index (GSI) of the Symptom Check List–90 (Derogatis, 1977), the authors showed an impact of the husbands' layoff, but only during the second year of follow-up; at 1 year follow-up, GSI scores were lower for both employed husband and laid-off husband groups. The elevated rates at two years were not different according to whether or not the husband was re-employed. Reports of cross-sectional results of unemployment among women suggest either no gender differences in impact (e.g., Ensminger & Celentano, 1990; Schaufeli & Van Yperen, 1992); somewhat stronger effects in women, particularly in the healthcare seeking area (D'Arcy, 1986); or somewhat weaker effects in women (Harding & Sewel, 1992).

Rural–urban differences in impact are also of interest. Dooley et al. (1981) failed to replicate in a nonmetropolitan community the effect of unemployment on depressed mood previously described for a metropolitan community. Harding and Sewel (1992), in their study of a Scottish island community, also suggest that the impact of unemployment in the rural setting may be weaker. Results from the Michigan study (Kasl & Cobb, 1982) also revealed differences in effects between the urban and the rural plant shutdowns. For example, the objective index of severity of job loss experience (number of weeks unemployed) showed substantial positive correlations with subjective indicators of job loss "stress" and with relative economic deprivation only in the urban setting, whereas in the rural setting the associations were nonsignificant and in the opposite direction. Furthermore, analyses of intraperson differences between occasions of employment and unemployment revealed the expected impact on mental health indicators in the urban setting, whereas in the rural setting, the impact was on work role deprivation scales (i.e., missing aspects of work and work-related activities). A Dutch study (Leeflang et al., 1992a, 1992b), however, did not find urban–rural differences in mental health impact.

Some studies are concerned with identifying possible *mediators* of the impact of unemployment on mental health and well-being. Financial strain is one strong candidate for mediating the effects (e.g., Frese & Mohr, 1987; Kessler et al., 1987b; Whelan, 1992). It appears likely that the mediating role is stronger for some outcomes (e.g., somatization) and weaker for other outcomes (e.g., anxiety). If one separates primary deprivation (e.g., food, heat, clothing) from secondary deprivation (e.g., holidays, telephone, car), one finds a more important mediating role for the former (Whelan, 1992). Similar findings were reported by Dooley and Catalano (1984), who identified "undesirable economic life events" as a mediator between the community unemployment rate and psychological symptoms.

The Kessler et al. (1987b) report examined other potential mediators, such as marital difficulty, affiliative interaction, and general life events, but these appeared to play a minor role. One interesting report, dealing with children's problem behavior (Elder & Caspi, 1988), showed that the impact of economic loss on children was mediated by paternal arbitrariness and marital conflicts.

Studies of possible *moderators* or *modifiers* of the impact of unemployment are more common inasmuch as there has been a growing interest in this issue (Fryer, 1992). Some of these modifiers have already been noted—for example, gender, rural versus urban setting, and the contextual effect of regional or community level of unemployment.

One frequently examined moderator is social support or related concepts such as social integration or presence of confidant. There is reasonable evidence for the benefits of social support (e.g., Brenner & Starrin, 1988; Broomhall & Winefield, 1990; Hammarstrom, 1994; Kessler et al., 1988; Mallinckrodt & Bennett, 1992; Turner et al., 1991; Winefield et al., 1993), although the findings are not straightforward. For example, pre-existing levels of support did not act as a moderator (Dew et al., 1987, 1992), but, *after* layoff, spousal levels of support ("crisis support") did moderate the impact (Dew et al., 1992). However, when the impact of husbands' layoff on wives' mental health was examined, pre-existing levels of social support (from relatives) did affect vulnerability (Penkower et al., 1988). Complex findings have also been reported from the Michigan study (Kasl & Cobb, 1982). For example, the role of social support may change depending on the phases of adaptation to the experience. In the early phases, men who found prompt re-employment showed a greater decrease in anxiety–tension (from the time of anticipation) if they scored low on support, rather than high. In the later phases, however, men who failed to find stable employment showed an increase in anxiety–tension under conditions of low support and a decrease under conditions of high support.

Several reports have also pointed to the benefits of social and leisure activities (e.g., Broomhall & Winefield, 1990; Warr et al., 1988; Winefield et al., 1992). Although this may require an interpretation similar to that for the benefits of social integration and social support, there is also a suggestion in these findings that purposeful and constructive use of spare time, aside from any social component, may be beneficial.

Among pre-existing psychological characteristics acting as modifiers, absence of psychiatric history (Penkower et al., 1988), sense of mastery (Brenner & Starrin, 1988), and positive self-concept (Kessler et al., 1988) have been identified. Additional analyses revealed that the self-concept variable operates primarily by attenuating vulnerability to other stressful life events (Turner et al., 1991). This is an important moderating process since the unemployment experience itself leaves the individual more vulnerable to the impact of other, unrelated life events (Kessler et al., 1987b).

The moderators listed above have applicability to a variety of stressful life events and their mental health impact. One moderator that is specific to the unemployment situation, however, is (nonfinancial) work commitment. There is reasonable consensus on its moderating role (Hammarstrom, 1994; Warr et al., 1988; for an exception, see Winefield et al., 1993): High work commitment aggravates the negative impact of becoming unemployed, but, among those going from unemployment to re-employment, high work commitment enhances the degree of recovery.

SUMMARY

There is extensive research literature on the impact of unemployment on health and well-being. With the exception of a very few controlled randomized intervention programs (e.g., Price, 1992; Vinokur et al., 1991), that research is based on observational (nonexperimental) designs. Potential and actual weaknesses of such designs lead to results that may be inconclusive, ambiguous, or biased. These limitations of observational data are aggravated by the fact that unemployment is a complex, multifaceted experience, richly embedded in a large matrix of other psychosocial variables and processes, and unlikely to have a uniform impact on all individuals.

The most important conceptual issue, linked to methodology, is the distinction between causation and selection: Does unemployment adversely influence health, or are individuals in poorer health (or with prior social and personal characteristics that lead to poor health) more likely to become unemployed? The evidence supports the existence of both processes, but several caveats are in order: (1) most studies do not explicitly examine selection but rather try to control for it, (2) the adequacy of such statistical controls is highly variable across studies, and (3) selection is better documented as an influence on re-employment than on the original unemployment. In particular, it is a rare study that attempts to examine both processes simultaneously. Thus an unanswered question remains: Do individuals who become unemployed because of prior poor health show a steeper decline in health status, attributable to unemployment, than individuals in comparably poor health who continue being employed?

The research evidence comes from a variety of study designs. Analyses of macroeconomic (aggregate, ecological) data involving business cycle information and fluctuations in national rates of various indicators (e.g., mortality, alcohol consumption) usually document an apparent negative impact but are too opaque to provide secure interpretations. The remainder of the evidence may be summarized as follows:

1. Unemployment appears to be associated with about a 20%–30% excess in total mortality, although a complete absence of an impact has also been observed. Cause-specific analyses suggest a greater impact for some conditions, such as suicide and, possibly, cardiovascular disease.

2. The impact of unemployment on physical morbidity is also evident, but the results are more variable and more difficult to interpret, because many indicators may reflect the influence of psychological distress and health care seeking rather than actual clinical morbidity.

3. Biological indicators of stress reactivity and disease risk provide rather good evidence of their acute sensitivity to some aspect of the unemployment experience (including anticipation), but chronic elevations in relation to enduring unemployment are seldom documented.

4. Behavioral and lifestyle risk factors, such as smoking or exercise, show sporadic evidence of impact, as well as considerable complexity of findings: Some of these variables seem implicated in selection rather than causation.

5. The documentation of impact on psychological distress is considerable, with only a small minority of studies being the exception. Furthermore, the increases in distress are typically reversible upon re-employment. It can also be noted that: (1) the impact varies in strength when examined across specific dimensions of distress/dysphoria; (2) the evidence is substantial for subclinical symptoms but not for an overt diagnosable disorder where little research has been conducted; (3) data on young adults leaving school also show an impact, but are more complicated because of the separate impact of other transitions and the importance of the nature of the first job; (4) evidence for gender differences in impact is limited, but rural–urban comparisons do suggest a greater impact in the latter group; (5) financial difficulties and additional life events are two likely mediators of impact of unemployment on mental health; and (6) moderators of impact include social support, social–leisure activities, pre-existing psychological characteristics (e.g., sense of mastery, self-esteem), and work commitment.

6. The impact of threatened job loss is much less adequately documented but can be inferred from different types of studies. The anticipation phase shortly

before a plant closes down is clearly associated with acutely elevated levels of biological variables (neuroendocrine, cardiovascular) and indicators of psychological distress. (The period of observation is too short for morbidity and mortality effects.) Longer periods of anticipated unemployment appear to be associated with enduring elevations of total cholesterol and low-density lipoproteins. High community levels of unemployment have an adverse impact on depressive symptoms of employed individuals (urban setting), an effect that can be interpreted as related to threatened job loss.

REFERENCES

Arber, S. (1987). Social class, non-employment, and chronic illness: Continuing the inequalities in health debate. *British Medical Journal, 294,* 1069–1073.

Arnetz, B. B., Wasserman, J., Petrini, B., et al. (1987). Immune function in unemployed women. *Psychosomatic Medicine, 49,* 3–12.

Bartley, M. (1988). Unemployment and health: Selection or causation—a false antithesis. *Sociology of Health and Illness, 10,* 41–67.

Beale, N., & Nethercott, S. (1987). The health of industrial employees from years after compulsory redundancy. *Journal of the Royal College of General Practitioners, 37,* 390–394.

Beale, N., & Nethercott, S. (1988a). The nature of unemployment morbidity. 1. Recognition. *Journal of the Royal College of General Practitioners, 38,* 197–199.

Beale, N., & Nethercott, S. (1988b). The nature of unemployment morbidity. 2. Description. *Journal of the Royal College of General Practitioners, 38,* 200–202.

Brenner, M. H. (1983). Mortality and economic instability: Detailed analyses for Britain and comparative analyses for selected industrialized countries. *International Journal of Health Services, 13,* 563–619.

Brenner, M. H. (1987a). Economic change, alcohol consumption, and heart disease mortality in nine industrialized countries. *Social Science and Medicine, 25,* 119–132.

Brenner, M. H. (1987b). Economic instability, unemployment rates, behavioral risk, and mortality rates in Scotland, 1952–1983. *International Journal of Health Services, 17,* 475–487.

Brenner, M. H. (1987c). Relation of economic change to Swedish health and social well-being, 1950–1980. *Social Science and Medicine, 25,* 183–195.

Brenner, M. H., & Monney, A. (1983). Unemployment and health in the context of economic change. *Social Science and Medicine, 17,* 1125–1138.

Brenner, S.-O., & Levi, L. (1987). Long-term unemployment among women in Sweden. *Social Science and Medicine, 25,* 153–161.

Brenner, S. O., & Starrin, B. (1988). Unemployment and health in Sweden: Public issues and private troubles. *Journal of Social Issues, 44,* 125–140.

Broomhall, H. S., & Winefield, A. H. (1990). A comparison of the affective well-being of young and middle-aged unemployed men matched for length of unemployment. *British Journal of Medical Psychology, 63,* 43–52.

Burchell, B. (1992). Towards a social psychology of the labour market: Or why we need to understand the labour market before we can understand unemployment. *Journal of Occupational and Organizational Psychology, 65,* 345–354.

Cahill, J. (1983). Structural characteristics of the macroeconomy and mental health: Implications for primary prevention research. *American Journal of Community Psychology, 11,* 553–571.

Catalano, R. (1991). The health effects of economic insecurity. *American Journal of Public Health, 81,* 1148–1152.

Catalano, R., Dooley, D., Wilson, G., et al. (1993). Job loss and alcohol abuse: A test using data from the Epidemiologic Catchment Area Project. *Journal of Health and Social Behavior, 34,* 215–225.

Charlton, J. R. H., Bauer, R., Thakhore, A., et al. (1987). Unemployment and mortality: A small area analysis. *Journal of Epidemiology and Community Health, 41,* 107–113.

Cobb, S. (1974). Physiologic changes in men whose jobs were abolished. *Journal of Psychosomatic Research, 18,* 245–258.

Cobb, S., & Kasl, S. V. (1977). *Termination: The consequences of job loss* [DHEW National Institute for Occupational Safety and Health (NIOSH) Publication No. 77-224]. Cincinnati.

Cohen, L. E., & Felson, M. (1979). On estimating the social costs of national economic policy: A critical examination of the Brenner study. *Social Indicators Research, 6,* 251–259.

Colledge, M. (1982). Economic cycles and health: Towards a sociological understanding of the impact of the recession on health and illness. *Social Science and Medicine, 16,* 1919–1927.

Cook, D. G. (1985). A critical view of the unemployment and health debate. *The Statistician, 34,* 73–82.

Cook, D. G., Cummins, R. O., Bartley, M. J., et al. (1982). Health of unemployed middle-aged men in Great Britain. *Lancet, 1,* 1290–1294.

Costa, G., & Segnan, N. (1987). Unemployment and mortality. *Lancet, 1,* 1550–1551.

Cullen, J. H., Ryan, G. M., Cullen, K. M., et al. (1987). Unemployed youth and health: Findings from the pilot phase of a longitudinal study. *Social Science and Medicine, 25,* 133–146.

D'Arcy, C. (1986). Unemployment and health: Data and implications. *Canadian Journal of Public Health, 77*(Suppl. 1), 124–131.

D'Arcy, C., & Siddique, C. M. (1985). Unemployment and health: An analysis of Canada Health Survey data. *International Journal of Health Services, 15,* 609–635.

Derogotis, L. R. (1977). *The SCL-90 Manual I: Scoring, administration and procedures for the SCL-90.* Baltimore: The Johns Hopkins University School of Medicine.

Dew, M. A., & Bromet, E. J., & Penkower, L. (1992). Mental health effects of job loss in women. *Psychological Medicine, 22,* 751–764.

Dew, M. A., Bromet, E. J., & Schulberg, H. C. (1987). A comparative analysis of two community stressors' long-term mental health effects. *American Journal of Community Psychology, 15,* 167–184.

Dooley, D., & Catalano, R. (1984). The epidemiology of economic stress. *American Journal of Community Psychology, 12,* 387–409.

Dooley, D., & Catalano, R. (1988). Recent research on psychological effects of unemployment. *Journal of Social Issues, 44,* 1–12.

Dooley, D., Catalano, R., & Hough, R. (1992). Unemployment and alcohol disorder in 1910 and 1990: Drift versus social causation. *Journal of Occupational and Organizational Psychology, 65,* 277–290.

Dooley, D., Catalano, R., Jackson, R., et al. (1981). Economic, life, and symptom changes in a nonmetropolitan community. *Journal of Health and Social Behavior, 22,* 144–154.

Dooley, D., Catalano, R., & Rook, K. S. (1988). Personal and aggregate unemployment and psychological symptoms. *Journal of Social Issues, 44,* 107–123.

Dooley, D., Catalano R., Rook, K., et al. (1989). Economic stress and suicide. *Suicide and Life Threatening Behavior, 19,* 321–336.

Elder, G. H., Jr., & Caspi, A. (1988). Economic stress in lives: Developmental perspectives. *Journal of Social Issues, 44,* 25–45.

Ensminger, M., & Celentano, D. O. (1988). Unemployment and psychiatric distress: Social resources and coping. *Social Science and Medicine, 27,* 239–247.

Ensminger, M. E., & Celentano, D. O. (1990). Gender differences in the effects of unemployment on psychological distress. *Social Science and Medicine, 30,* 469–477.

Eyer, J. (1977a). Does unemployment cause the death rate peak in each business cycle? A multifactor model of death rate change. *International Journal of Health Services, 7,* 625–663.

Eyer, J. (1977b). Prosperity as a cause of death. *International Journal of Health Services, 7,* 125–150.

Fleming, R., Baum, A., Reddy, D., et al. (1984). Behavioral and biochemical effects of job loss and unemployment stress. *Journal of Human Stress, 10,* 12–17.

Forbes, J. F., & McGregor, A. (1987). Male unemployment and cause-specific mortality in postwar Scotland. *International Journal of Health Services, 17,* 233–249.

Forcier, M. W. (1988). Unemployment and alcohol abuse: A review. *Journal of Occupational Medicine, 30,* 246–251.

Frese, M., & Mohr, G. (1987). Prolonged unemployment and depression in older workers: A longitudinal study of intervening variables. *Social Science and Medicine, 25,* 173–178.

Fryer, D. (1992). Editorial: Introduction to Marienthal and beyond. *Journal of Occupational and Organizational Psychology, 65,* 257–268.

Goldberg, D. P. (1978). *Manual for the General Health Questionnaire.* Windsor, Ontario, Canada: National Foundation for Educational Research.

Graetz, B. (1993). Health consequences of employment and unemployment: Longitudinal evidence for young men and women. *Social Science and Medicine, 36,* 715–724.

Gravelle, H. S. E., Hutchinson, G., & Stern, J. (1981). Mortality and unemployment: A critique of Brenner's time series analysis. *Lancet, 2,* 675–679.

Grayson, J. P. (1989). Reported illness after CGE closure. *Canadian Journal of Public Health, 80,* 16–19.

Hamilton, V. L., Broman, C. L., Hoffman, W. S., et al. (1990). Hard times and vulnerable people: Initial effects of plant closing on autoworkers' mental health. *Journal of Health and Social Behavior, 31,* 123–140.

Hammarstrom, A. (1994). Health consequences of youth unemployment—review from a gender perspective. *Social Science and Medicine, 38,* 699–709.

Hammer, T. (1992). Unemployment and use of drug and alcohol among young people: A longitudinal study in a general population. *British Journal of Addiction, 87,* 1571–1581.

Harding, L., & Sewel, J. (1992). Psychological health and employment status in an island community. *Journal of Occupational and Organizational Psychology, 65,* 269–275.

Iversen, L., Anderson, O., Andersen, P. K., et al. (1987). Unemployment and mortality in Denmark, 1970–80. *British Medical Journal, 295,* 879–884.

Iversen, L., & Sabroe, S. (1988). Psychological well-being among unemployed and employed people after a company closedown: A longitudinal study. *Journal of Social Issues, 44,* 141–152.

Iversen, L., Sabroe, S., & Damsgaard, M. T. (1989). Hospital admissions before and after shipyard closure. *BMJ, 299,* 1073–1076.

Jahoda, M. (1979). The impact of unemployment in the 1930s and the 1970s. *Bulletin of the British Psychological Society, 32,* 309–314.

Jahoda, M. (1992). Reflections on Marienthal and after. *Journal of Occupational and Organizational Psychology, 65,* 355–358.

Janlert, U., Asplund, K., & Weinehall, L. (1991). Unemployment and cardiovascular risk indicators. *Scandinavian Journal of Social Medicine, 20,* 14–18.

Kasl, S. V. (1979a). Changes in mental health status associated with job loss and retirement. In J. E. Barrett (Ed.), *Stress and mental disorder* (pp. 179–200). New York: Raven Press.

Kasl, S. V. (1979b). Mortality and the business cycle: Some questions about research strategies when utilizing macrosocial and ecological data. *American Journal of Public Health, 69,* 784–788.

Kasl, S. V. (1980). The impact of retirement. In C. L. Cooper, R. Payne, & J. Chichester (Eds.), *Current concerns in occupational stress* (pp. 137–186). New York: John Wiley & Sons.

Kasl, S. V. (1982). Strategies of research on economic instability and health. *Psychological Medicine, 12,* 637–649.

Kasl, S. V., & Cobb, S. (1970). Blood pressure changes in men undergoing job loss: A preliminary report. *Psychosomatic Medicine, 32,* 19–38.

Kasl, S. V., & Cobb, S. (1980). The experience of losing a job: Some effects on cardiovascular functioning. *Psychotherapy and Psychosomatics, 34,* 88–109.

Kasl, S. V., & Cobb, S. (1982). Variability of stress effects among men experiencing job loss. In L. Goldberger & S. Bresnitz (Eds.), *Handbook of stress* (pp. 445–465). New York: The Free Press.

Kasl, S. V., Cobb, S., & Brooks, G. W. (1968). Changes in serum uric acid and serum cholesterol in men undergoing job loss. *JAMA, 206,* 1500–1507.

Kasl, S. V., Gore, S., & Cobb, S. (1975). The experience of losing a job: Reported changes in health, symptoms, and illness behavior. *Psychosomatic Medicine, 37,* 106–122.

Kessler, R. C., House, J. S., & Turner, J. B. (1987a). Unemployment and health in a community sample. *Journal of Health and Social Behavior, 28,* 51–59.

Kessler, R. C., Turner, J. B., & House, J. S. (1987b). Intervening processes in the relationship between unemployment and health. *Psychological Medicine, 17,* 949–961.

Kessler, R. C., Turner, J. B., & House, J. S. (1988). Effects of unemployment on health in a community survey: Main, modifying, and mediating effects. *Journal of Social Issues, 44,* 69–85.

Kessler, R. C., Turner, J. B., & House, J. S. (1989). Unemployment, reemployment, and emotional functioning in a community sample. *American Sociological Review, 54,* 648–657.

Leeflang, R. L. I., Klein-Hesselink, D. J., & Spruit, I. P. (1992a). Health effects of unemployment—I. Long-term unemployed men in a rural and urban setting. *Social Science and Medicine, 34,* 341–350.

Leeflang, R. L. I., Klein-Hesselink, D. J., & Spruit, I. P. (1992b). Health effects of unemployment—II. Men and women. *Social Science and Medicine, 34,* 351–363.

Mallinckrodt, B., & Bennett, J. (1992). Social support and the impact of job loss in dislocated blue-collar workers. *Journal of Counseling Psychology, 39,* 482–489.

Martikainen, P. T. (1990). Unemployment and mortality among Finnish men, 1981–5. *BMJ, 301,* 407–411.

Mattiasson, I., Lindgarde, F., Nilsson, J. A., et al. (1990). Threat of unemployment and cardio-vascular risk factors: Longitudinal study of quality of sleep and serum cholesterol concentrations in men threatened with redundancy. *BMJ, 301,* 461–465.

Miles, I. (1987). Some observations on "unemployment and health" research. *Social Science and Medicine, 25,* 223–225.

Morrell, S., Taylor, R., Quine, S., et al. (1994). A cohort study of unemployment as a cause of psychological disturbance in Australian youth. *Social Science and Medicine, 38,* 1553–1564.

Morris, J. K., & Cook, D. G. (1991), A critical review of the effect of factory closures on health. *British Journal of Industrial Medicine, 48,* 1–8.

Morris, J. K., Cook, D. G., & Shaper, A. G. (1992). Non-employment and changes in smoking, drinking, and body weight. *BMJ, 304,* 536–541.

Morris, J. K., Cook, D. G., & Shaper, A. G. (1994). Loss of employment and mortality. *BMJ, 308,* 1135–1139.

Moser, K. A., Fox, A. J., & Jones, D. R. (1984). Unemployment and mortality in the OPCS Longitudinal Study. *Lancet, 2,* 1324–1328.

Moser, K. A., Fox, A. J., Jones, D. R., et al. (1986). Unemployment and mortality: Further evidence from the OPCS Longitudinal Study 1971–81. *Lancet, 1,* 365–367.

Moser, K. A., Goldblatt, P. O., Fox, A. J., et al. (1987). Unemployment and mortality: Comparison of the 1971 and 1981 longitudinal study census samples. *British Medical Journal, 294,* 86–90.

Penkower, L., Bromet, E. J., & Dew, M. A. (1988). Husbands' layoff and wives' mental health. *Archives of General Psychiatry, 45,* 994–1000.

Platt, S. (1984). Unemployment and suicidal behavior: Review of the literature. *Social Science and Medicine, 19,* 93–115.

Platt, S., Micciolo, R., & Tansella, M. (1992). Suicide and unemployment in Italy: Description, analysis, and interpretation of recent trends. *Social Science and Medicine, 34,* 1191–1201.

Price, R. H. (1992). Impact of preventive job search intervention on likelihood of depression among unemployed. *Journal of Health and Social Behavior, 33,* 158–167.

Robinson, D., & Pinch, S. (1987). A geographical analysis of the relationship between early childhood death and socio-economic environment in an English city. *Social Science and Medicine, 25,* 9–18.

Robinson, W. S. (1950). Ecological correlations and the behavior of individuals. *American Sociological Review, 15,* 352–357.

Schaufeli, W. B., & Van Yperen, N. W. (1992). Unemployment and psychological distress among graduates: A longitudinal study. *Journal of Occupational and Organizational Psychology, 65,* 291–305.

Schwefel, D. (1986). Unemployment, health, and health services in German-speaking countries. *Social Science and Medicine, 22,* 409–430.

Siegerist, J., Matschinger, H., Cremer, P., et al. (1988). Atherogenic risk in men suffering from occupational stress. *Atherosclerosis, 69,* 211–218.

Sogaard, J. (1992). Econometric critique of the economic change model of mortality. *Social Science and Medicine, 34,* 927–957.

Sorlie, P. D., & Rogot, E. (1990). Mortality by employment status in the National Longitudinal Mortality Study. *American Journal of Epidemiology, 132,* 983–992.

Spruit, I. P. (1982) Unemployment and health in macro-social analysis. *Social Science and Medicine, 16,* 1903–1917.

Starrin, B., Larsson, G., Brenner, S.-O., et al. (1990). Structural changes, ill health, and mortality in Sweden, 1963–1983: A macroaggregated study. *International Journal of Health Services, 20,* 27–42.

Stefansson, C.-G. (1991). Long-term unemployment and mortality in Sweden, 1980–1986. *Social Science and Medicine, 32,* 419–423.

Stern, J. (1983). The relationship between unemployment, morbidity, and mortality in Britain. *Population Studies, 37,* 61–74.

Turner, J. B., Kessler, R. C., & House, J. S. (1991). Factors facilitating adjustment to unemployment: Implications for intervention. *American Journal of Community Psychology, 19,* 521–542.

U.S. Department of Health and Human Services. (1988). *Health promotion and disease prevention, US 1985* [NCHS Series 10, No 163. DHHS Publication No (PHS) 88-1591]. Washington, DC.

Vinokur, A., van Ryn, M., Gramlich, E. M., et al. (1991). Long-term follow-up benefit-cost analysis of the JOBS program: A preventive intervention for the unemployed. *Journal of Applied Psychology, 76*, 213–219.

Wagstaff, A. (1985). Time series analysis of the relationship between unemployment and mortality: A survey of econometric critiques and replications of Brenner's studies. *Social Science and Medicine, 21*, 985–966.

Warr, P. B. (1987). *Work, unemployment, and mental health*. Oxford: Claredon Press.

Warr, P., Jackson, P., & Banks, M. (1988). Unemployment and mental health: Some British studies. *Journal of Social Issues, 44*(4), 47–68.

Westin, S. (1990a). The structure of a factory closure: Individual responses to job-loss and unemployment in a 10-year controlled follow-up study. *Social Science and Medicine, 31*, 1301–1311.

Westin, S. (1990b). *Unemployment and health: Medical and social consequences of a factory closure in a ten-year controlled follow-up study*. Troudheim: Faculty of Medicine, University of Troudheim.

Westin, S., Norum, D., & Schlesselman, J. J. (1988). Medical consequences of a factory closure: Illness and disability in a four-year follow-up study. *International Journal of Epidemiology, 17*, 153–161.

Westin, S., Schlesselman, J. J., & Korper, M. (1989). Long-term effects of a factory closure: Unemployment and disability during ten years' follow-up. *Journal of Clinical Epidemiology, 42*, 435–441.

Whelan, C. T. (1992). The role of income, lifestyle deprivation and financial strain in mediating the impact of unemployment on psychological distress: Evidence from the Republic of Ireland. *Journal of Occupational and Organizational Psychology, 65*, 331–344.

Winefield, A. H., Tiggemann, M., & Winefield, H. R. (1992). Sparetime use and psychological well-being in employed and unemployed young people. *Journal of Occupational and Organizational Psychology, 65*, 307–313.

Winefield, A. H., Tiggemann, M., Winefield, H. R., et al. (1993). *Growing up with unemployment*. London: Routledge.

Yuen, P., & Balarajan, R. (1986). Unemployment and patterns of consultation with the general practitioner. *British Medical Journal, 298*, 1212–1214.

8

Homelessness, Stress, and Psychopathology

Daniel B. Herman
Ezra S. Susser
Elmer L. Struening

Homelessness continues to be among the most visible and troubling social problems confronting the United States. The size of the homeless population is uncertain; estimates have ranged from about 200,000 to roughly 600,000 (Burt & Cohen, 1989; Dennis, 1991; Jahiel, 1992). The most recent research suggests however, that homelessness is not a rare experience (Culhane et al., 1994; Link et al., 1994). For example, using a telephone survey of a nationally representative probability sample of U.S. households, Link and associates estimated the 5 year prevalence (1985–1990) of literal homelessness at 3.1%, indicating that over 5 million Americans had experienced a homeless episode during this period.

Structural factors such as labor market changes, an inadequate supply of low-cost housing, and cuts in income assistance programs have all contributed to the increase in homelessness during the past 15 years (Rossi, 1989). Several likely individual-level risk factors for homelessness also have been identified. These include demographic factors such as poverty, gender (more males than females), ethnicity (more African-Americans

than other groups), and age (30–39 years old), as well as other characteristics such as adverse experiences during childhood (Herman et al., 1997), substance abuse, and mental disorder (Susser et al., 1993). Among these, mental disorder has generated the most research and the most controversy.

This chapter has three main purposes. First, we provide a brief overview of the association between homelessness and psychiatric disorder and consider questions about the direction of causality between these phenomena. Next, we assess homelessness as a stressor, placing it in the context of the body of work that relates stressful life events to psychiatric disorder. Finally, we explore the relationship between homelessness and depressive symptoms by making use of data collected in two large epidemiological surveys of residents of New York City's public shelters for homeless persons.

HOMELESSNESS AND PSYCHIATRIC DISORDER

The association between homelessness and psychiatric disorder is one of the most well-established findings in the research literature on homelessness. A number of studies conducted during the 1980s indicate that the lifetime prevalences of schizophrenia, bipolar disorder, depression, alcohol abuse, and drug abuse are more than twice as high among the homeless as in the general population. For schizophrenia and bipolar disorder, the lifetime prevalence is more than 5 times as high (Susser et al., 1993).

Extremely high current depressive symptoms, as measured by screening instruments such as the Center for Epidemiologic Studies for Depression measure (CES-D), have also been shown to be unusually common among homeless persons. For instance, most surveys of homeless people using the CES-D have found that the *average* score was over 16, the cutpoint that has traditionally been used to denote the need for treatment of depression in household samples (Burt & Cohen, 1989; Farr et al., 1986; LaGory et al., 1990; Robertson et al., 1985; Rossi et al., 1987; Susser et al., 1989b).

Although the evidence for an association is clear, the proper interpretation is uncertain. In particular, important questions remain regarding the direction of causality between homelessness and mental disorder. A significant weakness of most of these studies is their reliance on prevalent rather than incident samples of homeless persons. In prevalent samples, it is difficult to determine accurately whether the onset of a disorder preceded or followed the onset of homelessness (Susser et al., 1993).

For instance, although homelessness is clearly a stressor that would be expected to contribute to depressive symptoms, the findings on depressive symptoms are also consistent with the explanation that pre-existing psychological distress places individuals at risk of becoming or remaining homeless. The heterogeneity of the homeless experience, taken together with the fact that prevalent samples contain persons with widely varying degrees of homeless experience, confounds efforts to disentangle cause from effect. Another complication is that depressive symptoms and homelessness

could both be consequences of some other condition, such as substance abuse.

Moreover, legitimate questions can be raised about the meaning of depressive symptoms in an environmentally stressed population such as the homeless. It can be argued that depressive symptoms as measured by screening instruments such as the CES-D ought to be seen as reflecting a normal reaction to the overwhelmingly difficult conditions of homelessness. How many people, one might ask, would *not* develop symptoms of distress in the face of such circumstances? Based upon published data, it would appear to be atypical *not* to report depressive symptoms after exposure to homelessness. Given this, is it valid to consider such symptoms as indicators of psychopathology (Susser et al., 1989a)?

HOMELESSNESS AS A STRESSOR

For the purposes of our discussion, we define homelessness as sleeping in shelters or public places (Rossi et al., 1987). Despite the simplicity of this definition (or perhaps because of it), homelessness is difficult to categorize neatly within the context of the literature on stress and stressful life events, which typically distinguishes between acute life events and chronic stressors. Acute events, as conceptualized by Brown and Harris (1978), focus on conditions associated with significant life changes or dramatic events in a range of domains, including employment, health, housing, and relationships. Dohrenwend (1979) provides the examples of birth of a first child, serious physical illness or injury, and death of a loved one as typical stressful events that many individuals confront during their lives.

Stressful conditions that continue on a long-term basis have been classified as "persistent difficulties" by Brown and Harris (1989) or "ongoing situations" by Dohrenwend et al. (1987a). Examples of such chronic stressors include lack of social support, a dangerous living or work environment, or the conditions associated with severe poverty. In the body of work on the link between stress and psychopathology, a number of researchers have found both acute and chronic stressors to be associated with the onset of depression and depressive symptoms (Brown & Harris, 1989).

The experience of suddenly becoming homeless would clearly belong in the same category as the kinds of occurrences typically considered acute life events, such as job loss, divorce, and death of a loved one. In a review of issues in the measurement of stressors and stress, Wheaton (1994) notes the importance of distinguishing chronic stressors from acute stressors because this permits researchers to segregate the effects of a discrete event from the possible effects of the subsequent condition that the event has created (i.e., "distinguishing the effects of *getting* divorced from *being* divorced"). Similarly, we need to be able to differentiate the effects of *becoming* homeless from the effect of *being* homeless. Although losing one's home or entering a shelter is clearly an acute life event, the episode of homelessness that follows this loss would be seen as a chronic stressor.

Data we have published previously support the view that entering a shelter for the first time is indeed an acute event that generates considerable distress. In an incident sample of 223 men newly admitted to the New York City shelter system, 33% had CES-D scores of 30 or above, a rate over twice as high as we found in a comparison prevalent sample of shelter users (Susser et al., 1989b). The parsimonious interpretation is that a peak of depressive symptoms was provoked by entry into the shelter.

An acute event can, however, signal the onset of a chronic stressor, as when homelessness becomes long term. Furthermore, a chronic stressor can then generate further acute life events (McLean & Link, 1994), as when long-term homelessness increases the chances that affected individuals will experience specific life events such as becoming the victim of assault or robbery. Homelessness also could expose individuals to further chronic stressors associated with the conditions of homelessness, including poor nutri-

tion, sleep deprivation, or persistent health problems.

The particular living conditions that homeless persons are confronted with are characterized also by substantial variability. Living on streets, in subways, or in other public places, especially in harsh climates, would clearly generate a different set of difficulties and concerns than would staying in a large, institutional, public shelter or a small, church-based accommodation.

Another complicating factor with respect to categorizing homelessness as an acute stressor lies in the high degree of variability of circumstances surrounding individuals' entry into a homeless episode. In some cases, an individual may be rendered homeless as a result of a sudden occurrence outside of his or her control. A building fire, war damage, and a natural disaster are examples of such "fateful events" (Dohrenwend, 1979). In other cases, an individual may suddenly become homeless as a result of an event or series of events partially within his or her control, such as a tenant who is evicted for nonpayment of rent or a spouse forced to leave home by a partner as a result of interpersonal conflict. A young adult living with his parents might actually choose to leave the household to escape ongoing family conflict. In any of these types of conditions, the entry into homelessness would be abrupt and would therefore approximate the definition of an acute life event, but the event may be entirely fateful or not fateful at all. One might expect the event to have quite different meanings depending on these circumstances.

Some people who become homeless, however, have not experienced a precipitous fall into homelessness "from housing" but have become homeless from a setting that they do not perceive as a home at all. For instance, they may have been living in an institutional environment such as a hospital, prison, half-way house, or group home. For such individuals, whose residential histories could already be somewhat unstable, the entry into homelessness would likely not hold the same meaning as it would to those who had literally "lost their homes."

EXPLORING THE RELATIONSHIP BETWEEN HOMELESSNESS AND DEPRESSIVE SYMPTOMS

At present, we are not aware of any published data that clearly assess the degree to which homelessness can be implicated as a cause for any specific psychiatric disorder. However, the direction of causality between homelessness and psychiatric disorder could vary with respect to the disorder being considered. Schizophrenia, for example, could more often cause homelessness, because of poverty resulting from diminished social networks, cognitive and interpersonal difficulties, and reduced employment capacity, than be caused by homelessness. Nonetheless, stress associated with homelessness could contribute to the exacerbation of an already existing disorder of this type. Depression, in contrast, might more often be a result of stressors associated with homelessness rather than be the cause of homelessness.

In the following analysis we select one type of psychopathology—severe depressive symptoms—to begin an exploration of the nettlesome question of the degree to which homelessness causes mental disorder. We focus specifically on newly homeless individuals in an attempt to isolate the impact of the acute event of becoming homeless on depressive symptoms and to avoid the influence of both further acute events and additional chronic stressors to which homeless persons are exposed. We consider whether characteristics of individuals' pre-homeless circumstances mediate the risk that they will experience severe depressive symptoms following their entry into homelessness.

Homelessness, Loss, and Depression

The investigation of the association between acute life events and depression has been characterized by considerable controversy over both methodology and the interpretation of empirical findings (Brown, 1989; Dohrenwend et al., 1987a, 1987b; Harris &

Brown, 1989; Tennant & Bebbington, 1978; Tennant et al., 1981). Nonetheless, there appears to be some consensus that certain types of life events are more likely to lead to depression than are others. Although Bruce Dohrenwend's "pathogenic triad" of fateful loss events, physical illness and injury, and loss of social support (Dohrenwend, 1979) differs somewhat from George Brown's focus on events containing elements of loss, danger, and disappointment (Brown & Harris, 1993), both of these leading investigators implicate loss events as being particularly potent triggers of episodes of depression.

One set of conditions that would be expected to increase the prospect that a newly homeless person would become depressed is losing housing in combination with being rejected by his or her family. Brown proposes that danger, loss, and disappointment are key aspects of stressors that increase the likelihood that depression will ensue. He notes that "loss and disappointment can concern a person, role, or cherished idea" (Brown & Harris, 1993, p. 249), suggesting that the humiliation and rejection that would accompany being cast out of the home by one's family ought to be a particularly potent trigger of depressive symptoms. Following this logic, we hypothesized that persons for whom the event of becoming homeless coincided with extrusion from a family living arrangement would experience this event as a more severe stressor than would persons whose homelessness did not also involve loss of a family living arrangement. We therefore expected to observe higher levels of depressive symptoms in such individuals during the early stages of their initial homeless episodes.

Method

Subjects

The analysis we report below makes use of an unusually large sample of homeless men collected in two successive epidemiological surveys of New York City's public shelter system for homeless adults. The purpose of these surveys, conducted in 1985 and 1987, was to provide city and state government agencies with descriptive data on the shelter population so that the levels of need for specific housing, social, and health services could be estimated accurately. The interview protocol included a comprehensive range of measures of homeless persons' life experiences, demographic background, housing history, psychiatric status, and service needs.

The sampling procedure provided a reasonably representative sample of homeless people residing in all public shelters for single adults. We obtained 2523 completed interviews (1092 in 1985 and 1260 in 1987). Because the methods and results were essentially similar in both studies, we combined the data from both for the following analyses. Additional detail on these studies' methods and findings are available elsewhere (Herman et al., 1993; Struening, 1987, 1989; Struening & Padgett, 1990; Susser et al., 1989b). Because of the relatively small number of women interviewed, the present analysis used male subjects only ($n = 1738$).

Because our hypothesis concerned individuals whose onset of homelessness was relatively recent, we included in the analysis only those men who were in their initial homeless episode. In addition, the episode must have begun no longer than 90 days prior to their interview. This was achieved by computing the number of days between the interview date and the date of onset of initial homelessness provided by the respondent. After applying these criteria, 262 cases remained for whom complete data were available.

Measures

Depressive symptoms during the week preceding the interview were measured with a modified 20 item version of the self-report CES-D scale (Radloff, 1977; Weissman et al., 1977) that has demonstrated high internal consistency reliability (alpha coefficients between .86 and .90) in earlier studies of homeless shelter users (Struening, 1989;

Susser et al., 1989b). In accord with our previous reports on depression within this sample, CES-D scores of 30 and above were defined as severe depressive symptoms (Herman et al., 1994; Susser et al., 1988, 1989b).

Respondents were asked with whom they were living immediately before their initial homeless episode. Based upon their response to this question, we classified respondents into one of the following five groups: lived alone, lived with spouse, lived with parent(s), lived with other relative(s), and lived with nonrelative(s).

Data Analysis

We compared the prevalence of current severe depressive symptoms among men in each of the five groups indicating with whom they were living immediately preceding their initial homeless episode. We then collapsed the groups to compare the prevalence of depressive severe symptoms among those who lived with family with the prevalence among those who did not live with family. We tested the strength of this association by computing a relative risk (RR) ratio with 95% confidence intervals (CIs).

In a logistic regression analysis, we examined the association between prehomeless living situation (with family vs. not with family) and severe depressive symptoms after controlling for the following potential confounding variables: age; ethnicity (African-American vs. other); education (high school graduate or more vs. less than high school graduate); drug abuse (ever hospitalized for drug problems); alcohol abuse (ever hospitalized for alcohol problems); previous psychiatric hospitalization; and current psychoticism (two or more symptoms on a self-report seven-item scale adapted from the Psychiatric Epidemiology Research Instrument (Dohrenwend et al., 1980; Shrout et al., 1988).

Results

Consistent with previous studies of the homeless population, high levels of depres-

Table 8.1. Prevalence of current severe depressive symptoms (CES-D $\geq$ 30) by whom subject lived with immediately before initial homelessness ($n = 262$)

Severe depressive symptoms	Prehomeless living situation				
	Alone ($n = 75$)	Nonrelatives ($n = 41$)	Spouse ($n = 55$)	Parents ($n = 45$)	Other relatives ($n = 46$)
Yes	2	2	6	9	5
No	73	39	49	36	41
Prevalence rate (%)	2.7	4.9	10.9	20.0	10.9

sive symptoms were common overall. The mean CES-D score was 14.9, and 38.5% of respondents had scores of 16 or greater. Twenty-four of the 262 individuals (9.2%) had scores of 30 or greater, meeting our criteria for severe depressive symptoms among the homeless. The distribution of prehomeless living situations was as follows: 75 (28.6%) lived alone; 55 (21%) lived with a spouse; 45 (17.2%) lived with one or two parents; 46 (17.6%) lived with one or more other relatives; and 41 (15.6%) lived with nonrelatives. In total, 146 individuals (55.7%) reported that they were living with family members immediately prior to the onset of their initial homeless episode. As would be expected, the mean age of this group was significantly lower than that of the group that had not lived with relatives (30.7 vs. 36.4, $p < .001$); however, the two groups did not differ significantly on education, drug or alcohol problems, self-rated health status, previous psychiatric hospitalization, or current psychotic symptoms.

Table 8.1 compares the prevalence rates of severe depressive symptoms within each of these groups. As we hypothesized, subjects who were living with family before their homeless onset were more likely to report severe depressive symptoms than were subjects who were not living with family members. The highest rate of depressive symptoms was found in the group that had lived with parents—roughly 9 times higher than the rate among those living alone (RR = 9.1; 95% CIs = 1.9, 44.5). When we collapsed the groups and compared those living with relatives versus those not living with

relatives (Table 8.2), the with-relatives group was significantly more likely to report severe depressive symptoms (RR = 4.4; 95% CIs = 1.5, 13.4). This result was undiminished in the logistic regression analysis controlling for potential confounders.

DISCUSSION

These findings suggest that loss of social and emotional support could operate as a powerful cause of depression, even in the context of severe environmental stress associated with homelessness. Becoming homeless and entering a public shelter (by all accounts, a dangerous and intimidating place in which to live) must be viewed, in themselves, as highly stressful experiences. Such events would be expected to generate depressive symptoms in most persons unfortunate enough to experience them. This is supported by the findings of numerous surveys of homeless samples that have consistently found high levels of depressive symptoms to be quite common overall. Under these circumstances, it is perhaps surprising that the risk factor we considered—loss of family support—would appear to exert such a strong effect.

In his more recent work, Brown has begun to specify the relationship between particular types of stressful life events and various forms of psychopathology. He posits that depression is likely to result from psychologically meaningful events that involve loss, disappointment, and danger and has provided fairly strong empirical evidence for his assertion (Brown & Harris, 1993). Our

Table 8.2. Prevalence of current severe depressive symptoms (CES-D ≥ 30) by whether or not subject lived with family members immediately before initial homelessness ($n = 262$)[a]

Severe depressive symptoms	Lived with family	
	Yes ($n = 146$)	No ($n = 116$)
Yes	20	4
No	126	112
Prevalence rate (%)	13.7	3.4

[a]Relative risk = 4.4; 95% confidence interval = 1.5, 13.4.

findings are consistent with Brown's hypothesis in that, although many types of stressful events and conditions are associated with homelessness, it seems possible that some significant proportion of the depressive symptoms observed in this population could be attributed to the loss of family support that, for many, coincides with the onset of homelessness.

Although these data are consistent with such a hypothesis, there are other plausible explanations for the observed association between prehomeless living situation and depressive symptoms. Our model assumes that the elevated rates of severe depressive symptoms we observed in the group whose homelessness was preceded by living with family was in large part caused by the stressful event of becoming homeless and the associated loss of family support. As Dohrenwend points out, however, the impact of recent life events can be confounded with the stress associated with a stressful "ongoing situation" (Dohrenwend et al., 1987b). In this case, it is certainly possible that those men who were living with their family prior to homelessness may have been in the midst of ongoing difficulties and conflict with the very household members with whom they were living. If this were true, their elevated levels of depressive symptoms, possibly attributable to these difficulties, could have preceded their onset of homelessness or even have been relieved somewhat by becoming homeless. Without measures of depressive symptoms that precede the home-

less episode, such explanations cannot be definitively ruled out.

In addition, we have employed a rather limited proxy measure to identify those men whom we have categorized as having experienced the risk factor of emotional loss. Knowing little about the quality of their relationship with their family members and about the circumstances that led to their homelessness, our measure must be seen as only the roughest indicator that a serious loss occurred. No doubt there were cases in which men not living with family members prior to homelessness also experienced significant loss of social support from friends or other nonfamily sources of support. It is also plausible that some individuals who were living with relatives before the onset of homelessness experienced little or no emotional loss because the strength of their family relationships could have deteriorated markedly as a result of interpersonal problems, substance abuse, or other factors.

To explore these issues further, we examined the responses that subjects gave to a single open-ended question about their main reason for leaving the living arrangement that preceded their initial homeless episode. We then coded these responses into the following five categories: personal choice (i.e., wanted to leave, wanted to try something new); a fateful event (i.e., a fire or other building disaster); economic reasons (i.e., could not pay rent, evicted); interpersonal conflict (i.e., divorce, could not get along with family, conflict with friends);

and other (crowded conditions, violence in the building). In an attempt to control for the possibility that the elevated rate of depressive symptoms we observed in subjects whose homelessness coincided with family loss was actually attributable to family conflict that preceded their onset of homelessness, we removed from the analysis all cases in which the respondents said they left their residence because of interpersonal problems ($n = 61$). We then repeated the analysis with the remaining 185 subjects for whom this information was available. Within this subsample, 14 of 85 (16.5%) of those who lived with family before homelessness experienced severe depressive symptoms, while only 3 of 100 (3%) of those who did not live with family experienced such symptoms (RR = 6.4; 95% CIs = 1.8, 23). These results are essentially similar to those obtained in the original analysis.

We are aware that we cannot draw firm conclusions based upon these findings. Nonetheless, we have employed data on a sample that permits us to best approximate the impact of homelessness on psychopathology—that is, newly homeless men. We also note that, although we have focused on homelessness as a precipitant of pathology, it is likely to have an important impact on the course of existing disorder as well.

CONCLUSION

Although homelessness and psychiatric disorder are indeed associated, the nature of their relationship has yet to be investigated carefully. Many questions remain about the direction of causality between homelessness and specific psychiatric disorders such as schizophrenia and depression. Definitive answers to such questions must await further research, but the analysis we have described sheds some light on a potentially important mediating factor—separation from family members—that may be involved in the genesis of depressive symptoms among some homeless persons. Longitudinal research designs that follow cohorts of individuals at high risk for homelessness will be needed in

order to provide more conclusive evidence regarding these questions.

Acknowledgments: This study was supported in part by the following grants and contracts: a Scientist Development Award to Dr. Herman from the National Institute of Mental Health (NIMH) (K20 MH01204); a research grant from NIMH (RO1 MH46130; Elmer L. Struening, Prinicipal Investigator); and a contract with the New York City Department of Mental Health, Mental Retardation & Alcoholism Services (#NYC 92-206).

REFERENCES

Brown, G. (1989). Life events and measurement. In G. Brown & T. Harris (Eds.), *Life events and illness.* (pp. 3–45). New York: The Guilford Press.

Brown, G., & Harris, T. (1978). *The social origins of depression: A study of psychiatric disorder in women.* London: Tavistock Publications.

Brown, G., & Harris, T. (1989). Depression. In G. Brown & T. Harris (Eds.), *Life events and illness* (pp. 49–93). New York: The Guilford Press.

Brown, G., & Harris, T. (1993). Aetiology of anxiety and depressive disorders in an inner-city population. 1. Early adversity. *Psychological Medicine, 23,* 143–154.

Burt, M., & Cohen, B. (1989). *America's homeless: Numbers, characteristics, and programs that serve them.* Washington, DC: Urban Institute Press.

Culhane, D., Dejowski, E., Ibanez, J., Needham, E., & Macchi, I. (1994). Public shelter admission rates in Philadelphia and New York City: The implications of turnover on sheltered population counts. *Housing Policy Debate, 5,* 107–140.

Dennis, M. (1991). Changing the conventional rules: Surveying homeless people in nonconventional locations. *Housing Policy Debate, 2,* 701–732.

Dohrenwend, B. (1979). Stressful life events and psychopathology: Some issues of theory and method. In J. Barrett, R. Rose, & G. Klerman (Eds.), *Stress and mental disorder* (pp. 1–15). New York: Raven Press.

Dohrenwend, B., Levav, I., Shrout, P., Link, B., Skodol, A., & Martin, J. (1987a). Life stress and psychopathology: Progress on research begun with Barbara Snell Dohrenwend.

American Journal of Community Psychology,
15, 677–715.

Dohrenwend, B., Link, B., Kern, R., Shrout, P.,
& Markowitz, J. (1987b). Measuring life
events: The problem of variability within event
categories. In B. Cooper (Ed.), *The epidemi-*
ology of psychiatric disorders (pp. 103–118).
Baltimore: The Johns Hopkins University
Press.

Dohrenwend, B., Shrout, P., & Egri, G. (1980).
Nonspecific psychological distress and other
dimensions of psychopathology: Measures for
use in the general population. *Archives of*
General Psychiatry, 37, 12–36.

Farr, R., Koegel, P., & Burnam, A. (1986). *A*
study of homelessness and mental illness in the
skid row area of Los Angeles. Los Angeles: Los
Angeles County Department of Mental
Health.

Harris, T., & Brown, G. (1989). The LEDS findings in the context of other research: An overview. In G. Brown & T. Harris (Eds.), *Life*
events and illness (pp. 385–437). New York:
The Guilford Press.

Herman, D., Struening, E., & Barrow, S. (1993).
Self-rated need for mental health services
among homeless adults. *Hospital and Com-*
munity Psychiatry, 44, 1181–1183.

Herman, D., Susser, E., & Struening, E. (1994).
Childhood out-of-home care and current depressive symptoms among homeless adults.
American Journal of Public Health, 84, 1849–
1851.

Herman, D., Susser, E., Link B., & Struening,
E. (1997). Adverse childhood experiences: Are
they risk factors for adult homelessness?
American Journal of Public Health, 87, 249–
255.

Jahiel, R. (1992). The size of the homeless population. In R. Jahiel (Eds.), *Homelessness: A*
prevention-oriented approach (pp. 337–359).
Baltimore: The Johns Hopkins University
Press.

LaGory, M., Ritchey, F., & Mullis, J. (1990). Depression among the homeless. *Journal of*
Health and Social Behavior, 31, 87–101.

Link, B., Susser, E., Stueve, A., Phelan, J.,
Moore, R., & Struening, E. (1994). Lifetime
and five-year prevalence of homelessness in
the United States. *American Journal of Public*
Health, 84, 1907–1912.

McLean, D., & Link, B. (1994). Unraveling complexity: Strategies to refine concepts, measures, and research designs in the study of life
events and mental health. In W. Avison & I.

Gotlib (Eds.), *Stress and mental health: Con-*
temporary issues and prospects for the future
(pp. 15–42). New York: Plenum.

Radloff, L. (1977). The CES-D scale: A self-
report depression scale for research in the
general population. *Applied Psychological*
Measurement, 1, 385–401.

Robertson, M., Ropers, R., & Boyer, R. (1985).
The homeless in Los Angeles County: An empirical assessment. In *Federal response to the*
homeless crisis. Hearings before a Subcommit-
tee of the Committee on Government Opera-
tions, House of Representatives, Ninety-eighth
Congress (pp. 984–1108). Washington, DC:
U.S. House of Representatives.

Rossi, P. (1989). *Down and out in America: The*
origins of homelessness. Chicago: University of
Chicago Press.

Rossi, P., Wright, J., Fisher, G., & Willis, G.
(1987). The urban homeless: estimating composition and size. *Science, 235,* 1336–1341.

Shrout, P., Lyons, M., Dohrenwend, B., Skodol,
A., Solomon, M., & Kass, F. (1988). Changing
time frames on symptom inventories: Effects
on the Psychiatric Epidemiology Research Interview. *Journal of Consulting and Clinical*
Psychology, 56, 267–272.

Struening, E. (1987). *A study of residents of the*
New York City shelter system: Report to the
New York City Department of Mental Health,
Mental Retardation and Alcoholism Services.
New York: New York State Psychiatric Insti-
tute, Epidemiology of Mental Disorders Re-
search Department.

Struening, E. (1989). *A study of residents of the*
New York City shelter system for homeless
adults. New York: New York State Psychiatric
Institute, Epidemiology of Mental Disorders
Research Department.

Struening, E., & Padgett, D. (1990). Physical
health status, substance use and abuse, and
mental disorders among homeless adults.
Journal of Social Issues, 46, 65–81.

Susser, E., Conover, S., & Struening, E. (1988).
Homelessness and mental illness: Epidemiolog-
ical aspects. New York: New York State Psychiatric Institute, Epidemiology of Mental
Disorders Research Department.

Susser, E., Conover, S., & Struening, E. (1989a).
Problems of epidemiologic method in assessing the type and extent of mental illness
among homeless adults. *Hospital and Com-*
munity Psychiatry, 40, 261–265.

Susser, E., Moore, R., & Link, B. (1993). Risk
factors for homelessness. *American Journal of*
Epidemiology, 15, 546–556.

Susser, E., Struening, E., & Conover, S. (1989b). Psychiatric problems in homeless men. *Archives of General Psychiatry, 46,* 845–850.

Tennant, C., & Bebbington, P. (1978). The social causation of depression: A critique of the work of Brown and his colleagues. *Psychological Medicine, 8,* 565–575.

Tennant, C., Bebbington, P., & Hurry, J. (1981). The role of life events in depressive illness: Is there a substantial causal relation? *Psychological Medicine, 11,* 379–389.

Weissman, M., Pottenger, M., Prusoff, B., & Locke, B. (1977). Assessing depressive symptoms in five psychiatric populations: A validation study. *American Journal of Epidemiology, 106,* 203–214.

Wheaton, B. (1994). Sampling the stress universe. In W. Avison & I. Gotlib (Eds.), *Stress and mental health: Contemporary issues and prospects for the future* (pp. 77–114). New York: Plenum.

9

The Value and Limitations of Stress Models in HIV/AIDS

Suzanne C. Ouellette

It is not difficult to make the case that the concept of stress is a useful tool with which to perform research on human immunodeficiency virus (HIV) and acquired immunodeficiency syndrome (AIDS). In the very first published considerations of the psychological and social dimensions of HIV/AIDS, authors employed stress concepts to do all of the following: simply depict the phenomena requiring attention (Cassens, 1985; Deuchar, 1984), systematically propose a formal research agenda (Coates et al., 1984; Martin & Vance, 1984), and formally call for a multifaceted approach to intervention (Christ et al., 1986; Holland & Tross, 1985). Stress concepts provided an effective way to make the point that society needed to recognize and respond to the epidemic through more than biomedical means; stress concepts served to represent the political, institutional, cultural, historical, and psychological realities of HIV/AIDS.

STRESS MODELS AS FREQUENT ELEMENTS IN THE HIV/AIDS DISCOURSE

From the beginning, more than isolated concepts concerning stress and HIV/AIDS

were presented. As early as 1984, discussions began to appear in the literature on HIV/AIDS that applied the major components of elaborated stress models as well as the hypothesized relationships between components within those models. Most authors assumed a multifaceted conceptual framework that included all of the following factors: (1) HIV/AIDS-related stressors—the demands placed upon the person from both external and internal environments—as critical predictors of well-being; (2) the consequences of these stressors, which included a variety of mental as well as physical health outcomes; and (3) the function of a variety of moderators and mediators of the relationship between stressors and stress consequences in the lives of individuals with or at risk for HIV/AIDS.

Table 9.1 presents the major components of models familiar to stress researchers with examples of how those components have been represented in the HIV/AIDS literature. This table does not offer complete lists of documented HIV/AIDS stressors, moderators/mediators, and stress consequences; many more entries could be added to each of the columns. Instead, it provides an over-

Table 9.1. Major components of the stress process: examples of their use in HIV/AIDS research

Stressors	Stress moderators and mediators	Stress consequences
HIV testing	Income	Depressive symptoms
Presence and extent of HIV symptoms (e.g., neurological changes)	Education	Depressive disorder
	Social support	General distress
	Hope	AIDS-specific distress
Deaths of lovers, family, and friends	Active versus passive coping	Physical illness progression
Discrimination and stigmatization	Sense of control, hardiness	Change in immune function
	Low- versus high-risk sexual practices	

view of the kinds of stress-related issues that have been studied.

Stress Models in HIV/AIDS Research

Stressors

Relevant to the component "stressors," researchers often inquire about events connected with the illness experience itself, such as testing for HIV (Jacobsen et al., 1990) and the extent of symptomatology (Ostrow et al., 1989). Such factors have been documented to be predictors of mental health. There is also evidence for the health-damaging effects of stressful events that speak of the interpersonal and social demands of the illness—events such as the multiple loss through death of lovers, close friends, and family members (Goodkin et al., 1996; Martin & Dean, 1993). Interview studies have been conducted both with intravenous drug users (Demas et al., 1995) and with women who are HIV positive (Semple et al., 1993) for the purpose of identifying the HIV/AIDS stressors distinctive to the experience of the two groups. Results show that these groups, like groups of gay and bisexual men reported in the literature, experience multiple stressors, some of which are common to all groups. Among the common stressors are general symptoms of HIV, such as fatigue, uncertainty about the illness, and events involving other members of one's social network. Stressors that emerge as more group specific include the drug users' perception of a particular kind of social stigma and women's stressors that

involve gynecological problems (e.g., amenorrhea) and child and family needs.

Also among the stressors associated with HIV/AIDS are those of a "macro" or broad-based structural and political nature. These stressors include the occurrence (not simply the perception) of homophobia, marginalization of drug users, discrimination against women, and generalized stigmatization of persons living with HIV/AIDS (Bunting, 1996; Goldin, 1994; Kramer, 1989; Lawless et al., 1996), as well as actual stressful events that have resulted from the failures of many of society's institutions to provide for HIV/AIDS education, prevention, and care (Perrow & Guillen, 1990). Much speculation and a few qualitative studies have touched on the issues of discrimination and stigmatization, but essentially no large-scale quantitative investigations have attempted to document these sources of stress.

Stress Consequences

Numerous outcomes of the HIV/AIDS-related stressors are also presented in the literature. From the early years of the epidemic, there has been an emphasis on depression as a consequence of the stressors of AIDS, but also a recognition of other signs of threatened well-being. In their first paper on the psychosocial sequelae of AIDS, Holland and Tross (1985) listed, along with depression, all of the following: hopelessness, uncertainty, suicidal ideation, anxiety, intense anger, and guilt. The interest continues in assessing both specific clinical syndromes, such as the major psychotic, affective, and anxiety disorders, and generalized forms of distress (Maj, 1996).

Joining researchers focused on psychological outcomes of stressors in HIV/AIDS are investigators interested in identifying the biological consequences of stressors in persons living with HIV/AIDS. Kessler et al. (1991) hypothesized, but failed to find, a link between stressors and illness progression. Using a large longitudinal community sample of more than 1000 gay men and questionnaire assessments designed to tap their experiences of diagnoses and deaths resulting from HIV/AIDS and other major stressful life events, Kessler et al. found that stressors have no significant effect upon symptoms, with the latter represented by either a drop in T-helper lymphocyte (CD4) percent or onset of fever or thrush. In contrast, Goodkin et al. (1992a, 1992b), in a preliminary report based on 11 asymptomatic HIV-1 seropositive gay men, found significant associations between total lymphocyte count and both major life stressor impact over the past year and use of a passive coping style. A trend in the same direction exists for the relationship of stressors and coping with the T_4 cell count. This alternative picture is substantially supported by a prospective study by Leserman et al. (1996). These investigators monitored 66 HIV-positive gay men over a 2 year period, gathering assessments at 6 month intervals of severe stress, depressive symptoms, and immune measures. All of the men were asymptomatic at baseline. The researchers found that stress and depression were independently related to declines in $CD8^+$ T cells and $CD56^+$ and $CD16^+$ natural killer cell subsets, from baseline to 2 year followup. Research participants who scored near the median on both stress and depression were the ones most likely to show decreases in the immune measures that researchers speculate are related to disease progression.

Moderators and Mediators

Relevant to an understanding of the moderators and mediators of HIV/AIDS-related

stressors, one finds discussion of sociodemographic factors, psychosocial constructs representative of personality and interpersonal issues, and specific behaviors relevant to HIV risk. In using the term *moderators*, investigators are typically signifying an interest in variables that set the stage for either a strengthening or weakening of the relationship between stressors and stress consequences. Moderators set conditions; they buffer or amplify the negative consequences of stressors upon health. For example, many investigators assume that the relationship between stressful events and distress among HIV-positive gay men is often weak (see "The Overestimation of Psychopathology," later in this chapter) because of the moderating function of the relatively high education and income enjoyed by many of the men. That is, the impact of stressors such as being diagnosed HIV positive is thought to be buffered by the knowledge that one has medical and financial resources upon which to draw. *Mediators*, in contrast, are typically taken to represent the mechanisms or processes through which stressors lead to a worsening of health. For example, alcohol use in response to, or to cope with, the stressors of HIV/AIDS may serve as a stress mediator if, as suggested by Wang & Watson (1995), excessive alcohol use suppresses various types of immune response and thereby leaves the individual susceptible to infections and the quicker development of symptomatic AIDS.

Providing a broad look at demographic issues as moderators and mediators, Wallace (1993) offered a model of the sociogeographic network structure of a minority urban community at risk for HIV/AIDS. Through the model, he illustrated how externally applied stressors can cause the breakdown of formerly integrated groups and the associated disruption of economic opportunity, youth socialization, and mechanisms for social control. He argued that this breakdown can, in turn, limit the effectiveness of programs designed to curb the spread of HIV. Several papers with a more psychological orientation have reported the moderating and mediating roles of different forms of social support. For example, Hays et al., (1992) showed that gay and bisexual men's satisfaction with the informational support they receive moderates the negative effects of HIV symptoms; Lackner et al., (1993), in their longitudinal cohort study of both HIV-positive and -negative gay men, found that a subjective sense of integration in one's community remained a stable predictor of mental health over three testing periods. The picture of support is both complicated and enhanced by more recent studies. In a study of HIV-positive youth (Rotheram-Borus et al., 1996), investigators found that the high social support that the interviewed adolescents report receiving from parents, friends, and romantic partners—significant others who were also described as often engaging in sexual and substance use risk activities—did not lessen the youths' distress. These results stand in interesting contrast to those of a social support study with low-income, urban, drug-using mothers of young children (Black et al., 1994). In that research, HIV-positive mothers reported more positive attitudes and behaviors toward parenting and benefited more from social support—a home intervention support project—than did HIV-negative mothers.

Moderators of HIV/AIDS-related stressors that have to do with personality and coping issues also have been identified. Taylor et al. (1992) reported that, in a cohort of gay and bisexual men at risk for HIV/AIDS, dispositional optimism was associated with less distress. In addition, they, like other researchers, identified a health-protective role for active (versus passive) forms of coping. Elaborating on the significance of the coping aspect of stress models, Folkman and colleagues (1993) demonstrated through path analyses that (1) stress appraised as controllable is associated with involvement coping, which in turn is related to diminished depressed mood; and (2) stress associated with detachment forms of coping is associated with increased depressed mood. Thompson et al. (1994) found that, among

men living with HIV, those who report having primary control—that is, control over outcomes connected with their illness—are less likely to be depressed than those low in primary control. In a later study of HIV-positive men in a state prison, Thompson et al. (1996a) found that this relationship between primary control and distress holds only for the white inmates: HIV-positive African-American inmates reported comparable levels of control but no benefits from that kind of control for their mental health.

Last on our moderator and mediator list is evidence for the function of certain health-related behaviors. Martin and Dean (1989) reported links between the experience of stressors such as being HIV positive or the HIV/AIDS deaths of significant others and resorting to high-risk sex and drug and alcohol use, behaviors that are themselves correlated with negative changes in health. This configuration of stressors, risky behavior, and poorer health appears again in later research (Thompson et al., 1996b).

Stress Models in Community-Based HIV/AIDS Efforts

In addition to the popularity of stress concepts in formal social science research, one also finds—as early as the year that AIDS was first recognized in gay men in the United States—a practical use of stress notions by health care providers in community-based organizations. Individuals on the front lines of society's response to the epidemic conceived of ways to do their work that assumed a complex model of how AIDS stress might induce psychopathology *and* a complex model of how to counteract the process by which AIDS stress leads to pathology (Katoff & Dunne, 1988; Lopez & Getzel, 1984, 1987). Their conceptualization of what needed to be done appeared to be taken directly from the elaborate model for counteracting stress depicted by Barbara Dohrenwend in 1978. Although the majority of these health care providers may never have read Dohrenwend's paper, these early

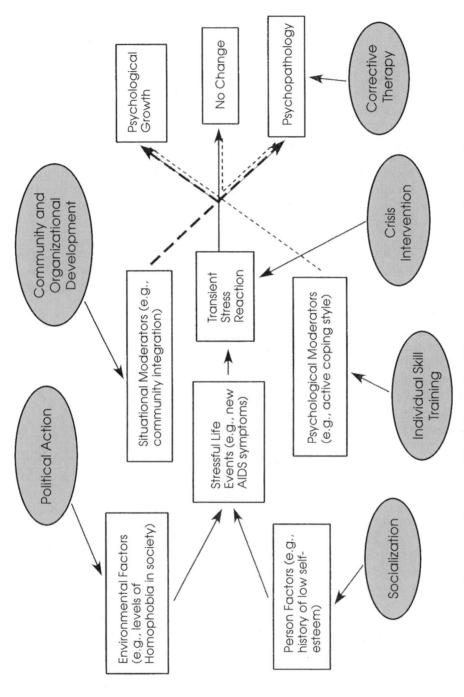

Figure 9.1. Adaptation of the Dohrenwend (1978) model of the process whereby stress induces pathology, and intervention efforts for counteracting that process.

advocates and caregivers for persons with HIV initiated a community-based response that is closer to realizing her model of intervention than is any other institutionalized effort to reduce pathology of which I am aware.

The boxes in Figure 9.1 represent the basic components of the process by which stress induces psychopathology, as they did in the original Dohrenwend depiction. They are filled in here with HIV/AIDS-related examples. The ovals represent the strategies Dohrenwend specified for counteracting the stress process. By bringing together the boxes and the ovals, Dohrenwend depicted strategies for moving directly from research findings to intervention. She described how a group interested in improving the social good (in her case, community psychologists) can use the observation of the significance of the relationships depicted by the arrows in this model to frame decisions about how best to interrupt the process. For example, if one finds a strong relationship between a transient stress reaction and psychopathology, one would want to influence that stress reaction process through crisis intervention. If the strong effect is in the buffering role of situational moderators (dashed line in Fig. 9.1), such that individuals with social support resources show no change following their experience of stressful life events while those without social support show heightened symptom reports, one would want to do something about increasing support across the community. If the link between extant environmental factors and stressful life events is most salient and determinative of pathology, one would choose to halt the occurrence of such factors and events (e.g., instances of antigay violence and stigmatization of those with HIV/AIDS) through means such as organized protest against the existing social order and demands for significant changes in legislation.

The early responders to the AIDS epidemic, in settings such as the Gay Men's Health Crisis (GMHC) Center in New York City, worked with the conviction that AIDS was a stressor with serious implications for mental health; equally important, their ac-

tions brought to life each of the counteracting strategies of the model (see Ouellette Kobasa, 1991). Gay men and their supporters who sat outside the New York mayor's office until he set up a special AIDS task force proved to be an effective form of "Political Action." HIV/AIDS activists in New York City continued their political action to include the diversity of groups subsequently affected (e.g., intravenous drug users, women) by the epidemic and prevented a second mayor from closing down critical AIDS service in the city. The founding and maintenance of complex social movement organizations like GMHC and ACT-UP are impressive examples of "Community and Organizational Development." "Crisis Intervention" is manifested in HIV hotlines; in group therapy sessions; between persons living with HIV/AIDS and their friends, patient advocates, and volunteer legal counsel; and through the many other innovative forms of broad-based health care delivery initiated by HIV/AIDS community-based organizations. Educating others in how to use safer sex techniques through neighborhood-based group meetings and informative, sexually explicit pamphlets are good examples of "Individual Skill Training."

Finally, "Socialization" to change the psychological predispositions of affected persons was instituted as the new community structures were developed in response to HIV/AIDS. In the case of gay men, these structures provided a new way of both taking social action and thinking about core identity issues (Altman, 1994; Kayal, 1993). Using terms popular among many current American and European social psychologists (Deaux, 1993), one can understand the HIV/AIDS epidemic as a basic socialization phenomenon that has provided a context for the development of new and more positive forms of social or collective identity among gay men. In the words of a research participant in a study of volunteers at GMHC (Ouellette Kobasa, 1991), "GMHC taught me new things about what it meant to be a gay man. I found a new kind of gay man there. I found cultured men, I found heros and saints working together to do what no one else was able to do." Without any formal training in psychiatric epidemiology, members of groups such as GMHC provided a remarkable model for how society might best respond to the epidemic as a psychosocial, cultural, and political—as well as biomedical—challenge.

Given the longstanding practice of applying stress concepts to phenomena of HIV/AIDS, within the health and research communities as well as in the popular arena, it seems appropriate now to ask: What have we learned from this frequent application of stress concepts and models? This question is most appropriately directed both to what we have learned about HIV/AIDS and to what we have learned about our stress models.

The rest of this chapter falls into three basic parts. In the first, guidelines are offered for the prospective HIV/AIDS researcher in the form of three basic decisions that must be made at the initiation of any new stress and HIV/AIDS research project. Next I turn to a consideration of some specific HIV and stress findings. Finally, I identify what is to be gained through *better* application of stress models and data-collection strategies. The basic point is that we have learned important things by approaching the phenomena of HIV/AIDS through stress models, but our data from these studies, as well as the more general observation of the epidemic, point up important ways in which stress and pathology models must be elaborated.

A CHECKLIST FOR THE NEW HIV/AIDS RESEARCHER

I want to highlight some of the ways in which investigators of HIV have used stress models. My aim is simply to provide prospective HIV and stress researchers with a short checklist of three important decisions that they will have to make as they enter this field: (*1*) whom to study, (*2*) where to place

HIV/AIDS in the model, and (3) what theory to use.

Whom Will I Study?

The first decision concerns the make-up of the group of research participants. Although I began my update of the HIV/AIDS and stress literature for this chapter with the assumption that the primary focus would be on those living with HIV/AIDS, I soon discovered that a large number of studies (if not the majority, when one includes conference presentations in the review) have been about people formally and informally caring for persons with HIV—not the HIV-positive people themselves. At the core of much of basic HIV/AIDS and stress research and the application of stress interventions has been the stress experienced by health care professionals, family and friends, and other caregivers (examples from the many studies are Armstrong et al., 1995; Bergeron & Handley, 1992; Eakin & Taylor, 1990; Miller & Gillies, 1996; Visintini et al., 1996).

New investigators must decide whether they will continue this focus on caregivers or return to those early concerns raised by researchers of gay and bisexual men about the stressors faced by people actually living with the illness. The need to look at the latter has certainly been confirmed and extended by research that documents the stress experience of women and drug users, groups now hit the hardest by HIV/AIDS (Demas et al., 1995; Semple et al., 1993). New investigators might also very choose a more complicated but compelling course for research that appears not to have been taken: the simultaneous observation of the person living with HIV/AIDS *and* the caregivers. If burnout among physicians working with HIV/AIDS patients is as much of a problem as articles in major newspapers as well as professional journals (e.g., Silverman, 1993) would have us believe, then it is time empirically to establish the direct impact of this burnout, not only on the physicians' well-being but on that of the many individuals for whom these physicians are caring. In other words, a viable next step in HIV/AIDS research is the kind of stress study that includes the caregivers' stressful life event experience and well-being as predictors of the mental health status of persons living with HIV/AIDS.

What is being suggested here is a conceptual shift from thinking strictly about isolated individuals caught in the stress process to an appreciation of the necessarily interpersonal and transactional nature of HIV/AIDS events. Studies of HIV/AIDS that take the family as the unit of analysis are just beginning to fill in some of this picture. For example, Drotar et al. (1997) compared the correlates of psychological distress in mothers of HIV-positive hemophiliac children with those of mothers of hemophiliac children without HIV. They found a significant interaction between children's HIV status and mothers' negative stressful life event experience in the prediction of mothers' psychological health. The presence of HIV in their children appeared to leave the mothers more vulnerable to the negative effect of the stressors they encountered.

Where Should HIV/AIDS Be Placed in the Model?

A second decision concerns where in the stress model—in what component(s)—HIV/AIDS is to appear as a construct. It is important to note that HIV/AIDS as a *research variable* appears in all of the major components of the model—as stressor, stress consequence or outcome of stressors, and as stress moderator or mediator.

Contrast the roles assigned to HIV/AIDS in the following studies. In the longitudinal cohort study of gay men at risk for HIV/AIDS in New York City led by John Martin until his death, HIV/AIDS was typically treated as a source of formidable stressors. For example, Martin and Dean (1993) showed that both having AIDS (or being HIV positive) and experiencing AIDS-related bereavement significantly increase levels of distress. In contrast, in the work by Kessler et al. (1991) and Goodkin et al.

(1992b), development of AIDS was examined as an outcome of general life stressors. Finally, in studies such as that by Taylor et al. (1992), HIV/AIDS emerges in the conceptualization of moderators of stress processes. These investigators focused on a form of optimism specific to AIDS and found that it is related to perceived control over AIDS and to engagement in active coping for gay and bisexual men who are seropositive for HIV/AIDS, but not those who are seronegative.

Typically, investigators placed HIV/AIDS in only one component of the stress model per research study, yet there are examples of the placement of HIV/AIDS in more than one component in a single stress report. Schneider et al. (1991) conceived of HIV/AIDS as both a stressor and a stress moderator as they examined the extent to which HIV status both directly predicts suicide intent and moderates the effects of other current AIDS-related stressors (deaths and illnesses of others and perceived AIDS risk) on suicide intent. The new investigator needs to (1) specify where in the stress model HIV/AIDS is to be placed, (2) take seriously the methodological challenges of each kind of placement, and (3) reconcile the problems of confounding that necessarily accompanying placement in more than one component.

What Theory to Use?

The prospective researcher also needs to appreciate the diversity of theoretical perspectives that have been relied upon in the application of stress models in the study of HIV/AIDS. These include the perspectives of stressful life event research (Martin & Dean, 1993), the transformational model of stress and coping as portrayed by Lazarus and Folkman (Folkman et al., 1993), psychoneuroimmunology (Goodkin et al., 1992b; Kiecolt-Glaser & Glaser, 1995), personality and social support moderator models (Blaney et al., 1992), and the social psychology of control and optimism (Taylor et al., 1992; Thompson et al., 1996a).

Especially intriguing is the extent to which HIV has provided the opportunity for the integration of two or more of these theoretical perspectives. For example, Goodkin et al. (1992a) used all but the last of the theoretical perspectives listed above in their report on the significant relationship between active coping style and natural killer cell cytotoxicity (NKCC) in asymptomatic HIV-1 seropositive gay men, and the trends toward a negative relationship of life stressors on NKCC and the buffer effect of social support.

New investigators need to decide early on what their theoretical commitments are, as well as what theoretical questions and even dilemmas might be resolved through stress research on HIV/AIDS. For Blaney et al. (1992), the study of HIV seropositive but asymptomatic gay men provided a means for considering the joint roles of personality hardiness and social support as predictors of distress and as moderators of life stress. In a regression analysis including both hardiness and social support, they found only main effects for life stressors and social support, and no interaction effects. Only when social support is dropped from the analysis do some hardiness effects emerge. These findings led Blaney et al. to conclude that additional research must examine hardiness as an influence on life event appraisals and on health practices using structural mediation models.

Another challenge that might be met through the deliberate combined application of a number of theoretical perspectives in future HIV/AIDS research is that of distinguishing between the psychopathology that derives from the disease process itself and the psychopathology that is secondary to or a reaction to the disease process. This "essentialist versus adaptational" view of distress emerges as a dilemma in the study of several serious illnesses, including systemic lupus erythematosus, Parkinson's disease, and cancer. If we can untangle the theoretical and methodological aspects of this dilemma, we can probably effectively apply our resolution to other illness situations.

Given the amount of research attention devoted to the assessment of neuropathology and cognitive deficits in persons with HIV/AIDS, the need for conceptual clarity is particularly compelling in the case of this illness (Skoraszewski et al., 1991). That progress can be made here is demonstrated in a study by Sewell et al. (1994). In a comparison of 20 HIV-infected men with new-onset psychosis with 20 HIV-infected nonpsychotic men matched on demographics and stage of HIV, they found that the psychotic patients tended to have greater global neuropsychological impairment, a higher mortality rate, and a higher lifetime prevalence of drug use. The data support the explanation that the psychosis is secondary to HIV encephalopathy, and do not confirm the hypotheses that psychosis is the result of brain damage from HIV-related infections or the result of stress from HIV.

INFORMATION ABOUT STRESS AND HIV/AIDS FROM STUDIES OF GAY AND BISEXUAL MEN

Most of the studies cited in this chapter have been based on the stress of groups consisting largely of white gay and bisexual men living in North America with HIV/AIDS or the threat of HIV/AIDS. Other groups contending with the illness—hemophiliacs, intravenous drug users, straight and lesbian women, persons representative of a diversity of races and ethnicities, and groups in nonindustrialized parts of the world—have been involved in remarkably fewer studies that take advantage of stress models and measures. Therefore, this section which presents generalizations drawn from published HIV/AIDS stress studies, focuses on data emerging from U.S.-based longitudinal studies of gay and bisexual men living with the threat of HIV, including HIV-negative men, HIV-positive but asymptomatic men, HIV-positive and symptomatic men, and men diagnosed with AIDS. These are not only the most plentiful studies but also, taken as a whole, the most methodologically sound examples of HIV/AIDS and stress research. These are also studies of individuals who generally possess a fair number of what are thought to be resources in our society. The serious implications of this characterization are discussed in the section "Elaborating Our HIV/AIDS and Stress Models" below. First, on the basis of data now available, there are three critical generalizations to be drawn.

The Overestimation of Psychopathology

Early commentators on stress and HIV/AIDS may have overestimated the extent to which psychological distress would be present in gay and bisexual men at risk for as well as living with HIV. Several convincing studies that typically take the form of comparisons of HIV-seropositive men and HIV-seronegative men, both with each other and with available norms, show low levels of anxiety, depression, and other forms of distress. These studies use structured diagnostic interviews and operational diagnostic criteria and/or self-report instruments. Joseph and colleagues (1990), who worked with a Midwestern cohort of 436 gay and bisexual men at risk for HIV/AIDS, reported no increase in psychiatric symptoms over a 3 year period of observation. Williams et al. (1991), using a standardized clinical assessment procedure, found that only 6% of 124 HIV-seropositive gay men they interviewed in New York had depressive disorder. Hays et al. (1992) reported that only 20% of their group of 257 HIV-seropositive gay and bisexual men in San Francisco scored above the clinically relevant cutoff of 16 on the Center for Epidemiologic Studies for Depression (CES-D) measure, with the mean score for the group at 9.99. Using survey data, Leserman et al., (1992) found that 52 asymptomatic HIV-positive gay men did not have noteworthy depressive symptoms or current major depression, and they scored low on denial. Looking across essentially all of the relevant studies now available, there appear to be no significant mental health differences between the seropositive and seronegative gay male groups, and current scores for both gay male groups show no differences with established community norms.

Perry (1994), a very early and consistent contributor to the psychiatric literature on HIV/AIDS until his death, usefully reviewed the work on depression that had been done during the first decade of systematic research. Taken chronologically, the literature shifted from articles in the early years of the epidemic that relied on clinical impressions and chart reviews to the more methodologically sound later work that used large samples and more reliable and valid data-collection strategies. That review also provided a picture of a sharp decline in levels of pathology associated with HIV/AIDS. Perry concluded that, consistent with studies on persons living with cancer, depressive disorders are the exception and not the rule among gay men with HIV/AIDS.

One lesson derived from the stress model shown in Figure 9.1 is the importance of recognizing that it depicts three outcome boxes and not just one. The "Stress Consequences" box, which represents increases in pathology, is accompanied by two others; one of these allows for the observation of no change in mental health status following the experience of stress; and the other allows for an improvement in mental state. Most of the studies done to date, both those comparing HIV-seropositive and -seronegative gay men and those comparing psychopathology scale scores of gay men at risk for HIV with normative data, suggest that the "No Change" box may be most appropriate for depicting the consequence of the stressor defined by being HIV-seropositive or the stressor of being at risk of being positive, at least when these stressors are assessed in isolation from other stresses in persons' lives.

There is also a group of studies that validate the "Positive Outcome" box in this stress model. Consistent with several theorists who propose positive outcomes of a variety of traumatic experiences (Holahan et al., 1996; O'Leary & Ickovics, 1995), Rabkin and Remien and their colleagues in New York City went beyond the documentation of "little sign of pathology" to the provocative observation of health and adjustment in 53 gay men who had been living with AIDS for at least 3 years and as long as 9 years (Rabkin et al., 1993; Remien et al., 1992). These men are actively involved in their medical care. They report satisfaction with their social relationships and jobs and, overall, find life to be worthwhile. The investigators attempted to capture the spirit of their research participants with the theme "psychological resilience and positive survival."

Further evidence for the seemingly positive consequences of HIV/AIDS is provided by Schwartzberg (1994, 1996). In intensive interviews, 7 of 19 HIV-positive gay men reported that they had successfully integrated HIV into their schema of beliefs about themselves and the world. According to Schwartzberg, despair had become a challenge, and a threat of psychopathology turned into a catalyst for psychological growth. Several characteristics typify those men who showed evidence of growth: they feel control over the meaning of the disease and can distance themselves from the it, enjoy a sense of community and belonging with other gay and HIV-positive men, live for the present, exhibit altruistic behavior, believe in an afterlife, and see HIV as conferring a degree of specialness upon their lives.

The Importance of the Full Stress Model

In the study of HIV/AIDS, as in that of other serious life stressors, investigators have been quick to move from the observation of little pathology in the group thought to be beset by the stressor to the investigation of the moderators and mediators of stress that may be responsible for keeping research participants healthy. The data collected to date on HIV/AIDS demonstrate the need to fill all of the boxes between stressors and stress consequences in

our stress model with a number of elements. In fact, review of the studies on stress and HIV/AIDS in gay and bisexual men in the United States shows the links between hypothesized moderators/mediators and outcomes to be more significant than the outcomes treated independently.

The earlier discussion of the popularity of stress models makes it clear that the following factors have been identified as positive determinants of well-being in gay and bisexual men living with HIV/AIDS or its threat:various forms of perceived social support, active and involved forms of coping, and dispositional characteristics such as optimism. Added to that list is the critical mediating role played by individuals' ability to remain hopeful, which was identified by Rabkin and colleagues (1990) in their sample of 208 HIV-seropositive and -seronegative gay men. Perceived support, the commitment dimension of hardiness, and internal health locus of control all correlate with hope—and hope correlates negatively with depression.

It is clear from this discussion that full stress models require elaborate conceptualization of stressors and examination of the link between stressors and outcomes. The studies on gay and bisexual men demonstrate that HIV status, taken in isolation, is not a compelling stressor, at least in the sense that there are generally no differences in the mental health status of HIV-positive and HIV-negative groups. A change in focus from the absolute level of depression or pathology to the relationship between pathology and HIV/AIDS reveals a firmer basis for the discussion of HIV/AIDS as a stressor. In their report on psychological distress in gay men studied longitudinally from 1985 to 1991, Martin and Dean (1993) concluded that research participants' knowledge that they are HIV positive or their experience of AIDS symptoms "represents the strongest, most consistent correlate of psychological distress we have found to date" (p. 102). In other words, there may not be a great deal of distress, but what is there is significantly related to HIV issues. Similarly, although Hays et al. (1992) reported no significant differences on depression between HIV-positive and -negative gay men and low mean CES-D scores in both groups, they did find that the number of HIV/AIDS symptoms experienced by seropositive men predicts depression concurrently and 1 year later. There are also sufficient data for the generalization that HIV/AIDS status and symptoms are best conceived of as stressors when observed in association with other stressful life events. The Martin and Dean longitudinal results, for example, show that, across all time periods, the groups of gay men with the highest levels of pathology are those who are HIV-positive and who have experienced the stressful life events associated with loss of lovers and close friends to AIDS.

A final comment that can be made on the importance of applying stress models in their fullest form, using the available data on gay men in the United States, involves a box at the far left-hand side of the stress model, "Extant Person Factors." Available results suggest placing in this box research participants' prior psychiatric status. In his review, Perry (1994) cited three studies that show "history of depression" and another study that shows "earlier personality disorder" to be significant risk factors for depression in the face of HIV/AIDS. Perry combined these findings with others to call for a multidisciplinary approach to understanding the causes of depression. He combined psychiatric risk with what he called the "strong predictor" of social support, the "moderate predictor" of severity of HIV symptoms, and the "weak predictors" of bereavement, early neuropsychiatric impairment, and knowledge of T-cell count and infection to claim that, in order to understand the link between HIV/AIDS and depression, "it may be less important what illness the person has and more important what person has the illness" (p. 229).

The Value of Longitudinal Studies

A third and final generalization justified by the available data is that stress investigators should consider components of their stress models as well as relationships between components at several points in time and over time. Longitudinal reports have demonstrated the value of looking at the stress of HIV/AIDS at times that differ in their interpersonal, social, and medical dimensions.

Most impressive are the data from the Martin and Dean (1993) study of gay men at risk for HIV in New York City. Their publication shows significant changes in how gay men are responding to the HIV/AIDS stressful life events of bereavement. Specifically, they report that men observed from 1985 to 1991 are increasingly less distressed in connection with the deaths of significant others. Although they found, through annual interviews with 746 gay men with or at risk for HIV/AIDS, a main effect for bereavement (death of close friend or lover within the previous 12 months) on pathology (assessed as depression, traumatic stress response, sedative use, and suicide ideation) for each year from 1985 to 1991, the intensity and duration of these bereavement effects diminish over time. Martin and Dean explained their findings in terms of an "adaptation hypothesis" and in terms of changes in the scientific and general understanding of HIV/AIDS that make knowing one's own status matter differently now than it did earlier in the epidemic. They called this explanation their "salience hypothesis."

Another good example of the value of longitudinal studies of HIV/AIDS phenomena is the Lackner et al. (1993) report on the role of social support in their Midwestern gay male cohort. Their data demonstrate that certain types of social support—but not all types—influence mental health, and, furthermore, that some associations between social support and mental health are stable over time and others are not. In this publication, they actually reversed a finding published in one of their earlier papers. In their first look at individuals' subjective sense of integration using 1985 data, they found that, the more connected their subjects felt with others, the more they reported distress. Their 1986 and 1987 data, however, show the reverse: the higher the subjective integration, the less the distress. They conclude that it is only social support conceived of as subjective integration—and not other forms of social support or coping strategies—that remains a stable and positive influence upon mental health. They suggest that there may be both methodological and substantive explanations for the discrepancy between their earlier and later interpretations of their data. The most interesting of these explanations relates to the possibility that, in 1985, gay men were without access to the collective gay-identified structures that developed later to form an important HIV/AIDS stress moderator in their lives.

ELABORATING OUR HIV/AIDS AND STRESS MODELS

For this part of the chapter we face the task of charting where to go next in HIV/AIDS research. We need keep in mind the three generalizations discussed in the previous section regarding what the available data from gay men tell us; at the same time, we need to include the changing societal context of the AIDS epidemic. The new challenges of HIV/AIDS require us to know about the lives of individuals about whom we now know relatively little.

Just as there are many opportunities for applying stress and stress-resistance models, so too there are many opportunities for changing those models. The apparent tension in this last sentence has to do with the notion that, although I have found stress models to be fairly powerful constructs for understanding a variety of human phenomena (Ouellette, 1993), I also think that, if science works in the way I believe it does, truly good models are those that push beyond themselves to the discovery of new ideas that cannot be contained within the conceptual frameworks established at the outset of our work. What emerges is the need to keep working with these models but also to revise them as contexts change.

Going Beyond the Groups Most Frequently Studied

It is time to use these models in their fullest forms in groups other than those consisting primarily of white gay and bisexual men living in the United States, with high levels of educational and material resources. At this point in the literature, there is certainly evidence for the claim that stress concepts and models will serve as useful tools for understanding the psychological and social dimensions of HIV/AIDS in a wide variety of groups. For example, in a comparison of 24 Hispanic and 49 non-Hispanic white HIV-positive men, no differences were found on most of the psychological factors assessed, but the Hispanic men did report more stressors (Ceballos et al., 1990). Similarly, in an examination of ethnic–racial differences among 48 Puerto Rican, 48 African-American, and 47 Caucasian HIV-positive gay men, Siegel and Epstein (1996) found that Puerto Rican and African-American men reported significantly more stressors related to the gay lifestyle than did Caucasian men. McClure et al. (1996) extended earlier research with middle-class gay white males to minority, heterosexual, and low-socioeconomic-status populations by showing that major life stress and perceived social support, along with extent of HIV symptomatology, significantly accounted for variance in depression scores.

As the research moves to include other groups such as women living with HIV/AIDS in the United States and men and women living outside Western industrialized countries, it is important that the stress models remain complex and capable of capturing all of the phenomena relevant to an understanding of well-being and the factors that influence it. Peterson et al., (1996) provide a good example. In their study of 139 African-American gay, bisexual, and heterosexual men, which employed both physical examinations and an interview, they found no association between depressed mood and HIV status or sexual orientation; however, they observed that psychosocial resources significantly mediated the effects on depressive mood of general stressful life events, hassles, and health symptoms. Unfortunately, there are signs that research with groups other than resourceful white gay men is not always as conceptually multifaceted as the study by Peterson and colleagues. In fact, some of that research employs very few of the behavioral and social science constructs available to stress researchers. For example, a study by Maj et al., (1994) reported on HIV/AIDS-related psychiatric findings from systematic assessments at five different geographic sites: Bangkok, Thailand; Kinshase, Zaire; Munich, Germany; Nairobi, Kenya; and São Paulo, Brazil. Care was taken in each country to enroll participants representing the broad population of HIV-infected persons. This study concluded that, in nonindustrialized, non-Western countries, there are more psychopathological consequences of HIV/AIDS than reported in the North American studies of gay men. Diagnostic interviews reveal that in two of the five sites (Bangkok and São Paulo), there are significant differences between HIV-positive and symptomatic individuals and HIV-negative controls in overall prevalence of current mental disorders. The self-report scale data show significant differences between the HIV-positive and symptomatic group and the HIV-negative group in all five locations.

Certainly, these data must be taken seriously. They convincingly confirm the speculation of many HIV/AIDS stress researchers (Perry, 1994; Rabkin et al., 1993) that studies would reveal greater pathology among groups lacking the many resources found in most published studies of gay men. Nonetheless, the data from groups beset by poverty, racism, and other forms of social oppression have not been taken seriously enough. What is missing critically from the report by Maj and colleagues (1994) is information relevant to most of the boxes in the stress model shown in Figure 9.1. For example, it seems that no systematic attention has been paid to (1) the impact of stressors that characterize the lives of the new research participants living with HIV/AIDS status and symptoms, (2) the socio-

demographic moderators, (3) the situational or psychological factors that might serve as stress moderators and mediators, or (4) prior psychiatric histories. A more broad-based concern with stress and fuller use of stress models is necessary to the study of such groups because it provides a better explanation of what is occurring. Vedhara and Nott's (1996) study confirmed what many other investigators have suggested. In their 12 month investigation of 61 gay men with HIV, it is measures of stressful life event frequency and *several mediators*, rather than a single mediator, that predict levels of emotional distress. The mediators they define include social support, personal self-esteem, and effective coping efforts. A broader and fuller approach also promises to offer direction on how to use the information we gather. All of the boxes *and* ovals of Figure 9.1 must be filled, to show ways one might intervene in the process through which stress leads to pathology.

Maj et al. (1994) concluded their paper with the statement that previous studies—those done in the United States with largely white and resourceful gay men— may have underestimated the significance of psychopathological consequences of living with HIV/AIDS. To bring this conclusion home, they present what is for them a very troubling finding. Of the 22 subjects who fulfilled the criteria for major depression in the *Diagnostic and Statistical Manual of Mental Disorders (Third Edition, Revised)* (American Psychiatric Association, 1987), only 2 were taking antidepressant medication. They close their paper rather solemnly with the sentence: "This is a finding on which clinicians dealing with HIV 1 seropositive persons should probably reflect" (p. 49). Such reflection may well be in order, but at the same time it is important to encourage those attempting to respond to the epidemic in Kinshasa, São Paulo, Bangkok, and other parts of the world to employ the kinds of intervention represented by the ovals in the Dohrenwend model. For example, on the streets of São Paulo, where many of those living with HIV/AIDS are young boys struggling to find their next meal, what is required goes far beyond prescribing medication; serious social, political, and economic intervention is essential. Indeed, Maj, in a later paper (1996) on HIV data collected in the five geographical sites, concluded that it is not only the biomedical aspects of AIDS but also the social rejection of HIV-positive persons that contributes to the prevalence of depression.

Better Elaboration and Measurement of the Boxes

Another direction for future research has to do with how we fill in the boxes in the stress model. Although from the very earliest discussions there was the assumption that many of the stressors of HIV/AIDS would have to do with socially based dimensions of the epidemic, there has not been sufficient development of ways of conceiving and systematically measuring cultural, political, and economic stressors or of observing them in interaction with those stressors that can be well measured, such as HIV status, number of symptoms, or general stressful life events experience. This need to fill out the stressor side of the model is particularly salient to research with women with HIV/AIDS. Many women in this country and other parts of the world are contending with the disease while also living in poverty and bearing primary responsibility within their families. A qualitative study in Australia well captures the complexity of the discrimination stressors that women also must endure (Lawless et al., 1996), yet, as this study points out, women and their distinctive concerns have been largely ignored in the HIV/AIDS research literature. When women are included as research participants, questions directed to them have often been limited to those about reproduction, with a focus on the fetus or infant. Large areas of women's lives have not been addressed.

There is additional work to be done with the stress outcomes sections of the models. More attention can be paid to what is called psychological growth, or the "Positive Outcome" box. In work such as that of Rabkin and Remien's group, it is clear that there are psychological changes accompanying HIV/AIDS that we should be able to articulate as being more than the absence of psychopathology. This lack of words for health brings one back to the gap pointed out many years ago by Aaron Antonovsky (1979). An important start on this task is a conceptual scheme proposed by Schaefer and Moos (1992) for understanding growth following life crises and transitions. They outlined three major kinds of personal growth that one can easily speculate are relevant to those living with the stressful life situation defined by HIV/AIDS: enhanced social resources (e.g., formation of new support networks), enhanced personal resources (e.g., empathy, altruism, and maturity); and development of new coping skills (e.g., problem-solving and help-seeking skills).

Another way of thinking about positive outcomes is suggested by data collected in a study of AIDS volunteers at the GMHC center. In this generally stress-resistant group, Ouellette et al. (1995) found not only few reports of demoralization and burnout but also signs of psychological growth represented by the volunteers' enactment of the stress intervention ovals (see Fig. 9.1). In other words, the volunteers display their successful responses to the many stressors of their HIV/AIDS work by becoming involved in "Community and Organizational Development," "Political Action," "Socialization" and the many other forms of intervention designed to both reduce the stressors associated with HIV/AIDS and enhance the moderators and mediators of those stressors. The behavior of the volunteers calls for a redrawing of the stress model to show that arrows can go from the "Positive Outcome" box to each of the ovals. Barbara Dohrenwend originally conceived of the ovals as descriptive of the work done by community psychologists for people beset by stressful life experiences. A development of this idea is that these forms of social change—of action within the world to reduce stress for oneself and for others—may be equally well understood as signs of psychological growth in those persons beset. In ongoing GMHC center interviews by

Ouellette and her colleagues, the so-called new clients at the GMHC center—clients who are likely not to be white middle-class gay men but women, straight men, and persons of Hispanic and African descent—often request the opportunity to volunteer at the center. A current task of this research group is to examine whether such involvement does indeed correlate with lessened distress in the lives of these clients.

CONCLUSION

A final important point must be made about where to go next. As the work on HIV/AIDS and stress is pursued, one needs seriously to ask on a regular basis, "What about this reliance on models and boxes?" The reminder that they are only models and boxes—or, better, only metaphors—is an important one. All of scientific knowledge is based in metaphors, analogues, and comparative thinking, and therefore we are always at risk of weakening the scientific enterprise by a failure to take into account the foundation in metaphor or a restriction of the view to that provided by a single metaphor. Nonetheless, in the case of HIV/AIDS, there is a particularly high risk of forgetting that one is engaged in a metaphorical discourse, of reifying the constructs, and of limiting our enterprise to too narrow a set of constructs.

Susan Sontag makes this point the most powerfully (cited in Kobasa, 1989). Metaphors are present in the study and discussion of HIV/AIDS because they protect us from the essential horror of AIDS. Metaphors are a way of containing and making manageable the grief. However, as one does this research and watches one's friends and collaborators die, one knows that at many points the boxes suddenly no longer protect us and fail to provide a way to organize and sustain our efforts. I would like to suggest that it is critical for us to stare into the reality that emerges in those events, that it is only by confronting that reality that we can continue to hope to do useful research in this area.

I find a complementary call in Jonathan Mann's (1993) editorial, written in response to the 1993 International Conference on AIDS. Instead of a guiding sense of meaning and common purpose, Mann found at the conference feelings of uncertainty and confusion among the researchers. He complained that, instead of a discussion of the large HIV/AIDS problems now confronting much of the world, he heard a preoccupation with what can be measured. Mann believes the solution and hope resides in HIV/AIDS researchers' looking beyond favorite constructs and measures, and their recognition of what to him is the basic insight gained from over a decade's worth of global struggle with the epidemic—the reality that vulnerability to HIV/AIDS is fundamentally linked to societal discrimination.

[T]o the extent that societies can reduce discrimination, they will be able to uproot the HIV/AIDS pandemic, rather than addressing only its surface features. The missing message in Berlin was that societal risk factors can be identified and reduced, and that this work will add the critical missing dimension to global efforts against HIV/AIDS and to public health efforts more broadly. (p. 10)

The stress researcher's job is to help us all better see what is in our world, even the most horrible of things, not to provide us with protective glasses that blur our vision.

Acknowledgments: Thanks to Sarah Carney and Eric Schrimshaw for their help in updating references, and for their own work that promises to elucidate the complexity and compellingness of experiences like those pursued in this paper.

REFERENCES

American Psychiatric Association. (1987). *Diagnostic and statistical manual of mental disorders* (3rd ed., rev.). Washington, DC: American Psychiatric Press.

Altman, D. (1994). *Power and community: Organizational and cultural responses to AIDS*. Bristol, PA: Taylor & Francis.

Antonovsky, A. (1979). *Health, stress, and coping*. San Francisco: Jossey-Bass.

Armstrong, K., Gorden, H., & Santorella G. (1995). Occupational exposure of health care workers (HCWS) to human immunodeficiency virus (HIV): Stress reactions and counseling interventions. *Social Work in Health Care, 21,* 61–80.

Bergeron, J. P., & Handley, P. R. (1992). Bibliography on AIDS-related bereavement and grief. *Death Studies, 16,* 247–305.

Black, M. M., Nair, P., & Harrington, D. (1994). Maternal HIV infection: Parenting and early child development. Special issue: The impact of parental health risks on pediatric populations. *Journal of Pediatric Psychology, 19,* 595–615.

Blaney, N. T., Goodkin, K., Morgan H. O., et al. (1992). A stress-moderator model of distress in early HIV-1 infection: Concurrent analysis of life events, hardiness and social support. *Journal of Psychosomatic Research, 35,* 297–305.

Bunting, S. M. (1996). Sources of stigma associated with women with HIV. *Advances in Nursing Science, 19,* 64–73.

Cassens, B. (1985). Social consequences of the acquired immunodeficiency syndrome. *Annals of Internal Medicine, 103,* 768–771.

Ceballos, C. A., Szapocznik, J., Blaney N. T., Morgan, H. O., Millon, C., & Eisdorger, C. (1990). Ethnicity, emotional distress, stress-related disruption, and coping among HIV positive gay males. *Hispanic Journal of Behavioral Science, 12,* 135–152.

Christ, G. H., Wiener, L. S., Moynihan, H. T. (1986). Psychosocial issues in AIDS. *Psychiatric Annals, 16,* 173–179.

Coates, T. J., Temoshok, L., & Mandel, J. (1984). Psychosocial research is essential to understanding and treating AIDS. *American Psychologist, 39,* 1309–1314.

Deaux, K, (1993). Reconstructing social identity. *Perspectives on Social Psychology Bulletin, 19,* 4–12.

Demas, P., Schoenbaum, E. E., Wills, T. A., Doll, L. S., & Klein, R. S. (1995). Stress, coping, and attitudes toward HIV treatment in injecting drug users: A qualitative study. *AIDS Education and Prevention, 7,* 429–442.

Deuchar, N. (1984). AIDS in New York City with particular reference to the psychosocial aspects. *British Journal of Psychiatry, 145,* 612–619.

Dohrenwend, B. S. (1978). Social stress and community psychology. *American Journal of Community Psychology, 6,* 1–14.

Drotar, D., Agle, D. P., Eckl, C. O., et al. (1997). Correlates of psychological distress among

mothers of children and adolescents with hemophilia and HIV infection. *Journal of Pediatric Psychology, 22,* 1–14.

Eakin, J. M., & Taylor, K. M. (1990). The psychosocial impact of AIDS on health workers. *AIDS, 4,* S257–S262.

Folkman, S., Chesney, M. A., Pollack, L., & Coates, T. J. (1993). Stress, control, coping, and depressive mood in human immunodeficiency virus-positive and -negative gay men in San Francisco. *Journal of Nervous and Mental Disease, 181,* 409–416.

Goldin, C. (1994). Stigmatization and AIDS: Critical issues in public health. *Social Science Medicine, 39,* 1359.

Goodkin, K., Blaney, N. T., Feaster, D., et al. (1992a). Active coping style is associated with natural killer cell cytotoxicity in asymptomatic HIV-1 seropositive homosexual men. *Journal of Psychosomatic Research, 36,* 635–650.

Goodkin, K., Blaney, N. T., Tuttle, R. S., et al. (1996). Bereavement and HIV infection. *International Review of Psychiatry, 8,* 201–216.

Goodkin, K., Fuchs, I., Feaster, D., et al. (1992b). Life stressors and coping style are associated with immune measures in HIV-1 infection: A preliminary report. *International Journal of Psychiatry in Medicine, 22,* 155–172.

Hays, H. B., Turner, H., & Coates, T. J. (1992). Social support, AIDS-related symptoms, and depression among gay men. *Journal of Consulting and Clinical Psychology, 60,* 463–469.

Holahan, C. J., Moos, H. H., & Schaefer, J. A. (1996). Coping, stress, resistance, and growth: Conceptualizing adaptive functioning. In M. Zeidner & N. S. Endler (Eds.), *Handbook of coping: Theory, research, application* (pp. 24–43). New York: John Wiley & Sons.

Holland, J. C., & Tross, S. (1985). The psychosocial and neuropsychiatric sequelae of the acquired immunodeficiency syndrome and related disorders. *Annals of Internal Medicine, 103,* 760–764.

Jacobsen, P. B., Perry, S. W., & Hirsh, D. A. (1990). Behavioral and psychological responses to HIV antibody testing. *Journal of Consulting and Clinical Psychology, 58,* 31–37.

Joseph, J. G., Caumartin, S. M., Tal, M., & Kirscht, J. (1990). Psychological functioning in a cohort of gay men at risk for AIDS: A three-year descriptive study. *Journal of Nervous and Mental Disease, 178,* 607–615.

Katoff, L. & Dunne, R. (1988). Supporting people with AIDS: The Gay Men's Health Crisis model. Special issue: AIDS. *Journal of Palliative Care, 4,* 88–95.

Kayal, P. M. (1993). *Bearing witness: Gay men's health crisis and the politics of AIDS.* Boulder, CO: Westview Press.

Kessler, R. C., Foster, C., Joseph, J. G., Ostrow, D., et al. (1991). Stressful life events and symptom onset in HIV infection. *American Journal of Psychiatry, 148,* 733–738.

Kiecolt-Glaser, J. K., & Glaser, H. (1995). Psychoneuroimmunology and health consequences: Data and shared mechanisms. *Psychosomatic Medicine, 57,* 269–274.

Kobasa, S. C. (1989). The what and why of AIDS metaphors. *Social Policy, 19,* 60–63.

Kramer, L. (1989). *Report from the Holocaust.* New York: St. Martin's Press.

Lackner, J. B., Joseph, J. G., Ostrow, D., & Eshleman, S. (1993). The effects of social support on Hopkins Symptom Checklist—assessed depression and distress in a cohort of human immunodeficiency virus-positive and -negative gay men: A longitudinal study at six time points. *Journal of Nervous and Mental Disease, 181,* 632–638.

Lawless, S., Kippax, S., & Crawford, J. (1996). Dirty, diseased, and undeserving: The positioning of HIV positive women. *Social Science and Medicine, 43,* 1371–1377.

Leserman, J., Perkins, D. O., & Evans, D. L. (1992). Coping with the threat of AIDS: The role of social support. *American Journal of Psychiatry, 149* 1514–1520.

Leserman, J., Petitto, J. M., Perkins, D. O., et al. (1996). Severe stress, depressive symptoms, and changes in lymphocyte subsets in human immunodeficiency virus-infected men: A 2 year follow-up study. *Archives of General Psychiatry, 54,* 279–285.

Lopez, D. & Getzel, G. S. (1984). Helping gay AIDS patients in crisis. *Social Casework, 65,* 387–394.

Lopez, D. & Getzel, G. S. (1987). Group work with teams of volunteers serving people with AIDS. *Social Work with Groups, 10,* 33–48.

Maj, M. (1996). Depressive syndromes and symptoms in subjects with human immunodeficiency virus (HIV) infection. *British Journal of Psychiatry. Supplement, A 30,* 117–122.

Maj, M., Janssen, R., & Starace, F. (1994). WHO neuropsychiatric AIDS study, cross-sectional phase I: Study design and psychiatric findings. *Archives of General Psychiatry, 51,* 39–49.

Mann, J. M. (1993). We are all Berliners: Notes from the Ninth International Conference on AIDS. *American Journal of Public Health, 83,* 10–11.

Martin, J. L., & Dean, L. (1993). Effects of AIDS-related bereavement and HIV-related illness on psychological distress among gay men: A 7-year longitudinal study, 1985–1991. *Journal of Consulting and Clinical Psychology, 61,* 94–103.

Martin J. L. & Dean, L. (1989). Risk factors for AIDS-related bereavement in a cohort of homosexual men in New York City. In B. Cooper & T. Helgason (Eds.), *Epidemiology and the prevention of mental disorders* (pp. 170–184). London: Routledge.

Martin, J. L., & Vance, C. S. (1984). Behavioral and psychosocial factors in AIDS: Methodological and substantive issues. *American Psychologist, 39,* 1303–1308.

McClure, J. B., Catz, S. L., Prejean, J., Brantley, P. J., & Jones, G. N. (1996). Factors associated with depression in a heterogeneous HIV infected sample. *Journal of Psychosomatic Research, 40,* 407–415.

Miller, D., & Gillies, P. (1996). Is there life after work? Experiences of HIV and oncology health staff. *AIDS Care, 8,* 167–182.

O'Leary, V. E., & Ickovics, J. H. (1995). Resilience and thriving in response to challenge: An opportunity for a paradigm shift in women's health. *Women's Health, 1,* 121–142.

Ostrow, D. G., Monjan, A., Joseph, J., et al. (1989). HIV-related symptoms and psychological functioning in a cohort of homosexual men. *American Journal of Psychiatry, 146,* 737–742.

Ouellette, S. C. (1993). Inquiries into hardiness. In L. Goldberger & S. Breznitz (Eds.), *Handbook of stress: Theoretical and clinical aspects* (2nd ed.) (pp. 77–100). New York: The Free Press.

Ouellette, S. C., Cassel, J. B., Maslanka, H., & Wong, L. M. (1995). GMHC volunteers and the challenges and hopes for the second decade of AIDS. *AIDS Education and Prevention, 7*(Suppl.), 64–79.

Ouellette Kobasa, S. C. (1991). AIDS volunteering: Links to the past and future prospects. In D. Nelkin, D. P. Willis, & S. V. Parris (Eds.), *A disease of society: Cultural and institutional responses to AIDS.* New York: Cambridge University Press.

Perrow, C., & Guillen, M. F. (1990). *The AIDS disaster: The failure of organizations in New York and the nation.* New Haven, CT: Yale University Press.

Perry, S. W. (1994). HIV-related depression in HIV, AIDS, and the brain. *Research Publications—Association for Research in Nervous and Mental Disease, 72,* 223–238.

Peterson, J. L., Folkman, S., & Bakeman, R. (1996). Stress,coping, HIV status, psychosocial resources, and depressive mood in African-American gay, bisexual, and heterosexual men. *American Journal of Community Psychology, 24,* 461–487.

Rabkin, J. G., Remien, R., Katoff, L., & Williams, J. B. W. (1993). Resilience in adversity among long-term survivors of AIDS. *Hospital and Community Psychiatry, 44,* 162–167.

Rabkin, J. G., Williams, J. B. W, Neugebauer, R., et al. (1990). Maintenance of hope in HIV-spectrum homosexual men. *American Journal of Psychiatry, 147,* 1322–1326.

Remien, R. H., Rabkin, J. G., & Williams, J. B. W. (1992). Coping strategies and health beliefs of AIDS long-term survivors. *Psychological Health, 6,* 335–345.

Rotheram-Borus, M. J., Murphy, D. A., Reid, H. M., & Coleman, C. L. (1996). Correlates of emotional distress among HIV+ youths: Health status, stress, and personal resources. *Annals of Behavioral Medicine, 18,* 16–23.

Schaefer, J. A., & Moos, R. H. (1992). Life crises and personal growth. In B. N. Carpenter (Ed.), *Personal Coping: Theory, research, and application* (pp. 149–170). Westport, CT: Praeger.

Schneider, S. F. (1991). Reflections on an epidemic. Special issue: AIDS and the community. *Journal of Community Psychology, 18,* 310–315.

Schwartberg, S. S. (1994). Vitality and growth in HIV-infected gay men. *Social Science and Medicine, 38,* 593–602.

Schwartberg, S. S. (1996). *A crisis of meaning: How gay men are making sense of AIDS.* New York: Oxford University Press.

Semple, S. J., Patterson, T. L., Temoshok, L. R., et al. (1993). Identification of psychobiological stressors among HIV-positive women. *Women and Health, 20,* 15–36.

Sewell, D. D., Jeste, D. V., Atkinson, J., et al. (1994). HIV-associated psychosis: A study of 20 cases. *American Journal of Psychiatry, 151,* 237–242.

Silverman, D. C. (1993). Psychosocial impact of HIV-related caregiving on health providers: A review and recommendations for the role of psychiatry. *American Journal of Psychiatry, 150,* 705–712.

Skoraszewski, M. J., Ball, J. D., & Mikulka, P. J. (1991). Neuropsychological functioning of HIV-infected males. *Journal of Clinical and Experimental Neuropsychology, 13,* 278–290.

Sontag, S. (1988). *AIDS and its receptors.* New York: Farrar, Straus, Giroux.

Taylor, S. E., Kemeny, M. E., Aspinwall, L. G., et al. (1992). Optimism, coping, psychological distress, and high-risk sexual behavior among men at risk for acquired immunodeficiency syndrome (AIDS). *Journal of Personality and Social Psychology, 63,* 460–473.

Thompson, S. C., Collins, M. A., Newcomb, M. D., & Hunt, W. (1996a). On fighting versus accepting stressful circumstances: Primary and secondary control among HIV-positive men in prison. *Journal of Personality and Social Psychology, 96,* 1307–1317.

Thompson, S. C., Nanni, C., & Levine, A. (1994). Primary versus secondary and disease versus consequence-related control in HIV-positive men. *Journal of Personality and Social Psychology, 67,* 540–547.

Thompson, S. C., Nanni, C., & Levine, A. (1996b). The stressors and stress of being HIV-positive. *AIDS Care, 8,* 5–14.

Vedhara, K., & Nott, K. H. (1996). Psychosocial vulnerability to stress: A study of HIV positive homosexual men. *Journal of Psychosomatic Research, 41,* 255–267.

Visintini, R., Campanini, E., Fossati, A., et al. (1996). Psychological stress in nurses' relationships with HIV-infected patients: The risk of burnout syndrome. *AIDS Care, 8,* 183–194.

Wallace, R. (1993). Social disintegration and the spread of AIDS II: Meltdown of sociogeographic structure in urban minority neighborhoods. *Social Science and Medicine, 37,* 887–896.

Wang, Y., & Watson, R. R. (1995). Is alcohol consumption a cofactor in the development of acquired immunodeficiency syndrome? *Alcohol, 12,* 105–109.

Williams, J. B. W., Rabkin, J. G., Remien, R. H., et al. (1991). Multidisciplinary baseline assessment of homosexual men with and without human immunodeficiency virus infection. II. Standardized clinical assessment of current and lifetime psychopathology. *Archives of General Psychiatry, 48,* 124–130.

10

Rape, Other Violence Against Women, and Posttraumatic Stress Disorder

Dean G. Kilpatrick
Heidi S. Resnick
Benjamin E. Saunders
Connie L. Best

Crime victimization, other traumatic events, and posttraumatic stress disorder (PTSD) are prevalent within the general population, with prevalence of exposure to traumatic events observed at rates ranging from 39% to approximately 80% (Breslau et al., 1991; Kilpatrick et al., 1987; Norris, 1992; Resnick et al., 1993; Kessler et al., 1995). Given exposure to such events, rates of lifetime PTSD ranging from approximately 18% to 28% (Breslau et al., 1991; Kilpatrick et al., 1987; Resnick et al., 1993) have been found. Most recently, within a sample of 5,877 men and women, Kessler et al. reported lifetime PTSD rates in association with traumatic event histories of 20.4 and 8.1 among women and men, respectively. Current rates of PTSD are approximately 7% across studies (Kilpatrick et al., 1987; Norris, 1992; Resnick et al., 1993). Because being a victim of violent crime increases the risk for PTSD (Norris, 1992; Kilpatrick et al., 1989; Resnick et al., 1993), it is particularly important that more sophisticated methods be used to address the complexity of this problem. In this introductory section, we outline several issues that are important in the study of the

history of violence in association with PTSD outcome in particular.

CRITICAL ISSUES IN RESEARCH ON VIOLENCE AGAINST WOMEN AND ITS MENTAL HEALTH IMPACT

Women's violence history, particularly rape, is difficult to measure (Kilpatrick, 1983; Koss, 1993; Resnick et al., 1991). This issue has been examined empirically by Koss, who found that most women with experiences that meet the legal definition of rape do not respond affirmatively to assessment questions that use the term *rape*. Both Kilpatrick and Koss have discussed factors involved in the underreporting of rape as a result of women's stereotypes about the characteristics that define typical rape incidents. Such factors as an unknown assailant and a high degree of physical injury are more likely to lead to reporting of incidents because they fit the stereotype for violent assault; however, typical incidents most often involve perpetrators known to the victim and do not usually include a high degree of physical injury. Use of behaviorally defined screening questions to assess for history of completed rape to counteract these biases rather than using the term *rape* itself, the meaning of which may vary across individuals, has been recommended (Kilpatrick, 1983; Resnick et al., 1991). As noted by Resnick et al. (1993), it is particularly important to assess history of rape within the context of PTSD or other outcome assessment, because this particular stressor has been consistently identified among the highest risk factors for PTSD across studies (Breslau et al., 1991; Resnick et al., 1993). Given the high prevalence of exposure to multiple traumatic events described below, Resnick et al. (1993) suggested that failure to assess rape history might lead to faulty inferences about risk factors for PTSD in cases where a positive rape history is undetected and PTSD is assessed with reference to other events such as disaster or accident.

Types of crime associated with elevated risk of PTSD cross a variety of crime types (Kilpatrick et al., 1989). Data on particular crime characteristics indicated that perception of threat to life and receipt of injury are associated with increased risk of PTDS (Kilpatrick et al., 1989).

In addition to the need to use sensitive screening for sexual assault and aggravated assault, it must be recognized that violence history is often complex, and many women have experienced multiple incidents of violence occurring throughout their lifetimes. For example, Breslau et al. (1991) found that 33% of a sample of men and women who had experienced at least one traumatic event had experienced multiple traumatic events. Kilpatrick et al. (1987) found that 54% of a community sample of women exposed to at least one crime had experienced multiple crime events. Similarly, Resnick et al. (1993) found that 52% of women exposed to crime had experienced more than one incident. More recently, Kessler et al. (1995) reported that 34% of men and 25% of women had experienced multiple traumatic events. Findings within populations of rape victims as well as in general population

samples of victims of a variety of crimes indicate that history of victimization is a significant risk factor for subsequent victimization (Koss & Dinero, 1989; Norris & Kaniasty, 1992; Sorenson et al., 1991; Steketee & Foa, 1987; Wyatt et al., 1992) as well as poorer mental health outcome following new victimization (Gidycz & Koss, 1991; Norris & Kaniasty, 1992; Wyatt et al., 1992). Therefore, comprehensive victimization history should be examined in research on PTSD outcome.

Other critical issues relate to evaluation of PTSD or other mental health outcome in association with trauma or crime victimization history. A major issue relates to the difficulty of sorting out the chronology of event history and mental health outcome without prospective designs and with methods that may lead to omission of significant trauma history incidents that may occur early in life, such as sexual assault. For example, Breslau et al. (1991) identified demographic, trait, and family history variables that increased risk of trauma exposure but noted that neuroticism, early separation from parents, preexisting history of anxiety or depression, and family history of anxiety were risk factors for PTSD. More recently, Breslau et al. (Chapter 15, this volume) found that several variables increased the risk for new traumatic events as evaluated at follow-up in a prospective study. Risk factors for new traumatic events that included injury to self were African-American race, history of prior traumatic events, history of major depression, history of drug or alcohol abuse, and personality measures of extroversion and neuroticism. However, the latter findings may require re-examination because rape and other sexual assault, which are most likely to occur in childhood and adolescence, were not assessed sensitively in the study. The order of onset of mental health problems and victimization history reported must be evaluated critically, as should other findings from this study about interrelationships between traumatic events, other Axis I diagnoses, and PTSD.

A final critical issue concerns the potential role of personality as a factor that might be related to risk of violent attack and/or to development of PTSD following violent attack. This issue must be approached with caution to avoid possible stigmatization of victims by those who might argue that certain of their personality traits make victims responsible for violent attacks. As long as we remain clear that perpetrators always bear the moral responsibility for violent attacks against victims, it is appropriate to investigate whether certain personality traits increase women's risk of being attacked.

One personality variable that merits such research attention is the trait of sensation seeking. As described in greater detail elsewhere (Hanson et al., 1995), there are several reasons for hypothesizing that sensation seeking might increase risk of violent assaults against women and/or of development of PTSD once such assaults have occurred. Zuckerman (1979, p. 10) states that "sensation seeking is a personality trait defined by the need for varied, novel, and complex sensations and experiences and the willingness to take physical and social risks for such experiences." Sensation seeking is inversely related to age and is higher among men than among women (Zuckerman, 1983); furthermore, there is some evidence that the sensation seeking trait is heritable (Eysenck, 1983). Zuckerman (1979, 1983) identifies several characteristics of high sensation seekers that might make them more vulnerable to assault: (1) they are more likely than low sensation seekers to engage in high-risk behaviors; (2) they appraise most situations as less risky than low sensation seekers; and (3) they are more adventuresome in phobic situations that make low sensation seekers anxious, fearful, and avoidant. Such behaviors might result in potential attackers having greater access to high-sensation-seeking women than to low-sensation-seeking women. Also, there is considerable evidence that sensation seeking increases risk of substance use and abuse (Brill et al., 1971; Carrol & Zuckerman, 1977; Kilpatrick et al., 1982, 1976). This could increase assault risk in the following ways: (1) visibly intoxicated people might be targeted by potential assailants; (2) substance use might reduce

judgment about degree of risk posed by given situations; and (3) some types of drug use might increase exposure to potentially violent members of the drug trade.

In summary, most existing research on violence and its mental health impact on women suffers from conceptual or methodological problems that include the following: (1) focus on one type of violence occurring at one time of life, perpetrated by one type of assailant; (2) failure to consider the potential impact of multiple violent events; (3) use of nonrepresentative samples; (4) use of univariate models that do not examine for complex relationships between violence risk factors and mental health impact risk factors; and (5) failure to establish the temporal sequence of violence, mental health functioning, and further violence. The National Women's Study study was designed to address most of these limitations:

1. Base rates of aggravated assault and rape cases from Wave 1 lifetime assessment were described, and detailed characteristics of these lifetime incidents were elicited using sensitive screening questions.

2. Descriptive characteristics of prospectively assessed cases of completed rape and aggravated assault incidents were assessed; such incidents are less likely to be affected by retrospective bias.

3. Lifetime history of rape and aggravated assault history as well as demographic variables and the proposed trait variable of sensation seeking were used in univariate and multivariate logistic regression analyses of risk factors for exposure to *prospectively* assessed completed rape or aggravated assault incidents.

4. Lifetime rape and aggravated assault history, assault history at follow-up, and demographic variables were used in univariate and multivariate logistic regression analyses to determine risk factors for current PTSD prospectively assessed at follow-up.

5. Within these analyses, we also included the Sensation Seeking Scale

(SSS; Zuckerman, 1984), a variable hypothesized to tap the construct of sensation seeking. This allowed us to further evaluate a potential factor that theoretically may relate to increased risk of future victimization.

NATIONAL WOMEN'S STUDY METHODOLOGY

Random digit dialing telephone survey methodology was used to interview a national household probability sample of 4008 adult women. Of this total, 2008 were a national probability household sample of U.S. female adults (age 18 and older), whereas the remaining 2000 women were an oversample of women ages 18 to 34. To correct for the effects of oversampling, the data were weighted by age and race to 1989 estimates of the distribution of these characteristics in the U.S. population of adult women. The mean age for the entire sample was 44.9 (standard deviation = 18.4). The majority of women were high school graduates (63.4%). The majority of the sample (63.7%) were married or cohabiting. Over half the sample reported household income between $15,001 and $50,000, with a substantial minority (27.3%) reporting incomes of no more than $15,000. For more detail on descriptive data from Wave 1 of the study, see Resnick et al. (1993).

Eighty-five percent of designated respondents completed Wave 1 interviews; 3359 women completed at least one of two follow-up interviews (83.8% of the original sample); 2892 (72.2%) completed both follow-up interviews. Sample selection and interviewing were done by female interviewers from Schulman, Ronca, and Bucuvalas, Inc., a New York City–based survey research firm. Lifetime prevalence of rape, aggravated assault, and PTSD was assessed at Wave 1. Descriptive information about lifetime rape and aggravated assault cases was collected at Wave 1 and about new victimization cases at Waves 2 and 3. The 3359 women with at least 1 year's follow-up data were separated into those with a new victimization in the follow-up period and those

without a new victimization. Current PTSD status was assessed at the time of both follow-up interviews.

OPERATIONAL DEFINITION OF VARIABLES

Assault Incidents

Rape

Rape was defined as nonconsensual assault using force or threat of force involving some type of sexual penetration of the victim's vagina, rectum, or mouth. Up to three incidents were assessed during Wave 1 (first, most recent, and worst—if distinct from first or most recent). Only one incident was assessed at each follow-up interview. The specific questions to assess rape used sensitive behaviorally specific phrasing following an orienting preface as follows:

Another type of stressful event that many women have experienced is unwanted sexual advances. Women do not always report such experiences to the police or discuss them with family or friends. The person making the advances isn't always a stranger, but can be a friend, boyfriend, or even a family member. Such experiences can occur anytime in a woman's life—even as a child. Regardless of how long ago it happened or who made the advances. . . .

> Has a man or boy ever made you have sex by *using force* or threatening to harm you or someone close to you? Just so there is no mistake, by sex we mean putting a penis in your vagina.

> Has anyone ever made you have oral sex by force or threat of harm? Just so there is no mistake, by oral sex we mean that a man or boy put his penis in your mouth or someone penetrated your vagina or anus with their mouth or tongue.

> Has anyone ever made you have anal sex by force or threat of harm?

> Has anyone ever put fingers or objects in your vagina or anus against your will by using force or threats?

An affirmative response to any of these questions indicated that a woman had been a victim of rape, defined as vaginal, anal, or oral penetration that occurred through the use of force or threat of force, whether or not the woman subjectively defined the incident(s) as rape or reported them to police or other authorities.

Aggravated Assault

Aggravated assault was defined as an attack with a weapon or without a weapon with intent to kill or seriously injure the victim. Descriptive data were gathered about a respondent's only or worst incident during Wave 1. Data were gathered on only one incident per follow-up assessment. Positive history of aggravated assault was defined as a positive response to either of the following questions:

Another type of stressful event women sometimes experience is being *physically* attacked by another person. Not counting any incidents already described to me, has anyone—including family members or friends—ever attacked you with a gun, knife or some other weapon, regardless of when it happened or whether you ever reported it or not?

Has anyone—including family members and friends—ever attacked you without a weapon, but with the intent to kill or seriously injure you?

History of Prior Victimization

The number of rapes or aggravated assaults occurring prior to Wave 1 interview was determined. The range of this variable was 0–4.

New Victimization

Whether a rape or aggravated assault occurred in the interval between Wave 1 and Waves 2 and 3 was assessed. This variable was scored dichotomously as negative (0) if no incidents had occurred or positive (1) if any incident was reported. In a small subset of cases in which a victimization occurred during both waves, analyses were based on data from the earliest follow-up assessment (Wave 2) for purposes of defining assault status and current PTSD status.

Current PTSD

This was measured at Wave 2 and Wave 3 interviews, using the National Women's Study (NWS) PTSD Module (Kilpatrick et al., unpublished manuscript; Resnick et al., 1993). PTSD status was scored dichotomously based on absence (0) or presence (1) of sufficient symptoms within the last 6 months to meet the diagnostic criteria in the *Diagnostic and Statistical Manual of Mental Disorders (Third Edition, Revised) (DSM-III-R*; American Psychiatric Association, 1987). Kappa's computed to assess reliabilities between the NWS PTSD module and the Structured Clinical Interview for DSM-III-R (Spitzer et al., 1987) were .77 for lifetime PTSD and .71 for current PTSD based on *DSM-IV* PTSD Field Trial data (Kilpatrick et al., in press). Further validity data relate to the consistent population- and event-specific rates of PTSD obtained with this instrument using the telephone assessment method employed in this study and those obtained using in-person structured clinical interviews (Resnick et al., 1993).

Sensation Seeking

A six-item short form of the Disinhibition-Intentions for the Future subscale of Zuckerman's SSS Form VI was use to measure this variable (Zuckerman, 1987). Scores ranged from 6 to 18. The scale asks respondents how likely they would be to engage in or consider engaging in the following activities sometime in the future: "doing something illegal but enjoyable; doing what feels good, regardless of the consequences; going out with someone just because they are physically exciting; going to wild, uninhibited parties; doing unconventional things, even if they are a little frightening; refusing to follow orders from someone in authority." Individual item scores in the present study were (1) "have no desire to do it"; (2) "have thought about, but wouldn't do it"; and (3) "probably would do it."

Percent

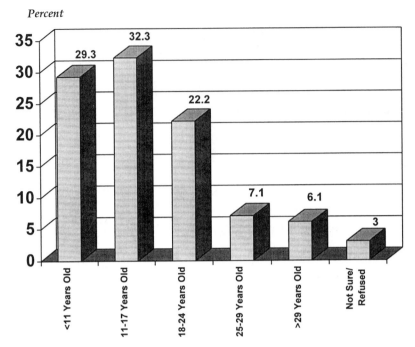

Figure 10.1. Age at time of rape among respondents in a national study cohort (*n* = 714 cases).

Demographic Variables

The following demographic data were collected:

Current age: measured in years at Wave 1

Race: African American, Asian, Hispanic, Native American, white; collapsed to white versus nonwhite for multivariate analyses based on population distribution and ease of interpretation of results

Education: less than high school graduate, high school graduate, college graduate; measured at Wave 1

Household income: subdivided for conceptual reasons into poverty level, defined as less than $10,000 in 1988; or above poverty level, defined as more than $10,000 in 1988; measured at Wave 1

Marital status: single, cohabiting, married, separated, divorced, widowed; collapsed to married versus nonmarried for multivariate analyses

SUMMARY OF WAVE 1 RESULTS

Prior to presentation and analysis of the longitudinal data, it is useful to consider some of the baseline findings about victimization and PTSD obtained at the Wave 1 interview. Lifetime history of at least one aggravated assault that was distinct from any sexual assault incidents was reported by 10.3% of women (*n* = 412), while 12.7% (*n* = 714) reported a history of completed rape. A total of 20% of the Wave 1 sample for whom follow-up data were available reported a history of rape or aggravated assault. Among this group, 33.5% reported having experienced more than one assault incident. Descriptive characteristics of all Wave 1 cases indicated that only about one in five rape (22%) and aggravated assault (21%) cases were perpetrated by strangers. Only 16% of rape cases and 46% of aggravated assault cases were reported to police. The lifetime prevalence of PTSD was 12.3%, and the past 6 months' prevalence was 4.6% at Wave 1 assessment.

Because of the thorough assessment of up to three Wave 1 rape cases, more comprehensive data about rape incidents than

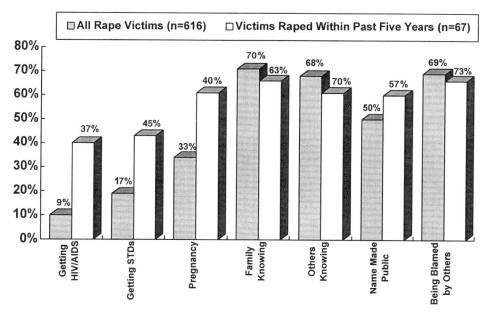

Figure 10.2. Important concerns of rape victims: all rapes versus recent rapes (based on data obtained from Wave 3 interviews).

about aggravated assault incidents are presented here. As can be seen in Figure 10.1, of the total of 714 cases described, almost one-third (29.3%) occurred before age 11, while approximately two-thirds occurred before the age of 18. Another substantial risk (22.2%) was observed for the age group between 18 and 24 years, after which the risk dropped steeply. These data on relationship with the perpetrator and age of assault indicate that it is particularly important to assess adequately incidents that may have occurred during childhood or adolescence and that may have involved assailants known to the victim.

Additional data from the NWS provide information documenting some of the potential difficulty in assessing history of completed rape. Figure 10.2 presents data from a subset of 616 lifetime rape cases on rape victim's concerns following rape incidents. Data are also displayed for cases restricted to the previous 5 year period to assess concerns about human immunodeficiency virus (HIV) and acquired immunodeficiency syndrome (AIDS) during a more relevant risk time frame. Results indicate that more rape

victims are concerned about disclosure issues than are concerned about major health problems, including pregnancy, sexually transmitted diseases, and HIV/AIDS infection. It is reasonable to assume that victims with such concerns would only disclose their rapes if considerable care was used to allay their concerns.

DESCRIPTIVE DATA ON NEW RAPE AND AGGRAVATED ASSAULT CASES

Among those completing at least one follow-up assessment period, 4.3% of this national probability sample of U.S. adult women experienced at least one rape or aggravated assault. Data on age at time of rape or aggravated assault are presented in Figure 10.3. These data indicate a somewhat different pattern for completed rape than for aggravated assault. Rape rates decrease as a function of increasing age, whereas the rate of aggravated assault almost doubles among those age 36 or older compared to those less than age 36.

Data on relationship with the perpetrator of rape and aggravated assault are presented

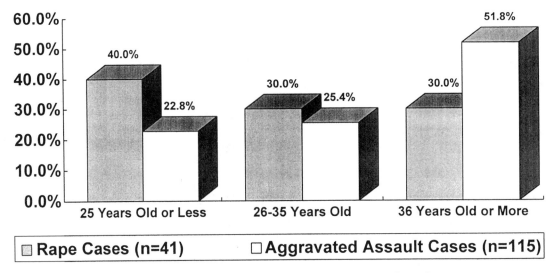

Figure 10.3. Age at time of assault in new rape and aggravated assault cases.

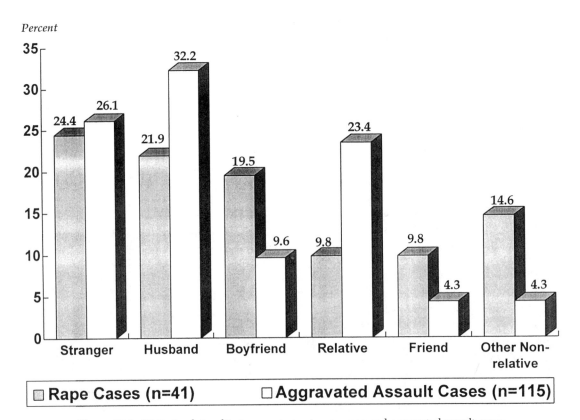

Figure 10.4. Victim's relationship to perpetrator in new rape and aggravated assault cases.

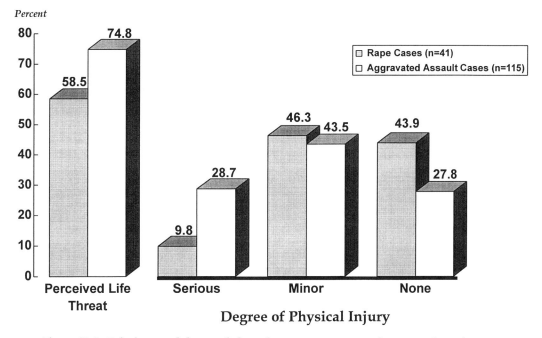

Figure 10.5. Life threat and degree of physical injury in new rape and aggravated assault cases.

in Figure 10.4. In the case of both types of assault, most incidents involve known perpetrators. Husbands and other relatives are more common perpetrators of adult aggravated assault incidents, while boyfriends, friends, and other nonrelatives are more common perpetrators of rape than aggravated assault incidents. Husbands constitute one-fifth of the rape perpetrators, exceeded only slightly by the rate of stranger perpetrators.

Reported rates of fear of death or serious injury and degree of actual injury suffered during rape and aggravated assault incidents are presented in Figure 10.5. For rape cases, only about 10% of victims reported the occurrence of serious physical injury, while over half (58.5%) feared serious injury or death. Higher rates of actual injury and fear were reported for aggravated assault incidents. However, these characteristics were also inherent in the criteria used to screen for such incidents. (Recall that the screening questions asked about attack with a weapon or without a weapon but with intent to kill or seriously injure the victim.)

Data were also gathered about rates of reporting to police by type of assault expe-

rienced. A higher percentage of aggravated assault cases (44%) than rape cases (29%) were reported to police or other authorities. It has been argued by Resnick et al. (1993) that rates of rape obtained in studies that use the term *rape* are likely to be similar to numbers of reported rapes, because these individuals can readily identify the incident using the legal term. Thus it is possible that at least two-thirds of all adult cases may be missed by using such a screening approach. Rates of reporting for child rapes were even lower in our sample, and it is likely that a much greater proportion of those cases would be missed with the use of legal terms in assessment approaches.

RELATIONSHIP BETWEEN PAST VICTIMIZATION AND NEW RAPES AND AGGRAVATED ASSAULTS DURING WAVES 2 AND 3

The distribution of number of Wave 1 assaults indicated that the majority of respondents (2686, or 80%) had no Wave 1 history of rape or aggravated assault. One prior as-

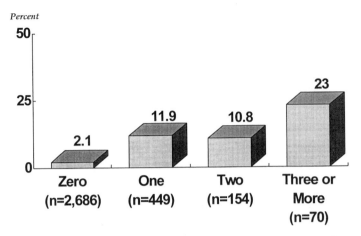

Figure 10.6. Risk of new rapes and aggravated assaults in Wave 2 and 3 interviews in relation to number of past incidents of victimization.

sault was reported by 449 women (13.4%), two incidents by 154 women (4.6%), and three or more incidents by 70 women (2.1%). Rates of new rape or aggravated assault in association with prior history of Wave 1 assaults are depicted in Figure 10.6. As can be observed, risk of new victimization increased with prior exposure to one (11.9% risk) or two (10.8% risk) assault in-

cidents, and jumped substantially in association with a history of three or more prior assaults (23% risk). The association between number of prior assaults and exposure to new assaults was significant (overall $\chi^2 = 171.81$; $p < .0005$). Further group comparisons indicated that the rate of new assault exposure was significantly lower in the group without prior history of assault than

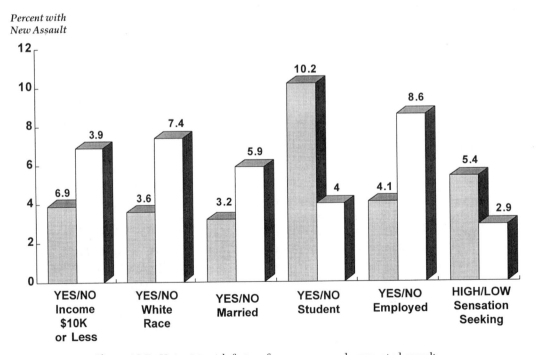

Figure 10.7. Univariate risk factors for new rape and aggravated assault.

the rates observed in all other groups (all p < .0005). Groups with previous history of either one or two assaults did not differ in rates of new assault exposure, but rates of new exposure in these groups were significantly less than the 23.0% rate observed among the group that had experienced at least three prior assaults (all p < .05).

Other univariate analyses were conducted to examine relationships between demographic characteristics and the trait variable of sensation seeking with new assault exposure. Variables identified as univariate risk factors for new rape and aggravated assault incidents based on significant chi-square associations are displayed in Figure 10.7. Findings indicated that those with household incomes below poverty level, who were nonwhite (17.8% of the sample), who were not married, who were students, who were unemployed, and who scored above the mean of 8.02 on the SSS classified as high sensation seeking had significantly higher rates of exposure to new assaults (all chi-square values with p < .005). Finally, those with new assaults were significantly younger than those without new assaults ($F_{1, 3347}$ = 18.37; p < .0005). Further analyses on the dichotomous demographic variables indicated that the employment, race, and marital status variables were all significantly associated with the poverty variable. These demographic variables were then tested in a block multiple logistic regression analysis to predict new victimization. Only age and student status remained significant in association with victimization. These two variables were retained along with predictor variables of prior number of assaults from Wave 1 and continuous score on the SSS in the final multiple logistic regression to predict new assaults at follow-up.

FINAL MULTIVARIATE LOGISTIC REGRESSION MODEL PREDICTING NEW VICTIMIZATION

Of the four variables entered into the model (age, student status, sensation seeking, prior

Table 10.1. Final multivariate logistic regression model predicting new victimization

Variable	Range	95% Confidence interval	Odds ratio
Sensation seeking	6–18	1.00–1.17	1.08
Student status	0–1	1.22–4.28	2.28
Prior victimization	0–3	1.99–2.83	2.37

number of assaults), all but age were significant predictors of new assaults in the final model that controlled for associations between all other variables in the model. The ranges associated with each significant predictor, odds ratios, and confidence intervals of the odds ratios are presented in Table 10.1. Odds increase geometrically with each unit change in the predictor variable. For example, those with prior history of one assault have increased odds of 2.4 of a new assault compared to those with no prior history, while the odds increase to 5.8 (2.4^2) for those with two versus no prior assaults or three versus one prior assault. Odds of new victimization increased positively as sensation seeking increased, and odds of new victimization were 2.3 times greater among women who were currently students than among women who were not students. Each of these three variables in the final model predicted new victimization, controlling for the effects of the other two.

CURRENT PTSD AS A FUNCTION OF PRIOR AND NEW ASSAULT HISTORY

Univariate Risk Factors for Current PTSD

The rate of current PTSD measured at follow-up assessment was 5.1%. Similar to the analyses conducted to predict new assault, relationships between current PTSD and demographics, prior history, sensation seeking, and new assault variables were examined using univariate followed by multivariate analyses.

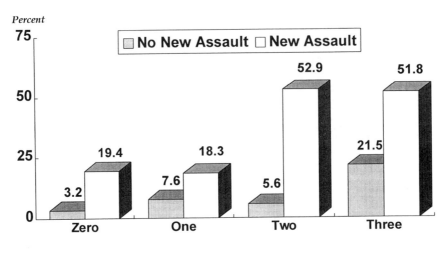

Figure 10.8. Rate of current PTSD as a function of prior and new assault history.

Number of prior assaults was significantly associated with past 6 months' prevalence of PTSD (overall χ^2 = 115.16; $p < .0005$). Further group comparisons indicated that the group with no prior history of assault had a significantly lower rate of current PTSD (3.6%) than the group with history of one prior incident (8.9%), the group with two prior incidents (10.7%), or the group with three prior assaults (28.5%) (all $p < .0005$).

Groups with either one or two prior assaults did not differ in rates of current PTSD, while both of these groups had lower rates of PTSD than that observed within the group with three prior assaults (both $p < .005$).

Current PTSD was also significantly associated with new assault exposure (4.3% of sample). Regardless of prior history of assault at Wave 1 assessment, the PTSD rate

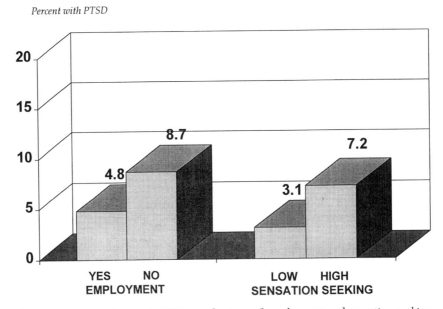

Figure 10.9. Rate of current PTSD as a function of employment and sensation seeking.

within the group that had experienced a new assault (26.5%) was higher than that within the group that had not experienced a new assault (4.2%; $\chi^2 = 141.27$; $p < .0005$). Rates of current PTSD associated with new assault crossed with number of prior assaults are presented in Figure 10.8. Age was significantly associated with current PTSD. As with exposure to new assault, those with current PTSD were significantly younger than those without current PTSD ($F_{1,3347} = 10.55$; $p < .005$). Those in the dysjunctive category unemployed *or* students also had a higher rate of current PTSD, as did those who were classified as high sensation seeking; both chi-square values were significant, with $p < .005$. Rates of PTSD associated with the latter two variables are displayed in Figure 10.9.

FINAL MULTIVARIATE LOGISTIC REGRESSION MODEL PREDICTING CURRENT PTSD

Prior to the final multivariate analysis, the two demographic variables of age and student *or* unemployed status were evaluated in a logistic regression. Only age remained a significant demographic predictor of PTSD, and the employment status variable was removed from further analyses. Of the four variables entered into the final model (age, sensation seeking, prior number of assaults, new assaults) only the two assault exposure variables and the sensation seeking variable were significant predictors of current PTSD in the final model that controlled for associations between all other variables. The ranges associated with each significant predictor and the associated odds ratios are presented in Table 10.2. Ranges of variables must be considered in evaluating increased odds associated with each. For example, a prior history of one assault is associated with increased odds of current PTSD of 1.75 compared to the odds of current PTSD with no prior assault history. A two-unit increase in number of prior assaults (from 0 to 2 or from 1 to 3) is associated with increased odds of 3.09, while a three-unit increase is

Table 10.2. Final multivariate logistic regression model predicting current PTSD

Variable	Range	95% Confidence interval	Odds ratio
Sensation seeking	6–18	1.04–1.19	1.12
Prior victimization	0–3	1.46–2.11	1.75
New victimization	0–1	4.16–10.33	6.56

associated with increased odds of current PTSD of 5.45. The 5.45 rate is comparable to the increased odds of current PTSD for those who have been exposed to a new assault. A final analysis was conducted to explore the possibility of an interaction between prior assault history and new assault exposure. No significant interaction was observed, indicating that these risk factors are additive. This relationship was depicted in Figure 10.8.

DISCUSSION

The lifetime prevalence and past 2 years' prevalence of rape and aggravated assault are substantial, suggesting that these types of violence are major problems for American women. Most rapes occur during childhood and adolescence, are not reported to police, involve perception of life threat but not physical injury, and are not perpetrated by strangers. Researchers and clinicians alike need to be aware of these characteristics when developing or choosing screening instruments designed to assess rape history. Questions geared toward stereotypical views of rape or global screening questions using the term *rape* are likely to be inadequate for assessment of the vast majority of actual rape cases. In addition, it must be emphasized that, although the majority of such cases do not involve serious injury, the majority of victims *do* report fear that they will be killed or seriously injured during such incidents. Therefore these incidents in childhood or adulthood clearly qualify as DSM IV PTSD Criterion A stressor events that may lead to PTSD (APA, 1994).

It is problematic that many studies examining the etiology of PTSD or other outcomes such as substance abuse appear to have failed to assess these critical events that most often occur during childhood. For example, results reported by Cottler et al. (1992) indicated that substance abuse precedes and is a risk factor for PTSD. Likewise, the study reported by Breslau et al. (Chapter 15, this volume) indicates that some forms of pre-existing psychopathology increased the risk of subsequent victimization. Assessment procedures in both of these studies have been criticized as vastly underestimating rape events or other significant traumatic event histories. Findings from studies that fail to assess these early potentially traumatic events adequately must be evaluated critically to ensure that significant etiological factors are not overlooked in assessment of relationships between stressor history and development of psychopathology, including PTSD and other mental health problems.

Results of the NWS indicated that most aggravated assaults happen to adults, not children, and are not perpetrated by strangers. They are more likely than rapes to be reported to police, to produce physical injuries, and to involve perception of life threat. These findings may also relate to the nature of our screening questions, which were written to reflect the legal definition of aggravated assault. It is possible that these questions may be less sensitive to incidents that may occur during childhood or cases that are less likely to be reported to police.

History of rape and/or aggravated assault increases risk that adult women will suffer additional rapes or assaults. The more victimizations a woman has had in the past, the greater the risk she will be victimized in the future. Many traditional predictors of new victimization of adult women (e.g., age and employment status) do not predict new victimization after controlling for the effects of prior victimization. Consistent with results reported by Breslau et al. (Chapter 15, this volume), women in the NWS with higher sensation seeking experienced increased risk of new victimization, even after controlling

for the effects of demographics and prior victimization. The significant relationship between prior victimization and new victimization is consistent with findings from several other studies, including a prospective study by Norris and Kaniasty (1992) and the results reported by Breslau et al. in this volume.

Risk of current PTSD is substantially increased by past victimization, new victimization, and high sensation seeking. Each of these variables independently contributed to current PTSD in the NWS sample, even after controlling for the other two variables. The finding of significant effects for both prior history of traumatic events and new assault exposure is also highly consistent with results of Norris and Kaniasty (1992).

Although certain factors may put women at higher risk for victimization, the perpetrators, not the victims, bear the sole responsibility for attacking vulnerable women. Hanson et al. (1995) address the issue of prevention of violent assaults and point out that the bulk of prevention approaches can be characterized as "opportunity reduction," which has been defined as "making a potential target of attack inaccessible or unattractive by making the attack itself dangerous or unprofitable to the criminal" (National Crime Prevention Institute, 1986). Major assumptions of opportunity reduction are: (1) potential victims must do things that reduce their vulnerability to attack, (2) actions victims can take are limited to things they can control in the environment, and (3) the environment we are trying to control is that of potential victims, not that of potential criminals.

As Hanson et al. (1995) note, even if potential victims make themselves "hard targets" who are unattractive to potential attackers, attackers generally turn their attention to "soft targets," thereby redistributing the object of violent assault, not preventing it. Moreover, the cost of opportunity reduction for women is often severe restrictions in their freedom. This focus on victim control makes it the potential victim's responsibility to avoid attack and makes it a woman's fault if she is attacked (McCall, 1993; Sparks & Bar On, 1985). One crime victim articulated this point extremely well in her testimony to the President's Task Force on Victims of Crime: "To blame victims for crime is like analyzing the cause of World War II and asking, 'What was Pearl Harbor doing in the Pacific, anyway?'" (1982, p. 2)

There may be many factors involved in increased risk of victimization and PTSD given prior assault history. These may include general impairment in functioning leading to economic or other psychosocial risk factors. Such factors may include neighborhood of residence, which could increase risk of exposure to assault. In addition, a lack of resources may impede recovery given new exposure. The sensation-seeking measure may also tap some correlates or changes in functioning associated with victimization history that also put women at subsequent risk. This measure was administered at Wave 1 and, although it is hypothesized as a trait measure because victimization by assault often occurred at young ages, this history could theoretically impact upon a trait measure. Thus, if traumatic events happen early and possibly repeatedly at critical stages in development, there may be an impact on development of stable behavior patterns representative of sensation seeking.

Victimization history is a significant risk factor for future crime victimization. In addition, multiple crime victimizations have additive effects in development of PTSD postcrime. Prevention strategies designed to reduce initial victimization risks and to interrupt the cycle of revictimization are needed. In addition, treatment approaches must be developed to address long-term psychosocial problems associated with chronic victimization, rather than those focused more exclusively on acute psychological distress.

Acknowledgments: This work was supported in part by the National Institute on Drug Abuse by (NIDA grant No. DA 05220-01A2).

REFERENCES

American Psychiatric Association. (1987). *Diagnostic and statistical manual of mental disorders* (3rd ed., rev.). Washington, DC: American Psychiatric Press.

Breslau, N., Davis, G., Andreski, P., Federman, B., & Anthony, J. C. (1998). Epidemiologic findings on posttraumatic stress disorder and comorbid disorders in the general population. In B. P. Dohrenwend (Ed.), *Adversity, stress and psychopathology* (pp. 319–330). New York: Oxford University Press.

Breslau, N., Davis, G. C., Andreski, P., & Peterson, E. (1991). Traumatic events and posttraumatic stress disorder in an urban population of young adults. *Archives of General Psychiatry, 48,* 216–222.

Brill, N. Q., Crumpton, E., & Grayson, H. M. (1971). Personality factors in marijuana use. *Archives of General Psychiatry, 24,* 163–165.

Carroll, E. N., & Zuckerman, M. (1977). Psychopathology and sensation seeking in "downers," "speeders," and "trippers": A study of the relationship between personality and drug choice. *International Journal of the Addictions, 12,* 591–601.

Cottler, L. B., Compton, W. M., Mager, D., Spitznagel, E. L., & Janca, A. (1992). Posttraumatic stress disorder among substance users from the general population. *American Journal of Psychiatry, 149,* 664–670.

Eysenck, H. J. (1983). A biometrical-genetical analysis of impulsive and sensation seeking behavior. In M. Zuckerman (Ed.), *Biological bases of sensation seeking, impulsivity, and anxiety* (pp. 1–36). Hillsdale, NJ: Lawrence Erlbaum Associates.

Gidycz, C. A., & Koss, M. P. (1991). Predictors of long-term sexual assault trauma among a national sample of victimized college women. *Violence and Victims, 6,* 175–190.

Hanson, R. F., Kilpatrick, D. G., Falsetti, S. A., & Resnick, H. S. (1995). Violent crime and psychosocial adjustment. In J. R. Freedy & S. E. Hobfoll (Eds.), *Traumatic stress: From theory to practice* (pp. 129–162). New York: Plenum.

Kessler, R. C., Sonnega, A., Bromet, E., Hughes, M., & Nelson, C. B. (1995). Posttraumatic stress disorder in the National Comorbidity Survey. *Archives of General Psychiatry, 52,* 1048–1060.

Kilpatrick, D. G. (1983). Rape victims: Detection, assessment, and treatment. *The Clinical Psychologist, 36,* 92–95.

Kilpatrick, D. G., McAlhany, D. A., McCurdy, R. L., Shaw, D. A., & Roitzsch, J. C. (1982). Aging, alcoholism, anxiety, and sensation seeking: An exploratory investigation. *Addictive Behaviors, 7,* 139–142.

Kilpatrick, D. G., Resnick, H. S., Freedy, J. F., Pelcovitz, D., Resick, P. A., Roth, S., & van der Kolk, B. (in press). The Post-traumatic Stress Disorder field trial: Emphasis on Criterion A and overall PTSD diagnosis. In *DSM-IV Sourcebook.* Washington, DC: American Psychiatric Press.

Kilpatrick, D. G., Saunders, B. E., Amick-McMullan, A., et al. (1989). Victim and crime factors associated with the development of crime-related post-traumatic stress disorder. *Behavior Therapy, 20,* 199–214.

Kilpatrick, D. G., Saunders, B. E., Best, C. L., et al. (1987). Criminal victimization: Lifetime prevalence, reporting to police, and psychological impact. *Crime & Delinquency, 33,* 479–489.

Kilpatrick, D. G., Sutker, P. B., & Smith, A. D. (1976). Deviant drug and alcohol use: The role of anxiety, sensation seeking, and other personality variables. In M. Zuckerman & C. Spielberger (Eds.), *Emotions and anxiety: New concepts, methods, and applications* (pp. 247–278). New York: Lawrence Erlbaum Associates.

Koss, M. P. (1993). Detecting the scope of rape: A review of prevalence and research methods. *Journal of Impersonal Violence, 8,* 198–222.

Koss, M. P., & Dinero, T. E. (1989). Discriminant analysis of risk factors for sexual victimization among a national sample of college women. *Journal of Consulting and Clinical Psychology, 57,* 242–250.

McCall, G. J. (1993). Risk factors and sexual assault prevention. *Journal of Interpersonal Violence, 8,* 223–255.

Norris, F. H. (1992). Epidemiology of trauma: Frequency and impact of different potentially traumatic events on different demographic groups. *Journal of Consulting and Clinical Psychology, 60,* 409–418.

Norris, F. H., & Kaniasty, K. (1992). A longitudinal study of the effects of various crime prevention strategies on criminal victimization, fear of crime, and psychological distress. *American Journal of Community Psychology, 20,* 625–648.

President's Task Force on Victims of Crime. (1982). *President's Task Force on Victims of Crime final report.* Washington, DC: Author.

Resnick, H. S., Kilpatrick, D. G., Dansky, B. S., et al. (1993). Prevalence of civilian trauma and post-traumatic stress disorder in a representative national sample of women. *Journal of Consulting and Clinical Psychology, 61,* 984–991.

Resnick, H. S., Kilpatrick, D. G., & Lipovsky, J. A. (1991). Assessment of related posttraumatic stress disorder: stressor and symptom dimensions in rape. *Psychological assessment. Journal of Consulting and Clinical Psychology, 3,* 561–572.

Sorenson, S. B., Sigel, J. M., Golding, J. M., et al. (1991). Repeated sexual victimization. *Violence and Victims, 6,* 299–308.

Sparks, C. H., & Bar On, B. A. (1985). *A social change approach to the prevention of sexual violence against women.* Unpublished manuscript, Stone Center for Developmental Services and Studies, Wellesley College.

Spitzer, R. L., Williams, J. B., & Gibbon, M. (1987). *Structured clinical interview for DSM-III-R—Nonpatient version (SCID-NP-V).* New York: New York State Psychiatric Institute, Biometrics Research Department.

Steketee, G., & Foa, E. B. (1987). Rape victims: Post-traumatic stress responses and their treatment: A review of the literature. *Journal of Anxiety Disorders, 1,* 69–86.

Wyatt, G. E., Guthrie, D., Notgrass, C. M. (1992). Differential effects of women's child sexual abuse and subsequent revictimization. *Journal of Consulting and Clinical Psychology, 60,* 167–173.

Zuckerman, M. (1979). *Sensation seeking and risk taking: Emotions in personality and psychopathology.* New York: Plenum.

Zuckerman, M. (Ed.). (1983). *Biological bases of sensation seeking, impulsivity, and anxiety.* Hillsdale, NJ: Lawrence Erlbaum Associates.

Zuckerman, M. (1984). Experience and desire: A new format for sensation seeking scales. *Journal of Behavioral Assessment, 6,* 101–114.

11

Psychiatric Disorder in the Context of Physical Illness

Mary Amanda Dew

The experience of serious physical illness is one from which few of us escape. However, the rapid development and growing success of high-technology biomedical procedures and treatments enable increasing numbers of persons to recover from serious illness. The availability of these procedures also guarantees that more persons will live for longer periods—perhaps the remainder of their lives—with physical illness and its chronic effects. These effects often extend well beyond the boundaries of physical capabilities and functioning, as is shown in the proliferation of studies documenting broad quality-of-life effects of physical illness in emotional, social role functioning, and occupational domains (Canadian Erythropoietin Study Group, 1990; Croog et al., 1986; Dew & Simmons, 1990; Dew et al., 1997; Israel et al., 1996; Kaplan et al., 1989; Stewart et al., 1989; Wilson & Cleary, 1995).

Mental health and well-being are integral components of overall life quality. The unique potential for adverse mental health consequences in the face of physical illness is well recognized clinically, no matter whether physical illness itself is conceived to be a biological or a psychosocial stressor— and it appears to act in both capacities.

From a research perspective, literally hundreds of studies have examined the association of physical illness and psychological status, and numerous reviews have summarized portions of this vast literature. The foci of these reviews include (*1*) specific psychiatric disorders, most notably depression, and their presentation across a broad array of physical illnesses (Cameron, 1987; Cassem, 1988, 1990; Cavanaugh & Wettstein, 1984; Hall, 1980a, 1980b; Klerman, 1981; Lyness et al., 1996; Rodin & Voshart, 1986; Rodin et al., 1991; Stoudemire, 1996; Strain & Fulop, 1992); (*2*) specific types and categories of physical illness (e.g., neurological or end-stage organ diseases) and the spectrum of psychiatric disorders associated with them (Beidel, 1987; Fava, 1994; Fogel, 1993; Moran, 1996; Shapiro, 1996; Starkstein & Robinson, 1989); and (*3*) diagnostic and methodologic issues in disentangling psychiatric from physical illness (Cameron, 1987; Cavanaugh, 1984; Cohen-Cole & Stoudemire, 1987; Endicott, 1984; Fulop & Strain, 1991; Goldberg & Bridges, 1987; Kathol et al., 1990; Koenig et al., 1995; Schulberg et al., 1987).

Study of these reviews and commentaries suggests the following. First, despite strong clinical and anecdotal evidence—the importance of which is not to be underestimated—the empirical magnitude of the physical illness–psychiatric disorder relationship remains unclear. The lack of clarity stems in part from diagnostic difficulties and from weaknesses in research methodology and study design, as discussed further below. Second, although numerous hypotheses have been proferred, there has been little examination of specific mechanisms by which physical illness produces adverse mental health consequences. The extent to which physical illness itself can be produced directly or indirectly by mental illness further complicates our understanding of its unique role as a stressor and the mechanism whereby it operates.

Two additional issues have received little attention either in previous original studies or integrative reviews. With very few exceptions (e.g., Weyerer, 1990), there has been no consideration of whether the nature or magnitude of the physical illness–psychiatric disorder relationship is generalizable beyond the treated samples described in most clinical reports. Thus, the extent to which Berkson's (1946) bias, for example, could account for the magnitude of the observed relationship is unclear. However, several investigations are now available that focus on community-based samples and provide important information on this issue; these are discussed further below. An additional omission in the physical illness–psychiatric disorder literature pertains to issues of risk and vulnerability for psychiatric disorder: There has been little attention to the issue of *which* persons are at greatest risk for adverse mental health consequences in the face of physical illness. Also, beyond examining such "main effects" (i.e., the direct contributions of potential risk factors such as gender and age for psychiatric disorder), investigators have rarely evaluated the possibility that premorbid risk factors *in combination with* physical illness lead to particularly deleterious mental health outcomes. The potential for "vulnerability," or diathesis–stress, effects (e.g., Dohrenwend & Dohrenwend, 1981; Kessler et al., 1985)

deserves examination in light of growing evidence from other research domains. This research suggests that the effects of many other life stressors are often magnified among persons with certain pre-existing demographic, psychiatric, or psychosocial characteristics (Alloway & Bebbington, 1987; Brown & Harris, 1978; Coyne & Downey, 1991).

The present review complements and extends previous reviews of the physical illness–psychiatric disorder relationship by marshalling both epidemiological and clinical research evidence to examine the nature, magnitude, and generalizability of this relationship. Because the assessment of psychiatric disorder in the context of physical illness presents unique difficulties, the present chapter first provides a brief overview of diagnostic and related methodological issues. It then summarizes the descriptive epidemiological studies of psychiatric disorder in physical illness in both community-based and patient samples; reviews potential biological and psychosocial pathways by which physical illness acts as a stressor; and evaluates evidence regarding major risk and vulnerability factors for psychiatric disorder in the context of physical illness.

DIAGNOSTIC ISSUES IN RESEARCH ASSESSMENT OF PSYCHIATRIC DISORDER DURING PHYSICAL ILLNESS

As in the general literature on the association of stressors with psychopathology (Dohrenwend & Dohrenwend, 1981; Kessler et al., 1985), much of the research on the role of physical illness has assessed psychopathology via nonclinical impairment ratings and symptom checklists (see Attkisson & Zich, 1990; Rodin et al., 1991, for reviews). Although the association between physical illness and psychiatric distress is often observed to be quite strong in these studies, the interpretation and substantive significance of this association is unclear. From a measurement standpoint, distress scale scores are not necessarily highly related to diagnosis of psychiatric disorder or highly specific for the psychiatric syndromes they are designed to assess (Breslau, 1985; Myers & Weissman, 1980). Conceptually, the clinical significance of the distress levels determined by such scales—e.g., their duration, their temporal variability—cannot easily be determined from such measures (Roberts, 1990; Rodin et al., 1991; Schulberg et al., 1987).

A difficulty more specific to the utilization of nonclinical scales in physically ill persons is that virtually all such scales include somatic items that may overlap considerably with physical illness symptomatology. Exclusion of the somatic items in order to obtain "purer" measures of distress may not be a suitable option, however, because this would be likely to alter the psychometric properties of the original scale, as well as cloud comparisons to other populations that received the full scale. An alternative has been to select measures with well-normed subscales, such as the Symptom Checklist-90 (Derogatis, 1983), and, rather than relying on the commonly used overall scale score (which incorporates a somatic symptom subscale), consider only certain subscales such as those pertaining to depression, anxiety, or anger–hostility (e.g., Dew et al., 1990). Alternatively, among the many scales that may be available for a particular type of distress (e.g., depression), investigators may select the measure that includes relatively few somatic items (e.g., the Center for Epidemiologic Studies Depression Scale or the Beck Depression Inventory, Mayou & Hawton, 1986). This strategy, for example, was applied for the selection of a depression measure in the Multicenter AIDS Cohort Study (Davidson et al., 1992; Ostrow et al., 1989).

Overall, however, the various difficulties associated with the interpretation of nonclinical measures of distress and symptomatology underscore the importance of bringing diagnostic techniques to bear when studying physical illness effects on mental health. With the development of several systematic, clinical interviewing tools employ-

ing standard diagnostic criteria, a number of studies reporting prevalence rates based on standardized assessments have appeared in recent years; their findings are detailed later under "Descriptive Epidemiology of Psychiatric Disorder in Physical Illness." However, conceptual issues in judging the significance of observed psychopathology, plus the continued potential for confounding the measurement of psychopathology with the measurement of physical illness, continue even with the adoption of standardized diagnostic assessments.

The first issue, cogently described by Klerman (1981), involves the continuing debate over whether some psychiatric syndromes, particularly those pertaining to depression and anxiety, are in fact "normal" reactions to the stress of physical illness and therefore neither require nor justify the assignment of a diagnosis. Yet, as Klerman points out, the boundary between apparently normal, understandable reactions to stress and clinical disorder is unclear. The result has been that there are few systematic guidelines to apply in clinical or research settings to judge the normality–abnormality distinction. Judgments as to whether cardinal symptoms for psychiatric syndromes, such as dysphoric mood in the case of depressive disorders, are "normal" reactions will determine whether patients are even eligible to meet criteria for a psychiatric diagnosis. Thus such judgments can dramatically affect estimates of the prevalence of psychiatric disorder in the physically ill. Differences in decisions about whether psychiatric symptoms are normal or expectable may account in part for the frequently observed underdiagnosis of psychiatric disorders by primary care and medical specialty care providers (Attkisson & Zich, 1990; Cassem, 1988; Schulberg, 1991).

Additional issues arise once a decision has been made that a given symptom or set of symptoms is, indeed, more extreme than a "normal" reaction. Is the symptom biologically induced by the physical illness, or is it a functional—or "psychogenic"—reaction? It is useful to consider depression, in particular, because it has received the most attention in this regard. On the basis of strict application of the *Diagnostic and Statistical Manual of Mental Disorders* (*DSM*), dysphoria and associated symptoms such as anorexia, anergy, insomnia, and fatigue should, in the presence of many physical illnesses, result in the assignment of Organic Affective Disorder [under the *DSM-III* (American Psychiatric Association, 1980) and the *DSM-III-R* (American Psychiatric Association, 1987)], or Mood Disorder Due to a Medical Condition [under the *DSM-IV* (American Psychiatric Association, 1994)]. Yet it has been argued strongly that, in both clinical and research practice, invoking the organic–functional distinction—as well as similar ones pertaining to secondary versus primary depression—may lack usefulness with respect to either understanding the phenomenology of depression during physical illness or prescribing optimal treatments (Cassem, 1990; Hall et al., 1987; Strain & Fulop, 1992). Strain and Fulop argue that the *DSM* requirement that symptoms caused by medical illness not contribute to the diagnosis of Axis I mood disorder "increases the specificity of the diagnosis at the expense of sensitivity and further sacrifices reliability, since raters' assessment of causality may differ. There is often no way to determine the origin of a symptom— whether it is the product of a psychological process, a physiological process, or both" (1992, p. 454). As a result of this dilemma, the pragmatic clinical and research approach often adopted in the context of physical illness is to proceed with a modified application of the *DSM*, in which the fact that organic factors must be excluded in order to make the diagnosis of major depression is ignored or minimized (Cassem, 1990; Kathol et al., 1990; Strain & Fulop, 1992). Cohen-Cole and Stoudemire (1987) refer to this as the "inclusive approach," which considers all symptoms of depression, even though either depression or the physical illness could have caused them.

Two other available alternatives are less extreme than either the inclusive approach or the *DSM* approach of exclusion of

somatic symptoms related to physical illness. Endicott (1984) proposed that a set of four items—social withdrawal, fearfulness, brooding, and nonreactive mood—be substituted for the appetite, sleep and fatigue and symptoms typically evaluated for the diagnosis of major depression (see Silverstone, 1996, for a review of studies adopting this approach). A modification of Endicott's strategy has involved assigning weights to each somatic symptom (rather than using substitution altogether), where determination of the weight depends on the symptom's likelihood of being confounded by the physical illness (Koenig et al., 1988). Alternatively, Cavanaugh (1983, 1984) has developed additional criteria specifying the conditions under which somatic symptoms can meaningfully contribute to a diagnosis of depression during physical illness: Such symptoms should be included in formulating the diagnosis only when these symptoms are clinically severe, disproportionate to the medical illness, and temporally related to the affective/cognitive symptoms of depression.

Although the strategies discussed above were developed specifically for the diagnosis of major depressive disorder, analogous approaches might be useful for the assessment of other areas of psychopathology commonly observed in physically ill persons, such as anxiety disorders. To date, however, the bulk of the literature on diagnostic dilemmas in the context of physical illness pertains to depression. Furthermore, the role and attribution of somatic complaints in the diagnosis of other disorders may be even more difficult to determine. Anxiety, for example, frequently has a marked somatic component, even in persons without physical disorder (Strain et al., 1981).

Difficult diagnostic issues have not prevented the empirical examination of the physical illness–psychiatric disorder relationship. However, they do suggest caution in interpreting both the nature and the magnitude of observed associations. In light of the preceding discussion, the data reviewed below concerning the prevalence of psychopathology in physically ill persons derive only from studies in which psychiatric disorder (rather than symptomatology and distress) has been assessed, and in which the assessments employed standardized interviews with established psychometric properties. The majority either adopted the "inclusive" approach to diagnosis described above, or employed the additional outlined strategies for evaluating the contribution of somatic symptoms to a given psychiatric disorder.

DESCRIPTIVE EPIDEMIOLOGY OF PSYCHIATRIC DISORDER IN PHYSICAL ILLNESS

Similar to the broad literature on the association of life stressors and psychopathology, the literature on the relationship of physical illness and psychiatric disorder falls into two major categories. Analogous to the multiple life events strategy of considering whether the occurrence and absolute number of events increases individuals' risk for adverse mental health outcomes, one approach to the study of physical illnesses' effects focuses on whether persons with one or more (usually chronic) physical illnesses are at elevated risk for psychiatric disorder. This is the primary approach adopted in community-based studies of physical illness, as described below. In contrast, the second strategy has been to focus on mental disorders in the context of single, specific types of life events—here, specific physical illnesses. Studies of treated populations, usually served in specialty medical settings, are most typical under this second approach. Under both of these broad approaches, the most common research design is a cross-sectional/retrospective one in which psychiatric data are collected via respondent interviews. Only rarely are identified cohorts followed longitudinally, and there are extremely few incidence studies of physically ill cohorts free of lifetime psychiatric disorder who are then followed prospectively to establish rates of first-onset disorder. Nevertheless, the extant investigations provide important data on the co-occurrence of physical illness and psychiatric disorder.

General Population and Primary Care Population Studies of Persons with One or More Physical Illnesses

Table 11.1 summarizes the eight community-based studies of the association between presence of physical illness and psychiatric disorder. Given extensive evidence that many factors unrelated to health affect whether individuals seek treatment, these studies are critical for evaluating the strength of the physical illness–psychiatric disorder association because they evaluated samples that were *not* selected on the basis of treatment-seeking for either psychiatric or physical illness reasons.

Most of the eight studies included adults of all ages. The five studies conducted in the United States relied on data from individual sites of the Epidemiological Catchment Area (ECA) program (Regier et al., 1984); of these, all but the Bruce and Hoff (1994) incidence study focused on 6 month prevalence rates of psychiatric disorder. The three additional studies examined European cohorts and report either 1 month or point prevalence rates.

In addition to providing descriptive information on study site, sample size, and nature of the physical and psychiatric disorder assessments, Table 11.1 shows the rate of psychiatric disorder among persons in each sample identified as having any physical illness, compared to the rate among those with no physical health conditions. The last column of the table shows the odds ratio indicating the increased risk of psychiatric disorder among persons with physical illness relative to those without illness.

In the U.S. studies, the presence of physical conditions was based on self-reported health problems, including heart disease, cancer, lung disease, arthritis, and the like. In contrast, the European studies augmented self-reports with the collection of

Table 11.1. General population studies of association between physical illness and psychiatric disorder

Authors	Site, sample	Measures[a] Physical illness	Measures[a] Mental disorder	Disorder	Persons with physical illness	Physically healthy persons	Odds ratio
George et al. (1986)	Piedmont region, NC ECA, ages 18+ (including oversample of elders 60+), n = 3,798	Determined from DIS interview	DIS/DSM-III 6 mo prevalence	Any disorder	22.9	12.1	2.16
				mood	8.5	3.3	2.71
				anxiety	14.6	6.6	1.96
				substance abuse/dep.	5.9	3.9	1.50
Wells et al. (1988, 1989)	Los Angeles, CA ECA, ages 18+, n = 2,554	Self-reported conditions	DIS/DSM-III 6 mo prevalence	Any disorder	24.7	17.5	1.41
				mood	9.4	5.6	1.68
				anxiety	11.9	6.0	1.98
				substance abuse/dep.	8.5	6.8	1.25
Kramer et al. (1989, 1992)	Baltimore, MD ECA, ages 18+, n = 3,481	Self-reported conditions	DIS/DSM-III 6 mo prevalence	Any disorder	27.8	20.3	1.50
				mood	6.0	3.7	1.62
				anxiety/somatization	18.2	11.8	1.54
				substance abuse/dep.	8.8	7.3	1.20
				schizophrenia	1.4	1.0	1.40
				antisocial personality	0.6	0.9	0.67
Bruce and Leaf (1989)	New Haven, CT ECA subsample ages 55+ (including oversample of elders 65+), n = 3,007	Self-reported conditions	DIS/DSM-III 6 mo prevalence	Major depression or bipolar disorder	1.7	0.7	2.13

Study	Sample	Measure	Condition			
Bruce and Hoff (1994)	New Haven, CT ECA, ages 18+ (including oversample of elders 65+), $n = 3,170$	Self-reported conditions in lifetime	DIS/DSM-III 12 mo incidence	Major depression	2.2	1.8	1.20
Dilling and Weyerer (1984)	Upper Bavaria, Germany, ages 16+, $n = 1,536$	Self-report to M.D. interviewer	CIS/ICD-8 point prevalence	Any disorder	31.7	13.7	2.31
Vazquez-Barquero et al. (1987)	Cantabria, Spain, ages 17+, $n = 1,223$	Consulted medical agency, diagnosis verified in med. records	PSE/ICD-9 1 mo prevalence	Any disorder	27.9	9.4	2.96
Aromaa et al. (1994)	Finland, national sample ages 40+, $n = 5,355$	Clinical exam and diagnosis; cardiovascular diseases only	PSE/ICD point prevalence	Age 40–64 depression Age 65+ depression	5.5[†] 6.2[†]	4.6 4.0	2.71[†] 1.68[†]

°DIS, Diagnostic Interview Schedule; CIS, Clinical Interview Schedule; ICD, International Classification of Diseases; PSE, Present State Examination.

[†]Median across reported cardiovascular diseases.

data from medical agencies (Vazquez-Barquero et al., 1987), or by utilizing physician interviewers to collect physical health history data from respondents (Aromaa et al., 1994; Dilling & Weyerer, 1984).

Across the studies, the observed proportions of physically ill persons with at least one psychiatric disorder range from approximately 23% to 32%, while only 9%–20% of persons reporting no physical illness had psychiatric disorders. It is noteworthy that, unlike the other studies reporting rates for "any disorder" in Table 11.1, the overall rate reported by Vasquez-Barquero et al. (1987) did not include diagnoses related to substance abuse/dependence and antisocial personality disorder, since the Present State Examination (PSE; Wing et al., 1974) does not generate these diagnoses. It is therefore surprising that the rates for overall disorder among both physically ill and healthy respondents were not lower in this report. Vazquez-Barquero et al. note, however, that the prevalence rates reported across their entire sample (regardless of physical health) are similar to rates observed in other community studies utilizing the PSE.

As shown in the last column of Table 11.1, the odds ratios (ORs) for increased risk of psychiatric disorder in the presence of physical illness range from 1.4 to almost 3.0. The European studies generally report higher ORs than the U.S. studies; this is due in part to the fact that the rates of psychiatric disorder in physically healthy persons in the European studies are lower than the corresponding rates in the U.S. studies. In contrast, the rates of psychiatric disorder in physically ill persons are more similar across studies.

As shown in the table, several of the studies also provided information about specific classes of psychiatric disorders. In general, mood disorders (encompassing major depression, dysthymia, and bipolar illness) show the strongest relationship to physical illness, followed by anxiety disorders [panic, phobias, generalized anxiety disorder (GAD), and obsessive–compulsive disorder (OCD)]. Given the link between psychiatric disorder (particularly depressive illness) and

suicide, it is also relevant to note that, in addition to the data in Table 11.1, there is a separate literature that has documented a strong relationship between the presence of physical illness and increased risk for suicide (see MacKenzie & Popkin, 1987, for a review).

The Kramer et al. (1989, 1992) and Wells et al. (1988, 1989) investigations (Table 11.1) also reported the associations of individual classes of chronic physical conditions with psychiatric disorder in their samples. As shown in Table 11.2, both found particularly elevated rates of recent psychiatric disorder among persons with arthritis, heart disease, and chronic lung diseases, relative to persons with no reported physical conditions. Wells et al. also examined and found elevated rates of disorder associated with cancer and neurological conditions. As for the associations with overall physical illness shown in Table 11.1, mood and anxiety disorders were most strongly related to the specific physical illness classes examined in Table 11.2.

Clearly, the physical illness categories considered in these population-based studies are crude. There has been little effort to date to examine more narrowly defined physical illnesses in nonpatient populations. However, two such studies, focusing on the relationship of history of migraine with mood and anxiety disorders in nontreated samples, suggest the potential importance of such work (Breslau & Davis, 1993; Moldin et al., 1993). Both studies found that history of migraine was strongly associated with a lifetime history of major depression; Breslau and Davis found that migraine history also strongly predicted incident major depression and panic disorder.

The large literature on psychiatric disorder in primary care populations is also potentially relevant to the present review. However, although these studies are critical for establishing prevalence of psychiatric disorders and evaluating physician detection skills in treated populations (Schulberg, 1991), they are less useful for directly evaluating the nature and extent of the relationship between physical illness and psychiatric

Table 11.2. Percentages of persons in U.S. community samples with psychiatric disorders in the past 6 months, according to self-reported current physical health condition

Physical condition	Kramer et al. (1989, 1992) Any mental disorder	Wells et al. (1988, 1989)			
		Any mental disorder	Mood disorder	Anxiety disorder	Substance abuse disorder
None	20.3	17.5	4.4	5.3	6.0
Arthritis	26.1	25.3	11.3	9.1	7.8
Cancer	—	30.3	—	—	—
Diabetes	23.7	22.7	9.6	15.7	5.7
Heart disease	28.0	34.6	14.2	15.3	13.8
Hypertension	26.2	22.4	11.3	15.1	12.7
Chronic lung disease	—	30.9	18.3	8.7	9.2
asthma	35.6				
breathing trouble	44.1				
Neurological disorder	—	37.5	—	—	—

Dashes indicate that rates were not reported for the condition or disorder.

disorder because (*1*) they usually do not establish which patients have physical illness and which do not, and (*2*) as Rodin et al. (1991) point out, the primary care patients with the highest levels of psychiatric symptomatology are often those who do not have a physical illness.

Only five investigations have reported the prevalence of diagnosable psychiatric disorder (assessed via a standardized interview) specifically among physically ill primary care patients. Lobo et al. (1988) studied 245 patients attending an internal medicine clinic in Zaragoza, Spain, of whom 176 were determined by the treating physician to have one or more (nonpsychiatric) physical conditions. Based on administration of the Clinical Interview Schedule (Goldberg et al., 1970), 40.9% (*n* = 72) of the 176 patients were found to have psychiatric disorder as diagnosed by the ninth revision of the *International Classification of Diseases* (World Health Organization, 1977). Van Hemert et al. (1993) similarly assessed 245 internal medicine clinic outpatients from Leiden, The Netherlands. Of these, 91 were determined by the investigators to have definite physical illnesses, based on a review of physician notes and laboratory tests performed

at the time of the patient's visit. The PSE, with *DSM-III-R* criteria, was used for the diagnosis of mood, anxiety, or psychotic disorders. Eleven cases (12.1% of the 91 persons) were identified, four with major depression and six with anxiety disorders. (The remaining case received a diagnosis of psychosis.) Bridges and Goldberg (1992) collected physician evaluations of 590 consecutive patients attending 15 general practices in greater Manchester, England. Among the 507 considered by the treating physician to have a definite physical illness, the investigators obtained a point prevalence rate of 27.8% for *DSM-III* mood and anxiety disorders, utilizing the Psychiatric Assessment Schedule (Dean et al., 1983). In a methodologically similar study, Kisely and Goldberg (1996) obtained physical evaluations of 428 patients from seven Manchester practices. Among the 27 patients with moderate to severe physical illness, 33.3% were determined to meet *DSM-III-R* criteria for major depression, and 6% met criteria for GAD. Finally, in a study of 179 inpatients with physical illness diagnoses in medical and surgical units in an Australian hospital, Clarke et al. (1993) found 37.9% (*n* = 68) to have concurrent *DSM-III-R* disorders, based on the Structured Clinical Interview for DSM-III-R (covering the full range of Axis I disorders). The most common disorders were major depression (22 cases), and anxiety disorders (5 with GAD, 4 with panic disorder, 12 with phobias, and 1 with OCD). There were 19 cases of substance abuse/dependence.

Bearing in mind the fact that two of the five primary care studies evaluated only a limited range of diagnostic categories (thus rendering comparisons of rates of "any disorder" across the studies difficult), the primary care studies nevertheless appear to show higher prevalence rates for psychiatric disorder in the context of physical illness than the community-based studies. As Wells et al. (1988) suggest, this may reflect a gradient in severity of physical illness: Persons receiving treatment may have more severe conditions that are associated with more secondary psychiatric disorder. In contrast, many physically ill persons identified in the community-based studies in Table 11.1 were not under care for their physical condition.

Studies of Treated Samples with Specific Physical Illnesses

Most research on the physical illness–psychiatric disorder relationship is based on patient populations treated in specialty medical settings in which the specific physical illnesses have been carefully defined and diagnosed. The gain in diagnostic specificity for physical condition is partially offset, however, by considerably weaker sampling procedures than in the studies reviewed in the previous section. The majority of patient studies rely on samples of convenience; with few exceptions (e.g., Dew et al., 1990; Folstein et al., 1983), they do not consider issues of sample representativeness or generalizability. However, these studies have generally evaluated potential correlates and risk factors for psychiatric disorder in the context of physical illness to a much greater extent than have community-based or primary care–based studies. Data regarding such correlates are reviewed later in this chapter.

Table 11.3 summarizes studies that employed standardized clinical interview schedules and specific diagnostic criteria to investigate psychiatric disorders in the context of several major physical health conditions. The health conditions included in the table were selected because they are relatively prevalent and they correspond generally to the major classes of physical conditions considered in the general population studies (Table 11.2). Human immunodeficiency virus (HIV) disease is included as a category in Table 11.3; it has not been considered in the population-based studies to date. The studies in Table 11.3 were retrieved via computerized literature searches using Medline, Current Contents, and Psychological Abstracts for the period 1980–1994. (Prior to this time, standardized diagnostic interviews that applied reliable clinical criteria such as those specified in *DSM-III* were generally not available.) In addition, the contents of individual issues of several journals where relevant articles often appear were reviewed (e.g., *American Journal of Psychiatry, International Journal of Psychiatry in Medicine, Journal of Psychosomatic Research, Psychological Medicine*).

For each study in Table 11.3, four categories of psychiatric diagnostic data are shown: the overall rate of psychiatric disorder of any type in the sample (when reported), rates for specific mood disorders and anxiety disorders, and rates for any other disorders assessed. Most of the studies report point prevalence rates. However, adding to the difficulty of comparing studies, some report rates for other recent periods and/or lifetime rates. Of these, lifetime rates are the most problematic to interpret because psychiatric disorder may have begun well prior to the onset of physical illness.

One important issue in considering the studies in Table 11.3 is whether—across the varied types of physical illnesses—the rates of psychiatric disorders among patient groups are higher than would be expected, based on population rates. Most of the studies consider one or more types of mood and anxiety disorders; these rates can be cautiously compared to 1 month prevalence rates from two other large-scale studies in the United States, the ECA Program and the National Comorbidity Survey (NCS; Blazer et al., 1994; Eaton et al., 1994; Kessler et al., 1994; Wittchen et al., 1994). The median point prevalence rate for major depression across the 33 studies reporting it in Table 11.3 is 14.0%, which is notably higher than the 1 month rates of 3.0% in the ECA studies, and 8.1% in the NCS. Among the most frequently assessed anxiety disorders, panic has a median of 4.5% across the 10 studies reporting it in Table 11.3, compared to the ECA rate of 0.53% and the NCS rate of 1.5%. GAD had a median of 2.2% across 14 studies reporting it, compared to the 1 month rates of 1.3% and 1.6% for these disorders in the ECA study and in the NCS, respectively.

The studies in Table 11.3 also allow some comparison of rates of psychiatric disorders between the various physical illnesses. Lifetime prevalence rates appear generally similar across the categories of physical conditions. This is likely to reflect the fact, noted earlier, that these rates cover many years in patients' lives in which they did not have the physical illness. Point prevalence rates are more variable across reports. To facilitate comparison of these rates, Table 11.4 summarizes the median point prevalence rates for the most frequently assessed psychiatric disorders in each of the physical illness categories considered in Table 11.3. Table 11.4 also shows the number of studies on which each median rate is based, since most studies assessed only selected diagnostic categories. The fact that many medians are based on only two to three studies indicates the need for cautious comparisons. Indeed, some psychiatric disorders have yet to be examined at all in the context of certain physical health conditions; others have been examined in only one study.

With these caveats, Tables 11.3 and 11.4 suggest that neurological conditions are often associated with particularly high point prevalence rates of psychiatric disorder. Although these high rates may be partially influenced by the generally greater difficulty

of disentangling psychiatric symptoms from other symptoms in the context of neurological disease, it is noteworthy that the studies involving patients with neurological conditions are among the most careful in attempting to address potential confounding of symptoms when assigning psychiatric diagnoses. As discussed further below, the particularly great likelihood of psychiatric disorder in the context of neurological problems is probably due to significant biological and psychosocial mechanisms linking the conditions, rather than only to a general confounding of symptomatology in these studies.

Among non-neurological conditions, Table 11.4 shows relatively higher point prevalence rates for mood and anxiety disorders in association with arthritis, diabetes, and heart and lung disease. Some disorders appear more prominent in some physical illnesses than others (e.g., panic in lung disease and GAD in heart disease). Although there is reason to believe, for example, that the association of panic with lung disease is robust (Karajgi et al., 1990), it is difficult to reach strong conclusions about the magnitude of this association based on only a single available study.

The variability in point prevalence rates of psychiatric disorder across various physical illnesses no doubt reflects true differences in the magnitude of the association as a function of the specific nature of the physical health problem. However, methodological dilemmas are also likely to have contributed to this variability. As noted above, the physical illnesses differ in the degree of associated difficulty in distinguishing and attributing somatic symptoms to psychiatric versus physical disorder, or a combination of both. Even within categories of physical illness (e.g., cancer or heart disease), individual studies differ in choice of psychiatric interview and diagnostic criteria for psychiatric disorder. Other factors contributing to the variability in rates are clinical differences between samples in severity, duration, and course of the physical illness under consideration, as well as demographic and psychosocial differences. The role of such var-

Table 11.3. Prevalence of psychiatric disorders in samples with specific physical illnesses

Author, Country	Physical illness[a]	Sample size	Instrument/diagnostic criteria[b]	Prevalence rates of psychiatric disorders[c,d,e]			
				Any	Mood	Anxiety	Other
Arthritis							
Frank et al. (1988), USA	Rheumatoid	137	DIS/DSM-III	—	MDD 16.8; dysthymia 40.1; either, lifetime 46.7	—	—
Kirmayer et al. (1988), Canada	Rheumatoid	23	DIS/DSM-III	—	Lifetime: MDD 8.7; dysthymia 13.0; no other disorder	Lifetime: social phobia 4.4; OCD 4.4; no other disorder	Lifetime: 0.0
Ahles et al. (1991), USA	Rheumatoid	33	Psychiatric Diagnostic Interview/DSM-III	57.6	MDD 39.4	Panic 6.1; phobia 21.2; OCD 3.0	Somatization 3.0
Kokkonen and Kokkonen (1993), Finland	Rheumatoid	35	PSE/ICD-8	—	Depression 17.1	Anxiety 14.3	Psychosis 0.0
Cancer							
Joffe et al. (1986), USA	Carcinoma of pancreas or stomach	21 + 16	SADS/RDC	—	MDD 23.8 ($n = 21$); MDD (12 mo) 24.3 ($n = 37$)	—	—
Weddington et al. (1986), USA	Sarcoma survivors	33	SADS/RDC	45.4	MDD 15.1, lifetime 24.2; minor depression 3.0	Panic 3.0, lifetime 6.1; phobia 3.0, lifetime 3.0	Alcoholism 3.0, lifetime 12.1
Dean (1987), UK	Breast (postmastectomy)	113	PSE/RDC	—	MDD 9.7; minor depression 17.7	GAD 0.9	—
Devlen et al. (1987), UK	Lymphoma	90	PSE/ICD	—	1 mo: depression 2.2; minor depression 6.6	1 mo: anxiety 3.3; minor anxiety 7.7	—
Hardman et al. (1989), UK	Various types	126	PSE/ICD	—	Depression 3.3	Anxiety 20.8	—
Razavi et al. (1990), Belgium	Various types	128	DIS/DSM-III	—	MDD 7.8	—	—

Study	Disease/type	N	Assessment/criteria		MDD and/or GAD		
Ibbotson et al. (1994), UK	Various types	513	Psychiatric Assessment Schedule/DSM-III	—		MDD and/or GAD 16.8	—
Hosaka et al. (1994), Japan	Hematological malignancies	31	SCID/DSM-III-R	—	MDD 6.4	No current disorder	—
Diabetes							
Lustman et al. (1986), USA	Types I, II	114	DIS/DSM-III	39.5 (12 mo) 71.1 (lifetime)	MDD: 12 mo 14.0, lifetime 32.5; lifetime dysthymia 17.5; mania, lifetime 2.6	Lifetime: panic 3.5; simple phobia 26.3; social phobia 26.3; GAD 40.9; OCD 0.9	Lifetime: alcohol abuse/dependence 22.8; drug abuse/dependence 7.9; schizophrenia 0.9; antisocial personality 5.3; somatization 1.8
Popkin et al. (1988), USA	Type I (pancreas transplant applicants)	78	DIS/DSM-III	—	MDD (6 mo) 10.7; no other recent disorder	6 mo: panic 1.3; phobia 20.3; GAD 17.1; OCD 1.3; no other recent disorder	6 mo: alcohol abuse/dependence 2.7; drug abuse/dependence 1.3; antisocial personality 1.3; no other recent disorder
Mayou et al. (1991), UK	Type I	113	PSE/ICD-9	—	Depression 11.0	Anxiety 5.0	—
Popkin et al. (1993), USA	Type I (pancreas transplant applicants)	140	DIS/DSM-III	—	Lifetime: MDD 19.3; dysthymia 5.7; bipolar 1.4	Lifetime: phobia 21.4; GAD 28.0; PTSD 2.8; other 1.4	Lifetime: alcohol abuse/dependence 13.6; drug abuse/dependence 7.1; antisocial personality 7.9; other 0.9
Kokkonen and Kokkonen (1993), Finland	Type I	63	PSE/ICD-8	—	Depression 14.3	Anxiety 1.6	Psychosis 1.6
Heart disease							
Carney et al. (1987, 1988), USA	Coronary artery disease	52	DIS/DSM-III	—	MDD 17.3	—	—

Table continued on following page

Table 11.3. Prevalence of psychiatric disorders in samples with specific physical illnesses—*Continued*

Author, Country	Physical illness[a]	Sample size	Instrument/diagnostic criteria[b]	Any	Mood	Anxiety	Other
Schleifer et al. (1989), USA	Post-MI	283	SADS/RDC	—	MDD 18.4; minor depression 26.9	—	—
Shapiro and Kornfeld (1989), USA	ESHD (transplant candidates)	23	SCID/DSM-III-R	—	MDD 4.3	Anxiety disorders 8.7	Personality disorders 43.5
Forrester et al. (1992), USA	Ischemic heart disease (post MI)	129	PSE/DSM-III	—	MDD 19.4; dysthymia 2.3	GAD 7.7	—
Magni and Borgherini (1992), Italy	ESHD (transplant candidates)	36	SADS/RDC	58.3	MDD 13.9; minor depression 2.8	Panic 2.8; GAD 25.0	Alcoholism 2.8
Frasure-Smith et al. (1993), Canada	Post-MI	222	DIS/DSM-III-R	—	MDD 15.8	—	—
Alexander et al. (1994), India	Ischemic heart disease	30	SADS/DSM-III-R	26.7	MDD 3.3; dysthymia 3.3; depression NOS 6.7	Panic 10.0; GAD 3.3	Alcohol dependence 3.3
Dew et al. (1994, 1996a), USA	ESHD (transplant recipients)	105	SCID/DSM-III-R	—	MDD: 12 mo 18.4, lifetime 22.1	GAD: 12-mo 0.0, lifetime 8.6	—
HIV disease							
Atkinson et al. (1988), USA	HIV, AIDS	45	DIS/DSM-III	84.4 (lifetime)	MDD: 6 mo 11.1, lifetime 28.9; no other recent or lifetime disorder	6 mo: panic 4.4, lifetime 4.4; phobia 0.0, lifetime simple phobia 4.4; lifetime social phobia 17.6; GAD 28.6, lifetime 40.5; OCD 0.0, lifetime 6.7; no other recent or lifetime disorder	6 mo: alcohol abuse/dependence 8.8, lifetime 31.1; drug abuse/dependence 6.7, lifetime 35.6; no other recent or lifetime disorder
Brown and Rundell (1990), USA	HIV, no AIDS	20	SCID/DSM-III-R	50.0	—	—	Alcohol abuse 5.0; substance abuse 0.0

Study	Group	N	Instrument	Prevalence (%)	Depression	Anxiety	Other
Perry et al. (1990), USA	HIV, no AIDS	51	SCID/DSM-III-R	31.4 56.9 (lifetime)	1 mo: MDD 3.9, lifetime 25.5; dysthymia 13.7; bipolar 0.0, lifetime 3.9	Anxiety disorders: 1 mo 5.9, lifetime 11.8	1 mo: alcohol dependence 5.9, lifetime 21.6; non-IV drug dependence 3.9, lifetime 11.8
Williams et al. (1991), USA	HIV, no AIDS	124	SCID/DSM-III-R	—	1 mo: MDD 4.0; dysthymia 2.4; bipolar 0.0, lifetime 0.8; no other current disorder	1 mo: Any anxiety disorder 1.6; panic, lifetime 4.0	1 mo: alcohol abuse/ dependence 2.4, lifetime 41.1; drug abuse/dependence 8.9, lifetime 55.6
Brown et al. (1992), USA	HIV, AIDS	884	SCID/DSM-III-R	38.7 69.7 (lifetime)	MDD 6.3, lifetime 22.4; dysthymia 2.5, lifetime 2.5; bipolar 1.1, lifetime 2.0	Panic 1.4, lifetime 2.5; simple phobia 4.1, lifetime 4.3; social phobia 3.8, lifetime 4.0; GAD 2.3, lifetime 2.3; OCD 1.4, lifetime 1.4	Alcohol abuse/ dependence 3.6; drug abuse/ dependence 1.6; no other current disorder
Catalan et al. (1992a), UK	HIV, AIDS	24	PSE/ICD	20.8	Depression 16.7	Anxiety 4.2	Psychosis 0.0
Catalan et al. (1992b), UK	Hemophiliacs with HIV, AIDS	37	PSE/ICD	10.8	Depression 5.4	Anxiety 5.4	Psychosis 0.0
Rosenberger et al. (1993), USA	HIV, no AIDS	121	SCID/DSM-III-R	19.0	MDD (2 mo) 19.0	—	—
Lipsitz et al. (1994), USA	HIV, no AIDS	124	SCID/DSM-III-R	—	1 mo: MDD 21.0; dysthymia 11.3	—	—
Maj et al. (1994), USA, Brazil, Zaire, Germany, Thailand	HIV, AIDS	602	CIDI/DSM-III-R	8.8 15.6 (lifetime)	1 mo: MDD 7.1, lifetime 12.0; dysthymia 1.0, lifetime 0.7; bipolar 0.0, lifetime 0.2	1 mo: Panic 0.0, lifetime 0.3; GAD 1.0, lifetime 2.0	1 mo: Schizophrenia 0.0, lifetime 0.0; schizophreniform 0.2, lifetime 0.3

Table continued on following page

Table 11.3. Prevalence of psychiatric disorders in samples with specific physical illnesses—*Continued*

Author, Country	Physical illness[a]	Sample size	Instrument/diagnostic criteria[b]	Prevalence rates of psychiatric disorders[c,d,e]			
				Any	Mood	Anxiety	Other
Perkins et al. (1994), USA	HIV, no AIDS	98	SCID/*DSM-III-R*	—	MDD: 1 mo 8.2, lifetime 28.6	1 mo: Panic 1.0, lifetime 2.0; phobia 2.0, lifetime 5.1; GAD 0.0, lifetime 0.0; OCD 0.0, lifetime 0.0	—
Pugh et al. (1994), UK	HIV, no AIDS	20	PSE/ICD	15.0	Depression 15.0	Anxiety 0.0	Psychosis 0.0
Bix et al. (1995), USA	HIV, AIDS	95	SCID/*DSM-III-R*	34.7 (6-mo)	6 mo: MDD 18.9; bipolar 1.1	Anxiety disorders (6 mo) 4.2	Substance abuse/ dependence (6 mo) 9.4
McDaniel et al. (1995), USA	HIV, AIDS	37	SCID/*DSM-III-R*	62.2 83.8 (lifetime)	MDD 32.4, lifetime 43.2; dysthymia 10.8, lifetime 0.0; no other disorder	Panic 2.7, lifetime 0.0; no other disorder	Alcohol abuse/ dependence 21.6, lifetime 40.5; any substance abuse/ dependence 32.4; schizoeffective 0.0, lifetime 5.4; no other disorder
Summers et al. (1995), USA	HIV, AIDS	171	SCID/*DSM-III-R*	12.1 71.9 (lifetime)	MDD: 1 mo 9.4, lifetime 49.6	1 mo: Panic 4.1, lifetime 3.5; GAD 1.2, lifetime 4.1	1 mo: Alcohol abuse/ dependence 6.4, lifetime 38.6; drug abuse/dependence 2.3, lifetime 39.8
Kidney disease							
Smith et al. (1985); Hong et al. (1987), USA	ESRD	60	SADS/*DSM-III*	—	MDD 5.0, lifetime 30.0	—	—
Craven et al. (1987), Canada	ESRD	99	DIS/*DSM-III*	—	MDD 8.1, lifetime 20.2; dysthymia 6.1; no other current disorder	—	—

Study	Disease	Instrument/Criteria	N	%	Depression	Anxiety	Other
House (1987), UK	ESRD	PSE/DSM-III	80	31.3	MDD 12.5; no other current disorder	Panic + agoraphobia 2.5; GAD 1.3; no other current disorder	Alcoholism (12-mo) 1.5; no other current disorder
Hinrichsen et al. (1989), USA	ESRD	SADS/RDC	124	—	MDD 6.5; minor depression 17.7	—	—
Lung disease							
Yellowlees and Ruffin (1989), Australia	Asthma (post life-threatening attack)	DIS/DSM-III	25	40.0	MDD 4.0; no other current disorder	Panic 28.0; PTSD 2.0; no other current disorder	No other current disorders
Karajgi et al. (1990), USA	COPD	SCID/DSM-III-R	50	36.0	MDD 6.0, lifetime 10.0; dysthymia 2.0; no other current disorder	Panic 8.0; no other current disorder; anxiety disorders, lifetime 16.0	Alcohol abuse 8.0; no other current disorder
Kokkonen and Kokkonen (1993), Finland	Asthma	PSE/ICD-8	108	—	Depression 9.3	Anxiety 9.3	Psychosis 0.9
Neurological disorder							
Brown and MacCarthy (1990), UK	Parkinson's	PSE/ICD-9	40	20.0	Depression 5.0	Anxiety 5.0	Psychosis 0.0
Starkstein et al. (1990), USA	Parkinson's	PSE/DSM-III	105	—	MDD 20.0	—	—
Stein et al. (1990), USA	Parkinson's	SADS/DSM-III-R	24	—	MDD 8.3, lifetime 45.8; hypomania 4.2; no other current disorder	Panic 16.7, lifetime 20.8; social phobia 16.7, lifetime 16.7; GAD 4.2; other anxiety disorders 4.2	Schizophrenia 0.0
Hantz et al. (1994), New Zealand	Parkinson's	SCID/DSM-III-R	73	6.8	MDD 2.7; no other current disorder	Panic 1.4; simple phobia 1.4; GAD 1.4; no other current disorder	No other current disorders

Table continued on following page

Table 11.3. Prevalence of psychiatric disorders in samples with specific physical illnesses—*Continued*

Author, Country	Physical illness[a]	Sample size	Instrument/diagnostic criteria[b]	Prevalence rates of psychiatric disorders[c,d,e]			
				Any	Mood	Anxiety	Other
Caine and Shoulson (1983), USA	Huntington's	24	SADS/DSM-III	75.0	MDD 20.8; dysthymia 25.0; no other current disorder	Anxiety disorders 8.3	Schizophrenia 12.5; other 20.8
Folstein et al. (1983), USA	Huntington's	88	DIS/DSM-III	90.9 (lifetime)	Lifetime: MDD 31.8; dysthymia 9.1; bipolar 9.1	(Not differentiated from 31.8% with "other" disorders)	Lifetime: substance abuse 10.0; schizophrenia 2.6; antisocial personality 1.8; other 31.8
King (1985), USA	Huntington's	42	DIS/DSM-III	—	—	—	Alcohol abuse/dependence 7.1, lifetime 16.7
Robinson et al. (1983), USA	Stroke	103	PSE/DSM-III	—	MDD 27.0; dysthymia 20.0	—	—
House et al. (1990), UK	Stroke	95	PSE/DSM-III	—	MDD 11.0; no other current disorder	Anxiety disorders 6.0	—
Fedoroff et al. (1991), USA	Stroke	205	PSE/DSM-III	—	MDD 22.4	—	—
Castillo et al. (1993), USA	Stroke	309	PSE/DSM-III-R	—	—	GAD 25.2	—
Schiffer et al. (1983), USA	MS	30	SADS/DSM-III	—	MDD since onset of MS 36.7	—	—

Study	Disease	N	Criteria	Prevalence	Depression	Anxiety	Other
Joffe et al. (1987), Canada	MS	100	SADS/RDC	72.0 (lifetime)	MDD 14.0, lifetime 47.0; minor dep 1.0, lifetime 9.0; hypomania 1.0, lifetime 2.0; bipolar 0.0, lifetime 13.0	Panic 1.0, lifetime 5.0; GAD 2.0, lifetime 3.0	Schizophrenia 0.0
Minden et al. (1987), USA	MS	50	SADS/RDC	84.0 (lifetime)	MDD: 12-mo 34.0, lifetime 54.0; minor depression, lifetime 52.0; hypomania, lifetime 16.0, mania, lifetime 2.0	GAD (lifetime) 16.0; no other disorder	Alcoholism, lifetime 2.0; schizoaffective, lifetime 2.0; other, lifetime 8.0
Moller et al. (1994), Germany	MS	25	SCID/DSM-III-R	—	MDD and/or dysthymia 24.0	—	—

aMI, myocardial infarction; ESHD, end-stage heart disease; HIV, human immunodeficiency virus; AIDS, acquired immunodeficiency syndrome; ESRD, end-stage renal disease; COPD, chronic obstructive pulmonary disease; MS, multiple sclerosis.

bDIS, Diagnostic Interview Schedule; PSE, Present State Examination; ICD, International Classification of Diseases; SADS, Schedule for Affective Disorders and Schizophrenia; RDC, Research Diagnostic Criteria; SCID, Structured Clinical Interview for DSM-III or DSM-III-R; CIDI, Composite International Diagnostic Interview.

cPoint prevalence rates are reported unless otherwise noted.

dDashes indicate that no rates were reported for disorders in the cateogry.

eMDD, major depressive disorder; GAD, generalized anxiety disorder; OCD, obsessive–compulsive disorder; PTSD, post-traumatic stress disorder; NOS, not otherwise specified.

Table 11.4. Median point prevalence rates of psychiatric disorders in persons with physical illness°

Physical illness	Median point prevalence rate of psychiatric disorder (No. of studies reporting rate)						
	Any disorder	Major depression	Dysthymia	Panic	Phobias	GAD	Alcohol abuse/dependence
Arthritis	57.6 (1)	17.1 (3)	40.1 (1)	6.1 (1)	12.8 (2)	0.0 (1)	0.0 (1)
Cancer	45.4 (1)	8.7 (6)	—	3.0 (1)	3.0 (1)	0.9 (1)	3.0 (1)
Diabetes	—	12.6 (2)	0.0 (1)†	1.3 (1)†	20.0 (1)†	17.1 (1)†	2.7 (1)†
Heart disease	26.7 (1)	15.8 (7)	2.8 (2)	6.4 (2)	—	7.7 (3)	3.1 (2)
HIV disease	20.8 (5)	8.2 (11)	10.8 (5)	2.0 (5)	2.0 (3)	1.0 (5)	5.0 (5)
Kidney disease	31.3 (1)	7.3 (4)	6.1 (1)	—	—	1.3 (1)	1.5 (1)
Lung disease	38.0 (2)	4.0 (3)	1.0 (2)	18.0 (2)	0.0 (2)	0.0 (2)	4.0 (2)
Neurological disease							
Parkinson's	20.0 (1)	6.2 (4)	—	9.1 (2)	9.1 (2)	3.8 (2)	—
Huntington's	75.0 (1)	20.8 (1)	25.0 (1)	—	—	—	7.1 (1)
Stroke	—	22.4 (3)	20.0 (1)	—	—	25.2 (1)	—
Multiple sclerosis	—	14.0 (1)	—	0.5 (2)	0.0 (1)	2.0 (1)	—

°Medians calculated from studies listed in Table 11.3. Dashes indicate that no studies reported point prevalence rates for these disorders.

†The only available study reported 6 month rates for these disorders.

iables has been explicitly examined in some reports; data in this regard are summarized below.

In summary, the descriptive epidemiology of psychiatric disorders in the context of physical illness provides convergent evidence that physical and mental health are related. This evidence comes from general population, primary care, and specialty medical populations, and is based on careful application of systematic interviews and reliable diagnostic criteria for psychiatric disorder. The physical illness–psychiatric disorder relationship appears to vary in strength depending on the specific physical illness and the specific psychiatric disorder under consideration, although few studies have provided detailed data on this issue. Such variability is likely to be influenced at least in part by methodological variability and by sample differences along other dimensions. Beyond this variability, however, the elevated rate of many psychiatric disor-

ders in the context of *any* physical illness—versus none—is quite striking. Physically ill persons in community samples are up to 3 times more likely to have psychiatric disorders than physically healthy persons in these samples (Tables 11.1 and 11.2); rates of specific psychiatric disorders in studies of physically ill persons in treated samples (Table 11.3) are up to 8.5 times higher than prevalence rates reported in large-scale epidemiological studies of community populations. Finally, rates of psychiatric disorder in these ill persons may be even higher in the context of specific physical illnesses, although the number of studies within specific illness categories remains small.

PATHWAYS TO PSYCHIATRIC DISORDER IN PHYSICAL ILLNESS

The physical illness–psychiatric disorder relationship has a number of potential explanations. The evidence discussed above strongly suggests that one possibility—that they co-occur by coincidence—is unlikely. The causal direction of the association, however, is more difficult to determine. The pathogenesis of most psychiatric disorders is unknown; it is equally poorly understood how and when psychiatric factors play an etiological role in physical illness. From a pragmatic perspective, it is therefore likely to be more useful to focus discussion on issues of risk and vulnerability.

There is growing longitudinal evidence that psychiatric disorder can increase risk for (1) *subsequent* physical morbidity and mortality (Aromaa et al., 1994; Bruce & Leaf, 1989; Carney et al., 1988; Frasure-Smith et al., 1993), and (2) intermediate outcomes, such as noncompliance, that ultimately affect physical health (Dew et al., 1996; Lustman et al., 1986; Strain & Fulop, 1992). Even so, the bulk of the clinical and research literature has focused on documenting the contribution of physical illness *to risk for* psychiatric disorder. Therefore, many of the studies summarized in Tables 11.1 and 11.3 not only report these variables to be related, but provide evidence that physical illness increases the risk for psychiatric disorder over and above the impact of other factors, including psychiatric disorder antedating the physical illness (Bruce & Hoff, 1994; Craven et al., 1987; Hong et al., 1987; Minden et al., 1987). Of course, the use of a cross-sectional retrospective methodology in the majority of these studies leaves room for uncertainty regarding actual timing of physical illness versus psychiatric disorder onset. However, the few longitudinal studies (Dean, 1987; Kokkonen & Kokkonen, 1993; Pugh et al., 1994), and the truly prospective investigation of incidence of psychiatric disorder (Bruce & Hoff, 1994) also indicate that physical illness is an important independent risk factor for subsequent psychiatric disorder. The increased risk appears to be conferred via both biological and psychosocial pathways. Furthermore, the size of the risk is influenced by a number of other demographic and psycho-social factors. Evidence regarding the potential pathways and other variables influencing those pathways is reviewed below.

Physical Illness as a Biological Stressor

Clinical epidemiological and subsequent laboratory work has firmly linked psychiatric disorders to certain infectious, nutritional, and metabolic abnormalities. Classic examples include pellagra-induced psychosis and the neuropsychiatric sequelae of infectious diseases of the central nervous system (CNS), such as syphilis (Cooper, 1993). HIV infection is a relatively recent example of a virus with the demonstrated capacity to provoke neuropathological changes and neuropsychiatric illness, although the precise mechanism remains unclear (Portegies, 1994). The evidence of particularly high rates of many psychiatric disorders among persons with chronic CNS disorders and diseases, as noted earlier, is also consistent with biological mechanisms. Some work has begun to examine the particular neurophysiological factors that may be involved. In stroke, for example, the occurrence of anxiety disorders is strongly related to the brain structures involved in the injury (Castillo et al., 1993). Lesion location and size also affect the likelihood and nature of poststroke mood disorders (Starkstein & Robinson, 1989).

For many other physical conditions, however, although biological mechanisms have been implicated in the production of psychiatric disorder, little direct evidence is available. Comprehensive lists of the physical conditions and medications that are likely to induce mood, anxiety, and psychotic disorders through biological pathways have been provided in a number of reviews (e.g., Hall, 1980a, 1980b; Klerman, 1981; Larson & Richelson, 1988). Major categories of physical conditions include (in addition to CNS disorders) endocrine, infectious, collagen, cardiovascular, and malignant diseases. Major drug categories include antihypertensives, antiparkinsonian agents, hormones, corticosteroids, and anticancer agents. Excellent discussions of the range of plausible biological mechanisms linking such categories of physical illness and medication with depression, in particular, are available (e.g., Rodin et al., 1991).

The biological pathways offered as most plausible in studies such as those in Table 11.3 usually involve either (1) a cascade of biological changes linking the physical condition to ultimate psychiatric disorder, or (2) a common underlying set of biological factors accounting for both the physical illness and the psychiatric disorder. Studies of psychiatric disorder in diabetes, for example, have invoked both explanations. On the basis of other laboratory studies, Lustman et al. (1992) proposed that the association they and others have documented between diabetes and major depression results from a series of effects, in which changes in cortisol activity produced by chronic hypoglycemia lead to mood changes in some diabetic patients. Alternatively, from the standpoint of common underlying factors, the association may result from similar neurotransmitter abnormalities present in both diabetes and depression. This latter view is consistent with family study data showing an elevated rate of depression in nondiabetic relatives of diabetic probands (Lustman et al., 1987).

In sum, with some notable exceptions, the evidence for the role of biological factors in explaining the physical illness–psychiatric disorder relationship is indirect, implicating but not testing these factors. However, for most disorders, it is unlikely that biological pathways—even if accurately specified— are the only explanations for the relationship. If the relationship were only biological, one might expect a dose–response effect between standard physiological indices of severity of physical illness and likelihood of psychiatric disorder. Such effects are often *not* observed. Frasure-Smith et al. (1993) found no relationship between physiological indices of degree of heart disease following myocardial infarction (e.g., left ventricular ejection fraction) and likelihood of major depression during recovery from myocardial infarction. Joffe et al. (1987) were unable to link level of neurological dysfunction to oc-

currence of psychiatric disorder in their sample of patients with multiple sclerosis. Popkin et al. (1988) reported no relationship between physiological indices of diabetes complications and rate of psychiatric disorders in patients with longstanding type 1 diabetes. Studies have yet to demonstrate a consistent linkage between clinical and laboratory measures of HIV disease progression (such as Centers for Disease Control and Prevention illness stage and levels of immune function) with the mood and anxiety disorders prominent in HIV-infected persons (e.g., Atkinson et al., 1988; Williams et al., 1991).

In contrast, a number of studies, discussed below, suggest that physiological severity may be less important in predicting psychiatric disorder than the severity of disease-related symptoms and disability that are evident to the ill individual. This suggests the importance of also considering psychosocial pathways linking physical illness and mental health.

Physical Illness as a Psychosocial Stressor

Stroke was cited above as an example of a physical condition for which there is relatively clear evidence for biological pathways to psychiatric disorder (even though the exact mechanism is not known). However, there is also evidence that—independent of neurophysiological damage—patients' degree of functional disability in the aftermath of stroke is an important predictor of psychiatric status, and disability becomes an increasingly strong correlate of mental health with the passage of time (Robinson et al., 1984; Starkstein & Robinson, 1989). Indeed, level of disability and the changes it may necessitate in daily life are core factors that contribute to making stroke such a devastating event for patients and their families. In this sense, stroke clearly constitutes a catastrophic life event to no lesser degree than other catastrophic nonhealth life stressors. More broadly, like stroke, most physical illnesses are major life stressors; each has the potential to influence mental health in the same way that other major life events have been observed to increase the likelihood of psychopathology (Coyne & Downey, 1991; Dohrenwend & Dohrenwend, 1981; Kessler et al., 1985).

Like the potential biological pathways between physical illness and psychiatric disorder, the psychosocial pathways by which illness—as a major life event—leads to psychopathology are poorly specified. For nonhealth life events, some features that have repeatedly been found to be important for the development of psychopathology are undesirability, uncontrollability, and magnitude (see Kessler et al., 1985, for a review). Physical illness is, virtually by definition, undesirable. Its initial occurrence is frequently uncontrollable. The magnitude of the illnesses considered in this review can vary but have often been life threatening in the samples included, for example, in Table 11.3. Although the precise roles of each of these features are not usually examined separately in studies of the physical health–psychiatric disorder association, they are—as in the general life events literature—frequently invoked as plausible means by which increased risk for disorder is conferred.

Pearlin et al. (1981) have proposed that life events may influence mental health by increasing the individual's exposure to chronic stressors. This possibility is of particular relevance for physical illness because, although the major physical illnesses discussed in this chapter may be acute stressors at the time of their onset or diagnosis, their long-term course often more closely resembles situations of chronic strain, involving a constellation of interrelated elements (Dew et al., 1996a). Some elements will be unique to specific illnesses, but some are more universal, including the presence of illness-related and treatment-related symptoms, resulting disability and impairment, and potential uncertainty regarding clinical course. Like the findings on mental health effects of nonhealth chronic stress, these ongoing strains of living with physical illness have been observed to correlate with—and often predict—the occurrence and duration of depressive disorders, anxiety disorders, and associated distress levels (e.g., Cassileth et al., 1984; Dew et al., 1994; Frank et al., 1988; Yellowlees & Ruffin, 1989).

One psychosocial pathway implicated in these chronic stressor effects involves recognition and appraisal of the stressor elements (Lazarus & Folkman, 1984). At the most extreme, for conditions such as HIV infection, awareness that one has a physical condition or belief that one has certain illness-associated symptoms often serves as a more powerful predictor of psychopathology than objective evidence of disease status (e.g., Ostrow et al., 1986). Similarly, it has been observed across a variety of physical conditions that perceived impairment—e.g., limitations in ability to perform activities of daily living; inability to leave one's home—increases risk for psychopathology. Such findings have been observed not only for nonclinical measures of distress, but also among studies focused on diagnosable disorder (Aromaa et al., 1994; Brown & MacCarthy, 1990; Bruce & Hoff, 1994; Minden et al., 1987). These associations with mental health have been found to be independent of the association of biological indices of disease status with mental health.

VULNERABILITY TO PSYCHIATRIC DISORDER IN THE CONTEXT OF PHYSICAL ILLNESS

Psychiatric disorder is not observed in all persons who are physically ill. Even as the definition of physical illness is progressively narrowed from general illness categories (e.g., heart disease) to specific conditions within those categories (e.g., transplant candidates: persons with end-stage heart disease for whom medical therapies have failed), we still fail to observe disorder prevalence rates of 100%. Aside from the litany of methodological reasons why this might be so, two other critical factors must be considered: individual differences in (1) patients' general risk for psychiatric disorder (regardless of their physical health), and (2) their unique vulnerability to disorder in the context of physical illness. The first sort of individual difference posits important "main effects" of individual difference variables on psychiatric disorder. The second posits "interactive" or synergistic effects of the individual difference variables with the stressor (here, physical illness). In other words, stressors such as physical illness may impair mental health in individuals who are vulnerable because they possess certain other characteristics (Dohrenwend & Dohrenwend, 1981). This vulnerability hypothesis has gained empirical support in a wide variety of other life stressor contexts (Brown & Harris, 1978, 1989; Cassel, 1976).

Major risk and vulnerability factors for psychiatric disorder in the context of physical illness are reviewed below. For each, its role as an independent variable with potential "main" effects is considered, as well as evidence, when available, concerning whether it acts as a vulnerability factor that magnifies the strength of the physical health–psychopathology relationship. Because of the dearth of evidence on these issues—particularly on vulnerability effects —the sections below depart from the convention adopted earlier in this review and include studies with nonclinical mental health outcomes (i.e., levels of psychological distress) as well as studies of diagnosable psychiatric disorder. It is also important to note that the majority of relevant studies examine the potential roles of risk and vulnerability factors utilizing cross-sectional/ retrospective designs. Although some potential risk factors clearly antedate both the physical illness stressor and any observed psychiatric outcome (e.g., gender), the temporal ordering of many others (e.g., social supports, coping styles) *vis-à-vis* the illness and the psychiatric status of the respondent is more difficult to determine. It is therefore possible, for example, that some putative vulnerability factors such as coping styles are at least in part influenced by the stressors and the outcomes that they are hypothesized to modify. The disentangling of temporal order among these variables is one of the primary tasks needed to further our understanding of the role of the potential risk and vulnerability factors discussed below. The very few studies that employed longitudinal designs in examining these factors are highlighted. Nevertheless, at this early stage in our knowledge about the roles of such variables, even the cross-sectional work provides much-needed data regarding vulnerability issues.

Gender

Although general population studies report men and women to have very similar overall rates of psychiatric disorder, many studies of physically ill persons report women to be at higher overall risk (Kokkonen & Kokkonen, 1993; Kramer et al., 1992; Vazquez-Barquero et al., 1987). However, this apparent difference is most likely explained by the fact that the psychiatric disorders most strongly associated with female gender— the mood and anxiety disorders—constitute a larger proportion of the disorders seen in physically ill persons than they do in the general population. In fact, the pattern of gender differences in prevalence of *specific* mental disorders among physically ill persons closely resembles that for the general population. Thus, physically ill women are at increased risk for depressive and anxiety-related symptomatology and diagnosable disorders, relative to ill men (Carney et al., 1987; Craven et al., 1987; Fava, 1994; Frank et al., 1988; Frasure-Smith et al., 1993; Karajgi et al., 1990; Kramer et al., 1992; Schleifer et al., 1989). Men with physical illnesses are at relatively increased risk for alcohol and other substance abuse/dependence, antisocial personality disorders, and suicide (King, 1985; Kramer et al., 1992; MacKenzie & Popkin, 1987; Popkin et al., 1988).

Over and above this "main effect," some evidence is available concerning whether gender selectively heightens vulnerability to psychiatric disorder in the context of physical illness. Although formal analyses were not performed, Kramer et al.'s (1992) data concerning gender–mental health associations among physically ill persons at the Baltimore ECA site do not suggest that these associations were any stronger than the gender effects found in the Baltimore sample overall, or the effects reported for other ECA sites (Myers et al., 1984). In contrast, Vazquez-Barquero et al. (1987) did find that the impact of gender on psychiatric disorder was stronger among physically ill than well persons. The differences in these studies' findings may be due in part to the fact that neither considered gender effects within specific physical illnesses, and the samples undoubtedly differed in proportions with various health conditions. This is important because there is some evidence that gender operates as a vulnerability factor selectively —and in varying directions—across specific physical illnesses. For example, Popkin et al. (1988) found that diabetic women were at increased risk to develop anxiety disorders, and that this gender effect was more pronounced than that observed in either the ECA samples or an additional comparison group of nondiabetic family members. In contrast, with respect to cardiovascular disease, Aromaa et al. (1994) report the surprising finding that ill men, rather than women, were at increased risk for major depression. Finally, there is epidemiological evidence that men's heightened risk for completed suicide—which is well established in general population studies—becomes even larger in the presence of physical illness (MacKenzie & Popkin, 1987).

Both biological and psychosocial mechanisms have been proposed to account for observed vulnerability effects of gender. Popkin et al. (1988), for example, hypothesized that female diabetics may have a heightened emotional sensitivity to the variability in hypoglycemia and autonomic disturbances associated with the diabetes, and that this fosters the development of anxiety disorders. With regard to suicide, speculation has focused on the notion that men (at least in Western culture) are less able emotionally to accept the passivity and feelings of helplessness often associated with physical illness (MacKenzie & Popkin, 1987). However, potential mechanisms for vulnerability effects of gender have received no empirical evaluation in physically ill cohorts.

Age

Given its importance as a risk factor for psychiatric disorder in the general population, it is surprising that many studies of persons with specific physical conditions do not consider age effects. Although this may sometimes be due to the nature of the physical disorder under study, which may be most prevalent in certain age groups (e.g., stroke), many other illnesses occur or continue across many decades of adult life (e.g., asthma, diabetes, heart disease). The limited collection of data on age effects is thus an important omission. When examined, age effects in the context of physical illness appear similar to such effects in the general population: at least for adults through approximately 70, age appears to be inversely related to psychiatric disorder during physical illness, with younger persons (generally less then 45 years old) at greater risk (Cassileth et al., 1984; Dew et al., 1996a; Fedoroff et al., 1991; George et al., 1986; Kramer et al., 1992; Pugh et al., 1994). This relationship holds for total rates of all psychiatric disorder, as well as for specific disorders, including mood and anxiety disorders. Even among illnesses where the typical age range is more narrow (e.g., stroke), there is evidence that age is inversely related to these disorders (e.g., Robinson et al., 1983).

Concerning potential vulnerability effects, there is limited and conflicting evidence regarding whether the physical illness– psychiatric disorder association is stronger among certain age groups. On the one hand, several studies found no evidence of such vulnerability effects for depressive or anxiety symptomatology (Dew et al., 1991), prevalence of affective and/or anxiety disorders (George et al., 1986), or incidence of major depression (Bruce & Hoff, 1994). On the other hand, George et al. did find that age moderated the relationship between substance abuse and physical illness: the link between illness and abuse was considerably stronger in persons under age 50. Aromaa et al. (1994) report similar moderating effects such that the relationship between cardiovascular disease and depression was strongest in younger persons. There is also some longitudinal evidence that, once significant psychiatric distress develops in physically ill individuals, younger age seems to prolong the duration of the distress, relative to its duration in older persons (Dew et al., 1994).

To the extent that age does serve as a vulnerability factor in the context of physical illness, it has been hypothesized to do so for several reasons. From a psychosocial perspective, it has been argued that younger persons are less experienced at coping with physical illness, and see physical illness as less expected and therefore psychologically more devastating than do older persons (Simmons et al., 1987). There may be biological factors operating as well. Flint (1994), for example, has argued that age-related neurochemical changes and specific patterns of cell loss within the brain reduce the older person's sensitivity to the effects of threatening events, be they medical illness or other life stressors. This appears to be particularly the case for certain disorders such as anxiety and depression; these biological changes may be one set of factors, therefore, that account for older persons' decreased propensity for developing anxiety in the face of physical illness and other stressors. Finally, it is likely that the selective survival of healthier persons (defined in terms of both physical and mental status) into old age influences the strength of the effects described above.

Ethnic Group

Although earlier studies reported that depressive and anxiety symptom levels were higher among younger, physically ill African-Americans than physically ill Caucasians (Cavanaugh, 1983; Schwab et al., 1967), ethnic group effects have received little consideration in more recent studies of diagnosable psychiatric disorder in physically ill cohorts. Kramer et al. (1992) did report that nonwhites were overrepresented among physically ill persons with psychiatric disorders, relative to their overall proportions

among persons with psychiatric disorders, at the Baltimore ECA site. However, whether this effect would have been maintained if the impact of social class had been controlled was not evaluated. Social class effects are themselves difficult to measure and have rarely been adequately assessed in population-based studies (Dohrenwend, 1990). In household surveys in the United States using crude measures of social class (respondents' education, income, current occupation), there are mixed findings concerning ethnic differences in the distributions of psychiatric disorders or distress levels (e.g., depressive symptomatology). The ECA study found few ethnic differences once the effects of social class had been taken into account (Robins et al., 1984). In contrast, the NCS reported a variety of black-white and Hispanic-non-Hispanic differences (Kessler et al., 1991a).

Regarding the role of ethnic group as a vulnerability factor, there are no data pertaining to effects on psychiatric disorder. However, with regard to psychiatric symptomatology, Kolody et al. (1986) found that the association of depression with severity of physical health complaints was stronger in Mexican-Americans than in non-Hispanic whites, even after controlling for a number of other demographic variables. Baron et al. (1990) report indirect evidence of vulnerability effects in a sample of Native Americans with chronic physical health conditions. Their sample had higher average levels of depressive symptomatology than that reported in other groups studied previously, including Caucasian-Americans with chronic illnesses and a general population sample selected without regard to physical health.

It is difficult to interpret ethnic group effects and the role of ethnic group as a vulnerability factor, because the manner of expression of psychiatric symptomatology—and the phenomenology of affective and anxiety disorders in particular—vary across ethnic groups. Roberts (1990), in an extended discussion of these issues, concludes that, although cross-national studies have considered such issues, we have little knowledge about how the cultural backgrounds of ethnic groups *within* specific countries, such as the United States, shape psychopathology in unique ways. This is especially the case in the context of physical illness.

Socioeconomic Status

It is well established (although poorly understood) that socioeconomic status (SES) is associated with health, including both physical and psychiatric morbidity, and mortality (Adler et al., 1994; Dohrenwend, 1990). As for gender and age, the effects of SES on psychiatric disorder *during* physical illness mirror its relationship to mental health in the general population: lower social class, and related proxy variables such as lower income, less education, and unemployment, are associated with higher rates of psychiatric disorder and symptomatology among the physically ill (Craven et al., 1987; Dean, 1987; Dew et al., 1991; Joseph et al., 1990; Kramer et al., 1992; Robinson et al., 1983). However, the direction of this association with disorder is unclear. Moreover, particularly in the context of physical illness, the SES–psychiatric disorder relationship may have a large spurious component because physical illness itself often influences patients' SES, through their ability to maintain employment or achieve a higher education level. Nevertheless, it has been argued that SES exerts its own effects on mental health during illness by, for example, increasing the ill individual's degree of social isolation (Bruce & Hoff, 1994). Social isolation and related features of social support, in turn, have received extensive consideration as risk factors for psychiatric disorder in the context of physical illness, as discussed below.

There has been virtually no examination of whether SES-related variables selectively heighten the physical illness–psychopathology relationship. In one relevant cross-sectional study, Dew et al. (1990) did find such vulnerability effects for level of education: infection with HIV was most strongly associated with depressive and anxiety-related symptomatology among persons with the least education. This effect may relate to differences in coping skills and resources available to persons with differing levels of education. The role of coping factors is discussed further below.

Personal Psychiatric History Prior to Physical Illness

Psychiatric history prior to onset or diagnosis of physical illness has been consistently documented as one of the strongest risk factors for psychiatric distress and disorder in the presence of physical illness (Atkinson et al., 1988; Carney et al., 1987; Craven et al., 1987; Dean, 1987; Dew et al., 1990, 1994, 1996a; Hardman et al., 1989; Minden et al., 1987; Perkins et al., 1994; Starkstein et al., 1990; Yellowlees & Ruffin, 1989). This finding is consistent with extensive clinical and psychiatric epidemiological literatures (see Coyne & Downey, 1991, for a review) that emphasize the power of psychiatric history in predicting the nature and degree of new episodes of psychiatric disorder in both chronically physically ill and physically healthy populations. Positive history of a given disorder, such as major depression, not only increases risk for recurrences of the same disorder but places physically ill persons at risk for new psychiatric disorders. For example, Dew et al. (1996a) found that, within a group of patients with end-stage heart disease, history of major depression increased risk for incident post-traumatic stress disorder.

There is some further evidence that a positive history of disorder not only exerts such "main effects" but also seems to confer a heightened vulnerability to new periods of distress and diagnosable psychiatric disorder specifically in the face of physical illness. In other words, the risk for disorder is substantially higher among persons with both a physical illness and a positive psychiatric history than would be expected based on the individual contribution of each of these risk factors alone (Dew et al., 1990, 1994). However, the role of psychiatric history as a vulnerability factor may be more important in some physical illnesses than others. Among persons with idiopathic inflammatory bowel diseases, for example, Tarter et al. (1987)

found that personal psychiatric history increased risk for the development of *DSM-III* disorder (based on the Diagnostic Interview Schedule) after the onset of Crohn's disease, while psychiatric history did not increase this risk among persons with ulcerative colitis.

Family Psychiatric History

With few exceptions (e.g., Hong et al., 1987; Yellowlees & Ruffin, 1989), this factor has rarely been considered in studies examining the unique impact of physical illness on mental health, despite two large bodies of relevant data. First, it is well established that there is familial aggregation of psychopathology of many types (Ciaranello & Ciaranello, 1991; Merikangas, 1987). Given the prominence of mood disorders in the context of physical illness, it is noteworthy that such familial aggregation has been repeatedly observed for major depression and related disorders (e.g., Weissman, 1987; Weissman et al., 1984).

Second, there is evidence that predisposition to psychiatric disorder—whether the mode of familial transmission of risk be sociocultural or genetic—may frequently require a trigger before psychiatric disorder is elicited in a specific individual (Merikangas, 1987). Physical illness may serve as such a trigger, much as other life stressors have been observed to act in this role *vis-à-vis* family history (e.g., Penkower et al., 1988). Thus, family history of depression and/or anxiety has been observed to create vulnerability for high psychiatric symptomatology in the face of HIV infection, even though it played no such role among a comparison sample of persons not infected with HIV (Dew et al., 1990). Furthermore, there is strong evidence that family history of bipolar disorder confers special vulnerability to mania following stroke, relative to likelihood of mania among persons with family history but no stroke (Starkstein & Robinson, 1989). Nevertheless, such vulnerability effects are not universally obtained. For example, in studying onset of major depression following onset of renal disease, Hong et al. (1987) found no evidence for unique vulnerability for disorder conferred by a positive family history of depression.

Undoubtedly, both psychosocial and biological mechanisms are at work in these synergistic effects of family psychiatric history and physical illness. Better understanding of these mechanisms might help to explain why—at least in the very few studies available—family history has been observed to create vulnerability in the face of physical illness in some samples but not in others.

Social Supports

Both one's specific connections with others (defined by marital status, living alone vs. with others) and the quality of those relationships have been widely demonstrated to affect risk for psychiatric disorder and symptomatology. There is evidence both for direct effects of supports on mental health and for their role as vulnerability factors (see Alloway & Bebbington, 1987; Cohen & Wills, 1985; Coyne & Downey, 1991; Kessler et al., 1985 for reviews). This evidence comes from cross-sectional work as well as from longitudinal and prospective investigations.

These effects have been documented not only in generally physically healthy populations but also in the context of physical illness (although virtually all relevant data in ill cohorts are cross-sectional). With respect to specific social connections, physically ill persons who are unmarried, those who live alone, and persons who live with nonrelatives rather than relatives are more likely to experience psychiatric disorders (e.g., Craven et al., 1987; Dean, 1987; Hong et al., 1987; Kramer et al., 1989). Levels of self-reported psychiatric symptomatology are generally higher in such persons as well (Frankel & Turner, 1983), and are also higher among persons lacking affiliation with a religious organization (Koenig et al., 1992) or having fewer numbers of social connections and routine contacts with friends and relatives (Dew et al., 1993; Robinson et al., 1983).

The quality of relationships with spouse, primary family caregiver, other family members, and friends has received little evaluation in terms of its impact on psychiatric *disorder* in the physically ill. However, two longitudinal studies suggest that relationship quality is critical: poor spousal support was a key predictor of psychiatric disorder among women with cancer (Dean, 1987); poor support from one's primary family caregiver (who was, in most cases, the spouse) was a strong predictor of major depression in heart transplant recipients (Dew et al., 1996a). Most work on support quality has focused on psychiatric symptomatology levels. Important effects have been found in such diverse populations as persons with end-stage renal disease (Christensen et al., 1989; House, 1987; Simmons et al., 1987); HIV infection and acquired immunodeficiency syndrome (Hays et al., 1992; Kurdek & Siesky, 1990), cancer (Fitzpatrick et al., 1988; Siegal et al., 1987), arthritis (Fitzpatrick et al., 1988), and heart disease (Dew et al., 1994; Fontana et al., 1989). These studies vary in whether they utilize cross-sectional designs (e.g., Christensen et al., 1989; Fitzpatrick et al., 1988), or a longitudinal approach in which social supports are clearly measured prior to psychiatric outcome (e.g., Dew et al., 1994; Hays et al., 1992). However, generally across both types of studies, spouse/caregiver support effects are the largest, followed by family and friend support.

The ability of social ties and supports to act specifically as vulnerability factors has not been examined with respect to diagnosable psychiatric disorder. Some cross-sectional data are available concerning vulnerability for psychiatric symptomatology. Christensen et al.'s (1989) work with end-stage renal disease patients and Dew et al.'s (1991) work in the context of HIV infection both indicated that the impact of physical illness on distress was stronger among persons with poor supports. Again, as for "main effects" of social support on mental health, the quality of the most intimate relationships (with spouse or family caregiver) appears particularly important as a vulnerability factor; such effects are less marked for family and friend support.

In sum, the findings regarding social support corroborate anecdotal and descriptive accounts emphasizing the significance of relationships with others in influencing and moderating patients' psychological adjustment following physical illness and life-threatening health events. Although the mechanisms for main and vulnerability effects of social supports are widely believed to be psychosocial, there have been biological mechanisms proposed as well, relating, for example, to possible neurohumoral responses to human contact (House et al., 1988).

Coping Strategies and Styles

In summarizing a relatively large and sometimes contradictory literature on coping in chronic illness, Taylor and Aspinwall (1993) conclude that "active coping efforts are more consistently associated with good adjustment [during chronic illness] than avoidant strategies, so long as aspects of the disease are amenable to active coping efforts" (p. 520). Thus, active behavioral strategies (e.g., seeking out information to solve specific problems) and active cognitive strategies (e.g., cognitive restructuring by concentrating on potential positive outcomes of having the illness) have been found to be associated both cross-sectionally and longitudinally with lower levels of distress in the context of daily life with many illnesses, including hypertension, heart disease, diabetes, rheumatoid arthritis, cancer, and HIV infection (Felton et al., 1984; Dew et al., 1994, 1996a; Kurdek & Siesky, 1990). In contrast, during periods of crisis, such as learning that one has a life-threatening disease or experiencing an acute, life-threatening complication—situations where individuals may have little choice as to their own behaviors—denial appears related to lower distress (e.g., Levine et al., 1988).

This literature, similar to broader research on coping with a wide variety of life stressors, has focused on psychiatric symptomatology and other measures of psychological adjustment, rather than on psychiatric disorder outcomes. The only two studies that could be located that examined coping in relation to diagnosable disorder appear to support the conclusions of Taylor and Aspinwall (1993) regarding situations where avoidance coping is harmful versus helpful. Dew et al. (1996a) found that, in the year following heart transplantation—during which individuals' own behavior can greatly affect their health status—recipients with a pre-existing style of avoidance coping for managing health problems were over 3 times more likely than other recipients to experience major depression. Alternatively, Dean (1987) found that women who coped with denial when they were first informed that they had breast cancer requiring immediate surgery were less likely to experience episodes of major depression in the next 3 months than those who used other forms of coping.

Although focusing less on specific coping strategies, several related literatures have documented positive psychological effects of other personal difference variables that relate to coping styles. These include, most prominently, religious coping (relying on beliefs and utilizing prayer and other religious practices) (Harris et al., 1995; Koenig et al., 1992; Pargament et al., 1990) and views of personal competence, including (1) dispositional optimism (Scheier et al., 1986), (2) hardiness (Kobasa et al., 1982; Pollock, 1985), (3) locus of control and personal sense of mastery (Burgess et al., 1988; Dew et al., 1990, 1994; Schleifer et al., 1989), and (4) self-esteem (Brown et al., 1990; Catalan et al., 1992a, 1992b; Dew et al., 1994; Schleifer et al., 1989; Simmons et al., 1987). Although studies examining these coping styles have focused almost exclusively on psychiatric symptomatology rather than diagnosable disorder, each of these variables has been found to predict and/or correlate with lower levels of distress in the face of physical illness and other life stressors. However, there is some evidence that the strength of these factors' effects may vary across physical illnesses. For example, Pollock (1985) found hardiness to be associated with positive psychological outcomes in diabetes but not in hypertension or rheumatoid arthritis. Furthermore, given the cross-sectional design of many studies examining coping style variables, it will be important to examine more closely the unique longitudinal effects of these variables in additional work.

Do coping strategy and coping style factors selectively increase vulnerability to distress and disorder in the face of illness? Sense of mastery, and the related notion of locus of control, appear to be among the most important of the coping style variables in this regard (Cohen & Edwards, 1989): a poor sense of mastery heightens the association of physical condition with psychiatric symptomatology. Moreover, in two reports that included an array of coping variables— mastery, self-esteem, use of active behavioral coping strategies, and use of avoidance coping strategies—mastery was the only characteristic to act as an independent vulnerability factor (Dew et al., 1990, 1996a).

Other Stressful Life Events

As noted throughout this review, stressful events and circumstances have been demonstrated to elevate an individual's risk of psychiatric disorder as well as nonclinical distress scale scores (Brown & Harris, 1989; Coyne & Downey, 1991; Kessler et al., 1985). Indeed, this review has considered physical illness to exemplify one such category of stressors. However, it is important to consider as well the role of nonhealth life events antedating or co-occurring with physical illness, and the extent to which they not only exert their own effects on the mental health of ill persons, but also act synergistically with illness to influence mental health.

With respect to life events history *prior* to the illness, reviews have concluded that a large minority of individuals—20%–40%— do not recover fully from major life stressors despite the passage of many years (Kessler et al., 1985). Extended stress effects have been primarily noted in the areas of somatic complaints and affective disorder and associated symptoms, and have been observed in the years following such diverse events as job loss, bereavement, exposure to interpersonal violence, and natural and human-made disasters (Breslau et al., 1991; Bromet & Dew, 1995; Dew et al., 1991, 1993; Mendes de Leon et al., 1994). It is possible, therefore, that by generating or provoking enduring psychiatric distress in an otherwise healthy individual, life events may thus indirectly increase risk for new psychiatric disorder, should that individual coincidentally go on to develop a physical illness—insofar as previous psychiatric history itself is well-established to predict new disorder following physical illness. In other words, life events in the remote past may have generated psychiatric disorder in the past; as discussed previously, this history of disorder itself is likely to serve as a risk factor for new psychiatric disorder in the presence of more recently developed physical illness.

Life events *co-occurring* with physical illness, even though they may be independent of it, may also play an important role in provoking and maintaining psychiatric distress and disorder. Life events involving loss (e.g., loss of important relationships with others through divorce, death, etc.) appear to be particularly potent in this regard, especially for future depression (Brown & Harris, 1978; Finlay-Jones & Brown, 1981; Paykel et al., 1969). With respect to loss events co-occurring with physical illness, Dew et al. (1990, 1994) have found that physically ill individuals who also experience loss events are at heightened risk for depressive and anxiety-related symptoms. Once such symptoms develop, the occurrence of new loss events appears to prolong symptom duration. The potential for such effects during physical illness has not yet been examined with respect to diagnosable disorder.

Summary

This section has considered major risk factors for psychiatric disorder that are essential to evaluate in studies examining the physical illness–psychopathology relationship. These risk factors also act in some circumstances as vulnerability factors that selectively heighten the likelihood of psychopathology during physical illness for some individuals. Their role in increasing overall risk (independent of physical illness) has received much more extensive examination than their status as vulnerability characteristics. Indeed, most of the data regarding the capacity of risk factors to increase vulnerability come from studies of distress and symptomatology, rather than diagnosable psychiatric disorder. Finally, many of the data regarding both risk and vulnerability are cross-sectional, and longitudinal and/or prospective data are now needed to more fully delineate the causal direction of observed effects. To date, evidence suggesting vulnerability effects is relatively stronger and more extensive for gender, age, personal psychiatric history, some aspects of social support, certain coping style variables, and the occurrence of additional nonhealth life events. There has been less attention to potential vulnerability effects of ethnic group, SES, family psychiatric history, and most coping strategies and styles.

GENERAL CONCLUSIONS AND FUTURE DIRECTIONS

To provide a backdrop for suggesting future directions for research and clinical applications, the following conclusions can be drawn from the present review:

- The nature and magnitude of the relationship between physical illness and psychiatric disorder historically has remained difficult to determine empirically. Until recently, few studies had applied standardized assessment techniques utilizing reliable psychiatric diagnostic criteria. Continuing difficulties unique to this topic stem from complex diagnostic issues in evaluating and attributing respondents' symptomatology, and lack of consensus on what constitute optimal strategies to approach the diagnostic discrimination of psychiatric versus physical disorders.

- Convergent evidence from a variety of samples suggests, nevertheless, that physical illness and psychiatric disorder are reliably associated. Although most work has examined the association in treated samples, studies of nonpatient, community-based samples indicate a robust relationship as well.

- The physical illness–psychiatric disorder relationship appears to vary in strength (1) depending on the specific physical illness and the specific psychiatric disorder under consideration and (2) as one moves from general population to primary care to specialty care medical populations. The data summarized in Tables 11.1–11.4 indicate that physically ill persons in community samples are up to 3 times more likely to have psychiatric disorders than physically healthy persons in these samples; rates of specific psychiatric disorders in studies of physically ill persons in treated samples are up to 8.5 times higher than prevalence rates reported in healthy, nonpatient populations. Finally, rates of psychiatric disorder may be very much higher within certain types of physical illnesses, although the number of studies available within specific physical illness categories is generally small.

- Although growing evidence indicates that psychiatric disorder serves as a risk factor for physical illness, the bulk of evidence focuses on the extent to which physical illness increases risk for subsequent psychiatric disorder and implicates both biological and psychosocial mechanisms. Direct evaluation of these proposed mechanisms remains in very early stages.

- A specific set of additional variables appear not only to act as risk factors for psychiatric disorder but under some circumstances to serve as vulnerability factors that selectively heighten the likelihood of psychopathology during physical illness for some individuals.

However, the dearth of longitudinal studies of these variables' effects limits our understanding of their potential roles *vis-à-vis* the physical illness–psychiatric disorder relationship.

In light of these conclusions, what directions are critical for future work in this field? Study of psychiatric disorder, as it is produced and maintained in the context of physical illness, will continue to be critical both for practical reasons and for reasons pertaining to conceptual understanding of processes by which life stressors are related to psychopathology. From a practical perspective, psychiatric disorder occurring during physical illness has already been shown to substantially increase expenditures for care of the physical illness itself, through prolonging hospitalization and treatment and increasing the rate of long-term physical morbidity and mortality (Carney et al., 1988; Frasure-Smith et al., 1993; Popkin et al., 1993, Saravay & Lavin, 1994). From conceptual and theoretical standpoints, continued study of psychiatric disorder in the context of physical illness will provide a prime situation for examining a complete biopsychosocial model of the stress process and its mental health consequences. Physical illness, as a major life stressor, is multifaceted: It almost invariably includes both acute and chronic components, and it is likely to operate most frequently through combinations of psychosocial and biological pathways. Furthermore, physical illness is so widely distributed across demographically, psychosocially, and culturally diverse groups that it provides multiple, varied opportunities for examining (1) its independent effects, relative to combinations of these other risk factors, and (2) circumstances under which its effects on mental health are either aggravated or ameliorated by other variables. Of course, the multifaceted nature and wide distribution of physical illness *vis-à-vis* other factors also make investigation of its relationship to psychiatric disorder quite difficult.

Consider this relationship itself, aside from the role of other factors. As noted above, the central concerns in examining the relationship to date have involved problems and strategies for assigning psychiatric diagnoses in the face of physical illness, and determination of the absolute strength of the association. Most studies have not been designed to examine the direction of, or pathways explaining, the relationship. Thus, one task for future research is to evaluate if not the causal, at least the predictive components of the link between physical illness and psychopathology. Additional work is needed to directly examine the biological and psychosocial pathways that have been repeatedly implicated in the relationship. These goals will require (1) more frequent use of longitudinal study designs capable of disentangling predictors of psychiatric disorder from the disorder and its consequences, and (2) wider application of quasi-experimental methods, with prospective data, to examine how much of the link between physical illness and psychopathology is due to a causal component (Kessler et al., 1985).

Other variables' roles in this process must be considered as well, either as risk factors in their own right or as factors with the capacity to create vulnerability for psychopathology in the context of physical illness. The inclusion of a full range of such factors within any given study is extremely rare. Moreover, work evaluating them specifically as vulnerability characteristics remains at a very early stage. Future research that builds causal, or at least predictive, models of the physical illness–psychopathology relationship will need to integrate more routinely hypothesized risk and vulnerability factors, including the factors reviewed above.

The evaluation of predictive models, based on longitudinal and/or prospective data with integration of risk and vulnerability factors, is critical from more than a conceptual viewpoint. From a pragmatic, public health perspective, the ability to predict psychiatric disorder in the face of physical illness, even if the pathogenesis of that psychiatric disorder is poorly understood, may enable us to gain some degree of preventive control over the occurrence and nature of

the disorder (Earls, 1987). Furthermore, control over the risk and vulnerability factors involved may also facilitate primary or secondary prevention of psychiatric disorder during physical illness (Dew & Bromet, 1993). Specifically, the risk/vulnerability factors reviewed above fall into two categories: some are fixed, unmodifiable features of an individual or that person's environment (gender, age, ethnicity, personal and family history of psychiatric disorder, major non-health life events); others are potentially more amenable to change (SES, social supports, coping strategies and styles). Prevention efforts in the case of unmodifiable factors may aim to alter other features or resources in the individual's environment so as to minimize the impact of these factors. In contrast, prevention efforts for modifiable factors may focus on changing the factors themselves through education, self-help groups and activities, and the development of formal comprehensive care programs that consider not only physical but psychiatric and psychosocial adjustment to illness as well. Although such prevention activities would not break any etiological link between physical illness and psychopathology, they may result in substantial reductions in the likelihood or persistence of psychopathology in the context of physical illness.

In summary, the research reviewed in this paper places us on the brink of new territory in the areas of conceptual understanding and preventive interventions for psychiatric disorder during physical illness. As Cassem (1990) has noted, "mind and body remain stubbornly one" (p. 609). Thus better understanding and prevention of psychiatric disorder during physical illness is likely, in turn, to influence the physical illness itself and its ultimate course. That possibility is an exciting one to entertain for the future.

REFERENCES

Adler, N. E., Boyce, T., Chesney, M. A., Cohen, S., Folkman, S., Kahn, R. L., & Syme, S. L. (1994). Socioeconomic status and health: The challenge of the gradient. *American Psychologist, 49*, 15–24.

Ahles, T. A., Khan, S. A., Yunus, M. B., Spiegel, D. A., & Masi, A. T. (1991). Psychiatric status of patients with primary fibromyalgia, patients with rheumatoid arthritis, and subjects without pain: A blind comparison of DSM-III diagnoses. *American Journal of Psychiatry, 148*, 1721–1726.

Alexander, P. J., Prabhu, S. G. S., Krishnamoorthy, E. S., & Hakatti, P. C. (1994). Mental disorders in patients with noncardiac chest pain. *Acta Psychiatrica Scandinavica, 89*, 291–293.

Alloway, R., & Bebbington, P. (1987). The buffer theory of social support—a review of the literature. *Psychological Medicine, 17*, 91–108.

American Psychiatric Association. (1980). *Diagnostic and statistical manual of mental disorders* (3rd ed.). Washington, DC: American Psychiatric Press.

American Psychiatric Association. (1987). *Diagnostic and statistical manual of mental disorders* (3rd ed., rev.). Washington, DC: American Psychiatric Press.

American Psychiatric Association. (1994). *Diagnostic and statistical manual of mental disorders* (4th ed.). Washington, DC: American Psychiatric Press.

Aromaa, A., Raitasalo, R., Reunanen, A., Impivaara, O., Heliovaara, M., Knekt, P., Lehtinen, V., Joukamaa, M., & Maatela, J. (1994). Depression and cardiovascular diseases. *Acta Psychiatrica Scandinavica. Supplementum, 377*, 77–82.

Atkinson, J. H., Grant, I., Kennedy, C. J., Richman, D. D., Spector, S. A., & McCutchan, J. A. (1988). Prevalence of psychiatric disorders among men infected with human immunodeficiency virus: A controlled study. *Archives of General Psychiatry, 45*, 859–864.

Attkisson, C. C., & Zich, J. M. (Eds.). (1990). *Depression in primary care: Screening and detection.* New York: Routledge.

Baron, A. E., Manson, S. M., Ackerson, L. M., & Brenneman, D. L. (1990). Depressive symptomatology in older American Indians with chronic disease: Some psychometric considerations. In C. C. Attkisson & J. M. Zich (Eds.), *Depression in primary care: Screening and detection* (pp. 217–231). New York: Routledge.

Beidel, D. C. (1987). Psychological factors in organ transplantation. *Clinical Psychology Review, 7*, 677–694.

Berkson, J. (1946). Limitations of the application of fourfold table analysis to hospital data. *Biometrics, 2*, 47–53.

Bix, B. C., Glosser, G., Holmes, W., Ballas, C., Meritz, M., Hutelmyer, C., & Turner, J. (1995). Relationship between psychiatric disease and neuropsychological impairment in HIV seropositive individuals. *Journal of the International Neuropsychological Society, 1*, 581–588.

Blazer, D. G., Kessler, R. C., McGonagle, K. A., & Swartz, M. S. (1994). The prevalence and distribution of major depression in a national community sample: The National Comorbidity Survey. *American Journal of Psychiatry, 151*, 979–986.

Breslau, N. (1985). Depressive symptoms, major depression, and generalized anxiety: A comparison of self-reports on CES-D and results from diagnostic interviews. *Psychiatry Research, 15*, 219–229.

Breslau, N., & Davis, G. C. (1993). Migraine, physical health, and psychiatric disorder: A prospective epidemiologic study in young adults. *Journal of Psychiatric Research, 27*, 211–221.

Breslau, N., Davis, G. C., Andreski, P., & Peterson, E. (1991). Traumatic events and posttraumatic stress disorder in an urban population of young adults. *Archives of General Psychiatry, 48*, 216–222.

Bridges, K. W., & Goldberg, D. P. (1992). Somatization in primary health care: Prevalence and determinants. In B. Cooper & R. Eastwood (Eds.), *Primary health care and psychiatric epidemiology* (pp. 341–350). London: Routledge.

Bromet, E. J., & Dew, M. A. (1995). A review of psychiatric epidemiologic research on disasters. *Epidemiologic Reviews, 17*, 113–119.

Brown, G. R., & Rundell, J. R. (1990). Prospective study of psychiatric morbidity in HIV-seropositive women without AIDS. *General Hospital Psychiatry, 12*, 30–35.

Brown, G. R., Rundell, J. R., McManis, S. E., Kendall, S. N., Zachaary, R., & Temoshok, L. (1992). Prevalence of psychiatric disorders in early stages of HIV infection. *Psychosomatic Medicine, 54*, 588–601.

Brown, G. W., Bifulco, A., & Andrews, B. (1990). Self-esteem and depression. III. Aetiological issues. *Social Psychiatry and Psychiatric Epidemiology, 25*, 235–243.

Brown, G. W., & Harris, T. O. (1978). *Social origins of depression: A study of psychiatric disorder in women.* London: Tavistock.

Brown, G. W., Harris, T. O. (Eds.). (1989). *Life events and illness*. New York: The Guilford Press.

Brown, R. G., & MacCarthy, B. (1990). Psychiatric morbidity in patients with Parkinson's disease. *Psychological Medicine, 20,* 77–87.

Bruce, M. L., & Hoff, R. A. (1994). Social and physical health risk factors for first-onset major depressive disorder in a community sample. *Social Psychiatry and Psychiatric Epidemiology, 29,* 165–171.

Bruce, M. L., & Leaf, P. J. (1989). Psychiatric disorders and 15-month mortality in a community sample of older adults. *American Journal of Public Health, 79,* 727–730.

Burgess, C., Morris, T., & Pettingale, K. W. (1988). Psychological response to cancer diagnosis—I. Evidence for coping styles (coping styles and cancer diagnosis). *Journal of Psychosomatic Research, 32,* 263–272.

Caine, E. D., & Shoulson, I. (1983). Psychiatric syndromes in Huntington's disease. *American Journal of Psychiatry, 140,* 728–733.

Cameron, O. G. (Ed.). (1987). *Presentations of depressions: Depressive symptoms in medical and other psychiatric disorders*. New York: John Wiley & Sons.

Canadian Erythropoietin Study Group. (1990). Association between recombinant human erythropoietin and quality of life and exercise capacity of patients receiving haemodialysis. *British Medical Journal, 300,* 573–578.

Carney, R. M., Rich, M. W., Freedland, K. E., Saini, J., teVelde, A., Simeone, C., & Clark, K. (1988). Major depressive disorder predicts cardiac events in patients with coronary artery disease. *Psychosomatic Medicine, 50,* 627–633.

Carney, R. M., Rich, M. W., teVelde, A., Saini, J., Clark, K., & Jaffe, A. S. (1987). Major depressive disorder in coronary artery disease. *American Journal of Cardiology, 60,* 1273–1275.

Cassel, J. (1976). The contribution of the social environment to host resistance. *American Journal of Epidemiology, 104,* 107–123.

Cassem, E. H. (1988). Depression secondary to medical illness. In A. J. Frances & R. E. Hales (Eds.), *Review of psychiatry* (Vol. 7, pp. 256–273). Washington, DC: American Psychiatric Press.

Cassem, E. H. (1990). Depression and anxiety secondary to medical illness. *Psychiatric Clinics of North America, 13,* 597–612.

Cassileth, B. R., Lusk, E. J., Strouse, T. B., Miller, D. S., Brown, L. L., Cross, P. A., & Tenaglia, A. N. (1984). Psychosocial status in chronic illness: A comparative analysis of six diagnostic groups. *New England Journal of Medicine, 311,* 506–511.

Castillo, C. S., Starkstein, S. E., Fedoroff, J. P., Price, T. R., & Robinson, R. G. (1993). Generalized anxiety disorder after stroke. *Journal of Nervous and Mental Disease, 181,* 100–106.

Catalan, J., Klimes, I., Bond, A., Day, A., Garrod, A., & Rizza, C. (1992a). The psychosocial impact of HIV infection in men with haemophilia: Controlled investigation and factors associated with psychiatric morbidity. *Journal of Psychosomatic Research, 36,* 409–416.

Catalan, J., Klimes, I., Day, A., Garrod, A., Bond, A., & Gallwey, J. (1992b). The psychosocial impact of HIV infection in gay men: A controlled investigation and factors associated with psychiatric morbidity. *British Journal of Psychiatry, 161,* 774–778.

Cavanaugh, S. (1983). The prevalence of emotional and cognitive dysfunction in a general medical population: Using the MMSE, GHQ, and BDI. *General Hospital Psychiatry, 5,* 15–24.

Cavanaugh, S. (1984). Diagnosing depression in the hospitalized patient with chronic medical illness. *Journal of Clinical Psychiatry, 45,* 13–16.

Cavanaugh, S., & Wettstein, R. M. (1984). Prevalence of psychiatric morbidity in medical populations. In L. Grinspoon (Ed.), *Psychiatry update* (Vol. 3, pp. 187–215, 279–281). Washington, DC: American Psychiatric Press.

Christensen, A. J., Turner, C. W., Slaughter, J. R., & Holman, J. M. (1989). Perceived family support as a moderator of psychological well-being in end-stage renal disease. *Journal of Behavioral Medicine, 12,* 249–265.

Ciaranello, R. D., & Ciaranello, A. L. (1991). Genetics of major psychiatric disorders. *Annual Review of Medicine, 42,* 151–158.

Clarke, D. M., Smith, G. C., & Herman, H. E. (1993). A comparative study of screening instruments for mental disorders in general hospital patients. *International Journal of Psychiatry in Medicine, 23,* 323–337.

Cohen, S., & Edwards, J. R. (1989). Personality characteristics as moderators of the relationship between stress and disorder. In R. W. J. Neufeld (Ed.), *Advances in the investigation of psychological stress* (pp. 235–283). New York: John Wiley & Sons.

Cohen, S., & Wills, T. A. (1985). Stress, social support, and the buffering hypothesis. *Psychological Bulletin, 98,* 310–357.

Cohen-Cole, S. A., & Stoudemire, A. (1987). Major depression and physical illness. *Psychiatric Clinics of North America, 10*, 1–17.

Cooper, B. (1993). Single spies and battalions: The clinical epidemiology of mental disorders. *Psychological Medicine, 23*, 891–907.

Coyne, J. C., & Downey, G. (1991). Social factors and psychopathology: Stress, social support, and coping processes. *Annual Review of Psychology, 42*, 401–425.

Craven, J. L., Rodin, G. M., Johnson, L., & Kennedy, S. H. (1987). The diagnosis of major depression in renal dialysis patients. *Psychosomatic Medicine, 49*, 482–492.

Croog, S. H., Levine, S., Testa, M. A., Brown, B., Bulpitt, C. J., Jenkins, C. D., Klerman, G. L., & Williams, G. H. (1986). The effects of antihypertensive therapy on the quality of life. *New England Journal of Medicine, 314*, 1657–1664.

Davidson, S., Dew, M. A., Penkower, L., Becker, J. T., Kingsley, L., & Sullivan, P. F. (1992). Substance use and sexual behavior among homosexual men at risk for HIV infection: Psychosocial moderators. *Psychology and Health, 7*, 259–272.

Dean, C. (1987). Psychiatric morbidity following mastectomy: Preoperative predictors and types of illness. *Journal of Psychosomatic Research, 31*, 385–392.

Dean, C., Surtees, P., & Sashidharan, S. (1983). Comparisons of research diagnostic systems in an Edinburgh community sample. *British Journal of Psychiatry, 142*, 247–256.

Derogatis, L. R. (1983). *SCL-90R administration, scoring and procedures manual–II* (2nd ed.). Towson, MD: Clinical Psychometrics Research.

Devlen, J., Maguire, P., Phillips, P., & Crowther, D. (1987). Psychological problems associated with diagnosis and treatment of lymphomas. II. Retrospective study. *British Medical Journal, 295*, 953–954.

Dew, M. A., & Bromet, E. J. (1993). Epidemiology. In A. Bellack & M. Hersen (Eds.), *Psychopathology in adulthood: An advanced text* (pp. 21–40). New York: Pergamon.

Dew, M. A., Bromet, E. J., & Penkower, L. (1992). Mental health effects of job loss in women. *Psychological Medicine, 22*, 751–764.

Dew, M. A., Kormos, R. L., Roth, L. H., Armitage, J. M., Pristas, J. M., Harris, R. C., Capretta, C., & Griffith, B. P. (1993). Life quality in the era of bridging to cardiac transplantation: Bridge patients in an outpatient setting. *ASAIO Journal, 39*, 145–152.

Dew, M. A., Penkower, L., & Bromet, E. J. (1991). Effects of unemployment on mental health in the contemporary family. *Behavior Modification, 15*, 501–544.

Dew, M. A., Ragni, M. V., & Nimorwicz, P. (1990). Infection with human immunodeficiency virus and vulnerability to psychiatric distress: A study of men with hemophilia. *Archives of General Psychiatry, 47*, 737–744.

Dew, M. A., Roth, L. H., Schulberg, H. C., Simmons, R. G., Kormos, R. L., Trzepacz, P. T., & Griffith, B. P. (1996a). Prevalence and predictors of anxiety-related disorders during the year after heart transplantation. *General Hospital Psychiatry, 18*, 48S–61S.

Dew, M. A., Roth, L. H., Thompson, M. E., & Griffith, B. P. (1996b). Medical compliance and its predictors in the first year after heart transplantation. *Journal of Heart and Lung Transplantation, 15*, 631–645.

Dew, M. A., & Simmons, R. G. (1990). The advantage of multiple measures of quality of life. *Scandinavian Journal of Urology and Nephrology, 131*(Suppl.), 23–30.

Dew, M. A., Simmons, R. G., Roth, L. H., Schulberg, H. C., Thompson, M. E., Armitage, J. M., & Griffith, B. P. (1994). Psychosocial predictors of vulnerability to distress in the year following heart transplantation. *Psychological Medicine, 24*, 929–945.

Dew, M. A., Switzer, G. E., Goycoolea, J. M., Allen, A. S., DiMartini, A., Kormos, R. L., & Griffith, B. P. (1997). Does transplantation produce quality of life benefits? A quantitative review of the literature. *Transplantation, 64*, 1261–1273.

Dilling, H., & Weyerer, S. (1984). Prevalence of mental disorders in the small-town–rural region of Traunstein (Upper Bavaria). *Acta Psychiatrica Scandinavica, 69*, 60–79.

Dohrenwend, B. P. (1990). Socioeconomic status (SES) and psychiatric disorders: Are the issues still compelling? *Social Psychiatry and Psychiatric Epidemiology, 25*, 41–47.

Dohrenwend, B. S., & Dohrenwend, B. P. (1981). Life stress and illness: Formulation of the issues. In B. S. Dohrenwend & B. P. Dohrenwend (Eds.), *Stressful life events and their context* (pp. 1–27). New York: Prodist.

Earls, F. (1987). Toward the prevention of psychiatric disorders. In R. E. Hales & A. J. Francis (Eds.), *Psychiatry update* (Vol. 6, pp. 664–675). Washington, DC: American Psychiatric Press.

Eaton, W. W., Kessler, R. C., Wittchen, H. U., & Magee, W. J. (1994). Panic and panic disorder in the United States. *American Journal of Psychiatry, 151,* 413–420.

Endicott, J. (1984). Measurement of depression in patients with cancer. *Cancer, 53,* 2243–2249.

Fava, G. A. (1994). Affective disorders and endocrine disease: New insights from psychosomatic studies. *Psychosomatics, 35,* 341–353.

Fedoroff, J. P., Starkstein, S. E., Parikh, R. M., Price, T. R., & Robinson, R. G. (1991). Are depressive symptoms nonspecific in patients with acute stroke? *American Journal of Psychiatry, 148,* 1172–1176.

Felton, B. J., & Revenson, T. A. (1984). Coping with chronic illness: A study of illness controllability and the influence of coping strategies on psychological adjustment. *Journal of Consulting and Clinical Psychology, 52,* 343–353.

Finlay-Jones, R., & Brown, G. W. (1981). Types of stressful life event and the onset of anxiety and depressive disorders. *Psychological Medicine, 11,* 803–815.

Fitzpatrick, R., Newman, S., Lamb, R., & Shipley, M. (1988). Social relationships and psychological well-being in rheumatoid arthritis. *Social Science and Medicine, 27,* 399–403.

Flint, A. J. (1994). Epidemiology and comorbidity of anxiety disorders in the elderly. *American Journal of Psychiatry, 151,* 640–649.

Fogel, B. S. (1993). Parkinson's disease: Recent developments of psychiatric interest. In A. Stoudemire & B. S. Fogel (Eds.), *Medical-psychiatric practice* (Vol. 2, pp. 447–469). Washington, DC: American Psychiatric Press.

Folstein, S. E., Abbott, M. H., Chase, G. A., Jensen, B. A., & Folstein, M. F. (1983). The association of affective disorder with Huntington's disease in a case series and in families. *Psychological Medicine, 13,* 537–542.

Fontana, A. F., Kerns, R. D., Rosenberg, R. L., & Colonese, K. L. (1989). Support, stress, and recovery from coronary heart disease: A longitudinal causal model. *Health Psychology, 8,* 175–193.

Forrester, A. W., Lipsey, J. R., Teitelbaum, M. L., DePaulo, J. R., Andrzejewski, P. L., & Robinson, R. G. (1992). Depression following myocardial infarction. *International Journal of Psychiatry in Medicine, 22,* 33–46.

Frank, R. G., Beck, N. C., Parker, J. C., Kashani, J. H., Elliott, T. R., Haut, A. E., Smith, E., Atwood, C., Brownlee-Duffeck, M., & Kay, D. R. (1988). Depression in rheumatoid arthritis. *Journal of Rheumatology, 15,* 920–925.

Frankel, B. G., & Turner, R. J. (1983). Psychological adjustment in chronic disability: The role of social support in the case of the hearing impaired. *Canadian Journal of Sociology, 8,* 273–291.

Frasure-Smith, N., Lesperance, F., & Talajic, M. (1993). Depression following myocardial infarction: Impact on 6-month survival. *JAMA, 270,* 1819–1825.

Fulop, G., & Strain, J. J. (1991). Diagnosis and treatment of psychiatric disorders in medically ill inpatients. *Hospital and Community Psychiatry, 42,* 389–394.

George, L. K., Landerman, R., Blazer, D., & Melville, M. L. (1986). Concurrent morbidity between physical and mental illness: An epidemiologic examination. In L. L. Carstensen & J. M. Neale (Eds.), *Mechanisms of psychological influence on physical health, with special attention to the elderly* (pp. 9–22). New York: Plenum.

Goldberg, D. P., & Bridges, K. (1987). Screening for psychiatric illness in general practice: The general practitioner versus the screening questionnaire. *Journal of the Royal College of General Practitioners, 37,* 15–18.

Goldberg, D. P., Cooper, B., Eastwood, M. R., Kedward, H. B., & Shepherd, M. (1970). A standardized psychiatric interview for use in community surveys. *British Journal of Preventive and Social Medicine, 24,* 18–23.

Hall, R. C. W. (1980a). Anxiety. In R. C. W. Hall (Ed.), *Psychiatric presentations of medical illness* (pp. 13–35). New York: Spectrum Publications.

Hall, R. C. W. (1980b). Depression. In R. C. W. Hall (Ed.), *Psychiatric presentations of medical illness* (pp. 37–63). New York: Spectrum.

Hall, R. C. W., Beresford, T. P., & Blow, F. C. (1987). Depression and medical illness: An overview. In O. G. Cameron (Ed.), *Presentations of depressions: Depressive symptoms in medical and other psychiatric disorders* (pp. 401–414). New York: Wiley.

Hantz, P., Caradoc-Davies, G., Caradoc-Davies, T., Weatherall, M., & Dixon, G. (1994). Depression in Parkinson's disease. *American Journal of Psychiatry, 151,* 1010–1014.

Hardman, A., Maguire, P., & Crowther, D. (1989). The recognition of psychiatric morbidity on a medical oncology ward. *Journal of Psychosomatic Research, 33,* 235–239.

Harris, R. C., Dew, M. A., Lee, A., Amaya, M., Buches, L., Reetz, D., & Coleman, G. (1995). The role of religion in heart transplant recipients' long-term health and well-being: Implications for health care professionals. *Journal of Religion and Health, 34,* 17–32.

Hays, R. B., Turner, H., & Coates, T. J. (1992). Social support, AIDS-related symptoms, and depression among gay men. *Journal of Consulting and Clinical Psychology, 60,* 463–469.

Hinrichsen, G. A., Lieberman, J. A., Pollack, S., & Steinberg, H. (1989). Depression in hemodialysis patients. *Psychosomatics, 30,* 284–289.

Hong, B. A., Smith, M. D., Robson, A. M., & Wetzel, R. D. (1987). Depressive symptomatology and treatment in patients with end-stage renal disease. *Psychological Medicine, 17,* 185–190.

Hosaka, T., Aoki, T., & Ichikawa, Y. (1994). Emotional states of patients with hematological malignancies: Preliminary study. *Japanese Journal of Clinical Oncology, 24,* 186–190.

House, A. (1987). Psychosocial problems of patients on the renal unit and their relation to treatment outcome. *Journal of Psychosomatic Research, 31,* 441–452.

House, A., Dennis, M., Warlow, C., Hawton, K., & Molyneux, A. (1990). Mood disorders after stroke and their relation to lesion location: A CT scan study. *Brain, 113,* 1113–1129.

House, J. S., Landis, K. R., & Umberson, D. (1988). Social relationships and health. *Science, 241,* 540–545.

Ibbotson, T., Maguire, P., Selby, P., Priestman, T., & Wallace, L. (1994). Screening for anxiety and depression in cancer patients: The effects of disease and treatment. *European Journal of Cancer, 30A,* 37–40.

Israel, E., Cohn, J., Dube, L., & Drazen, J. M. (1996). Effect of treatment with zileuton, a 5-lipoxygenase inhibitor, in patients with asthma—a randomized clinical trial. *JAMA, 275,* 931–936.

Joffe, R. T., Lippert, G. P., Gray, T. A., Sawa, G., & Horvath, Z. (1987). Mood disorder and multiple sclerosis. *Archives of Neurology, 44,* 376–378.

Joffe, R. T., Rubinow, D. R., Denicoff, K. D., Maher, M., & Sindelar, W. F. (1986). Depression and carcinoma of the pancreas. *General Hospital Psychiatry, 8,* 241–245.

Joseph, J. G., Caumartin, S. M., Tal, M., Kirscht, J. P., Kessler, R. C., Ostrow, D. G., & Wortman, C. B. (1990). Psychological functioning in a cohort of gay men at risk for AIDS: A three-year descriptive study. *Journal of Nervous and Mental Disease, 178,* 607–615.

Kaplan, R. M., Anderson, J. P., Wu, A. W., Mathews, W. C., Kozin, F., & Orenstein, D.

(1989). The Quality of Well-being Scale: Applications in AIDS, cystic fibrosis, and arthritis. *Medical Care, 27,* 27–43.

Karajgi, B., Rifkin, A., Doddi, S., & Kolli, R. (1990). The prevalence of anxiety disorders in patients with chronic obstructive pulmonary disease. *American Journal of Psychiatry, 147,* 200–201.

Kathol, R. G., Noyes, R., Williams, J., Mutgi, A., Carroll, B., & Perry, P. (1990). Diagnosing depression in patients with medical illness. *Psychosomatics, 31,* 434–440.

Kessler, R. C., McGonagle, K. A., Zhao, S., Nelson, C. B., Hughes, M., Eshelman, S., Wittchen, H., & Kendler, K. S. (1994). Lifetime and 12-month prevalence of DSM-III-R psychiatric disorders in the United States. *Archives of General Psychiatry, 51,* 8–19.

Kessler, R. C., Price, R. H., & Wortman, C. B. (1985). Social factors in psychopathology: Stress, social support, and coping processes. *Annual Review of Psychology, 36,* 531–572.

King, M. (1985). Alcohol abuse in Huntington's disease. *Psychological Medicine, 15,* 815–819.

Kirmayer, L. J., Robbins, J. M., & Kapusta, M. A. (1988). Somatization and depression in fibromyalgia syndrome. *American Journal of Psychiatry, 145,* 950–954.

Kisely, S. R., & Goldberg, D. P. (1996). Physical and psychiatric comorbidity in general practice. *British Journal of Psychiatry, 169,* 236–242.

Klerman, G. L. (1981). Depression in the medically ill. *Psychiatric Clinics of North America, 4,* 301–317.

Kobasa, S. C., Maddi, S. R., & Kahn, S. (1982). Hardiness and health: A prospective study. *Journal of Personality and Social Psychology, 42,* 168–177.

Koenig, H. G., Cohen, H. J., Blazer, D. G., Pieper, C., Meador, K. G., Shelp, F., Goli, V., & DePasquale, B. (1992). Religious coping and depression among elderly, hospitalized medically ill men. *American Journal of Psychiatry, 149,* 1693–1700.

Koenig, H. G., Meador, K. G., Cohen, H. J., & Blazer, D. G. (1988). Depression in elderly hospitalized patients with medical illness. *Archives of Internal Medicine, 148,* 1929–1936.

Koenig, H. G., Pappas, P., Holsinger, T., & Bachar, J. R. (1995). Assessing diagnostic approaches to depression in medically ill older adults: How reliably can mental health professionals make judgments about the cause of symptoms? *Journal of the American Geriatrics Society, 43,* 472–478.

Kokkonen, J., & Kokkonen, E. R. (1993). Prevalence of mental disorders in young adults with chronic physical diseases since childhood as identified by the Present State Examination and the CATEGO program. *Acta Psychiatrica Scandinavica, 87,* 239–243.

Kolody, B., Vega, W., Meinhardt, K., & Bensussen, G. (1986). The correspondence of health complaints and depressive symptoms among Anglos and Mexican Americans. *Journal of Nervous and Mental Disease, 174,* 221–228.

Kramer, M., Simonsick, E., Lima, B., & Levav, I. (1989, June). *The epidemiological basis for primary care: A case for action.* Paper presented at the International Symposium on Primary Health Care and Psychiatric Epidemiology, Section of Epidemiology and Community Psychiatry of the World Psychiatric Association, Toronto, Canada.

Kramer, M., Simonsick, E., Lima, B., & Levav, I. (1992). The epidemiological basis for mental health care in primary health care: A case for action. In B. Cooper & R. Eastwood (Eds.), *Primary health care and psychiatric epidemiology* (pp. 69–98). London: Routledge.

Kurdek, L. A., & Siesky, G. (1990). The nature and correlates of psychological adjustment in gay men with AIDS-related conditions. *Journal of Applied Social Psychology, 20,* 846–860.

Larson, E. W., & Richelson, E. (1988). Organic causes of mania. *Mayo Clinic Proceedings, 63,* 906–912.

Lazarus, R. S., & Folkman, S. (1984). *Stress, appraisal, and coping.* New York: Springer-Verlag.

Levine, M. N., Guyatt, G. H., Gent, M., De Pauw, S., Goodyear, M. D., Hryniuk, W. M., Arnold, A., Findlay, B., Skillings, J. R., Bramwell, V. H., Levin, L., Bush, H., Abu-Zahra, H., & Kotalik, J. (1988). Quality of life in stage II breast cancer: An instrument for clinical trials. *Journal of Clinical Oncology, 6,* 1798–1810.

Lipsitz, J. D., Williams, J. B. W., Rabkin, J. G., Remien, R. H., Bradbury, M., el Sadr, W., Goetz, R., Sorrell, S., & Gorman, J. M. (1994). Psychopathology in male and female intravenous drug users with and without HIV infection. *American Journal of Psychiatry, 151,* 1662–1668.

Lobo, A., Perez-Echeverria, M. J., Artal, J., Rubio, L., Escolar, M. V., Gonzalez-Torrecillas, J. L., Morera, B., Dia, J. L., & Miranda, M. (1988). Psychiatric morbidity among medical out-patients in Spain: A case for new methods of classification. *Journal of Psychosomatic Research, 32,* 355–364.

Lustman, P. J., Clouse, R. E., Carney, R. M., & Griffith, L. S. (1987). Characteristics of depression in adults with diabetes. In *Proceedings of NIMH Conference on Mental Disorders in General Health Care Settings* (Vol. 1, pp. 127–129). Seattle: The Foundation for Group Health Cooperative of Puget Sound.

Lustman, P. J., Gavard, J. A., & Clouse, R. E. (1992). Depression in adults with diabetes. *Diabetes Care, 15,* 1631–1639.

Lustman, P. J., Griffith, L. S., Clouse, R. E., & Cryer, P. E. (1986). Psychiatric illness in diabetes mellitus: Relationship to symptoms and glucose control. *Journal of Nervous and Mental Disease, 174,* 736–742.

Lyness, J. M., Bruce, M. L., Koenig, H. G., Parmelee, P. A., Schulz, R., Lawton, M. P., & Reynolds, C. F., III. (1996). Depression and medical illness in late life: Report of a symposium. *Journal of the American Geriatrics Society, 44,* 198–203.

MacKenzie, T. B., & Popkin, M. K. (1987). Suicide in the medical patient. *International Journal of Psychiatry in Medicine, 17,* 3–22.

Magni, G., & Borgherini, G. (1992). Psychosocial outcome after heart transplantation. In P. J. Walter (Ed.), *Quality of life after open heart surgery* (pp. 457–465). Dordrecht, The Netherlands: Kluwer Academic Publishers.

Maj, M., Janssen, R., Starace, F., Zaudig, M., Satz, P., Sughondhabirom, B., Luabeya, M. K., Riedel, R., Ndetei, D., Calil, H. M., Bing, E. G., St. Louis, M., & Sartorius, N. (1994). WHO Neuropsychiatric AIDS Study, cross-sectional phase I: Study design and psychiatric findings. *Archives of General Psychiatry, 51,* 39–49.

Mayou, R., & Hawton, K. (1986). Psychological disorder in the general hospital. *British Journal of Psychiatry, 149,* 172–190.

Mayou, R., Peveler, R., Davies, B., Mann, J., & Fairburn, C. (1991). Psychiatric morbidity in young adults with insulin-dependent diabetes mellitus. *Psychological Medicine, 21,* 639–645.

McDaniel, J. S., Fowlie, E., Summerville, M. B., Farber, E. W., & Cohen-Cole, S. A. (1995). An assessment of rates of psychiatric morbidity and functioning in HIV disease. *General Hospital Psychiatry, 17,* 346–352.

Mendes de Leon, C. F., Kasl, S. V., & Jacobs, S. (1994). A prospective study of widowhood and changes in symptoms of depression in a community sample of the elderly. *Psychological Medicine, 24,* 613–624.

Merikangas, K. R. (1987). Genetic epidemiology of psychiatric disorders. In R. E. Hales & A. J. Francis (Eds.), *Psychiatry update* (Vol. 6, pp. 625–646). Washington, DC: American Psychiatric Press.

Minden, S. L., Orav, J., & Reich, P. (1987). Depression in multiple sclerosis. *General Hospital Psychiatry, 9,* 426–434.

Moldin, S. O., Scheftner, W. A., Rice, J. P., Nelson, E., Knesevich, M. A., & Akiskal, H. (1993). Association between major depressive disorder and physical illness. *Psychological Medicine, 23,* 755–761.

Moller, A., Wiedemann, G., Rohde, U., Backmund, H., & Sonntag, A. (1994). Correlates of cognitive impairment and depressive mood disorder in multiple sclerosis. *Acta Psychiatrica Scandinavica, 89,* 117–121.

Moran, M. G. (1996). Psychiatric aspects of rheumatology. *Psychiatric Clinics of North America, 19,* 575–588.

Myers, J. K., & Weissman, M. M. (1980). Use of a self-report symptom scale to detect depression in a community sample. *American Journal of Psychiatry, 137,* 1081–1084.

Myers, J. K., Weissman, M. M., Tischler, G. L., Holzer, C. E., III, Leaf, P. J., Orvaschel, H., Anthony, J. C., Boyd, J. H., Burke, J. D., Kramer, M., & Stoltzman, R. (1984). Six-month prevalence of psychiatric disorders in three communities. *Archives of General Psychiatry, 41,* 959–967.

Ostrow, D. G., Joseph, J., Monjan, A., Kessler, R., Emmons, C., Phair, J., Fox, R., Kingsley, L., Dudley, J., Chmiel, S., & Van Raden, M. (1986). Psychosocial aspects of AIDS risk. *Psychopharmacology Bulletin, 22,* 678–683.

Ostrow, D. G., Monjan, A., Joseph, J., VanRaden, M., Fox, R., Kingsley, L., Dudley, J., & Phair, J. (1989). HIV-related symptoms and psychological functioning in a cohort of homosexual men. *American Journal of Psychiatry, 146,* 737–742.

Pargament, K. I., Ensing, D. S., Falgout, K., Olsen, H., Reilly, B., Van Haitsma, K., & Warren, R. (1990). God help me: (I): Religious coping efforts as predictors of the outcomes to significant negative life events. *American Journal of Community Psychology, 18,* 793–824.

Paykel, E. S., Myers, J. K., Dienelt, M. N., Klerman, G. L., Lindenthal, J. J., & Pepper, M. P. (1969). Life events and depression: A con-

trolled study. *Archives of General Psychiatry, 21,* 753–760.

Pearlin, L. I., Lieberman, M. A., Menaghan, E. G., & Mullen, J. T. (1981). The stress process. *Journal of Health and Social Behavior, 22,* 337–356.

Penkower, L., Bromet, E. J., & Dew, M. A. (1988). Husbands' layoff and wives' mental health. *Archives of General Psychiatry, 45,* 994–1000.

Perkins, D. O., Stern, R. A., Golden, R. N., Murphy, C., Naftolowitz, D., & Evans, D. L. (1994). Mood disorders in HIV infection: Prevalence and risk factors in a nonepicenter of the AIDS epidemic. *American Journal of Psychiatry, 151,* 233–236.

Perry, S., Jacobsberg, L. B., Fishman, B., Frances, A., Bobo, J., & Jacobsberg, B. K. (1990). Psychiatric diagnosis before serological testing for the human immunodeficiency virus. *American Journal of Psychiatry, 147,* 89–93.

Pollock, S. E. (1985). Human responses to chronic illness: Physiologic and psychosocial adaptation. *Nursing Research, 35,* 90–95.

Popkin, M. K., Callies, A. L., Colon, E. A., Lentz, R. D., & Sutherland, D. E. (1993). Psychiatric diagnosis and the surgical outcome of pancreas transplantation in patients with type I diabetes mellitus. *Psychosomatics, 34,* 251–258.

Popkin, M. K., Callies, A. L., Lentz, R. D., Colon, E. A., & Sutherland, D. E. (1988). Prevalence of major depression, simple phobia, and other psychiatric disorders in patients with long-standing type I diabetes mellitus. *Archives of General Psychiatry, 45,* 64–68.

Portegies, P. (1994). AIDS dementia complex: A review. *Journal of Acquired Immune Deficiency Syndromes, 7*(Suppl. 2), S38–S49.

Pugh, K., Riccio, M., Jadresic, D., Burgess, A. P., Baldeweg, T., Catalan, J., Lovett, E., Hawkins, D. A., Gruzelier, J., & Thompson, C. (1994). A longitudinal study of the neuropsychiatric consequences of HIV-1 infection in gay men. II: Psychological and health status at baseline and at 12-month follow-up. *Psychological Medicine, 24,* 897–904.

Razavi, D., Delvaux, N., Farvacques, C., & Robaye, E. (1990). Screening for adjustment disorders and major depressive disorders in cancer in-patients. *British Journal of Psychiatry, 156,* 79–83.

Regier, D. A., Myers, J. K., Kramer, M., Robins, L. N., Blazer, D. G., Hough, R. L., Eaton, W. W., & Locke, B. Z. (1984). The NIMH Epidemiologic Catchment Areas Program: Historical context, major objectives, and study population characteristics. *Archives of General Psychiatry, 41,* 934–941.

Roberts, R. E. (1990). Special population issues in screening for depression. In C. C. Attkisson & J. M. Zich (Eds.), *Depression in primary care: Screening and detection* (pp. 183–216). New York: Routledge.

Robins, L. N., Helzer, J. E., Weissman, M. M., Orvaschel, H., Gruenberg, E., Burke, J. D., Jr., & Regier, D. A. (1984). Lifetime prevalence of specific psychiatric disorders in three sites. *Archives of General Psychiatry, 41,* 949–958.

Robinson, R. G., Starr, L. B., Kubos, K. L., & Price, T. R. (1983). A two-year longitudinal study of post-stroke mood disorders: Findings during the initial evaluation. *Stroke, 14,* 736–741.

Robinson, R. G., Starr, L. B., Lipsey, J. R., Rao, K., & Price, T. R. (1984). A two-year longitudinal study of post-stroke mood disorders: Dynamic changes over the first six months of follow-up. *Stroke, 15,* 510–517.

Rodin, G., Craven, J., & Littlefield, C. (1991). *Depression in the medically ill: An integrated approach.* New York: Brunner/Mazel.

Rodin, G., & Voshart, K. (1986). Depression in the medically ill: An overview. *American Journal of Psychiatry, 143,* 696–705.

Rosenberger, P. H., Bornstein, R. A., Nasrallah, H. A., Para, M. F., Whitacre, C. C., Fass, R. J., & Rice, R. R., Jr. (1993). Psychopathology in human immunodeficiency virus infection: Lifetime and current assessment. *Comprehensive Psychiatry, 34,* 150–158.

Saravay, S. M., & Lavin, M. (1994). Psychiatric comorbidity and length of stay in the general hospital. *Psychosomatics, 35,* 233–252.

Scheier, M. F., Weintraub, J. K., & Carver, C. S. (1986). Coping with stress: Divergent strategies of optimists and pessimists. *Journal of Personality and Social Psychology, 51,* 1257–1264.

Schiffer, R. B., Craine, E. D., Bamford, K. A., & Levy, S. (1983). Depressive episodes in patients with multiple sclerosis. *American Journal of Psychiatry, 140,* 1498–1500.

Schleifer, S. J., Macari-Hinson, M. M., Coyle, D. A., Slater, W. R., Kahn, M., Gorlin, R., & Zucher, H. D. (1989). The nature and course of depression following myocardial infarction. *Archives of Internal Medicine, 149,* 1785–1789.

Schulberg, H. C. (1991). Mental disorders in the primary care setting: Research priorities for the 1990s. *General Hospital Psychiatry, 13,* 156–164.

Schulberg, H. C., McClelland, M., & Burns, B. J. (1987). Depression and physical illness: The prevalence, causation, and diagnosis of comorbidity. *Clinical Psychology Review, 7,* 145–167.

Schwab, J. J., Bialow, M., Brown, J. M., & Holzer, C. E. (1967). Diagnosing depression in medical inpatients. *Annals of Internal Medicine, 67,* 695–707.

Shapiro, P. A. (1996). Psychiatric aspects of cardiovascular disease. *Psychiatric Clinics of North America, 19,* 613–629.

Shapiro, P. A., & Kornfeld, D. S. (1989). Psychiatric outcome of heart transplantation. *General Hospital Psychiatry, 11,* 352–357.

Siegal, B. R., Calsyn, R. J., & Cuddihee, R. M. (1987). The relationship of social support to psychosocial adjustment in end-stage renal disease patients. *Journal of Chronic Disease, 40,* 337–344.

Silverstone, P. H. (1996). Concise Assessment for Depression (CAD): A brief screening approach to depression in the medically ill. *Journal of Psychosomatic Research, 41,* 161–170.

Simmons, R. G., Marine, S. K., & Simmons, R. L. (1987). *Gift of life: The effect of organ transplantation on individual, family, and societal dynamics.* New Brunswick, CT: Transaction Books.

Smith, M. D., Hong, B. A., & Robson, A. M. (1985). Diagnosis of depression in patients with end-stage renal disease: Comparative analysis. *American Journal of Medicine, 79,* 160–166.

Starkstein, S. E., Preziosi, T. J., Bolduc, P. L., & Robinson, R. G. (1990). Depression in Parkinson's disease. *Journal of Nervous and Mental Disease, 178,* 27–31.

Starkstein, S. E., & Robinson, R. G. (1989). Affective disorders and cerebral vascular disease. *British Journal of Psychiatry, 154,* 170–182.

Stein, M. B., Heuser, I. J., Juncos, J. L., & Uhde, T. W. (1990). Anxiety disorders in patients with Parkinson's disease. *American Journal of Psychiatry, 147,* 217–220.

Stewart, A. L., Greenfield, S., Hays, R. D., Wells, K., Rogers, W. H., Berry, S. D., McGlynn, E. A., & Ware, J. E., Jr. (1989). Functional status and well-being of patients with chronic conditions: Results from the Medical Outcomes Study. *JAMA, 262,* 907–913.

Stoudemire, A. (1996). Epidemiology and psychopharmacology of anxiety in medical patients. *Journal of Clinical Psychiatry*, 57(Suppl. 7), 64–75.

Strain, J. J., & Fulop, G. (1992). Mood disorders and medical illness. In A. Tasman & M. B. Riba (Eds.), *Review of psychiatry* (Vol. 11, pp. 453–476). Washington, DC: American Psychiatric Press.

Strain, J. J., Liebowitz, M. R., & Klein, D. F. (1981). Anxiety and panic attacks in the medically ill. *Psychiatric Clinics of North America*, 4, 333–350.

Summers, J., Zisook, S., Atkinson, J. H., Sciolla, A., Whitehall, W., Brown, S., Patterson, T., & Grant, I. (1995). Psychiatric morbidity associated with acquired immune deficiency syndrome-related grief resolution. *Journal of Nervous and Mental Disease*, 183, 384–389.

Tarter, R. E., Switala, J., Carra, J., & Edwards, K. L. (1987). Inflammatory bowel disease: Psychiatric status of patients before and after disease onset. *International Journal of Psychiatry in Medicine*, 17, 173–181.

Taylor, S. E., & Aspinwall, L. G. (1993). Coping with chronic illness. In L. Goldberger & S. Breznitz (Eds.), *Handbook of stress* (2nd ed., pp. 511–531). New York: The Free Press.

Van Hemert, A. M., Hengeveld, M. W., Bolk, J. H., Rooijmans, H. G. M., & Vandenbroucke, J. P. (1993). Psychiatric disorders in relation to medical illness among patients of a general medical out-patient clinic. *Psychological Medicine*, 23, 167–173.

Vazquez-Barquero, J. L., Diez-Manrique, J. F., Pena, C., Aldama, J., Samaniego Rodriquez, C., Menendez Arango, J., & Mirapeix, C. (1987). A community mental health survey in Cantabria: A general description of morbidity. *Psychological Medicine*, 17, 227–241.

Weddington, W. W., Segraves, K. B., & Simon, M. A. (1986). Current and lifetime incidence of psychiatric disorders among a group of extremity sarcoma survivors. *Journal of Psychosomatic Research*, 30, 121–125.

Weissman, M. M. (1987). Advances in psychiatric epidemiology: Rates and risks for major depression. *American Journal of Public Health*, 77, 445–451.

Weissman, M. M., Prusoff, B. A., Gammon, G. D., Merikangas, K. R., Leckman, J. F., & Kidd, K. K. (1984). Psychopathology in the children (aged 6–18) of depressed and normal parents. *Journal of the American Academy of Child Psychiatry*, 23, 78–84.

Wells, K. B., Golding, J. M., & Burnam, M. A. (1988). Psychiatric disorder in a sample of the general population with and without chronic medical conditions. *American Journal of Psychiatry*, 145, 976–981.

Wells, K. B., Golding, J. M., & Burnam, M. A. (1989). Affective, substance use, and anxiety disorders in persons with arthritis, diabetes, heart disease, high blood pressure, or chronic lung conditions. *General Hospital Psychiatry*, 11, 320–327.

Weyerer, S. (1990). Relationships between physical and psychological disorders. In N. Sartorius, D. Goldberg, G. de Girolamo, J. Costa e Silva, Y. Lecrubier, & H.-U. Wittchen (Eds.), *Psychological disorders in general medical settings* (pp. 34–46). Toronto: Hogrefe and Huber Publishers.

Williams, J. B. W., Rabkin, J. G., Remien, R. H., Gorman, J. M., & Ehrhardt, A. A. (1991). Multidisciplinary baseline assessment of homosexual men with and without human immunodeficiency virus infection: II. Standardized clinical assessment of current and lifetime psychopathology. *Archives of General Psychiatry*, 48, 124–130.

Wilson, I. B., & Cleary, P. D. (1995). Linking clinical variables with health-related quality of life: A conceptual model of patient outcomes. *JAMA*, 273, 59–65.

Wing, J. K., Cooper, J. E., & Sartorius, N. (1974). *The description and classification of psychiatric symptoms: An instruction manual for the PSE and CATEGO system*. London: Cambridge University Press.

Wittchen, H.-U., Zhao, S., Kessler, R. C., & Eaton, W. W. (1994). DMS-III-R generalized anxiety disorder in the National Comorbidity Survey. *Archives of General Psychiatry*, 51, 355–364.

World Health Organization. (1977). *Manual of the international statistical classification of diseases, injuries, and causes of death* (9th rev.). Geneva: Author.

Yellowlees, P. M., & Ruffin, R. E. (1989). Psychological defenses and coping styles in patients following a life-threatening attack of asthma. *Chest*, 95, 1298–1303.

12

Divorce and Psychopathology

Martha L. Bruce

Divorce ranks high on most lists of life stressors, from those found in tabloids to those used in scientific research. The hypothesis that divorce leads to mental health problems seems almost a truism and is consistent with studies in psychiatric epidemiology that report disproportionately high rates of depression, depressive symptoms, and other mental health problems among separated and divorced adults in many epidemiological samples (e.g., Blazer et al., 1994; Robins & Regier 1991; Srole et al., 1962; Warheit et al., 1976; Weissman & Myers, 1978). These results from cross-sectional epidemiological research find further support from numerous longitudinal and case–control studies (Aseltine & Kessler, 1993; Briscoe et al., 1973; Bruce & Kim, 1992; Menaghan & Lieberman, 1986).

This proliferation of evidence suggesting that divorce may affect the risk of psychopathology obscures how little is known either about the direction of any causal relationships between divorce and psychiatric disorders or about their underlying mechanisms. Three aspects of the divorce–psychopathology relationship underline the complexity of the problem: (1) *divorce* is a single term representing a long process generally characterized by multiple stressful events and chronic strains; (2) while most

epidemiological studies address the impact of divorce on psychopathology, there is also evidence suggesting that psychopathology can itself affect (as well be affected by) any or all of the components of the divorce process, and (3) the impact of divorce on psychopathology can be direct or indirect and affects not only the divorcing spouses but also their children.

The purpose of this chapter is twofold: (1) to describe what is known about the relationship between divorce and psychopathology—in terms both of the effect psychiatric problems can have on the risk of divorce and of the effect of marital instability on the risk and course of psychopathology—and (2) to articulate some of the challenges that remain in understanding the nature of the connections between psychopathology and divorce and the mechanisms underlying those connections. The chapter first describes the divorce process and then examines the causal relationship between divorce and psychiatric status among involved adults and children.

BACKGROUND

Once relatively rare in the population, divorce has become almost commonplace. In the United States, divorce rates rose slowly but steadily from the mid-19th century, when approximately 5% of marriages would ultimately end in divorce, to the mid-1960s when approximately one-third of all marriages were estimated to end in divorce. The yearly incidence rate of divorce then rose sharply over the following 15 years, doubling from 10.6/1000 in 1964 to 22.8/1000 in 1978. Demographers generally believe that the divorce rate is no longer rising but has steadied to a point where approximately 40%–50% of today's marriages are expected to end in divorce (Furstenberg, 1994).

Divorce statistics enumerate the moment when a marriage is legally ended. This legal moment is only one of many points in the process of marital disruption, involving marital discord, separation, filing for a divorce, divorce proceedings, and being divorced. Because each of these events and the circumstances surrounding them may fit the notion of "stressor," a wider assessment than the legal decree is needed to understand the relationship of divorce to psychopathology.

The process of marital disruption and divorce begins in many often imperceptible ways, from gradual distancing on the part of both partners to overt fighting. Awareness of marital problems may be shared equally by both spouses over time, or one spouse may be surprised by the other's expressed (verbally or otherwise) desire to end the marriage. Ironically, the legal event of finalizing a divorce often may be less stressful than the events and circumstances leading up to that moment. The relative insignificance of this event has become apparent in an ongoing case–control study of life events and major depression conducted with colleagues at Yale. Using Dohrenwend and colleagues's structured event probe and narrative rating method (SEPRATE); (Dohrenwend, Raphael, Schwartz, et al., 1993) to rate the magnitude of reported events, we have found that the "event" of a divorce being finalized often has little bearing on the day-to-day lives of the divorcing spouses. The disruptions have already occurred with, for example, the changes in residence, withdrawal of intimacy, reorganization of family finances, and restructuring of time with chil-

dren. A notable exception to this generalization is when some element of the divorce, such as child custody, has been contested in court and the parent experiences loss at that time.

Research on circumstances following divorce suggests some common patterns (Holden & Smock, 1991; Seltzer, 1994; Smock, 1993). On average, the ways in which marital disruption affects their daily living differ for men and women, although both face demands in both time and money, especially if children are involved. Divorcing mothers are granted custody of the children more often than fathers, and thus bear the responsibilities of being a single parent— although, of course, many mothers serve as de facto single parents during the divorce proceedings and possibly prior to formal marital separation. Divorcing fathers, in contrast, often must learn how to live alone and how to restructure relationships with nonresident children.

The economic problems associated with divorce are not trivial. Because the incomes of the former spouses must now support two households rather than one, both men and women often experience declines in their standards of living, at least over the short term, and household incomes decline on average 30% (Hoffman & Duncan, 1988). The marked reductions in family income are often long term for women unless they remarry (Smock, 1993). For mothers, the economic effects are gravest. Separation and divorce are responsible for the majority of mother-only families (Bianchi & Spain, 1986), and almost half of women and children living as single-parent families live below the poverty level (U.S. Bureau of the Census, 1989). Men, in contrast, generally rise in postdivorce economic well-being over the long term.

In summary, the process of divorce generally entails dramatic change in many aspects of a person's daily life while also representing a major loss in terms of self-definition and future aspirations. This description of the divorce process is consistent with two separate conceptualizations of a life event in the research literature (McLean

& Link, 1994). One, articulated earlier by Holmes & Rahe (1967), is based on the notion of change: The magnitude of a life event is defined by the amount of life change expected as a consequence of the experience. The other, the basis of work by Brown and colleagues (Brown & Harris, 1978), focuses more on the psychological meaning attached to the events. From either perspective, divorce and the process of marital disruption meet the conceptual criteria of a severe stressful life event. As a profound and negative life event, divorce is expected to have a strong effect on the risk of psychiatric outcomes. However, in order to assess this effect, the role of psychopathology in the risk of divorce must be disentangled.

EFFECTS OF PSYCHOPATHOLOGY ON DIVORCE

There is little question that divorce is not a random event but one predicted by numerous social and psychological factors characterizing each of the spouses and their interaction (Gottman & Levenson, 1992; Morgan & Rindfuss, 1985). In their review of the literature, Karney and Bradbury (1995) critique the four major theoretical perspectives underlying much of the extant research on marital stability. These include, first, social exchange theory, which posits that marital success or failure depends upon the balance in each spouse's weighing of the attractiveness of the marriage (e.g., as a source of emotional fulfillment, economic security), the perceived barriers to leaving the marriage (e.g., religious prohibitions, financial constraints); and potential alternatives to the marriage (e.g., other partners or lifestyles). Second, behavioral theory attributes stable marriages to the ability of couples to interact in a mutually rewarding manner, especially in dealing with disagreements. In contrast to the first two theories, which address ongoing interpersonal aspects of marriage, attachment theory directs attention to the contribution of each spouse's personal history. In particular, attachment theory fo-

cuses on the role of childhood relationships in developing adult attachment needs and relationship styles, with successful marriages characterized by successful meshing of the attachment styles of both partners. Finally, crisis theory adds the perspective of external challenges to marriage, with stable marriages being those in which the partners deal successfully with the stressful events that confront the marriage.

After evaluating more than 100 longitudinal studies of marital quality and stability, Karney and Bradbury (1995) offer a model that integrates the personal, interpersonal, and external perspectives of the four different theoretical models of divorce. Briefly, in their "vulnerability–stress–adaptation" model, each spouse's enduring vulnerabilities (e.g., attribution needs as well as other characteristics a person brings to a marriage, such as personality, social status, and prior experiences) affect both the occurrence of stressful events in a marriage and the ability of the marriage partners to adapt successfully to those crises. Behaviors leading to successful adaption are reinforced both by improved marital quality and by reduced risk of additional stressors, a feedback loop resulting in even greater marital stability.

Karney and Bradbury's (1995) model provides a framework for describing the numerous ways in which psychiatric problems might affect marital stability. A history of psychopathology falls within the broad definition of "enduring vulnerabilities" and may affect both the risk of acute or chronic stressors in a marriage as well as the capacity of the couple to adapt successfully to those stressors. During marriage, psychiatric symptoms and their functional sequelae may themselves be conceptualized as ongoing stressors while potentially undermining the ability to cope with these problems. Furthermore, both the experience of stressors and the inability of couples to cope with the stressors might increase the risk of mental health problems, further exacerbating marital instability.

Although psychopathology clearly could affect marital stability and the divorce process in many ways, even an observed association between psychopathology and sub-sequent divorce in longitudinal data does not eliminate the possibility that additional factors associated with the risk of divorce also increase the risk of psychiatric disorders (i.e., are confounding factors). A simple example of possible confounding is the relationship of younger age with the risk of divorce and with the risk of many psychiatric disorders. In analyzing the impact of divorce on psychiatric status, one needs to be sure that any observed effect is not accounted for by the psychological problems related to the age of the people experiencing divorce. A more complicated example might be when a married couple experience other stressful life events, such as job loss. Job loss can add considerable stress to a marriage, especially in terms of finances and role responsibility, and the impact of job loss could increase the risk of divorce in an already weak marriage. Job loss could also directly increase the risk of a depressive reaction in one or both spouses. In this scenario, any observed relationship between divorce and depression would be confounded by job loss. As suggested by Karney and Bradbury's (1995) model, however, the relationships among life events such as job loss, divorce, and depression would most likely be far more complex. For example, depression might be expected to exacerbate the effects of job loss on divorce, and the negative impact of unemployment on marital quality might exacerbate the risk of depression.

The complicated and drawn-out nature of marriage–divorce processes (beginning with selection into marriage and continuing with marital difficulties, marital separation, divorce proceedings, divorce, and living as a formerly married person) also poses huge difficulties in attempting to assess the role of psychological states. The challenge is to obtain sufficient detail at multiple time points in a sample whose biases from the general population are minimal or can be quantified. At minimum, regardless of the study design or source of sample, accurate dating of psychiatric episodes (onset and duration of episodes) and of marital events is needed.

Because of problems in cost and access to relevant populations, the kinds of data used to investigate the effect of psychological factors on the risk of divorce rarely meet this goal. One common compromise is the decision to measure the divorce process as single event rather than as individual units (i.e., series of events and chronic strains). The trade-off involved in this decision is the loss of specificity when aggregating the different stages into a single stressor versus the loss of statistical power when disaggregating them. Other constraints apply to the choice of measures used to assess mental status and the source of cases. Community-based samples tend to be less biased than patient samples, but rates of episodes of particular types of psychopathology and the incidence of divorce in community-based samples are generally very low at any particular time, making adequate sample sizes and provision of sufficiently long-term follow-up prohibitively costly. Self-report symptom scales are economical of time and money and allow for more statistical power but do not generate the kind of data on psychiatric history needed to understand causality. All retrospective data, including cohort and case–control, suffer from potential recall bias regarding the timing and sequencing of psychiatric and marital events.

Despite the limitations of existing data sources, in aggregate they strongly suggest that psychopathology does influence the risk of divorce. For example, case–control studies affirm the poorer marital functioning of depressed spouses (Paykel & Weissman, 1973), while studies of couples have documented an additive effect of psychopathology in each spouse on marital functioning (Merikangas et al., 1985). These studies indicate that pre-existing psychopathology can increase both marital conflict and the inability to cope with conflict in a marriage. Similarly, in their comparisons of divorced versus married adults, Briscoe and Smith (1973) reported not only a very high association between divorce and depression, but also that at least 20% of the divorced cases who reported depression also reported first onset as prior to their marriage, suggesting that the risk of divorce in at least a few cases may have been exacerbated by pre-existing depression. Another source of data implicating depression psychopathology in the risk of divorce is Kandel and Davies's (1986) 9 year follow-up of adolescents. In this study, children with high levels of depressive symptoms were not only more likely to report depressive symptomatology at follow-up but, among girls, to have already experienced divorce.

One study that contradicts the general findings from this body of research is Menaghan's (1985) analysis of 4 year follow-up data on a community-based sample. In these data, baseline depressive symptoms did not predict subsequent divorce. One interpretation of these conflicting findings is that the relationship between depression and divorce is restricted to the diagnosis of depression. This interpretation makes sense, given the contribution of functional disability in domains like marital functioning to the diagnostic criteria for major depressive disorder. Another explanation for the contradictory findings may be that the 4 year follow-up period is too long a period of risk relative to the assessment of current depressive symptoms. Studies of depressed patients report that marital impairment can last long after the episode of depression ends (Bothwell & Weissman, 1977). The total effect of depression on subsequent divorce would be underestimated if respondents with past histories of depression, who may have impaired functioning and who are at greater risk for future episodes, are grouped in the analysis with respondents without a history of depression.

Because few studies have assessed the relationship of psychiatric diagnoses to subsequent divorce in a longitudinal community-based sample, data from the Epidemiological Catchment Area (ECA) study are instructive. Table 12.1 compares the likelihood of experiencing marital separation or divorce over a 1 year period by lifetime history at baseline of several psychiatric disorders assessed using the Diagnostic Interview Schedule (DIS; Robins et al., 1981). Although DIS assessments of life-time diagnoses have low reliability (Bromet et al., 1986; Parker, 1987), the effort to examine psychiatric history in a community-based sample is arguably an important step toward understanding the causal relationships in divorce and psychopathology.

These panel data come from all five sites of the ECA (for a description of methods, see Eaton & Kessler, 1985; Robins & Regier, 1991). Table 12.1 includes only respondents (ages 18–64) who were married at their initial interview and excludes married respondents whose spouses died during the follow-up period. Lifetime psychiatric history was defined as meeting criteria during the respondent's lifetime for an episode of the disorder in question (1) at the baseline interview, or (2) at follow-up, reporting an age of onset younger than the baseline age. The outcome variable combines marital separation with divorce, a common strategy in community-based studies used to represent the divorce process and to enhance statistical power. This approach, however, perpetuates the problems in disregarding the heterogeneity within the divorce process.

In these ECA data, 3.6% of respondents who were married at baseline separated from or divorced their spouses during the follow-up period. Marital disruption was twice as likely to occur among respondents with a history of one or more of the disorders presented. The risk of separation or divorce varied by specific type of psychiatric disorder and was highest among respondents with a history of schizophrenia, major depression, or anxiety disorder. Because of the risk associated with varied disorders and the high level of psychiatric comorbidity among respondents with a history of at least one disorder, logistic regression models were used to estimate the odds of divorce associated with each disorder, adjusting for history of other psychiatric disorders. These data indicate that respondents with a history of major depression were 70% more likely than those without major depression to experience marital separation or divorce in the upcoming year ($p < .02$). History of anxiety increased the risk by 50% ($p < .02$), and the estimated odds ratio of 2.0 for schizophre-

Table 12.1. Marital separation or divorce within one year among married individuals by lifetime psychiatric history[*]

	Number at risk	Separated/divorced		Adjusted odds ratio[†]	(p)
		No.	%		
Total married respondents	5106	185	3.6		
Any psychiatric disorder history[‡]					
Yes	1861	100	5.4	2.0	(<.01)
No	3245	85	2.6		
Past history of major depression					
Yes	382	28	7.3	1.7	(<.02)
No	4721	157	3.3		
Past history of alcohol abuse/dependency					
Yes	739	32	4.3	1.3	(<.25)
No	4291	149	3.5		
Past history of drug abuse					
Yes	267	19	7.1	1.2	(<.44)
No	4815	166	3.4		
Past history of anxiety					
Yes	1038	58	5.6	1.5	(<.02)
No	4056	127	3.1		
Past history of schizophrenia					
Yes	69	8	11.6	2.0	(<.10)
No	5022	177	3.5		

[*]Five-site ECA data, ages 18–64, married at baseline interview. Ns do not always add up to 5106 because of missing data for specific disorders.

[†]Adjusted for sex, age, and history of other psychiatric disorders at baseline.

[‡]Any disorder is an aggregate measure of major depression, anxiety, alcohol or drug abuse/dependence, and schizophrenia. The "yes" category includes respondents who met criteria for one to four different disorders. Past history refers to lifetime diagnoses.

nia, although not reaching statistical significance, also suggests that a history of this disorder predisposed to marital disruption. One-fourth of the respondents with a psychiatric history met criteria for more than one disorder. Comorbidity increased the risk of marital disruption. When psychiatric history is represented by a count of the total number of disorders, each disorder increased the risk by 49% ($p < .001$; not shown in Table 12.1).

Table 12.1 is illustrative both for what it does tell us and what it does not. Although it is clear that a number of psychiatric disorders are associated with subsequent marital disruption, one cannot tell from these data whether (1) the psychiatric disorders contributed to the problems in the marriage that resulted in divorce; (2) given problems in the marriage, a history of the disorder increased a person's vulnerability to divorce; (3) the reported psychiatric episode was a reaction to marital problems that also resulted in divorce, or (4) the psychiatric reaction to marital problems increased the likelihood that those problems would prompt divorce. Hence, psychiatric problems may "cause" divorce, but they also may be a side effect of the divorce process or a factor exacerbating the process.

A closer look at the limited data available on the timing of psychiatric episodes and marital history in the ECA indicates support for a variety of patterns. For example, among the married respondents who both had a history of depression at baseline and subsequently experienced marital separation or divorce ($n = 28$), 13 (46%) reported their first depressive episode as occurring more than 10 years prior to their divorce, including 5 whose first onset was during childhood (ages 6–18). For this subgroup, the long history of depression suggests that depression may have contributed to the marital disruption. In contrast, 5 of the 28 cases (18%) reported a first-onset episode of major depression within 2 years of the baseline interview. For these men and women, depression may have been a reaction to problems in the marriage that ultimately led to divorce or separation (or a reaction to the separation that ultimately led to divorce). Regardless of age of onset, more than half of the 28 respondents who both had a history of depression and experienced marital disruption reported their most recent depressive episode within 1 year of the baseline interview. The predominance of recent episodes suggests both that some of these depressions are reactions to ongoing marital problems and that depressive reactions to marital strain may exacerbate the likelihood that marital problems lead to divorce.

EFFECTS OF DIVORCE ON PSYCHOPATHOLOGY

Numerous studies have associated divorce with a wide range of negative psychological and behavioral outcomes (e.g., car accidents, suicide, homicide, death, drinking problems) (Bloom et al., 1978). Determining the causal relationships between divorce and the presumed outcomes from these studies is difficult, however, given the many methodological weaknesses, including reliance on retrospective reports of past behavior or emotional states, selective samples, poor response rates, and lack of comparison groups. Studies also provide evidence of positive outcomes, such as relief from conflictual or abusive relationships (Chiriboga & Cutler, 1978; Spanier & Thompson, 1986) and increased self-confidence (Nelson, 1989). A number of researchers hypothesize that the type of outcome associated with marital disruption depends upon both the point in the process used to predict the outcome and the amount of time passed between the predicting event and the outcome assessment (Booth & Amato, 1991; Doherty et al., 1989; Jacobs, 1982; Wilcox, 1986). For example, one pattern observed among fathers who separate from their families is immediate despair, followed by a period of busy social activity, followed by depression and apathy (Jacobs, 1982).

Briscoe and colleagues' case–control study of divorced adults was among the first to document the range of psychiatric disorders associated with divorce and to date the onset of these disorders relative to the timing of events in the divorce process as an approach to disentangling the causal relationship (Briscoe & Smith 1973; Briscoe et al., 1973). In these data, 78% of divorced women compared with 18% of controls, and 68% of divorced men, compared with 34% of controls, had a past or current psychiatric disorder. Unipolar depression was the most predominant disorder, but rates were also elevated for antisocial personality in both men and women. There was no association between divorce and hysteria, anxiety, alcoholism, or bipolar disorder. Although, as described earlier, about 20% of the divorced–depressed cases had their first episode prior to marriage, approximately one-third of the women and more than half the men had their onset episode within 6 months of their separation or later. For this subgroup of cases, it is likely that the depression was at least partially a result of marital disruption.

Only a few community-based studies have assessed psychiatric disorders or symptoms before and after reported marital separation and divorce. These studies consistently report increased psychiatric symptoms or episodes with marital disruption (Aseltine & Kessler, 1993; Booth & Amato, 1991; Bruce & Kim, 1992; Menaghan & Lieberman,

1986). In keeping with the predominance of depression reported by Briscoe et al.'s study, the most common outcome assessed is depressive disorder or symptoms. A problem with all of these studies is that the baseline assessment aggregates people at different points in the divorce process.

Assessment of psychiatric history in community samples makes it possible to differentiate the effect of divorce on first versus recurrent episodes of psychiatric disorders. This strategy is important, first, as a means of identifying an at-risk group for whom it is possible to test the hypothesis that divorce is associated with first onset of psychopathology. This strategy is also useful for investigating hypotheses, such as Post's (1992), that the effect of stressful life events on the risk of depression will be different in direction or magnitude for adults without a history of depression (i.e., first-onset depression) compared with those with a history (i.e., recurrent episodes).

The relationship between marital disruption and first versus recurrent episodes of psychiatric disorders is described in Table 12.2 among ECA respondents ages 18–64 who were married at the baseline interview. The table assesses the risk of five specific types of psychiatric episodes—major depression, alcohol abuse/dependence, drug abuse/dependence, anxiety (i.e., phobia, panic, obsessive–compulsive disorder), and schizophrenia-related disorders (schizophrenia and schizophreniform)—and an aggregate measure of all five types. Within each diagnostic group, the percentage experiencing an episode during the follow-up period is compared between respondents who became separated or divorced during this period and those who remained married. This approach, common to those studies of the effects of divorce on psychiatric outcomes, assumes that the onset of the psychiatric episode is a reaction to the marital disruption during this period. This assumption cannot be rigorously tested with available data sets (and the temporal processes that characterize divorce most likely make it difficult to date "onset" in any event). However, the relatively short follow-up period (one year)

increases the likelihood that the index episode does not "cause" the marital disruption.

In accordance with the strategy described above, the relationship between marital disruption and each type of psychiatric episode is stratified by whether or not the respondent reported a past history of the outcome in question. The last column in Table 12.2 estimates the effect of marital disruption on the outcome from a logistic regression model that adjusts for age, sex, and whether the respondent had a history of at least one of the other psychiatric disorders assessed.

The first outcome examined in Table 12.2 is an aggregate measure of whether any of the five specific disorders was present or not. Among men and women with a history of at least one of the psychiatric disorders, marital disruption is associated with a small but significantly increased likelihood of another psychiatric episode or perpetuation of an episode present at the baseline interview [47%. vs. 34%, adjusted odds ratio (OR) = 1.6; p = .03]. With regard to specific disorders, divorce increases the risk of recurrent depressive (OR = 1.8; p < .01), anxiety (OR = 1.5; p < .01), and schizophrenic (OR = 8.6; p = .03) episodes, with history of other psychiatric disorders controlled. Increased risk of recurrent substance abuse (alcohol or drugs), by contrast, is explained by history of comorbid depression or anxiety.

Very few respondents without a history of psychopathology experience a first-onset psychiatric episode during the 1 year follow-up period (58/3245; 1.8%). Nonetheless, the observed effect of marital disruption on the risk of first-onset psychiatric disorder is much stronger than estimated for recurrent episodes. Among the newly separated or divorced without a psychiatric history, 9/85 (10.6%) experienced first-onset psychopathology compared with 49/3160 (1.6%) of their married counterparts (age- and sex-adjusted OR = 6.2; p < .01). Among the 9 newly separated or divorced individuals with a first onset disorder, the majority (6/9; 66.7%) had major depression. Major depression was less prominent the first-onset

Table 12.2. Psychiatric episodes during one year follow-up period by separation/divorce and lifetime psychiatric history[°]

	Number at risk	Number with outcome	Percentage with outcome	Adjusted odds ratio[†]	(p)
Any disorder[‡]					
Past history					
Newly separated/divorced	100	47	47.0	1.6	(<.03)
Married	1761	598	34.0		
No past history					
Newly separated/divorced	85	9	10.6	6.2	(<.01)
Married	3160	49	1.6		
Major depression					
Past history					
Newly separated/divorced	28	13	46.4	1.8	(<.01)
Married	354	99	28.0		
No past history					
Newly separated/divorced	157	13	8.3	18.1	(<.01)
Married	4558	21	0.5		
Alcohol abuse/dependence					
Past history					
Newly separated/divorced	32	12	37.5	1.3	(<.22)
Married	675	183	27.1		
No past history					
Newly separated/divorced	149	1	0.7	2.7	(.34)
Married	4142	13	0.3		
Drug abuse/dependence					
Past history					
Newly separated/divorced	19	7	36.8	1.4	(.23)
Married	248	39	15.7		
No past history					
Newly separated/divorced	166	1	0.6	1.8	(.52)
Married	4649	8	0.2		
Anxiety					
Past history					
Newly separated/divorced	58	20	34.5	1.5	(.01)
Married	980	312	31.8		
No past history					
Newly separated/divorced	127	3	2.4	1.8	(.32)
Married	3929	42	1.1		
Schizophrenia					
Past history					
Newly separated/divorced	8	4	50.0	8.6	(.03)
Married	61	14	23.0		
No past history					
Newly separated/divorced	177	1	0.6	20.7	(.04)
Married	4844	1	0.9		

[°]Five-site ECA data, ages 18–64, married at baseline interview. Respondents who were widowed during follow-up were omitted. Ns within disorder types do not always add up to 5106 because of missing data.

[†]Adjusted for sex, age, and history of other psychiatric disorders at baseline using logistic regression.

[‡]Any disorder is an aggregate measure of major depression, anxiety, alcohol or drug abuse/dependence, and schizophrenia. Past history refers to lifetime diagnoses.

disorders in the married group (13/49; 26.5%).

Disorder-specific analyses affirm the importance of depression as an outcome of divorce. Among respondents without a history of major depression, 13/157 (8.3%) of those experiencing marital disruption reported first-onset depression, compared with only 21/4558 (0.5%) of the married group at risk. The number of divorced–depressed cases is larger in the depression at-risk group than in the any disorder at-risk group (13 vs. 6) because some of the first onset depressive cases reported a lifetime history of a different disorder. As a side note, this rate of first-onset depression among the newly divorced (8.3%) is substantially higher than the 1.9% one year incidence rate reported by Anthony and Petronis (1991) for ECA respondents who reported their marital status as being divorced at the start of the study. The comparison between the incidence rates affirms the difference between experiencing divorce process and occupying the social status of a divorced person. Put differently, the data suggest that depressive reactions to marital disruption are both immediate and of short duration, although they may increase the risk for additional depressive episodes in the future.

Adjusting for age, sex, and baseline history of other psychiatric disorders, the effect of marital separation and divorce on first-onset major depression is very large (OR = 18.1; $p < .01$). The only other disorder affected significantly by divorce is schizophrenia (adjusted OR = 20.7; $p < .04$), although the total number of first-onset cases is extremely small ($N = 2$). The estimated effects of separation or divorce on the other disorders are positive and small to moderate in magnitude, but again the numbers of new cases, especially among the newly divorced group, are small and there is little statistical power.

Longitudinal studies of changes in depressive symptoms associated with intervening divorce have more statistical power than the ECA research on diagnoses, allowing for an assessment of factors that mediate the relationships between divorce and increased

depressive symptoms (Aseltine & Kessler, 1993; Booth & Amato, 1991; Menaghan & Lieberman, 1986). In these studies, there is some evidence that at least some of the effect of separation and divorce on psychological symptoms is mediated through the effect of marital disruption on financial strain and time pressures. Some of the remaining unexplained effect may reflect an intrapsychic reaction to loss similar to grief in marital bereavement. Indeed, rates of depressive episodes (without employing the bereavement exclusion) are similar in the New Haven ECA data for respondents experiencing separation or divorce and those experiencing marital bereavement (Bruce & Kim, 1992; Bruce et al., 1990).

THE IMPACT OF DIVORCE ON THE MENTAL HEALTH OF CHILDREN

Divorce is a major stressor not only in the lives of the spouses but also in the lives of their children (Erel & Burman, 1995). Like adults, children exposed to divorce generally experience not a single but a series of stressful events (e.g., parental arguments, parental separation, relocation, restricted access to the father and paternal grandparents, change in financial resources). These events are often emotionally charged and characterized by a dramatic changes in family structure and circumstances.

A diverse literature has implicated parental divorce in numerous childhood and adult outcomes. As reviewed by Seltzer (1994), the most frequently documented childhood mental health outcomes of the divorce process are depressed mood, anxiety, and disruptive behavior. In the longer term, children of divorced parents achieve less education, marry younger, and, if they do marry, have a higher risk of experiencing divorce themselves than do children whose parents remain stably married. These findings suggest that the ECA analyses would have benefited from information on childhood experiences of parental divorce if those question had been asked.

A number of studies have also documented long-term mental health effects of divorce on children. Two studies (McLeod, 1991; Rodgers, 1994) reported higher rates of depressed mood in women with divorced parents but not men. In McLeod's analysis, the effect of parental divorce on depressive symptoms in offspring was mediated by the offspring's own poorer marital functioning, suggesting an intergenerational transmission of marital behavior and coping styles. Because neither of these studies had access to parental psychiatric history, it is unknown the extent to which (1) parental divorce has an effect independent from parental psychopathology on the risk of psychopathology in adult offspring, (2) parental divorce mediates the effect of parental psychopathology, (3) parental divorce is confounded by parental psychopathology, or (4) parental divorce exacerbates the effects of psychopathology. Without well-documented psychiatric histories of the offspring in these studies, one also does not know the contribution of prior episodes of depression or other disorders independent from or in conjunction with the experience of parental separation and divorce. The literature on the short-term effects of divorce on children suggests that a sizable proportion of the adult offspring who scored high in depressive symptoms in both McLeod's and Rodgers's studies had experienced depressive episodes in childhood. As noted earlier, Kandel & Davies's (1986) 9 year follow-up of adolescents found an increased risk of both depressive symptoms and divorce associated with baseline depressive symptoms.

In their twin study of women, Kendler and colleagues (1992, 1993) report that residential separation from at least one parent for a year or more during childhood (92% of these separations were due to divorce) was associated with adult major depression, generalized anxiety disorder, and panic disorder. As noted by the authors, childhood separation from parents may also be a proxy measure for living in a home characterized by marital discord or conflict and experiencing the process of disruption. Controlling for genetic effects measured by twins' zygosity status, separation from parents accounted for a significant but small proportion of the variation in these disorders. Path models of the longitudinal twin data indicated that the effect of childhood loss (including parental separation) on major depressive episodes during the follow-up period was mediated primarily by earlier depressions and reported recent long-term difficulties.

Together, these data implicate parental divorce in the development of psychopathology during childhood and adulthood. As with the relationship of divorce to the mental health of the divorcing spouses, however, important questions remain. One set of questions involves the relative impact of divorce per se on the mental health of children compared to long-term exposure to parental conflict leading up to and following divorce. The hypothesis that children of stable but unhappy marriages, compared to children who experience parental divorce, are at comparable—if not greater—risk for psychosocial problems and adult psychopathology remains inadequately tested.

As noted by Kendler and colleagues (1992), however, a more complicated issue is the role of parental psychopathology in the risk of the mental health attributed to the parents' divorce. The increased risk of numerous disorders in offspring of affected parents is well documented (e.g., Merikangas et al., 1994; Weissman et al., 1992). To the extent that this increased risk can be attributed to genetic factors, the observed association between parental divorce and psychopathology in children (during childhood or adulthood) may be confounded by the contribution of parental disorders both to the risk of divorce and to the risk of children's mental health problems. Even the nongenetic components of family history may confound the association, because exposure to affected parents may predate the divorce process but already have influenced psychiatric vulnerability.

The complexity in these questions is evident in a study by Weissman and colleagues (1992), who document that children of depressed parents are disproportionately exposed to parental divorce. In this study, parental psychiatric history was associated with significantly higher 2 year incidence of depression and anxiety disorders (but not substance abuse or conduct disorder) in the offspring during childhood. In contrast, there was no increased risk of depression or anxiety associated with coming from a divorced household. Even this study, with its relative richness in measures of child and parent factors, needs additional data to clarify the full contribution of marital separation and divorce to depression in children. The kinds of data needed to measure the outcomes of divorce on the divorcing spouses (e.g., data on the timing of depressive episodes relative to timing of marriage, marital conflict, marital separation, and marital divorce) are also needed to assess the childhood and adult effects of parental divorce on the offspring.

CONCLUSION

As noted in the beginning of this chapter, divorce has become almost commonplace in the United States and many other parts of the world. In the face of this high prevalence, the effects of divorce on a number of negative outcomes in children are particularly disturbing. Equally important, however, is Seltzer's (1994) observation that most children survive divorce emotionally intact. The same point should be made for married couples who divorce. Because most research on divorce and psychopathology has not been conducted from the perspective of resilience, it may be useful to approach this question by examining whether psychological and social factors that are protective against divorce are also protective against the negative effects of divorce (Karney & Bradbury, 1995). Because there is so much evidence both that marital disruption is a devastating event (and process) to the individuals involved and that the impact can be severe, the adults and children who survive the experience intact may offer clues to more generic protective factors for mental health. Indeed, one might expect that any protective factors identified from

the divorce experience might be particularly robust.

At the same time, the magnitude and intergenerational nature of the negative effects of marital disruption on the risk and recurrence of psychopathology underscore the importance of learning more about how to prevent or ameliorate some of these effects. Divorce has become commonplace, but there is no evidence to suggest that the increased frequency has led to any reduction in the impact of divorce on the lives of the people involved. The multiple routes through which parental divorce may affect the mental health of children both as youth and through adulthood is particularly troublesome. Although some of the short-term effects may be unavoidable for either child or parent, preventing the long-term outcomes may be the most effective means of intervention.

REFERENCES

Anthony, J. C., & Petronis, K. R. (1991). Suspected risk factors for depression among adults 18–44 years old. *Epidemiology, 2*, 123–132.

Aseltine, R. H., & Kessler, R. C. (1993). Marital disruption and depression in a community sample. *Journal of Health and Social Behavior, 34*, 187–284.

Bianchi, S. M., & Spain, D. (1986). *American women in transition.* New York: Sage.

Blazer, D. G., Kessler, R. C., McGonagle, K. A., et al. (1994). The prevalence and distribution of major depression in a national community sample: The National Comorbidity Survey. *American Journal of Psychiatry, 151*, 979–986

Bloom, B. L., Asher, S. J., & White, S. W. (1978). Marital disruption as a stressor: a review and analysis. *Psychological Bulletin, 85*, 867–894.

Booth, A., & Amato, P. (1991). Divorce and psychological stress. *Journal of Health and Social Behavior, 32*, 396–407.

Bothwell, S., & Weissman, M. M. (1977). Social impairments four years after an acute depressive episode. *American Journal of Orthopsychiatry, 49*, 231–237.

Briscoe, C. W., & Smith, J. B. (1973). Depression and marital turmoil. *Archives of General Psychiatry, 29,* 811–817.

Briscoe, C. W., Smith, J. B., Robins, E., et al. (1973). Divorce and psychiatric disease. *Archives of General Psychiatry, 29,* 119–125.

Bromet, E. J., Dunn, L. O., & Connell, M. M. (1986). Long-term reliability of diagnosing lifetime major depression in a community sample. *Archives of General Psychiatry, 43,* 435–440.

Brown, G. W., & Harris, T. O. (1978). *Social origins of depression: A study of psychiatric disorder in women.* London: Tavistock.

Bruce, M. L., & Kim, K. M. (1992). Differences in the effects of divorce on major depression in men and women. *American Journal of Psychiatry, 149,* 914–917.

Bruce, M.L., Kim, K. M., Leaf, P. J., et al. (1990). Depressive episodes and dysphoria resulting from conjugal bereavement in a prospective community sample. *American Journal of Psychiatry, 147,* 608–611.

Chiriboga, D. A., & Cutler, L. (1978). Stress response among divorcing men and women. *Journal of Divorce, 1,* 95–106.

Doherty, W. J., Su, S., & Needle, R. (1989). Marital disruption and psychological well-being: A panel study. *Journal of Family Issues, 10,* 72–85.

Dohrenwend, B. S., Raphael, K. G., Schwartz, S., et al. (1993). The structured event probe and narrative rating meathod for measuring stressful life events. In L. Goldberg & S. Bresnitz (Eds), *Handbook of Stress: Theoretical and Clinical Aspects* (pp. 174–199). New York: The Free Press.

Eaton, W. W., & Kessler, L. G. (Eds). (1985). *The NIMH Epidemiological Catchment Area program.* New York: Academic Press.

Erel, O., & Burman, B. (1995). Interrelatedness of marital realtions and parent-child relation: A meta-analytic review. *Psychological Bulletin, 118,* 108–132.

Furstenberg, F. F. (1994). History and current status of divorce in the United States. *Children and Divorce, 4,* 29–43.

Gottman, J. M., & Levenson, R. W. (1992). Marital processes predictive of later dissolution: Behavior, physiology, and health. *Journal of Personality and Social Psychology, 63,* 221–233.

Hoffman, S., & Duncan, G. (1988). What are the economic consequences of divorce? *Demography, 25,* 641–645.

Holden, K. C., & Smock, P. J. (1991). The economic costs of marital dissolution: Why do women bear a disproportionate cost? *Annual Review of Sociology, 17,* 51–78.

Holmes, T. H., & Rahe, R. H. (1967). The Social Readjustment Rating Scale. *Journal of Psychosomatic Research, 11,* 213–218.

Jacobs, S. W. (1982). The effect of divorce on fathers: An overview of the literature. *American Journal of Psychiatry, 139,* 1235–1241.

Kandel, D. B., & Davies, M. (1986). Adult sequelae of adolescent depressive symptoms. *Archives of General Psychiatry, 43,* 255–262.

Karney, B. R., & Bradbury, T. N. (1995). The longitudinal course of marital quality and stability: A review of theory, method, and research. *Psychological Bulletin, 118,* 3–34.

Kendler, K. S., Kessler, R. C., Neale, M. C., et al. (1993). The prediction of major depression in women: Toward an integrated etiologic model. *American Journal of Psychiatry, 150,* 1139–1148.

Kendler, K. S., Neale, M. C., Kessler, R. C., et al. (1992). Childhood parental loss and adult psychopathology in women: A twin study perspective. *Archives of General Psychiatry, 49,* 109–116.

McLean, D. E., & Link, B. G. (1994). Unraveling complexity. Strategies to refine concepts, measures, and research designs in the study of life events and mental health. In R. R. Avison & I. H. Gotlib (Eds.), *Stress and mental health* (pp. 15–42). New York: Plenum.

McLeod, J.D. (1991). Childhood parental loss and adult depression. *Journal of Health and Social Behavior, 32,* 205–220.

Menaghan, E. G. (1985). Depressive affect and subsequent divorce. *Journal of Family Issues, 6,* 295–306.

Menaghan, E. G., Lieberman, M. A. (1986). Changes in depression following divorce: A panel study. *Journal of Marriage and Family, 48,* 319–328.

Merikangas, K. R., Prusoff, B. A., Kupfer, D. J., et al. (1985). Marital adjustment in major depression. *Journal of Affective Disorders, 9,* 5–11.

Merikangas, K. R., Risch, N. J., Weissman, M. M. (1994). Comorbidity and cotransmission of alcoholism, anxiety and depression. *Psychological Medicine, 24,* 69–80.

Morgan, S. P., & Rindfuss, R. R. (1985). Marital disruption: Structural and temporal dimensions. *American Journal of Sociology, 90,* 1055–1077.

Nelson, G. (1989). Life strains, coping and emotional well-being: A longitudinal study of recently separated and married women. *American Journal of Community Psychology*, *17*, 459–483.

Parker, G. (1987). Are the lifetime prevalence estimates in the ECA study accurate? *Psychological Medicine*, *17*, 275–282.

Paykel, E. S., & Weissman, M. M. (1973). Social adjustment and depression. *Archives of General Psychiatry*, *28*, 659–663.

Post, R. M. (1992). Transduction of psychosocial stress into the neurobiology of recurrent affective disorder. *American Journal of Psychiatry*, *149*, 999–1010.

Robins, L. N., Helzer, J. E., Croughan, J., et al. (1981). National Institute of Mental Health Diagnostic Interview Schedule: Its history, characteristics, and validity. *Archives of General Psychiatry*, *38*, 381–389.

Robins, L., & Regier, D. (Eds.). (1991). *Psychiatric disorders in America*. New York: The Free Press.

Rodgers, B. (1994). Pathways between parental divorce and adults depression. *Journal of Child Psychology Psychiatry and Allied Disciplines*, *35*, 1289–1308.

Seltzer, J. A. (1994). Consequences of marital dissolution for children. *Annual Review of Sociology*, *20*, 235–266.

Shrout, P. E., Link, B. G., Dohrenwend, B. P., et al. (1989). Characterizing life events as risk factors for depression: the role of fateful loss events. *Journal of Abnormal Psychology*, *98*, 460–467.

Smock , P. J. (1993). The economic costs of marital disruption for young women over the past two decades. *Demography*, *30*, 353–371.

Spanier, G. B., & Thompson, L. (1986). Relief and distress after marital separation. *Journal of Divorce*, *7*, 31–49.

Srole, L., Langer, T. S., Michael, S. T., et al. (1962). *Mental health in the metropolis: The Midtown Manhattan Study*. New York: McGraw-Hill.

U.S. Bureau of the Census. (1989). *Poverty in the United States, 1987* (Current Population Reports, Series P-60, No. 163). Washington. DC: U.S. Dept. of Commerce.

Warheit, G. J., Holzer, C. E., III, Bell, R. A., et al. (1976). Sex, marital status, and mental health: A reappraisal. *Social Forces*, *55*, 459–470.

Weissman, M. M., Fendrich, M., Warner, V., et al. (1992). Incidence of psychiatric disorder in offspring of high and low risk for depression. *Journal of American Academy of Child Adolescent Psychiatry*, *31*, 640–648.

Weissman, M. M., & Myers, J. K., (1978). Rates and risks of depressive symptoms in a United States urban community. *Acta Psychiatrica Scandinavica*, *34*, 854–862.

Wilcox, B. L. (1986). Stress, coping, and the social milieu of divorced women. In S. E. Hobfull (Ed.), *Stress, social support, and women* (pp. 115–133). Washington, D.C.: Hemisphere.

III

EPIDEMIOLOGICAL AND CASE–CONTROL STUDIES

Evelyn J. Bromet
Bruce P. Dohrenwend

Epidemiological research on the effects of stress has been an expanding enterprise since the 1960s, following the introduction of feasible methods for obtaining data on both stress and psychological symptoms. This part reports results from some major recent studies.

In a comprehensive updating of analyses of epidemiological studies of the true prevalence of psychiatric disorders in general population samples, Kohn, Dohrenwend, and Mirotznik show that demographic characteristics remain powerful correlates of mental illness. These results raise and re-raise many questions about the role of adversity as it may relate to social statuses such as gender and socioeconomic status (SES). Dohrenwend and his colleagues expand upon and describe in detail their quasi-experimental investigation of one of these questions, the classic social causation–social selection issue posed by inverse relations between SES and various types of psychiatric disorder and psychological distress. Stueve, Dohrenwend, and Skodol remind us of the power of case–control designs by examining the differing relation of fateful events to episodes of two impor-

tant and very different types of psychiatric disorder that are inversely related to SES; major depression and schizophrenia. Brown focuses on one of these disorders, depression. The report from his important program of research analyzes in depth and in detail the role of events involving loss in episodes of depression.

Robins and Robertson present some interesting analyses of longitudinal data from their epidemiological research in St. Louis. They show that life events on the one hand and substance abuse and antisocial behavior on the other tend to be linked in complicated and fascinating ways, even when the types of events appear to be fateful and apparently independent of the behavior of the respondents. Their checklist measures of life events are very different from those used in the studies by Stueve et al. and by Brown, and caution is warranted about the problems of interpretation that can arise in attempts to classify life events on the basis of checklist data rather than on the basis of more intensive information about the details of the events. The questions they raise, however, are of major importance and require further investigation with a variety of measures of the "fatefulness" of stressful events.

Both critical exposures to adversity and the development of psychiatric problems often occur early in life. It is extremely important, therefore, to have prospective data such as that of Breslau and her colleagues on post-traumatic stress disorder (PTSD). These investigators point out the perils of possible recall biases in retrospective data that can distort the picture of adverse effects. Breslau and co-workers also remind us that specifying the psychiatric impact of adversity requires data on prior psychiatric condition, because antecedent disorder increases the likelihood that PTSD or other disorders subsequently will occur. These lessons go in tandem with those from Robins and Robertson's research.

Epidemiological methods, including case–control, longitudinal, and prospective designs, provide powerful tools for descriptive, analytical, and intervention studies of the effects of adversity and stress on health. In any specific investigation, special methodological problems will inevitably arise and challenge our ingenuity. As Robins and Robertson point out, we cannot conduct human experiments on the effects of adversity. An ideal design that is both ethical and practical is something to be approximated rather than achieved. Although the epidemiological approach demonstrates that there is no such thing as a simple question or a simple, unconditional answer, the six chapters in this part illustrate the tremendous potential of epidemiological research for formulating or clarifying important questions and fully exploring the answers our data have to offer.

13

Epidemiological Findings on Selected Psychiatric Disorders in the General Population

Robert Kohn
Bruce P. Dohrenwend
Jerrold Mirotznik

Psychiatric epidemiology has undergone three generations of methodological advancement (Dohrenwend & Dohrenwend, 1981). Each generation has differed in its psychiatric nosology and methods of data collection.

The first generation, from the turn of the century to World War II, relied mainly on key informants and agency records to identify cases within the community (Dohrenwend & Dohrenwend, 1974). The second generation, following World War II, used an expanded definition of psychiatric disorders. In addition, community residents were directly interviewed, usually by a single psychiatrist or a team headed by a psychiatrist. Except for a few North American studies (Leighton et al., 1963; Srole et al., 1962), these interviews typically did not employ standardized data collection procedures (Lin, 1953). Case identification in the second-generation studies was made by psychiatrists following evaluation of protocols collected from the interview data.

The second generation of psychiatric epidemiology also used screening scales comprising symptom items. These scales attempted to distinguish cases from noncases using cutoff scores. Examples of these screening instruments include the Midtown or 22-item Langner Scale (Langner, 1962); the Center for Epidemiological Studies Depression Survey (CES-D; Radloff, 1977); the General Well-Being Schedule (GWB; Dupuy, 1974); and the Symptom Checklist 90 (SCL-90; Derogatis, 1977).

The third and current generation emerged with the development of explicit diagnostic criteria and structured clinical interview schedules, both of which contribute to improved diagnostic reliability. The predominant instruments employed include the Present State Examination (PSE; Wing et al., 1977) geared to the International Classification of Diseases (ICD) criteria (World Health Organization, 1978); the Schedule for Affective Disorders and Schizophrenia (SADS; Endicott & Spitzer, 1978), which generates Research Diagnostic Criteria (RDC; Spitzer et al., 1978) for establishing diagnoses; and the Diagnostic Interview Schedule (DIS; Robins et al., 1981), which uses *Diagnostic and Statistical Manual of Mental Disorders (Third Edition) (DSM-III)* criteria (American Psychiatric Association, 1980). More recently, new third-generation instruments have been developed. The Standardized Psychiatric Examination (SPE) (Romanoski & Chahal, 1981), which uses ICD or *DSM-III* criteria, is largely based on the PSE. The Composite International Diagnostic Interview (CIDI; Robins et al., 1988), which assess both ICD-10 (World Health Organization, 1992) and *DSM-III-R* (American Psychiatric Association, 1987) disorders, derives from the PSE and DIS.

As methodology and diagnostic reliability have evolved with each subsequent generation of psychiatric epidemiology, researchers have been better able to test the association between sociodemographic variables and specific mental disorders. This chapter focuses on the relationship between socioeconomic status (SES) and gender and schizophrenia, major depression, anxiety disorders, alcohol abuse/dependence, and personality disorders. Findings from the two earlier generations of studies also are discussed, including those related to nonspecific distress, providing a historical context for more recent research.

METHODS

The third-generation studies presented focused on community-based representative probability samples and used reliable diagnostic instruments. Table 13.1 summarizes the different studies included in this chapter. To facilitate comparisons between studies with regard to the role of SES, prevalence rates and ratios for the highest and lowest strata are presented in the remaining tables in this chapter. Significance tests refer to the differences between those two strata unless otherwise stated. For analyses of both SES and gender, the published odds or risk

ratios are presented, if available. Ratios and significance tests are based on rates unadjusted for other demographic factors, unless otherwise indicated. If a ratio is not published, we calculated one using the prevalence data. If a p value is not given, but the investigators clearly indicate that a statistically significant relationship exists, a p value of 0.05 is assumed and noted in the remaining tables. Significance tests should be interpreted in the context of the prevalence of the disorder and the study's sample size; it is possible that insufficient power exists in some studies to detect a relationship between the risk factor and diagnosis under consideration, although a clear trend may exist. Results of studies that publish data on SES and gender stratified by other demographic variables are included in the review but not in the remaining tables.

The median ratio across all studies for low versus high SES and gender is provided. For the median ratios, the Epidemiologic Catchment Area (ECA) study is considered as a whole and not by individual sites. The median ratios are calculated for lifetime prevalence and the prevalence rate closest to 1 year. If a study uses more than one measure for SES, these are averaged in calculating the median ratios.

SOCIOECONOMIC STATUS

Overall Psychopathology

A consistent inverse relationship between SES and overall rates of psychopathology has been demonstrated in the first two generations of psychiatric epidemiology research. Neugebauer et al.'s (1980) review, an update of two earlier reviews (Dohrenwend & Dohrenwend, 1969, 1974), found that 17 of 20 true prevalence studies reported higher rates of psychopathology in the lowest compared to the highest social class. Across all these studies, mental disorders, on average, were 2.6 times more prevalent among individuals in the lowest than in the highest socioeconomic stratum. In the

Table 13.1. Methods used in third-generation studies reviewed

Study	Instrument	Diagnostic criteria	Sample size	Methods
USA ECA	DIS	*DSM-III*	19,182	Five study sites: New Haven, Baltimore, St. Louis, Los Angeles, and Durham, NC. Household sampling and 10% from institutions; ages 18+. Results weighted for oversampling bias and weighted for age, sex, and racial distribution of the whole United States based on the 1980 census.
New Haven ECA°	DIS	*DSM-III*	3058	Household sample not including institutions. Weighted for oversampling elderly and census.
			5034	Household sample and institutionalized.
Baltimore ECA	DIS	*DSM-III*	3481	Household sample not including institutions. Weighted for oversampling elderly and census.
St. Louis ECA	DIS	*DIS-III*	3004	Household sample not including institutions. Weighted for oversampling blacks and census.
Piedmont, NC, ECA	DIS	*DSM-III*	3798	Household sample not including institutions. Weighted for oversampling elderly and census.
Los Angeles ECA	DIS	*DSM-III*	2947	Household sample not including institutions. Weighted for oversampling Hispanics and census.
Puerto Rico	DIS	*DSM-III*	1513	Household sample including interviews with those away in institutions. Ages 18–64; age 17 was included but excluded from the analysis. Weighted to the 1980 USA Puerto Rican census for age and sex and household size.
Beirut, Lebanon	DIS	*DSM-III*	658	Collected during war. Ages 18–65; four communities of Lebanese Christians surveyed using psychologists.
Edmonton, Canada	DIS	*DSM-III*	3258	Household sample; ages 18+. Weighted for household size and the 1981 census for age and sex.
Hong Kong	DIS	*DSM-III*	7229	Two-phase study of Shatin. Screening stage with Self-Reporting Questionnaire (SRQ). 25% of "nonflagged" interviewed and all "flagged" with DIS. Ages 18–64. Sample obtained from census data.
Iceland	DIS	*DSM-III*	862	Interviewed half those alive born in 1931 (ages 55–57).
Korea	DIS	*DSM-III*	5100	All members of household ages 18–65. A rural sample (*n* = 1966) and Seoul sample (*n* = 3134) obtained.
Lesotho	DIS	*DSM-III*	456	Random families interviewed from entire village. Abbreviated DIS.
Lima, Peru	DIS	*DSM-III*	815	Residents of Independencia by household, selected families and then one member of household, ages 18+.

Table continued on following page

Table 13.1. Methods used in third-generation studies reviewed—*Continued*

Study	Instrument	Diagnostic criteria	Sample size	Methods
Munich, Germany	DIS	*DSM-I7II*	483	Follow-up of a 1974 general population sample (*n* = 1952) receiving Clinical Self Rating Scale (CRS). DIS phase only ages 18–52, and no IQ less 85. DIS sample stratified by CRS. Weighted back to original sample.
New Zealand	DIS	*DSM-III*	1498	Household stratified sample ages 18–64 from the Christchurch area. Weighted for sampling design.
Taiwan	DIS	*DSM-III*	11,004	Multistaged stratified sample ages 18+ of Taipei (*n* = 5005), two towns (*n* = 3004) and six villages (*n* = 2995). The three groups were analyzed individually.
Baltimore EBMHS	SPE	*DSM-III*	810	ECA participants from the Baltimore site who were positive on BIS, General Health Questionnaire, or Mini-Mental State Examination were interviewed by a psychiatrist using SPE. Also, interviewed 17% of ECA sample regardless of whether positive on measures.
France (town)	DIS/CIDI	*DSM-III-R*	749	Household sample ages 18+ using modified abbreviated DIS/CIDI. Only major depression *DSM-III* diagnosis.
USA NCS	CIDI	*DSM-III-R*	8098	Stratified multistage probability sample of noninstitutionalized persons ages 15–54; 48 states. Weighted for non-responders, selection of households, and age, sex, race, marital status, education, living arrangements, region, and urbanicity from 1989 U.S. National Health Interview Survey.
Ontario	CIDI	*DSM-III-R*	9953	Household respondents from the Ontario Health Survey, ages 15–64. Oversampled 15–24-year-olds.
Concepcíon, Chile	CIDI	*DSM-III-R*	800	Household sample ages 15+. CIDI included parts of DIS.
Santiago, Chili	CIDI	*DSM-III-R*	1363	Household sample ages 15+. CIDI included parts of DIS.
Camberwell/Brown	PSE	Brown & Harris	220	Random sample of women ages 18–64. Diagnosed depression by Brown & Harris criteria, similar to Feighner criteria. The 1978 Camberwell study used an enlarged sample of 458.
Outer Hebrides	PSE	Brown & Harris	355	Random sample of women ages 18–64. Diagnosed depression by Brown & Harris criteria, similar to Feighner criteria.
Athens	PSE	CATEGO	489	Household sample of two boroughs. Weighted to census data on the population of Athens.

Table continued on next page

Table 13.1. *Continued*

Study	Instrument	Diagnostic criteria	Sample size	Methods
Buenos Aires, Argentina	PSE	CATEGO	3410	Household sample stratified by districts. Ages 17–55+.
Camberwell, England	PSE	CATEGO	800	Two-stage sample from electoral register of women ages 18–64 using shortened 40-item PSE and the full PSE on 228 respondents meeting severity criteria.
Canberra, Australia	PSE	CATEGO	756	Two-stage design in Australia with screening using General Health Questionnaire and then PSE. Sample from electoral roles, ages 18+ and weighted back.
Cantabria, Spain	PSE	CATEGO	1223	Two-stage study of a rural community in Spain. Screening stage was with the General Health Questionnaire and other instruments. All who screened positive and a random sample of negatives were interviewed with the PSE. Weighted to original population. Sample was ages 17+.
China	PSE	ICD-9	1000	Five hundred urban and 500 rural households selected in 12 study areas to undergo a screening interview. Positives and 10% of screened negatives had a diagnostic interview. Diagnoses using Chinese criteria. Ages 15+.
Finland	PSE	CATEGO	742	Follow-up of a population register sample from 1975, ages 30–80. Weighted to original stratified sample.
Great Britain	PSE	CATEGO	3322	Follow-up of 5362 persons born in 1946 (age 36) from Scotland, Wales, and England. Used a shortened version of the PSE.
Mexico	PSE	CATEGO	1984	Household survey with additional items from the SRQ and CES-D. Ages 18–64.
New Zealand	PSE	CATEGO	1516	Two samples of women from electoral roles, one urban and the other rural, from the province of Otago, in a two-stage screening study using the General Health Questionnaire. A weighted sampling by screening status was in 244 measure may also tap some correlates or terviewed with a shortened version of the PSE.
Zimbabwe	PSE	CATEGO	172	Randomly selected women from a township underwent a screen, of which 30% of the negatives received. Bedford College criteria used.

Table continued on following page

Table 13.1. Methods used in third-generation studies reviewed—*Continued*

Study	Instrument	Diagnostic criteria	Sample size	Methods
Nijmegen, Holland	PSE	CATEGO	3232	Two-stage study, ages 18–64, using the General Health Questionnaire in a screening stage. Only those who scored above the threshold on the screen were interviewed with the PSE (one-eighth of the sample). Weighted to original sample.
Sardinia	PSE	CATEGO	374	Household sampling with the short version of the PSE, ages 25+. Done by psychiatrists.
Uganda	PSE	CATEGO	237	All residents of two Ugandan villages ages 18–65.
Edinburgh, Scotland	PSE	CATEGO RDC Bedford College	576	Women ages 18–64 from electoral registrations using PAS, a diagnostic instrument combining questions from SADS and PSE. Taped interviews received consensus ratings for diagnosis using CATEGO, RDC, and Bedford College Criteria.
Florence, Italy	SADS	*DSM-III*	1110	Random sample from six general practitioner registrars. Most people are registered. Modified abbreviated SADS-L to make *DSM-III* diagnoses. Ages 14+.
Indian village, USA	SADS	*DSM-III-R*	131	A 25% sample of a U.S. Indian Village, modified SADS. Re-interview of 1969 sample and 33 new.
Israel	SADS	RDC	4914	Ten-year birth cohort (1949–58) of Israeli-born offspring of European and North African immigrants. Full probability sample, screened with the Psychiatric Epidemiology Research Interview. All positives and one-fifth of negatives interviewed with SADS, by psychiatrists. Weighted to original population.
Lancaster, PA	SADS	RDC	8186	Amish population. Field informants provided data on emotional problems. Those identified given SADS-L.
New Haven, CT	SADS	RDC	511	Re-interview of an earlier household sample ages 18+.
Great Britain	CIS-R	ICD-10	10,108	Households selected from the Postcode Address File of England, Wales, and Scotland. The Kish grid method was used to select a single person in each household, ages 16–64. Lay interviewers, except substance abuse was determined with a self-administered questionnaire. Weighted to represent national population structure.
Zurich, Switzerland	SPIKE	*DSM-III*	4547	Two-stage cohort. Representative sample from a canton, ages 19–20, screened with SCL-90; 591 randomly selected and given a diagnostic semi-structured interview (SPIKE).

Table continued on next page

Table 13.1. *Continued*

Study	Instrument	Diagnostic criteria	Sample size	Methods
Brazil	Checklist	*DSM-III*	6470	Cluster samples from three cities (Brasilia, *n* = 2345; São Paulo, *n* = 1742; Pôrto Alegra, *n* = 2384) using QMPA as a screen. Thirty percent of probable cases and 10% of noncases psychiatric interview by psychiatrists using *DSM-III* Symptom Checklist interviewed by psychiatrists and psychologists. Results weighted. Ages 15+.

ECA, Epidemiologic Catchment Area; CATEGO; CIS-R, Clinical Interview Schedule–Revised; SPIKE, Structured psychopathological interview and rating of the social consequences of psychic disturbances for epidemiology; QMPA, Questionáno de Morbidade P. siquiátrica de Adultos.

°Robins et al. (1984) does not include the institutionalized; Leaf et al. (1986) includes the institutionalized.

Dohrenwends' 1974 review, they similarly found that 28 of 33 studies had the highest rates of psychopathology in the lowest SES class.

Fifteen epidemiological studies in the third generation have provided published data on SES and overall rates of psychopathology (Table 13.2). Several publications resulting from the ECA studies confirm that lower SES has higher rates of psychopathology. Regier et al. (1993) pooled the data on 1 month prevalence rates for approximately 18,000 respondents who were interviewed across the five ECA sites. The Nam criteria (Nam & Powers, 1965), which combine household income, education, and occupation, were used to measure SES. Adjusting for age, sex, marital status, site, and ethnicity, the lowest socioeconomic level had a statistically significant odds ratio of 2.6 compared with the highest. A significant difference was found whether or not cognitive impairment, substance abuse, and antisocial personality were included in the definition of all disorders.

Using a similar definition of SES and examining 6 month prevalence (excluding phobias and cognitive impairment), Holzer et al. (1986) found a relative risk of 2.9 for the lowest class in contrast to the highest class, controlling for sex and age. That study

also examined psychopathology rates stratified by gender and age, and in each stratum the highest SES had the lowest rates. ECA 1 year and lifetime prevalence rates exhibited a similar pattern with SES measured by education, employment status, or receiving public financial assistance (Robins et al., 1984, 1991a). The SES relationship using Nam criteria and 6 month and lifetime prevalence rates from the pooled ECA sites were also examined stratified by gender and race controlled for age (Williams et al., 1992). Regardless of gender or race, SES exhibited a significant inverse relationship with 6 month prevalence. However, lifetime prevalence showed a more complex pattern; the inverse relationship held only for white men and black women. Analyses restricted to the New Haven ECA site (Leaf et al., 1984) also found a significant inverse relationship between 6 month prevalence and years of education, personal income, and employment status.

A DIS-based study from Canada found unemployed individuals in comparison to employed individuals to have a statistically significant odds ratio of 2.8 for lifetime rates of any disorder (Bland et al., 1988). Another study using the DIS in Puerto Rico (Canino et al., 1987) found a statistically significant inverse relationship between educational at-

Table 13.2. Overall psychopathology: Third-generation studies and SES

First author	Year	Site	Instrument & prevalence	Measure of SES	Low (%)	High (%)	Ratio	p <
Regier	1993	ECA five sites	DIS 1 month	Nam criteria[†]	11.0	21.6	2.6	0.003
Holzer	1986	ECA five sites	DIS 6 month	Nam criteria[†]	11.5	7.6	2.9	0.001
Robins	1991	ECA five sites	DIS 1 year	Education	23	18	1.3	0.001
				Financial dependence	31	18	1.7	0.001
				Occupational status	29	14	2.1	0.001
			DIS lifetime	Education	36	30	1.2	0.001
				Financial dependence	47	31	1.5	0.001
				Occupational status	48	30	1.6	0.05
Leaf	1984	ECA New Haven	DIS 6 month	Education	18.0	15.4	1.3	0.001[‡]
				Income	20.4	13.7	1.5	0.003[‡]
				Employment	18.4	16.3	1.1	0.04
Robins	1984	ECA New Haven	DIS lifetime	Education	30.2	25.1	1.2	0.01
		ECA Baltimore	DIS lifetime	Education	38.7	30.9	1.3	0.01
		ECA St. Louis	DIS lifetime	Education	31.9	25.6	1.2	0.05
Bland	1988	Edmonton, Canada	DIS lifetime	Employment	59.6	34.8	2.8	0.001
Canino	1987	Puerto Rico	DIS 6 month	Education	22.7	10.6	2.1	0.01[‡]
Kessler	1994	USA	CIDI 1 year	Income			1.9	0.05
				Education			2.3	0.05
			CIDI lifetime	Income			1.5	0.05
				Education			1.2	NS
Goering	1996	Ontario, Canada	CIDI 1 year	Education	34.1	24.2	1.4	0.0001
Bebbington	1981	Camberwell, England	PSE 1 month	Employment				0.0001
				Hope-Goldthorpe				0.005
				Middle v. working class				NS
Mavreas	1986	Athens, Greece	PSE 1 month	Education	24.0	9.3	2.6	NS[‡]
				Employment				0.0001

Author	Year	Location	Instrument	Variable				Significance
Vázquez-Barquero	1987	Cantabria, Spain	PSE 1 month	Education				0.01
Hodiamont	1987	Nijmegen, Holland	PSE 1 month	Education				0.01[†]
Lehtinen	1990	Finland	PSE 1 month	Education	6.5	9.7	0.7	NS[‡]
				Social class	39.6	4.3	9.2	0.001
				Employment	10.9	7.4	1.5	NS
Romans-Clarkson	1988	New Zealand	PSE current	Employment	10.1	5.9	1.7	0.005
				Occupational status	14.2	6.7	2.1	0.005
Rodgers	1991	Great Britain	PSE current	Financial hardship				0.001
				Personal income				NS
				Occupational status				NS
Surtees	1983	Edinburgh, Scotland	PAS-CATEGO current	Middle v. working	12.3	5.2	2.4	0.01
				Employment	14.8	6.1	2.4	0.01
			PAS-RDC current	Middle v. working	19.1	9.1	2.1	0.001
				Employment	21.9	10.3	2.1	0.001
			Bedford current	Middle v. working	5.5	1.8	3.1	0.05
				Employment	8.9	1.7	5.2	0.001
Weissman	1980	New Haven	SADS-PD point	Hollingshead	22.8	15.4	1.5	NS[‡]
Levav	1993	Israel	SADS-D 6 month*	Education	37.0	15.2	2.4	0.001
			SDS-PD 6 month*	Education	49.3	28.0	1.8	0.001
			SADS-D 1 year*	Education	37.6	16.0	2.4	0.001
			SADS-PD 1 year*	Education	50.5	28.8	1.8	0.001
			SADS-D lifetime*	Education	61.3	41.3	1.5	NS
			SADS-PD lifetime*	Education	75.9	56.1	1.6	NS

NS, not significant; SADS-PD, SADS-RDC Probable and Definite; SADS-D, SADS-RDC Definite.

*Unpublished data obtained from the author; all RDC categories, including "Other."

[†]Adjusted for other sociodemographic covariates.

[‡]Significance based on education as a continuous variable, not high versus low SES.

tainment with 6 month prevalence for any disorder.

The National Comorbidity Survey (NCS), (Kessler et al., 1994) which used the CIDI in a national probability sample of individuals ages 15–54 in the United States, found higher rates of psychopathology in the lowest stratum defined in terms of income and education. For lifetime rates, the NCS had a significant odds ratio of 1.5 for the lowest income and a nonsignificant odds ratio of 1.2 for the lowest educational group, using the highest income and highest educational groups as the base. However, the two middle educational groups had significantly higher rates of psychopathology than the highest educational group. The lowest educational and lowest income groups had significant odds ratios, in contrast to the highest groups, for the 1 year prevalence rates (2.3 and 1.9, respectively). The Ontario based CIDI study (Goering et al., 1996) had a 1 year prevalence rate of 34.1% among participants who completed primary school and a rate of 24.2% in those who completed postsecondary education.

An earlier study using the SADS-RDC conducted in New Haven (Weissman & Myers, 1980) also found an inverse relationship between the point prevalence of overall psychopathology, defined in terms of probable and definite cases, and Hollingshead's two-factor index of social position. This relationship, however, was not statistically significant.

Outside of North America, only studies using the PSE and SADS have investigated SES formally. The Camberwell Study in England (Bebbington et al., 1981) examined various measures of SES using the PSE in women and men separately. In comparing middle-class to working-class individuals, there were no significant differences in rates of 1 month prevalence of disorder when men and women were analyzed separately (men: 3.8% vs. 9.1%; women: 11.1% vs. 17.5%) or combined. However, when the investigators compared the three lowest Hope-Goldthorpe classes of occupational prestige (Goldthorpe & Hope, 1974) to the higher classes, the lowest classes had higher

rates for both sexes combined and for men (24.3% vs. 3.8%), but not women (21.2% vs. 12.8%). Being unemployed also was associated with higher prevalence of disorder for both genders (men: 13.6% vs. 5.5%; women: 25.4% vs. 9.6%).

A study conducted on a population from Athens (Mavreas et al., 1986), using PSE-CATEGO diagnoses, found education to be inversely associated with overall rates of disorder for both men (lowest 13.1% vs. highest 5.4%) and women (lowest 27.4% vs. highest 6.7%) separately and combined. Similarly, overall the unemployed compared to the employed had higher rates. However, when each gender was examined separately, the association between employment and disorder did not reach statistical significance (men: 16.7% vs. 6.8%; women: 25.7% vs. 15.4%). Defining working and middle classes by occupational prestige, working-class women were found to have significantly higher rates than middle-class women (29.2% vs. 11.5%); men had a similar, but not statistically significant, pattern (10.3% vs. 5.7%).

A two-stage PSE-CATEGO study in the region of Cantabria, Spain, examined several measures of SES by gender (Vázquez-Barquero et al., 1987). No clear trend between 1 month prevalence of psychopathology and occupational prestige was found for women (low 21.3% vs. high 27.7%), but a significant inverse relationship was found for men (low 11.7% vs. high 2.9%). Similarly, employed compared to unemployed men (15.8% vs. 4.8%) had significantly more mental illness, but no association was found in women (22.2% vs. 19.2%). Both sexes demonstrated a significant inverse relationship between low compared with high educational attainment and psychopathology (men: 9.7% vs. 2.1%; women: 23.2% vs. 11.3%).

Occupational status, employment, and education, and their relationship to overall current rates of CATEGO psychiatric disorder using logistic regression, were also examined in a Dutch PSE study of the Nijmegen area (Hodiamont et al., 1987). The rates of current disorders for men were significantly higher among those who were unemployed, had less education, and were in occupations of lower prestige. A similar pattern appeared for women, except that prevalence of disorders did not vary with employment status.

A fifth PSE study, from Finland (Lehtinen et al., 1990), found CATEGO-derived psychiatric disorders to have a significant inverse relationship with an undefined measure of social class. When stratified by gender, however, the association was found to hold for men but not women (men: lowest 23.5%, highest 3.4%; women: lowest 36.8%, highest 5.7%). Education, type of occupation, and employment status were found to be unrelated to overall psychopathology.

Two additional community-based studies, using a shortened version of the PSE, provided mixed results on the relationship between SES and rates of overall psychiatric disorder. The first study, conducted in Great Britain, found occupational status to be related to disorders in women but not men, and personal income to have no association for either sex (Rodgers, 1991). Employment was found to be a significant factor as a predictor of disorder in men but not women. Both men and women who were in financial hardship had significantly higher rates of disorder. The second study (Romans-Clarkson et al., 1988), investigating women in New Zealand, found a significant inverse relationship between SES based occupational and employment status. This study also examined urban versus rural differences (Romans-Clarkson et al., 1990). Occupational status was inversely related to SES for both urban and rural women; however, paid employment was inversely associated with caseness for urban but not rural women.

A study restricted to women was conducted in Edinburgh, Scotland (Surtees et al., 1983), with the Psychiatric Assessment Schedule (PAS) using current diagnoses with CATEGO, RDC, and Bedford College criteria. This investigation found a significant inverse relationship between psychiatric morbidity, regardless of diagnostic criteria, and socioeconomic status using a modified version of the Hope-Goldthorpe schema and also employment status.

A SADS-RDC study was conducted in Israel (Levav et al., 1993). Unlike the DIS studies, this Israeli cohort sample, ages 24–33, were interviews by psychiatrists rather than lay interviewers using the SADS. The 6 month prevalence rates from this study also exhibited significant differences according to education as a measure of SES. A ratio of 1.8 at the probable and definite case level and a ratio of 2.4 at the definite level were found comparing those who did not graduate high school to college graduates. One year prevalence rates also demonstrated this relationship.

In summary, regardless of the definition used for SES, the type of prevalence rate, or the type of case-identification instrument, an inverse relationship has been found to exist between SES and overall psychopathology. The median ratio, comparing the low to high socioeconomic levels, for the prevalence period closest to 1 year was 2.1, and that for lifetime prevalence was 1.4. Does this inverse relationship hold for specific disorders?

Schizophrenia

The first- and second-generation studies also documented an inverse relationship between SES and psychosis. A review of the true prevalence studies between 1950 and 1980 (Neugebauer et al., 1980) found six studies that reported higher rates in the lowest class, one that reported approximately the same rate in both the highest and lowest classes, and one that claimed that psychosis was more frequent in the highest class. The review stated that those studies that failed to find an inverse relationship had small sample sizes, raising questions about the instability of the rates. The average low- to high-class ratio in these studies was 2.1. In Dohrenwend and Dohrenwend's (1974) review, the SES distribution of psychosis was not as clear, with only 7 of 15 studies reporting higher rates in the lowest class compared to other than the lowest class.

More recent studies, using current and more specific diagnostic criteria, have examined the rates for schizophrenia and its related disorders, with less likelihood of confounding from other psychotic disorders, especially affective psychoses (Table 13.3). The different ECA reports demonstrate a statistically significant inverse relationship with SES defined by the Nam criteria. Regier et al. (1993) used a broad definition of schizophrenia that included schizophreniform disorders. The odds ratio for the lowest compared to the highest 1 month prevalence across all sites, adjusted for age, sex, marital status, site, and ethnicity, was 8.1. Using a more restricted definition of schizophrenia excluding schizophreniform disorders, Holzer et al. (1986) found a relative risk for 6 month prevalence (Holzer et al., 1986), adjusted for age and sex, of 7.9. Keith et al. (1991), using a definition that included schizophreniform disorders and adjusting for age, sex, race, and marital status, calculated the lifetime odds ratio to be a statistically significant 9.7. The unadjusted ratios for lifetime and 1 year prevalence were 5.0 and 4.8, respectively (Keith et al., 1991). This inverse relationship was confirmed in the North Carolina site examining education and 6 month prevalence of schizophrenia and schizophreniform disorder controlled for urbanicity, sex, age, and marital status, which calculated an odds ratio of 1.8 (Blazer et al., 1985). The ECA study also found that individuals with a lifetime diagnosis of schizophrenia were more likely to be unemployed, to not have graduated college, and to be on public financial assistance (Keith et al., 1991; Robins et al., 1984).

In the Canadian DIS study (Bland et al., 1988), a statistically significant odds ratio of 3.8 comparing unemployed versus employed individuals with schizophrenia was obtained. The Puerto Rican DIS study did not find a relationship between education as a measure of SES and lifetime or 6 month prevalence rates of schizophrenia (Canino et al., 1987).

The NCS study examined the rates of schizophrenia or schizophreniform disorder using a structured clinical re-interview fol-lowing administration of the CIDI. A statistically significant odds ratio was found between the lowest and highest educated groups, as well as the lowest and highest income groups (Kendler et al., 1996).

The SADS-RDC study conducted in Israel, consistent with most DIS studies, found the 6 month and 1 year prevalences at both the probable and definite and the definite levels of diagnosis to be significantly higher among those individuals with less education (Dohrenwend et al., 1992; Levav et al., 1993). A nonsignificant trend was found for lifetime prevalence. In Weissman and Myers' (1980) ECA study in New Haven, Connecticut, using the SADS and probable and definite point prevalence, only the two lowest social classes had cases of schizophrenia.

In summary, the literature is consistent in demonstrating an inverse relationship between SES and schizophrenia. The median low- compared with high-SES ratio was 3.4 for the prevalence period closest to 1 year and 2.4 for lifetime prevalence.

Major Depression

Few studies conducted during the first two generations of research presented data on the prevalence of specific affective disorders. Second-generation studies, however, do provide data on dysphoric mood and other depressive symptoms contained in some screening scales. These studies consistently find an inverse linear association between screening scale scores and SES. Link and Dohrenwend (1980) reviewed eight studies published between 1950 and 1980 that provided data on screening scales and SES. Interpreting symptom scores as a measure of demoralization, they observed that, across six of the studies, the lowest socioeconomic stratum had a median demoralization rate of 36.4% and the highest stratum 9.2%. This consistent inverse relationship was also found in another independent review of eight studies dating from 1967 to 1976 (Kessler, 1982).

Since these reviews, numerous additional reports focusing on measures of psycholog-

Table 13.3. Schizophrenia: Third-generation studies and SES

First author	Year	Site	Instrument & prevalence	Measure of SES	Low (%)	High (%)	Ratio	p <
						SES prevalence rate		
Regier	1993	ECA five sites	DIS 1 month	Nam criteria[†]	1.2	0.3	8.1	0.003
Holzer	1986	ECA five sites	DIS 6 month	Nam Criteria[†]	1.3	0.3	7.9	0.001
Keith	1991	ECA five sites	DIS 1 year	Nam criteria	1.9	0.4	4.8	
			DIS lifetime	Nam criteria[†]	2.5	0.5	9.7	0.0001
Blazer	1985	ECA Durham, NC	DIS 6 month	Education[†]			1.8	0.01[‡]
Robins	1984	ECA New Haven	DIS lifetime	Education	2.5	0.5	5.0	0.01
		ECA Baltimore	DIS lifetime	Education	1.7	0.6	2.8	NS
		ECA St. Louis	DIS lifetime	Education	1.1	0.6	1.8	NS
Bland	1988	Edmonton, Canada	DIS lifetime	Employment	1.4	0.4	3.8	0.05
Canino	1987	Puerto Rico	DIS 6 month	Education	1.8	0.9	2.0	NS[‡]
			DIS lifetime	Education	2.2	0.9	2.4	NS[‡]
Kendler	1996	USA	CIDI lifetime	Education			2.2	0.05
				Income			1.1	0.05[‡]
Weissman	1980	New Haven	SADS-PD point	Hollingshead	0.8	0.0	2.0[°°]	NS[‡]
Levav	1993	Israel	SADS-D 6 month	Education	1.4	0.3	4.7	0.05
			SADS-PD 6 month	Education	1.5	0.3	5.0	0.05
Dohrenwend	1992	Israel	SADS-D 1 year	Education	1.4	0.3	4.5	0.05
			SADS-PD 1 year	Education	1.5	0.3	5.0	0.05
			SADS-D lifetime	Education	1.4	0.8	1.6	NS
			SADS-PD lifetime	Education	1.5	0.8	1.7	NS

NS, not significant; SADS-PD, SADS-RDC Probable and Definite; SADS-D, SADS-RDC Definite.

[†]Adjusted for other sociodemographic covariates.

[‡]Significance based on education or income as a continuous variable, not high versus low SES.

[°°]Ratio of lowest versus highest where a cell does not contain zero.

ical distress using various instruments have confirmed this finding. The CES-D has been one of the most widely used measures in various community studies in the United States and other countries. In most studies, the CES-D has consistently demonstrated an inverse relationship with various measures of SES (Aneshensel et al., 1982; Berkman et al., 1986; Eaton & Kessler, 1981; Frerichs et al., 1981; Fuhrer et al., 1992; Neff & Husaini, 1987; Noll & Dubinsky, 1985; Radloff & Locke, 1986). Similar results have been obtained using the Langner Scale and SES measured in terms of occupational and employment status (Cochrane & Stopes-Roe, 1980), as well as education and income (Cockerham, 1990). A British study using the Symptom Rating Test (Kellner & Sheffield, 1973) found increased psychological disturbance in the unemployed compared to the employed in a community-based sample from five British towns (Cochrane & Stopes-Roe, 1981). The Psychiatric Epidemiology Research Instrument Demoralization Scale has been shown to have an inverse relationship with education in Israeli populations (Dohrenwend et al., 1987). Studies in the United States (Neff & Husaini, 1987) and Canada (Hay, 1988) using the Health Opinion Survey (MacMillan, 1957) have also obtained an inverse relationship with measures of socioeconomic status. A Finnish cohort study using the Zung Depression Scale found an inverse relationship between depressive symptoms in women but not men (Rajala et al., 1994). Indeed, only two studies were located that failed to document an inverse SES–demoralization relationship, one using the General Health Questionnaire (Goldberg, 1978) and the other using the GWB (Andrews et al., 1978; Romans-Clarkson et al., 1988). Thus, although the first two generations of psychiatric epidemiological research do not provide any direct information on SES and major depression, second-generation studies contain data that suggest an inverse relationship.

One of the first third-generation studies including the issue of SES and major de-

pression in the analyses was Brown et al.'s (1975; Brown & Prudo, 1981) PSE studies of random samples of women living in London (Camberwell) and Outer Hebrides, Scotland (Table 13.4). The 1975 London study found working class women to have a significantly higher 3 month prevalence rate of depression than middle class women (25% vs. 5%, respectively), with a relative risk of 5.0 (Brown et al., 1975). In a subsequent study, using a larger sample, Brown and Harris (1978) found that working-class women, as defined by the Hope-Goldthorpe measure, were 3.8 times more likely than middle-class women to have had a diagnosis of depression 3 months prior to interview. The relative risk for 1 year prevalence was 3.0 (Brown & Prudo, 1981). In a study of a sample of women from the Outer Hebrides, an area of rural islands off the coast of Scotland, Brown and Prudo (1981) found no association between 1 year prevalence rates for depression and SES.

A more recent PSE in Italy (Carta et al., 1991) found unemployed men to have significantly higher 1 month prevalence rates for depression (odds ratio of 3.8), but not women (odds ratio 1.8). However, education was inversely related, with those having less than 9 years of schooling at a higher risk than those with over 10 years of education. A study conducted in Lesotho, Africa (Hollifield et al., 1990) had a risk ratio of 2.3 between the lowest and highest educated groups. Another African study conducted in Zimbabwe found that women with depression were more likely to be unemployed, have lower incomes, and have less education (Abas & Broadhead, 1997).

The New Haven, Connecticut, ECA study, using point and lifetime prevalence rates at the probable and definite level of diagnosis for major depression, did not find an inverse relationship with Hollingshead's two-factor index of social position, a summary score of education and occupation; this relationship was not linear (Weissman & Myers, 1978). However, a reanalysis of the point prevalence results (P. E. Shrout, personal communication, 1980) did find a statistically significant inverse relationship, despite the fact that the relative risk for the lowest to the highest SES level was 2.3.

The various reports from the ECA study have resulted in different conclusions about the relationship of SES to major depression. The 1 month prevalence report (Regier et al., 1993) found no significant association, although the highest socioeconomic stratum had the lowest rates. Holzer et al.'s (1986) report on 6 month prevalence found a significant inverse association with SES. Although not formally tested, the relationship appeared to hold for women but not men. Weissman et al. (1991) reported no significant association between 1 year prevalence and education, income, or occupation. However, the risk of major depression was significantly greater among those subjects on public financial assistance. Also, education was not related to major depression in the lifetime prevalence data of the five sites combined (Robins et al., 1984), nor in the North Carolina site using 6 month prevalence (Blazer et al., 1985).

A separate analysis of the New Haven ECA site using a 6 month prevalence rate that included institutionalized individuals was conducted by Leaf et al. (1986). This study found major depression to have a curvilinear relationship with education uncontrolled for age and sex. Personal income had a significant inverse relationship with depression; however, this did not hold when controlled for age and sex. Household income had no consistent relationship. Unemployed subjects, however, were significantly more likely than employed subjects to be diagnosed with major depression, even after adjusting for age and sex. The Williams et al. (1992) report on gender–race differences and SES found an inverse SES 6 month prevalence relationship for whites but not blacks. Lifetime prevalence rates exhibited no significant association with SES regardless of race or gender.

Three other studies using the DIS contain information on social class. Comparing unemployed and employed respondents using lifetime rates, Bland et al. (1988) found a significant risk for major depression among the unemployed, with an odds ratio of 2.0. However, no association with major depression and education was found examining 6 month or lifetime prevalence rates in Puerto Rico (Canino et al., 1987). The study conducted in Taiwan had mixed results: a significant inverse relationship with education for 1 year prevalence but not lifetime prevalence (Hwu et al., 1996).

An offshoot from the Baltimore ECA study, the Eastern Baltimore Mental Health Study (EBMHS), examined *DSM-III* diagnoses of major depression made by psychiatrists using the SPE (Romanoski et al., 1992). Despite having odds ratios as high as 8.0, they found no significant inverse relationship between current major depression and socioeconomic status as measured by education, employment, or receiving public support after adjusting for sex, race, age, and marital status. This finding held when men and women were examined separately.

In the NCS, odds ratios for SES were calculated for affective disorder in general (Kessler et al., 1994). Major depression, however, represented the vast majority of those disorders (i.e., about 91% for 1 year and 89% for lifetime prevalence). The NCS found 1 year prevalence to be inversely related with SES as measured by education and income. Lifetime rates from this study demonstrated no relationship with education, but income level was inversely related and significant for the lowest income group in contrast to the highest. A follow-up report presented the SES relationship for 30 day prevalence of major depression, and demonstrated an inverse relationship for both income and education (Blazer et al., 1994).

Another study using the CIDI, conducted in Ontario (Offord et al., 1994), compared 1 year prevalence rates of unemployment, public assistance, low income, and completion of high school among individuals with any affective disorder to individuals with no psychiatric diagnosis. Among those with an affective disorder, 16% were unemployed, 8% received public assistance, 14% had low income, and 26% did not complete high

Table 13.4. Major depression: Third-generation studies and SES

First author	Year	Site	Instrument & prevalence	Measure of SES	SES prevalence rate			
					Low (%)	High (%)	Ratio	$p <$
Regier	1993	ECA five sites	DIS 1 month	Nam criteria[†]	2.2	1.3	2.2	NS
Holzer	1986	ECA five sites	DIS 6 month	Nam criteria[†]	2.2	1.7	1.8	0.05
Weissman	1991	ECA five sites	DIS 1 year	Employment[†]	3.4	2.2	1.5	0.001
				Occupational status[†]	1.7	2.5	1.1	NS
				Income[†]	2.9	1.8	1.4	NS
				Education[†]	2.6	2.8	1.2	NS
Leaf	1986	ECA New Haven	DIS 6 month	Education	1.5	2.4	0.6	NS
				Personal income	3.9	1.7	2.3	0.05
				Household income	3.9	1.9	2.1	NS
				Employment	8.0	2.2	3.6	0.03
Blazer	1985	ECA Durham, NC	DIS 6 month	Eduation[†]			1.0	NS[†]
Robins	1984	ECA New Haven	DIS lifetime	Education	6.6	7.1	0.9	NS
		ECA Baltimore	DIS lifetime	Education	3.6	5.5	0.7	NS
		ECA St. Louis	DIS lifetime	Education	5.7	4.6	1.2	NS
Bland	1988	Edmonton, Canada	DIS lifetime	Employment	13.9	7.5	2.0	0.001
Canino	1987	Puerto Rico	DIS 6 month	Education	1.9	1.6	1.2	NS[†]
			DIS lifetime	Education	3.8	4.5	0.8	NS[†]
Hwu	1996	Taiwan	DIS 1 year	Education	1.0	0.4	2.5	0.05
			DIS lifetime	Education	1.3	1.2	1.1	NS
Romanoski	1992	EBMHS Baltimore	SPE current	Education	2.4	0.3	8.0	NS[†]
				Employment	1.4	0.8	1.8	NS
				Public support	1.7	0.8	2.1	NS
Blazer	1994	USA	CIDI 1 month	Income			2.0	0.05
				Education			3.3	0.05
Kessler	1994	USA	CIDI 1 year	Income	1.7		1.7	0.05
				Education	1.8		1.8	0.05
			CIDI lifetime	Income	1.6		1.6	0.05
				Education	1.0		1.0	NS

Author	Year	Location	Instrument	SES measure				Significance
Goering	1996	Ontario, Canada	CIDI 1 year	Education	30.8	26.0	1.2	
Brown	1975	Camberwell, England	PSE 3 month	Occupation/education	25.0	5.0	5.0	0.001
Brown	1978	Camberwell, England	PSE 3 month	Hope-Goldthorpe	23.0	6.0	3.8	
Brown	1981	Camberwell, England	PSE 1 year	Hope-Goldthorpe	24.0	8.0	3.0	
		Hebrides, Scotland	PSE 1 year	Hope-Goldthorpe	10.0	14.0	0.7	NS
				Education	11.0	10.0	1.1	NS
Hollifield	1990	Lesotho	PSE 1 month	Education	0.2	0.1	2.3	
Carta	1991	Sardinia, Italy	PSE 1 month	Employment	16.7	8.6	1.8	NS
				Education	12.2	2.0	7.4	0.05
Abas	1997	Zimbabwe	PSE 1 year	Income	40	22	2.2	0.02
			PSE 1 year	Employment	35.0	15.0	2.9	0.02
			PSE 1 year	Education	39.0	16.0	3.5	0.01
Weissman	1978	New Haven	SADS-PD current	Hollingshead	4.1	1.5	2.7	NS
			SADS-PD lifetime	Hollingshead	15.6	21.5	0.7	NS
Levav	1993	Israel	SADS-D 6 month	Education	3.6	2.2	1.6	NS
			SADS-PD 6 month	Education	5.1	2.7	1.9	NS
Dohrenwend	1992	Israel	SADS-D 1 year	Education	4.4	2.6	1.7	NS
			SADS-PD 1 year	Education	7.0	3.5	2.0	NS
			SADS-D lifetime	Education	17.5	11.9	1.5	NS
			SADS-PD lifetime	Education	27.5	15.7	2.4	0.01
Meltzer	1995	Great Britain	CIS-R 1 week	Employment	5.6	1.1	5.1	0.01
				Occupational status	3.5	0.9	3.9	NS
				Education	1.3	2.9	1.7	0.01

NS, not significant; SADS-PD, SADS-RDC Probable and Definite; SADS-D, SADS-RDC Definite.

[a] Adjusted for other sociodemographic covariates.

[b] Significance based on education as a continuous variable, not high versus low SES.

school. This is in contrast to 6%, 3%, 9%, and 24%, respectively, for healthy individuals. A subsequent report (Goering et al., 1996) found a significant difference in 1 year prevalence rates between those who completed primary school (26.0%) and individuals who completed postsecondary education (30.8%).

The Israel study, examining 6 month prevalences of both probable and definite and definite RDC diagnoses, found a trend for major depression being highest in the lowest educational group level. These analyses were not controlled for gender, ethnicity, or age (Levav et al., 1993). A more detailed analysis was conducted by Dohrenwend et al. (1992) of 1 year and lifetime diagnoses. An inverse relationship between SES and major depression was found for all groups with the exception of North African women; those who graduated from college showed unusually high rates.

A report the Office of Population Census and Survey (OPCS) in Great Britain examined social class by employment status, occupational prestige, and educational attainment (Meltzer et al., 1995). Using the Clinical Interview Schedule–Revised (CIS-R) to make psychiatric diagnoses for the previous week, they found that unemployed women with depressive disorders (5.6%) had higher rates than employed women (1.1%). A similar result was obtained for men (2.7% among the unemployed; 1.2% among the employed). Comparing the lowest to the highest social class based on occupational status for both men and women, the lowest SES group had the higher risk for depressive disorder, but for neither gender was this a clearly linear relationship. Overall, an inverse relationship appeared to exist for educational attainment and the rate of depressive disorders; however, this was not the case for women.

The results of these various studies indicate that the relationship between SES and depression is more complex than originally suggested from the earlier studies of nonspecific distress. There is some evidence to suggest that this relationship may vary across gender, urbanicity, and ethnicity.

Among children, interestingly, parental SES is only significant for girls (Liu & Cohen, 1994). A further consideration is the possibility that the diagnostic instruments themselves, in particular the DIS, may bias against finding a stronger inverse association between major depression and SES. The median low- compared with high-SES ratio was 2.4 for the prevalence period closest to 1 year and 1.1 for lifetime prevalence.

Anxiety Disorders

Anxiety disorders in the first- and second-generation studies were included in a broad category known as "neurosis." A review of true prevalence studies examining "neurosis" found no trend with SES. Five of the studies reported higher rates in the lowest level, while four reported higher rates in the highest level (Neugebauer et al., 1980). Dohrenwend and Dohrenwend's (1974) review similarly found no trend; seven studies had higher rates for the lowest SES level and eight for other than the lowest level. The development of formal diagnostic classification systems resulted in the elimination of "neurosis" and the creation of specific disorders within the rubric of anxiety. Each of these individual disorders potentially varies in its relationship to SES.

Panic Disorder

Panic disorder and its relationship to SES has been investigated in the ECA, Edmonton, Israel, NCS, New Haven, OPCS, Lesotho, and Puerto Rico studies (Table 13.5). Regier and colleagues (1993), using Nam criteria for SES and examining 1 month prevalence data pooled across the five ECA sites, found the lowest stratum to have significantly more disorder (odds ratio of 11.6) than the highest stratum. Eaton et al. (1991) examined the relationship of 1 year prevalence of panic disorder to education, Nam criteria, and public financial dependence separately by gender. No consistent relationship was found except for those receiving financial aid having higher rates (men: yes, 1.9%; no, 0.4%; women: yes, 3.2%; no,

Table 13.5. Panic disorder: Third-generation studies and SES

First author	Year	Site	Instrument & prevalence	Measure of SES	SES prevalence rate			
					Low (%)	High (%)	Ratio	$p <$
Regier	1993	ECA five sites	DIS 1 month	Nam criteria[†]	1.2	0.2	11.6	0.003
Von Korff	1985	ECA New Haven	DIS 6 month	Education	2.8	6.0	0.5	NS[‡]
		ECA Baltimore	DIS 6 month	Education	13.2	7.5	1.8	0.01[‡]
		ECA St. Louis	DIS 6 month	Education	20.7	7.8	2.7	0.01[‡]
Robins	1984	ECA New Haven	DIS lifetime	Education	1.4	1.6	0.9	NS
		ECA Baltimore	DIS lifetime	Education	1.5	1.1	1.4	NS
		ECA St. Louis	DIS lifetime	Education	1.7	0.5	3.4	0.05
Bland	1988	Edmonton, Canada	DIS lifetime	Employment	2.1	1.2	1.8	NS
Canino	1987	Puerto Rico	DIS 6 month	Education	0.6	0.4	1.5	NS[‡]
			DIS lifetime	Education	1.4	0.9	1.6	0.05[‡]
Eaton	1994	USA	CIDI 1 month	Income			1.0	NS
			CIDI 1 month	Education			10.4	0.05
Weissman	1980	New Haven	SADS-PD point	Hollingshead	1.6	0.0		NS
Levav	1993	Israel	SADS-D 6 month	Education	0.6	0.0°°	6.0	0.01
			SADS-PD 6 month	Education	0.9	0.1	9.0	0.01
			SADS-D 1 year°	Education	0.6	0.0°°	6.0	0.01
			SADS-PD 1 year°	Education	1.1	0.1	5.5	0.01
			SADS-D lifetime°	Education	1.2	0.2	2.9	0.001
			SADS-PD lifetime°	Education	2.9	0.8	3.6	0.05
Hollifield	1990	Lesotho	PSE 1 month	Education	0.2	0.1	3.0	NS
Meltzer	1995	Great Britain	CIS-R 1 week	Employment	1.1	0.7	1.6	NS
				Occupational status	1.2	0.1	12.0	NS
				Education	1.1	1.1	1.0	NS

NS, not significant; SADS-PD, SADS-RDC Probable and Definite; SADS-D, SADS-RDC Definite.

°Unpublished data obtained from the author.

[†]Adjusted for other sociodemographic covariates.

[‡]Significance based on education as a continuous variable, not high versus low SES.

°°Ratio of lowest versus highest where a cell does not contain zero.

1.0%). Lifetime data from the St. Louis ECA site indicated college graduates had significantly higher rates of panic disorder than noncollege graduates, a finding not supported by results from New Haven or Baltimore (Robins et al., 1984). Analyses of 6 month prevalence from the New Haven, Baltimore, and St. Louis ECA sites found Baltimore and St. Louis to have a consistent inverse relationship with education as a continuous measure (Von Korff et al., 1985).

The DIS study done in Edmonton, Canada, found no significant difference in lifetime rates between unemployed and employed individuals (Bland et al., 1988). In Puerto Rico's DIS study (Canino et al., 1987) lifetime prevalence rates, but not 6 month prevalence rates, showed a significant inverse relationship with education. The NCS study (Eaton et al., 1994) found a significant inverse relationship with 1 month prevalence rates of panic disorder and education (odds ratio of 10.4) for less than 12 years compared to greater than 16 years of education, but no relationship for income level. Cases of panic disorder were found only in the lowest socioeconomic stratum in the New Haven SADS-RDC study (Weissman & Myers, 1980). The Israel study using the SADS found a significant inverse relationship with education at all prevalence periods and diagnostic levels for panic disorder (Levav et al., 1993). The Lesotho study found a risk ratio of 3.0 for 1 month prevalence using the PSE between those with no education and high school graduates (Hollifield et al., 1990). The British OPS study reported no significant relationship between 1 week prevalence of panic disorder and education, employment status, or occupational prestige (Meltzer et al., 1995). The median ratio of low compared with high SES was 5.6 for the prevalence period closest to 1 year and 1.9 for lifetime prevalence.

Phobic Disorder

Data on phobic disorders were also reported in several of the studies cited above (Table 13.6). The 1 month prevalence in the pooled ECA data using Nam criteria found a sig-

nificant inverse association (Regier et al., 1993), with an odds ratio of 2.3, as did the analysis for 6 month prevalence (Holzer & Shea, 1990), with an odds ratio of 2.5. Boyd et al. (1990) examined the 1 month prevalence rates between SES and phobias using Nam Criteria and found an inverse relationship for each of the ECA sites, although for two of the sites, Los Angeles and St. Louis, the association failed to reach statistical significance. Examining simple phobia, the Robins et al. (1984) lifetime report of the ECA results found college graduates to have significantly lower rates than others in New Haven and Baltimore, but not in St. Louis. Two reports from the ECA study have focused on social phobia. The first (Schneier et al., 1992) found that individuals with social phobia were significantly more likely to be of lower SES, using Nam Criteria, and of lower education than those without social phobia. The subsequent report (Wells et al., 1994) similarly found an inverse relationship; less than college education was associated with more than twice the risk of college education, with a relative risk of 2.3.

The NCS (Magee et al., 1996) found a negative relationship with education but not income for simple phobia, while social phobia was negatively correlated to education and income for 30 day prevalence. When examining the highest versus the lowest stratum, statistically significant odds ratios were obtained with education and income for both disorders. The Puerto Rico DIS study suggested a nonsignificant inverse trend with education (Canino et al., 1987). Employment was not significantly related to phobic disorders according to the Canadian DIS study (Bland et al., 1988), and no consistent relationship was found in the New Haven SADS study (Weissman & Myers, 1980). As with panic disorder, the Israel study found a significant inverse relationship with phobic disorders and education using the SADS-RDC (Levav et al., 1993). A statistically significant relationship was found between phobic disorders and high and low employment status, but not educational attainment or occupational status, in the British OPCS study (Meltzer et al., 1995). The

Table 13.6. Phobic disorder: Third-generation studies and SES

First author	Year	Site	Instrument & prevalence	Measure of SES	SES prevalence rate			p <
					Low (%)	High (%)	Ratio	
Boyd	1990	ECA five sites	DIS 1 month	Nam criteria[†]			1.8	0.0001
		ECA New Haven	DIS 1 month	Nam criteria[†]			2.4	0.05
		ECA Baltimore	DIS 1 month	Nam criteria[†]			2.5	0.01
		ECA St. Louis	DIS 1 month	Nam criteria[†]			2.3	NS
		ECA Durham, NC	DIS 1 month	Nam criteria[†]			1.8	0.05
		ECA Los Angeles	DIS 1 month	Nam criteria[†]			1.6	NS
Regier	1993	ECA five sites	DIS 1 month	Nam criteria[†]	8.6	3.6	2.3	0.003
Holzer	1990	ECA five sites	DIS 6 month	Nam criteria[†]	12.5	5.1	2.5	0.001
Robins	1984	ECA New Haven	DIS lifetime	Education	7.2	3.8	1.9	0.01
		ECA Baltimore	DIS lifetime	Education	21.4	12.8	1.7	0.001
		ECA St. Louis	DIS lifetime	Education	7.2	5.1	1.4	NS
Bland	1988	Edmonton, Canada	DIS lifetime	Employment	10.6	9.5	1.1	NS
Camino	1987	Puerto Rico	DIS 6 month	Education	6.7	5.9	1.1	NS[‡]
			DIS lifetime	Education	14.8	9.1	1.6	NS[‡]
Weissman	1980	New Haven	SADS-PD point	Hollingshead	0.8	0.8	0.3[°°]	NS[‡]
Levav	1993	Israel	SADS-D 6 month	Education	5.4	1.1	4.9	0.001
			SADS-PD 6 month	Education	8.0	3.0	2.7	0.01
			SADS-D 1 year[°]	Education	5.4	1.1	4.9	0.001
			SADS-PD 1 year[°]	Education	8.0	3.3	2.4	0.05
			SADS-D lifetime[°]	Education	7.5	1.4	5.4	0.001
			SADS-PD lifetime[°]	Education	10.2	4.8	2.1	0.05
Meltzer	1995	Great Britain	CIS-R 1 week	Employment	1.9	0.5	3.1	0.01
				Occupational status	1.3	0.2	6.5	NS
				Education	1.4	0.6	2.3	NS

NS, not significant; SADS-PD, SADS-RDC Probable and Definite; SADS-D, SADS-RDC Definite.

[°]Unpublished data obtained from the author.

[†]Adjusted for other sociodemographic covariates.

[‡]Significance based on education as a continuous variable, not high versus low SES.

[°°]Ratio of lowest versus highest where a cell does not contain zero.

median ratio of low compared with high SES was 2.5 for the prevalence period closest to 1 year and 1.6 for lifetime prevalence.

Obsessive–Compulsive Disorder

No consistent pattern emerged from studies that examined SES and obsessive–compulsive disorder (Table 13.7). The Regier et al. (1993) pooled ECA analysis, controlling for age, sex, marital status, race, and site, found an inverse relationship between 1 month prevalence and SES measured in terms of Nam criteria, with an odds ratio of 2.9. Analyses of 1 year prevalence in the pooled data also found obsessive–compulsive disorder to be significantly higher among welfare recipients (Karno & Golding, 1991). However, this same study did not find any consistent association with educational attainment or income. An earlier analysis controlling for site, sex, age, marital status, and ethnicity in a logistic regression found that unemployed compared to employed individuals had significantly higher rates for both lifetime and 6 month prevalences (Karno et al., 1988). Job status had a significant inverse relationship with the 6 month prevalence rate of obsessive–compulsive disorder but not the lifetime rate. Individual analysis of the Baltimore, New Haven, and St. Louis sites of the ECA found no relationship between closeness, compulsive disorder, and education (Robins et al., 1984). Controlled for urban setting, gender, marital status, and age, data from the North Carolina ECA site showed a significant inverse relationship between education and 6 month prevalence, with an odds ratio of 1.6 (Blazer et al., 1985). In contrast, three of the studies conducted outside the United States failed to find a relationship with SES (Bland et al., 1988; Canino et al., 1987; Levav et al., 1993). The British OPCS study found unemployed compared to employed individuals to be at higher risk, but it showed no relationship between education or occupational prestige and obsessive–compulsive disorder (Meltzer et al., 1995). The median low- compared with high-SES ratio of obsessive–compulsive disorder was 1.7 for

the prevalence period closest to 1 year and 1.3 for lifetime prevalence.

Generalized Anxiety Disorder

As for generalized anxiety disorder, limited data are available (Table 13.8). The report from the ECA study contained no tests of significance and also indicated mixed results, depending on the site and the socioeconomic status measure used (Blazer et al., 1991). The NCS found an inverse relationship with income, which disappeared when controlled for other covariates (Wittchen et al., 1994). The Lesotho study (Hollifield et al., 1990) had a 1.7 risk for those with no education compared to those with a high school education. The Israel (Levav et al., 1993) and the New Haven SADS (Weissman & Myers, 1980) studies found little evidence of an association with SES as measured by educational level. The British OPCS study (Meltzer et al., 1995) found unemployed compared to employed individuals to have higher rates of generalized anxiety disorder. The OPCS study did not find a relationship with occupational prestige or education for 1 week prevalence. The median low- compared with high-SES ratio was 1.7 for the prevalence period closest to 1 year and 1.0 for lifetime prevalence.

Summary

The current evidence suggests that there may be an inverse relationship between SES and panic and phobic disorders. The picture is far less clear for obsessive–compulsive and generalized anxiety disorders. However, as suggested by the ECA study (Regier et al., 1990), the NCS study (Kessler et al., 1994), and the Ontario Health Survey (Offord et al., 1994), there does seem to be an inverse relationship between anxiety disorders as a group and SES. For example, in the ECA study the 1 month prevalence for the upper Nam quartile was 4.6% and for the lowest quartile 10.5%. The NCS had significant odds ratios for both education and income for 1 year (2.8 and 2.1, respectively) and lifetime (1.86 and 2.0, respectively)

Table 13.7. Obsessive–compulsive disorder: Third-generation studies and SES

First author	Year	Site	Instrument & prevalence	Measure of SES	SES prevalence rate			
					Low (%)	High (%)	Ratio	p <
Regier	1993	ECA five sites	DIS 1 month	Nam criteria[†]	2.1	1.0	2.9	0.003
Karno	1988	ECA five sites	DIS 6 month	Employment[†]			2.0	0.001
				Occupational status[†]			1.0	0.05
			DIS lifetime	Employment[†]			1.6	0.01
				Occupational status[†]			1.0	NS
Karno	1991	ECA five sites	DIS 1 year	Welfare	3.3	1.5	2.2	0.05
Blazer	1985	ECA Durham, NC	DIS 6 month	Education[†]			1.6	0.05[‡]
Robins	1984	ECA New Haven	DIS lifetime	Education	2.6	2.7	1.0	NS
		ECA Baltimore	DIS lifetime	Education	3.1	1.9	1.6	NS
		ECA St. Louis	DIS lifetime	Education	1.9	2.1	0.9	NS
Bland	1988	Edmonton, Canada	DIS lifetime	Employment	4.1	2.7	1.5	NS
Canino	1987	Puerto Rico	DIS 6 month	Education	2.3	1.9	1.2	NS[‡]
			DIS lifetime	Education	3.3	2.6	1.3	NS[‡]
Levav	1993	Israel	SADS-D 6 month	Education	1.5	1.7	0.9	NS
			SADS-PD 6 month	Education	2.5	2.1	1.2	NS
			SADS-D 1 year[°]	Education	1.5	1.6	0.9	NS
			SADS-PD 1 year[°]	Education	2.5	2.1	1.2	NS
			SADS-D lifetime[°]	Education	1.5	4.4	0.3	NS
			SADS-PD lifetime[°]	Education	2.5	4.7	0.5	NS
Meltzer	1995	Great Britain	CIS-R 1 week	Employment	1.9	0.9	2.1	0.01
				Occupational status	1.2	0.1	1.2	NS
				Education	2.1	0.6	3.5	NS

NS, not significant; SADS-PD, SADS-RDC Probable and Definite; SADS-D, SADS-RDC Definite.

[°]Unpublished data obtained from the author.

[†]Adjusted for other sociodemographic covariates.

[‡]Significance based on education as a continuous variable, not high versus low SES.

Table 13.8. Generalized anxiety disorder: Third-generation studies and SES

First author	Year	Site	Instrument & prevalence	Measure of SES	SES prevalence rate			
					Low (%)	High (%)	Ratio	$p <$
Blazer	1991	ECA Durham, NC	DIS 1 year	Nam criteria	8.5	1.6	5.3	
				Income	7.5	0.0		
				Education	4.2	1.7	2.5	
				DIS lifetime	Education	6.8	4.1	1.7	
		ECA Los Angeles	DIS 1 year	Nam criteria	3.5	1.0	3.5	
				Income	4.0	3.0	1.3	
				Education	1.8	2.7	0.7	
		ECA St. Louis	DIS lifetime	Education	3.3	6.4	0.5	
			DIS 1 year	Education	2.4	2.7	0.9	
			DIS lifetime	Education	5.5	7.8	0.7	
Wittchen	1994	USA	CIDI lifetime	Income			2.1	0.05
Weissman	1980	New Haven	SADS-PD point	Hollingshead	2.5	1.5	1.7	NS
Levav	1993	Israel	SADS-D 6 month	Education	4.6	0.8	5.8	0.001
			SADS-PD 6 month	Education	6.9	4.2	1.6	NS
			SADS-D 1 year°	Education	4.9	3.1	1.6	NS
			SADS-PD 1 year°	Education	7.5	6.6	1.1	NS
			SADS-D lifetime°	Education	13.7	15.7	0.9	NS
			SADS-PD lifetime°	Education	18.9	21.7	0.9	NS
Hollifield	1990	Lesotho	PSE 1 month	Education	0.2	0.1	1.7	
Meltzer	1995	Great Britain	CIS-R 1 week	Employment	5.4	2.4	2.2	0.01
				Occupational status	3.1	2.3	1.3	NS
				Education	4.4	3.1	1.4	NS

NS, not significant; SADS-PD, SADS-RDC Probable and Definite; SADS-D, SADS-RDC Definite.

°Unpublished data obtained from the author.

prevalence rates. The Ontario Health Survey found that 8% of persons with a 1 year prevalence of anxiety disorders were on public assistance, 15% had low income, and 29% failed to graduate high school, compared with 3%, 9%, and 24% of healthy individuals, respectively. However, the rates of unemployment for those with anxiety disorders and those with no psychiatric disorder were similar (7% and 6%, respectively).

Personality Disorder

Few studies in the earlier generations of psychiatric epidemiology examined a wide array of specific personality disorders. Usually what was included under this heading was antisocial behavior and problems with alcohol, or both combined. However, these studies did suggest that "personality disorders" occurred more frequently among the lower socioeconomic level groups. Neugebauer et al. (1980) found this to be true in six of seven studies included in their review. An average low- to high-SES ratio of 1.8 was found—an underestimation according to the investigators. An earlier review (Dohrenwend & Dohrenwend, 1974) found 11 of 14 studies to have higher rates in the lowest stratum as compared with other than the lowest stratum.

Antisocial personality is the most widely studied specific personality disorder included in community-based epidemiological surveys (Table 13.9). Regier et al. (1993), using the pooled ECA data and the Nam criteria for SES, found a higher risk for this disorder among the lowest as compared to the highest strata. Although Blazer and associates (1985) report an inverse relationship between education and antisocial personality, the ECA studies do not show a smooth inverse association (Robins et al., 1984, 1991b). Robins et al. (1991b) concluded that no relationship between antisocial personality and earnings, job level, or current unemployment for men ages 30–64 could be found. The NCS study found a significant inverse relationship between education, income level, and antisocial personality (Kessler et al., 1994). Another U.S.

study that addressed this issue found cases only in the lowest stratum (Weissman & Myers, 1980).

The Canadian DIS study (Bland et al., 1988) found a marked difference with regard to employment, with unemployed individuals having very high rates of antisocial personality (odds ratio of 6.2). Seventeen percent of the individuals with antisocial personality disorder, compared with 6% of healthy individuals, were found to be unemployed in the Ontario Health Survey (Offord et al., 1994). Those with antisocial personality were more likely to be in the low income group (24% vs. 9% in those without psychiatric disorders). Failure to graduate from high school was more common among people exhibiting antisocial behavior than among healthy individuals (35% and 24%, respectively). Similarly, in Israel (Dohrenwend et al., 1992; Levav et al., 1993) education was found to have a significant inverse relationship to antisocial personality for definite and also probable and definite levels of RDC diagnoses.

Most third-generation studies examining this issue have found that antisocial personality is more prevalent in the lower socioeconomic levels. The median low- compared with high-SES ratio for lifetime prevalence was 7.7. However, education may not be the best indicator of SES for antisocial personality; in contrast with other disorders, antisocial personality begins at age 8 or 9, not after education is completed (Robins et al., 1991b).

Only three studies examining *other personality disorders* and SES were identified. These studies used ECA subjects to make a *DSM-III* diagnosis of a specific personality disorder. From the Baltimore site, histrionic personality (Nestadt et al., 1990) and compulsive personality disorder (Nestadt et al., 1991) were investigated in a second-stage study (EBMHS) using a semistructured interview schedule (the SPE), administered by psychiatrists. No relationship with education was found for histrionic personality disorder. However, compulsive personality was significantly more prevalent in the highest social stratum compared with the lowest,

Table 13.9. Personality disorders: Third-generation studies and socioeconomic status (SES)

First author	Year	Site	Instrument & prevalence	Measure of SES	SES prevalence rate			p <
					Low (%)	High (%)	Ratio	
Antisocial Personality								
Regier	1993	ECA five sites	DIS 1 month	Nam criteria[1]	0.9	0.2	9.4	0.003
Blazer	1985	ECA Durham, NC	DIS 6 month	Education[1]			1.8	2.1[1]
Robins	1984	ECA New Haven	DIS lifetime	Education	2.5	0.9	2.8	NS
		ECA Baltimore	DIS lifetime	Education	2.7	1.5	1.8	NS
		ECA St. Louis	DIS lifetime	Education	3.4	2.3	1.5	NS
Bland	1988	Edmonton, Canada	DIS lifetime	Employment	15.1	2.8	6.2	0.001
Kessler	1994	USA	CIDI lifetime	Income			3.0	0.05
				Education			14.1	0.05
Weissman	1980	New Haven	SADS-PD point	Hollingshead	0.8	0.0		NS[2]
Levav	1993	Israel	SADS-D lifetime	Education	2.4	0.0**	17.1	0.001
			SADS-PD lifetime	Education	5.5	0.0**	6.9	0.001
Borderline Personality								
Swartz	1990	ECA Durham, NC	DIS/DIB	Education/income				NS
				Education				NS
Compulsive Personality								
Nestadt	1991	EBMHS Baltimore	SPE	Employment	0.5	3.3	0.2	0.05
				Income	0.4	4.1	0.1	0.05
				Education	0.9	4.5	0.2	0.05
Histrionic Personality								
Nestadt	1990	EBMHS Baltimore	SPE	Education	1.3	1.3	1.0	NS

NS, not significant; SADS-PD, SADS-RDC Probable and Definite; SADS-D, SADS-RDC Definite.

[1] Adjusted for other sociodemographic covariates.

[2] Significance based on education as a continuous variable, not high versus low SES.

** Ratio of lowest versus highest where a cell does not contain zero.

as measured by education, employment, and income. In examining a wide range of personality disorders that met *DSM-III* criteria, the Baltimore study found no overall significant relationship with education or income, although higher prevalence rates were noted in those with more education and among those earning less money (Samuels et al., 1994). Borderline personality disorder was studied in the North Carolina site using a DIS module called the Diagnostic Interview for Borderlines (DIB); no significant relationship was found with the Nam criteria of either SES or education (Swartz et al., 1990). These data suggest that these three specific types of personality disorders may have a differential relationship with SES. However, replication of the above-cited results is needed before a firm conclusion can be drawn.

Alcoholism

Numerous sociological surveys examining the rates of alcohol use in community samples have been conducted (e.g., Cahalan, 1970; Clark & Midanik, 1982; Mulford, 1968) that suggest socioeconomic variations. Unfortunately, these studies did not define the prevalence of alcoholism as a specific disorder. Rather, alcoholism was measured by such proxy indicators as mortality from cirrhosis, volume of alcohol beverage sales, or drinking patterns. These studies have provided ambiguous information on the prevalence of alcoholism (Warheit & Auth, 1985). This review therefore is limited to investigations conducted using structured diagnostic instruments from the third generation of psychiatric epidemiology.

A number of studies using the DIS examining alcohol abuse/dependence and SES have been conducted throughout the world (Table 13.10). The ECA study found in general, a downward trend in lifetime prevalence with higher education (Helzer et al., 1991), but this was a saw-toothed curve. Helzer and colleagues described the results as follows: "Regardless of final level of attainment, those who finish an educational program and go no farther have lower rates

of alcoholism than those who begin the next higher level but drop out" (p. 101). No consistent relationship between 1 year rates of alcoholism and occupational prestige was found for women; however, an inverse relationship with occupational prestige was noted for men (Helzer et al., 1991). For men, a strong and statistically significant negative correlation was found between income and both 1 year and lifetime prevalence rates (-0.9 for both); a weaker correlation was seen for women (-0.1 and -0.6, respectively) (Helzer et al., 1991).

Regier et al.'s (1993) 1 month prevalence study, which controlled for age, sex, race, site, and marital status, found a consistent inverse relationship with SES as defined by the Nam criteria. The lowest level had a significant odds ratio of 2.5 compared to the highest level. A similar but more striking result was found for 6 month prevalence, with an odds ratio of 3.6 for the lowest SES level (Holzer et al., 1986). The North Carolina ECA site also found a significant inverse relationship for 6 month prevalence and SES divided into quartiles (Blazer et al., 1987), as well as education (Blazer et al., 1985). In another ECA report examining lifetime rates from New Haven, Baltimore, and St. Louis, only the New Haven site found that college graduates had significantly less alcohol abuse/dependence (Robins et al., 1984). Williams et al. (1992) found an inverse relationship between SES by Nam criteria and 6 month and lifetime rates of alcohol abuse for both black and white men and women.

In the Puerto Rico DIS study, education did not exhibit a consistent relationship with the 6 month prevalence rates of alcohol abuse/dependence (Canino et al., 1987). The lowest educational level, however, did have higher rates for alcohol abuse/dependence than the highest educational level for both 6 month and lifetime prevalence rates. In the Canadian DIS study, the unemployed were significantly more likely to abuse or depend on alcohol, with an odds ratio of 2.7 (Bland et al., 1988). A study using the DIS in Taiwan failed to find significantly higher rates for the lowest educational levels, ex-

Table 13.10. Alcoholism: Third-generation studies and SES

First author	Year	Site	Instrument & prevalence	Measure of SES	Low (%)	High (%)	Ratio	$p <$
Regier	1993	ECA five sites	DIS 1 month	Nam criteria[†]	3.0	2.3	2.5	0.003
Holzer	1986	ECA five sites	DIS 6 month	Nam criteria[†]	5.3	3.3	3.6	0.001
Helzer	1991	ECA five sites	DIS lifetime	Education	16.3	10.0	1.6	NS[‡]
Blazer	1985	ECA Durham, NC	DIS 6 month	Education[†]			1.5	0.01[‡]
Blazer	1987	ECA Durham, NC	DIS 6 month	Education/income[†]			20.0	0.01[‡]
Robins	1984	ECA New Haven	DIS lifetime	Education	12.2	9.5	1.3	0.05
		ECA Baltimore	DIS lifetime	Education	13.8	12.1	1.1	NS
		ECA St. Louis	DIS lifetime	Education	15.9	15.3	1.0	NS
Bland	1988	Edmonton, Canada	DIS lifetime	Employment	39.2	19.1	2.7	0.001
Canino	1987	Puerto Rico	DIS 6 month	Education	6.2	1.8	3.4	NS[‡]
			DIS lifetime	Education	13.6	7.6	1.8	0.01[‡]
Yeh	1992	Taiwan — Taipei	DIS lifetime	Education	3.1	2.9	1.1	NS
		Taiwan — towns	DIS lifetime	Education	7.8	5.0	1.6	NS
		Taiwan — villages	DIS lifetime	Education	5.9	5.9	1.0	NS
Anthony	1994	USA	CIDI lifetime	Income			1.6	0.05
			CIDI lifetime	Education			1.5	0.05
Weissman	1980	New Haven	SADS-D current	Hollingshead	3.3	0.0[°°]	2.5	NS
			SADS-PD current	Hollingshead	4.1	1.5	2.7	
			SADS-D lifetime	Hollingshead	10.7	3.1	3.5	
			SADS-PD lifetime	Hollingshead	10.7	3.1	3.5	
Levav	1993	Israel	SADS-D 6 month	Education	1.5	0.2	7.5	0.01
			SADS-PD 6 month	Education	2.2	0.2	11.0	0.001
			SADS-D 1 year°	Education	1.5	0.2	7.5	0.001
			SADS-PD 1 year°	Education	2.4	0.2	12.0	0.001
			SADS-D lifetime°	Education	1.5	0.2	7.5	0.01
			SADS-PD lifetime°	Education	2.2	0.2	11.0	0.001
Meltzer	1995	Great Britain	CIS-R 1 year	Employment	2.9	5.4	0.5	NS
				Occupational status	7.3	3.3	2.2	NS
				Education	3.3	4.4	0.8	NS

NS, not significant; SADS-PD, SADS-RDC Probable and Definite; SADS-D, SADS-RDC Definite.

°Unpublished data obtained from the author.

°°Ratio of lowest versus highest where a cell does not contain zero.

†Adjusted for other sociodemographic covariates. ‡Significance based on education as a continuous variable, not high versus low SES.

cept in metropolitan men (Yeh & Hwu, 1992). A number of other studies using the DIS have been conducted around the world that provide data on SES. However, rather than utilizing diagnostic categories, these studies limited their analyses to the proportion of all drinkers who are heavy drinkers or the proportion of heavy drinkers who are alcoholics (Helzer & Canino, 1992). These studies as a group usually found an inverse relationship with measures of SES.

The NCS study found a significant inverse relationship between alcohol dependence and education, as well as income, using lifetime prevalence (Anthony et al., 1994). Unfortunately, the Ontario CIDI (Offord et al., 1994) study did not separate out alcoholism from substance abuse. The rates of low income, unemployment, and receiving public assistance appeared to be increased among those with 1 year prevalence of anxiety disorders compared to healthy individuals (16%, 8%, and 14% vs. 6%, 3%, and 9%, respectively). No difference existed in the rate of failing to graduate from high school (26% for those with 1 year prevalence vs. 24% for those without).

The British OPCS study (Meltzer et al., 1995) did not find a statistically significant relationship between 1 year prevalence of alcohol dependence and three measures of SES: educational attainment, employment status, and occupational prestige. Two SADS-RDC studies have examined alcoholism. The New Haven study (Weissman et al., 1980) found an inverse relationship with SES as defined by the Hollingshead two-factor index of social position. However, no formal test was conducted on the strength of the inverse relationship. The Israeli SADS-RDC study found a significant inverse relationship between educational attainment and alcoholism at the probable and definite and also the definite levels of diagnoses for 6 month, 1 year, and lifetime prevalence rates (Dohrenwend et al., 1992; Levav et al., 1993).

Most studies suggest that an inverse relationship exists between alcoholism and SES. The median low- compared with high-SES ratio was 3.4 for the prevalence period

closest to 1 year and 1.6 for lifetime prevalence. This relationship, however, is often not seen if education alone is the measure of SES. Also, the inverse relationship appears to be more pronounced among men.

GENDER

Overall Psychopathology

Research from the earlier generations of psychiatric epidemiology led to considerable debate as to whether men or women had higher rates of psychopathology. Studies conducted before World War II suggested that rates were higher for men; the opposite gender relationship was suggested following the war. In their 1974 review, Dohrenwend and Dohrenwend found overall rates of psychopathology to be higher for men in seven of nine pre–World War II studies; overall rates for women were higher in 18 of 19 post–World War II studies. These findings led to debates on the changing role of women and psychopathology (Gove & Tudor, 1973). However, others (Dohrenwend & Dohrenwend, 1974) argued that methodological changes between the earlier and later studies, such as the expansion of the nomenclature, could account for the sex differences in rates.

Examination of the results from third-generation studies may address some of these issues (Table 13.11). Only a small number of the DIS reports found men to have higher overall lifetime rates of psychopathology (Lee et al., 1990; Robins et al., 1991a). In contrast, a somewhat larger number of PSE studies found higher rates for women (Bebbington et al., 1981; Carta et al., 1991; Hodiamont et al., 1987; Larraya et al., 1982; Mavreas et al., 1986; Rodgers, 1991; Vázquez-Barquero et al., 1987). Very likely, this difference can be explained by the failure of PSE studies to include male-predominant disorders, such as alcoholism and antisocial personality. Only three DIS studies, those done in St. Louis, Puerto Rico, and Edmonton, Canada, found men to

Table 13.11. Overall psychopathology: Third-generation studies and gender

First author	Year	Site	Instrument & prevalence	Gender prevalence rate			
				Female (%)	Male (%)	Ratio	$p <$
Regier	1993	ECA five sites	DIS 1 month[1]	16.6	14.0	1.1	NS[1]
Robins	1991	ECA five sites	DIS 1 year	20.0	20.0	1.0	NS
			DIS lifetime	30.0	36.0	0.8	0.001
Robins	1984	ECA New Haven	DIS lifetime	27.3	30.6	0.9	NS
		ECA Baltimore	DIS lifetime	36.7	39.6	0.9	NS
		ECA St. Louis	DIS lifetime	25.7	37.0	0.7	0.001
Bland	1988	Edmonton, Canada	DIS 6 month	15.3	18.9	0.8	0.05
			DIS lifetime	26.8	40.7	0.7	0.001
Canino	1987	Puerto Rico	DIS 6 month	13.4	18.7	0.7	0.05
			DIS lifetime	22.8	34.0	0.7	NS
Wittchen et al.	1992	Munich, Germany	DIS lifetime	33.6	30.3	1.1	NS
Stefánsson	1994	Iceland	DIS 1 month	17.1	15.7	1.1	NS
			DIS 1 year	23.3	24.7	0.9	NS
Stefánsson	1991	Iceland	DIS lifetime	54.9	59.2	0.9	NS
Oakley-Brown	1989	New Zealand	DIS 6 month	27.8	28.0	1.0	NS
Wells	1989	New Zealand	DIS lifetime	68.5	63.0	1.1	NS
Hwu	1989	Taiwan—Taipei	DIS lifetime	15.4	17.2	0.9	NS
		Taiwan—towns	DIS lifetime	26.5	29.3	0.9	NS
		Taiwan—villages	DIS lifetime	18.3	24.1	0.8	NS
Lee	1990a	Korea—Seoul	DIS lifetime	17.6	47.5	0.4	0.001
Chen	1993	Hong Kong	DIS lifetime	18.3	19.5	0.9	NS
Kessler	1994	USA	CIDI 1 year	31.2	27.7	1.1	NS
			CIDI lifetime	47.3	48.7	1.0	NS
Offord	1996	Ontario, Canada	CIDI 1 year	19.4	17.9	1.1	NS
Henderson	1979	Canberra, Australia	PSE 1 month	11.0	7.0	1.6	
Bebbington	1981	Camberwell, England	PSE 1 month	14.9	6.1	2.4	0.005
Larraya	1982	Buenos Aires, Argentina	PSE current	28.9	20.0	1.4	0.05
Mavreas	1986	Athens, Greece	PSE 1 month	22.6	8.6	2.6	0.0001
Vázquez-Barquero	1987	Cantabria, Spain	PSE 1 month	20.6	8.1	2.5	0.001
Hodiamont	1987	Nijmegen, Holland	PSE 1 month	7.5	7.2	1.0	NS
Lehtinen	1990	Finland	PSE 1 month	12.4	6.9	1.8	0.01
Carta	1991	Sardinia, Italy	PSE 1 month	19.6	10.5	1.9	0.05
Rodgers	1991	Great Britain	PSE current	8.6	3.8	2.3	
Weissman	1980	New Haven	SADS-PD point	16.4	18.9	0.9	NS
Levav	1993	Israel	SADS-D 6 month°	24.8	23.6	1.1	NS
			SADS-PD 6 month°	38.3	37.9	1.0	NS
			SADS-D 1 year°	27.2	24.3	1.1	NS
			SADS-PD 1 year°	40.3	39.1	1.0	NS
			SADS-D lifetime°	53.2	44.2	1.2	NS
			SADS-PD lifetime°	68.4	61.9	1.1	NS
Filho	1992	Brasilia, Brazil	Checklist 1 year	41.2	27.0	1.5	
		Pôrto Alegre, Brazil	Checklist 1 year	33.0	34.5	0.9	
		São Paulo, Brazil	Checklist 1 year	20.0	18.0	1.1	
		Brasilia, Brazil	Checklist lifetime	53.8	47.0	1.1	
		Pôrto Alegre, Brazil	Checklist lifetime	49.4	35.0	0.7	
		São Paulo, Brazil	Checklist lifetime	28.8	32.7	0.9	

NS, not significant; SADS-PD, SADS-RDC Probable and Definite; SADS-D, SADS-RDC Definite.

°Unpublished data obtained from the author, all RDC categories including "Other."

[1]Adjusted for other sociodemographic covariates.

[1]See Regier 1988 for additional 1-month gender analysis from the ECA.

have a greater risk for psychopathology (Bland et al., 1988; Canino et al., 1987; Robins et al., 1984). However, as indicated in Table 13.11, the third wave of psychiatric epidemiologicl studies demonstrates no evidence of a gender difference in rates of overall mental disorders between men and women. The median female-to-male ratio was 1.1 for the prevalence period closest to 1 year and 0.9 for lifetime prevalence.

Schizophrenia

The 1980 review by Neugebauer et al., found no trend for either psychoses or schizophrenia to be more predominant in men or women. They reviewed 17 studies reporting rates for psychoses; rates were higher in men in 8 studies and in women in 9. Of the 11 studies reporting rates of schizophrenia, rates were higher in men in 5 studies and in women in 6. An earlier report analyzing six studies conducted prior to 1950 (Dohrenwend & Dohrenwend, 1974) also found psychosis/schizophrenia to be evenly divided between the genders.

Similarly, no gender trend was found in the 22 third-generation studies examined (Table 13.12). Only the New Haven ECA found lifetime prevalence of DIS-diagnosed schizophrenia significantly higher for women (Robins et al., 1984). The median female-to-male ratio was 0.8 for the prevalence period closest to 1 year and 1.0 for lifetime prevalence. None of the studies had statistically significantly higher rates for men.

Major Depression

In 1977, a comprehensive review of the literature of the preceding 40 years concerning gender and rates of major depression was published by Weissman and Klerman. This review examined evidence from clinical observations of patients coming for treatment, surveys of persons not under treatment, studies of suicide and suicide attempts, and studies of grief and bereavement. Limiting the data analyses to community surveys, all but 1 of the 14 studies found higher rates of depression in women

(Weissman & Klerman, 1977). A later review limited to true prevalence studies of affective psychosis (Neugebauer et al., 1980) found an average female-to-male ratio of 3.0, with two studies having higher rates for men, six for women, and three with no gender difference. In their analysis, Link and Dohrenwend (1980) found demoralization to be higher among women in all seven studies examined. In an update to Weissman and Klerman's 1977 paper, Boyd and Weissman (1981) also found an increased risk for depression in women. Specifically, they found women at an increased risk for depressive symptoms or nonspecific distress in six studies examining symptom scales. In addition, they found rates to be higher for women in six of seven community-based studies examining point prevalence, in all three lifetime prevalence studies, in the single incidence study, in two of three studies surveying general practitioners, and in all four case registry studies.

Almost every community-based study conducted since 1979 has found women to have significantly higher rates of major depression than men (Table 13.13). These findings are consistent with an international comparison of gender and major depression (Weissman et al., 1993). The median female-to-male ratio in the studies listed in Table 13.13 was 1.9 for the prevalence period closest to 1 year as well as for lifetime prevalence.

Anxiety Disorders

Studies from the earlier generations of psychiatric epidemiology examining neurosis have consistently found higher rates among women. All 18 studies examined by Neugebauer and colleagues (1980) found rates to be higher among women, with an average female-to-male ratio of 2.9. Two of three pre-1950 studies had higher rates for women (Dohrenwend & Dohrenwend, 1974).

In the third wave of epidemiological studies, panic disorder has generally been found to be more prevalent among women (e.g., Canino et al., 1987; Weissman & Myers,

Table 13.12. Schizophrenia: Third-generation studies and gender

| First author | Year | Site | Instrument & prevalence | Gender prevalence rate | | | |
				Female (%)	Male (%)	Ratio	$p <$
Regier	1993	ECA five sites	DIS 1 month[†]	0.7	0.7	0.8	NS
Keith	1991	ECA five sites	DIS 1 year	1.1	0.9	1.2	NS
			DIS lifetime	1.7	1.2	1.4	NS
Blazer	1985	ECA Durham, NC	DIS 6 month[†]			0.9	NS
Myers	1984	ECA New Haven	DIS 6 month	1.6	0.7	2.3	NS
		ECA Baltimore	DIS 6 month	1.6	0.7	2.3	NS
		ECA St. Louis	DIS 6 month	0.4	0.9	0.4	NS
Robins	1984	ECA New Haven	DIS lifetime	2.6	1.2	2.2	0.01
		ECA Baltimore	DIS lifetime	1.9	1.2	1.6	NS
		ECA St. Louis	DIS lifetime	1.1	1.0	1.1	NS
Bland	1988	Edmonton, Canada	DIS 6 month	0.2	0.4	0.5	NS
			DIS lifetime	0.6	0.5	1.2	NS
Canino	1987	Puerto Rico	DIS 6 month	1.1	2.0	0.6	NS
			DIS lifetime	1.2	1.9	0.6	NS
Stefánsson	1994	Iceland	DIS 1 month	0.0	0.5	0.0	NS
			DIS 1 year	0.0	0.5	0.0	NS
Stefánsson	1991	Iceland	DIS lifetime	0.0	0.7	0.0	NS
Oakley-Brown	1989	New Zealand	DIS 6 month	0.3	0.0		NS
Wells	1989	New Zealand	DIS lifetime	0.4	0.3	1.3	NS
Hwu	1989	Taiwan—Taipei	DIS lifetime	0.3	0.3	1.0	NS
		Taiwan—towns	DIS lifetime	0.3	0.2	1.5	NS
		Taiwan—villages	DIS lifetime	0.1	0.4	0.3	NS
Lee	1990a,b	Korea—Seoul	DIS lifetime	0.2	0.4	0.5	NS
		Korea—rural	DIS lifetime	0.4	0.7	0.6	NS
Chen	1993	Hong Kong	DIS lifetime	0.1	0.1	1.0	NS
			CIDI lifetime	1.7	0.8	2.1	NS
Kessler	1994	USA	CIDI 1 year	0.6	0.5	1.2	NS
			CIDI lifetime	0.8	0.6	1.3	NS
Vicente	1994	Santiago, Chile	CIDI 6 month	0.9	0.0		NS
Rioseco	1994	Santiago, Chile	CIDI lifetime	1.4	0.5	2.8	NS
Vázquez-Barquero	1987	Cantabria, Spain	PSE 1 month	0.3	0.9	0.3	NS
Caraveo-Anguaga	1996	Mexico	PSE 1 month	0.7	0.7	1.0	NS
Cooper	1996	China	PSE current	0.7	0.4	1.6	0.01
			PSE lifetime	0.7	0.4	1.6	0.01
Weissman	1980	New Haven	SADS-PD point	0.0	0.9	0.0	NS
Levav	1993	Israel	SADS-D 6 month	0.4	1.0	0.4	NS
			SADS-PD 6 month	0.4	1.0	0.4	NS
Dohrenwend	1992	Israel	SADS-D 1 year	0.4	1.0	0.4	NS
			SADS-PD 1 year	0.4	1.0	0.4	NS
			SADS-D lifetime	0.5	1.0	0.5	NS
			SADS-PD lifetime	0.6	1.0	0.6	NS

NS, not significant; SADS-PD, SADS-RDC Probable and Definite; SADS-D, SADS-RDC Definite.

[†]Adjusted for other sociodemographic covariates.

Table 13.13. Major depression: Third-generation studies and gender

First author	Year	Site	Instrument & prevalence	Gender prevalence rate Female (%)	Male (%)	Ratio	$p <$
Regier	1993	ECA five sites	DIS 1 month[†]	2.9	1.6	1.8	NS
Weissman	1991	ECA five sites	DIS 1 year	4.0	1.4	2.9	0.001
			DIS lifetime	7.0	2.6	2.7	0.001
Blazer	1985	ECA Durham, NC	DIS 6 month[†]			2.7	0.05
Weissman	1984	ECA New Haven	DIS 2 weeks	2.4	1.2	2.0	0.05
			DIS 1 month	2.7	1.5	1.8	0.05
			DIS 1 year	4.9	2.1	2.3	0.001
Myers	1984	ECA New Haven	DIS 6 month	4.6	2.2	2.1	0.05
		ECA Baltimore	DIS 6 month	3.0	1.3	2.3	0.05
		ECA St. Louis	DIS 6 month	4.5	1.7	2.6	0.05
Leaf	1986	ECA New Haven	DIS 6 month	3.9	1.5	2.6	0.001
Robins	1984	ECA New Haven	DIS lifetime	8.7	4.4	2.0	0.001
		ECA Baltimore	DIS lifetime	4.9	2.3	2.1	0.001
		ECA St. Louis	DIS lifetime	8.1	2.5	3.2	0.001
Karam	1991	Beirut, Lebanon	DIS lifetime	23.1	14.7	1.6	
Bland	1988	Edmonton, Canada	DIS 6 month	3.9	2.5	1.6	0.05
			DIS lifetime	11.4	5.9	1.9	0.001
Wittchen et al.	1992	Munich, Germany	DIS lifetime	13.6	4.0	3.4	
Canino	1987	Puerto Rico	DIS 6 month	3.3	2.4	1.4	NS
			DIS lifetime	5.5	3.5	1.6	NS
Stefánsson	1994	Iceland	DIS 1 month	2.9	0.9	3.2	0.05
			DIS 1 year	4.0	1.8	2.2	NS
Stefánsson	1991	Iceland	DIS lifetime	7.8	2.9	2.7	0.001
Oakley-Brown	1989	New Zealand	DIS 6 month	7.1	3.4	2.1	0.01
Wells	1989	New Zealand	DIS lifetime	16.3	8.8	1.9	0.001
Hwu	1989	Taiwan—Taipei	DIS lifetime	1.0	0.7	1.4	NS
		Taiwan—towns	DIS lifetime	2.5	1.0	2.5	0.001
		Taiwan—villages	DIS lifetime	1.4	0.6	2.3	0.05
Lee	1990a,b	Korea—Seoul	DIS lifetime	4.1	2.4	1.7	0.01
		Korea—rural	DIS lifetime	4.1	2.9	1.4	0.01
Hollifield	1990	Lesotho	DIS 1 month	14.5	8.8	1.6	NS
Chen	1993	Hong Kong	DIS lifetime	2.4	1.3	1.8	0.05
Romanoski	1992	Baltimore EBMHS	SPE current	0.9	1.4	0.6	NS
Lepine	1989	France (town)	DIS/CIDI 6 month	3.6	1.5	2.4	NS
			DIS/CIDI lifetime	21.9	8.5	2.6	0.05
Vicente	1992	Concepcíon, Chile	CIDI lifetime	7.9	7.4	1.1	NS
Blazer	1994	USA	CIDI 1 month	5.9	3.8	1.6	0.05
Kessler	1993	USA	CIDI 1 year	12.9	7.7	1.7	0.05
			CIDI lifetime	21.3	12.7	1.7	0.05
Vicente	1994	Santiago, Chile	CIDI 6 month	9.8	3.0	3.7	NS
Rioseco	1994	Santiago, Chili	CIDI lifetime	15.4	5.5	2.8	0.05
Offord	1996	Ontario, Canada	CIDI 1 year	5.4	2.8	1.9	
Orley	1979	Uganda	PSE 1 month	22.6	20.0	1.1	NS
Henderson	1979	Canberra, Australia	PSE 1 month	6.7	2.6	2.6	
Bebbington	1981	Camberwell, England	PSE 1 month	9.0	4.8	1.9	

Table continues on following page

Table 13.13. Major depression: Third-generation studies and gender—*Continued*

First author	Year	Site	Instrument & prevalence	Female (%)	Male (%)	Ratio	p <
				Gender prevalence rate			
Mavreas	1986	Athens, Greece	PSE 1 month	2.7	1.3	2.1	
Vázquez-Barquero	1987	Cantabria, Spain	PSE 1 month	7.8	4.3	1.8	0.05
Lehtinen	1990	Finland	PSE 1 month	6.5	2.4	2.7	0.006
Carta	1991	Sardinia, Italy	PSE 1 month	12.5	7.5	1.8	NS
Weissman	1978	New Haven	SADS-PD current	5.2	3.2	1.6	NS
			SADS-PD lifetime	25.8	12.3	2.1	0.001
Egeland	1983	Lancaster, PA	SADS point			1.0	NS
Faravelli	1990	Florence, Italy	SADS point	4.1	1.3	3.2	
			SADS 1 year	8.8	3.5	2.5	
Kinzie	1992	Indian village, USA	SADS point	6.3	2.2	2.9	
			SADS lifetime	26.2	17.0	1.4	
Levav	1993	Israel	SADS-D 6 month	3.4	2.6	1.3	NS
			SADS-PD 6 month	4.5	3.8	1.2	NS
Dohrenwend	1992	Israel	SADS-D 1 year	4.9	3.1	1.6	NS
			SADS-PD 1 year	6.4	4.8	1.3	NS
			SADS-D lifetime	20.0	9.9	2.0	0.001
			SADS-PD lifetime	29.1	15.3	1.9	0.001
Meltzer	1995	Great Britain	CIS-R 1 week	2.5	1.7	1.5	NS
Filho	1992	Brasília, Brazil	Checklist 1 year	2.9	1.1	2.6	
		Pôrto Alegre, Brazil	Checklist 1 year	7.6	5.9	1.3	
		São Paulo, Brazil	Checklist 1 year	2.6	0.0		
		Brasília, Brazil	Checklist lifetime	3.8	1.9	2.0	
		Pôrto Alegre, Brazil	Checklist lifetime	14.5	5.9	2.5	
		São Paulo, Brazil	Checklist lifetime	3.8	0.0		
Angst	1992	Zurich, Switzerland	SPIKE lifetime	36.7	20.6	1.8	

NS, not significant; SADS-PD, SADS-RDC Probable and Definite; SADS-D, SADS-RDC Definite.

[†]Adjusted for other sociodemographic covariates.

1980) (Table 13.14), although in many reports the difference did not reach statistical significance. The median female-to-male ratio was 2.0 for the prevalence period closest to 1 year and 2.1 for lifetime prevalence, suggesting a strong female predominance.

A clearer gender pattern emerges for phobic disorders (Table 13.15). All studies had higher rates for women, and virtually all found the female-to-male difference in rates statistically significant. The median female-to-male ratio was 2.4 for the prevalence period closest to 1 year and 2.1 for lifetime prevalence.

Regarding obsessive–compulsive disorder, only three studies demonstrated a sig-

nificant gender difference (Table 13.16), indicating a greater lifetime prevalence among women (Chen et al., 1993; Robins et al., 1984; Wells et al., 1989). In an international comparison, Weissman et al. (1994) standardized obsessive–compulsive disorder rates by age for the DIS studies in Edmonton, Puerto Rico, Munich, Taiwan, Korea, and New Zealand using the U.S. study as the standard to examine gender differences. They found the lifetime prevalence rate of obsessive–compulsive disorder generally to be higher in women as compared with men, with the female-to-male ratio ranging from 1.2 to 3.8 except for Munich, where men had a higher rate (female-to-male ratio 0.8).

Table 13.14. Panic disorder: Third-generation studies and gender

| First author | Year | Site | Instrument & prevalence | Gender prevalence rate | | | |
				Female (%)	Male (%)	Ratio	p <
Eaton	1991	ECA five sites	DIS 1 month	0.7	0.4	1.8	NS
			DIS 1 year	1.2	0.6	2.0	NS
			DIS lifetime	2.1	1.0	2.1	NS
Myers	1984	ECA New Haven	DIS 6 month	0.9	0.3	3.0	0.05
		ECA Baltimore	DIS 6 month	1.2	0.8	1.5	NS
		ECA St. Louis	DIS 6 month	1.0	0.7	1.4	NS
Robins	1984	ECA New Haven	DIS lifetime	2.1	0.6	3.5	0.001
		ECA Baltimore	DIS lifetime	1.6	1.2	1.3	NS
		ECA St. Louis	DIS lifetime	2.0	0.9	2.2	NS
Bland	1988	Edmonton, Canada	DIS 6 month	1.0	0.4	2.5	NS
			DIS lifetime	1.7	0.8	2.1	0.05
Canino	1987	Puerto Rico	DIS 6 month	0.9	1.2	0.8	NS
			DIS lifetime	1.9	1.6	1.2	NS
Wittchen et al.	1992	Munich, Germany	DIS lifetime	2.9	1.7	1.7	
Stefánsson	1994	Iceland	DIS 1 month	0.7	0.2	3.5	NS
			DIS 1 year	1.4	0.7	2.0	NS
Stefánsson	1991	Iceland	DIS lifetime	3.1	1.1	2.8	0.001
Oakley-Brown	1989	New Zealand	DIS 6 month	1.7	0.5	3.4	NS
Wells	1989	New Zealand	DIS lifetime	3.4	0.9	3.8	0.01
Hwu	1989	Taiwan — Taipei	DIS lifetime	0.3	0.1	3.0	NS
		Taiwan — towns	DIS lifetime	0.4	0.3	1.3	NS
		Taiwan — villages	DIS lifetime	0.2	0.1	2.0	NS
Lee	1990a,b	Korea — Seoul	DIS lifetime	1.8	0.3	6.0	0.001
		Korea — rural	DIS lifetime	4.4	0.8	5.5	0.001
Hollifield	1990	Lesotho	DIS 1 month	15.5	3.7	4.2	0.01
Chen	1993	Hong Kong	DIS lifetime	0.3	0.2	1.5	NS
Lepine	1989	France (town)	DIS/CIDI 6 month	1.6	0.8	2.0	NS
			DIS/CIDI lifetime	3.1	2.3	1.3	NS
Eaton	1994	USA	CIDI 1 month	2.0	0.8	2.5	0.001
Vicente	1992	Concepcíon, Chili	CIDI lifetime	1.2	1.1	1.1	NS
Kessler	1994	USA	CIDI 1 year	3.2	1.3	2.5	0.05
			CIDI lifetime	5.0	2.0	2.5	0.05
Vicente	1994	Santiago, Chile	CIDI 6 month	0.8	0.8		NS
Rioseco	1994	Santiago, Chile	CIDI lifetime	0.8	0.4	2.0	NS
Offord	1996	Ontario, Canada	CIDI 1 year	1.5	0.0		
Faravelli	1989	Florence, Italy	SADS unknown			14.0	
Kinzie	1992	Indian village, USA	SADS point	1.1	0.0		
			SADS lifetime	1.1	0.0		
Weissman	1980	New Haven	SADS-PD point	0.3	0.5	0.6	NS
Levav	1993	Israel	SADS-D 6 month	0.2	0.2	1.0	NS
			SADS-PD 6 month	0.5	0.4	1.3	NS
			SADS-D 1 year°	0.2	0.2	1.0	NS
			SADS-PD 1 year°	0.5	0.5	1.0	NS
			SADS-D lifetime°	1.6	0.3	5.3	NS
			SADS-PD lifetime°	2.5	0.9	2.8	NS
Meltzer	1995	Great Britain	CIS-R 1 week	0.9	0.8	1.1	NS
Angst	1985	Zurich, Switzerland	SPIKE 1 year	2.2	1.5	1.5	

NS, not significant; SADS-PD, SADS-RDC Probable and Definite; SADS-D, SADS-RDC Definite.

°Unpublished data obtained from the author.

Table 13.15. Phobic disorder: Third-generation studies and gender

First author	Year	Site	Instrument & prevalence	Gender prevalence rate Female (%)	Male (%)	Ratio	$p <$
Eaton	1991	ECA five sites	DIS 1 month	8.9	4.2	2.1	0.5
			DIS 1 year	12.9	6.3	2.0	0.05
			DIS lifetime	17.7	10.4	1.7	0.05
Myers	1984	ECA New Haven	DIS 6 month	8.0	3.4	2.4	0.05
		ECA Baltimore	DIS 6 month	17.5	8.6	2.0	0.05
		ECA St. Louis	DIS 6 month	7.7	2.8	2.8	0.05
Robins	1984	ECA New Haven	DIS lifetime	8.5	3.8	2.2	0.001
		ECA Baltimore	DIS lifetime	25.9	14.5	1.8	0.001
		ECA St. Louis	DIS lifetime	9.4	4.0	2.4	0.001
Bland	1988	Edmonton, Canada	DIS 6 month	6.7	3.5	1.9	0.001
			DIS lifetime	11.7	6.1	1.9	0.001
Canino	1987	Puerto Rico	DIS 6 month	8.2	4.1	2.0	NS
			DIS lifetime	14.3	9.9	1.4	0.01
Wittchen et al.	1992	Munich, Germany	DIS lifetime	10.4	5.5	1.9	
Stefánsson	1994	Iceland	DIS 1 month	5.0	3.0	1.7	NS
			DIS 1 year	7.1	3.9	1.8	0.05
Stefánsson	1991	Iceland	DIS lifetime	16.4	10.7	1.5	0.05
Oakley-Brown	1989	New Zealand	DIS 6 month	10.4	4.4	2.4	0.001
Wells	1989	New Zealand	DIS lifetime	12.8	3.4	3.8	0.001
Hwu	1989	Taiwan—Taipei	DIS lifetime	5.7	2.7	2.1	0.001
		Taiwan—towns	DIS lifetime	8.9	2.7	3.3	0.001
		Taiwan—villages	DIS lifetime	5.0	2.2	2.3	0.001
Lee	1990a,b	Korea—Seoul	DIS lifetime	8.6	2.9	3.0	0.001
		Korea—rural	DIS lifetime	9.7	2.3	4.2	0.001
Chen	1993	Hong Kong	DIS lifetime	3.7	1.3	2.8	0.05
Kessler	1994	USA	CIDI 1 year	13.2	4.4	3.0	0.05
			CIDI lifetime	15.7	6.7	2.3	0.05
Vázquez-Barquero	1987	Cantabria, Spain	PSE 1 month	6.1	0.2	30.5	0.001
Faravelli	1989	Florence, Italy	SADS unknown			6.0	
Kinzie	1992	Indian village, USA	SADS point	1.1	0.0		
			SADS lifetime	1.1	0.0		
Weissman	1980	New Haven	SADS-PD point	1.7	0.9	1.9	NS
Levav	1993	Israel	SADS-D 6 month	4.2	1.5	2.8	0.01
			SADS-PD 6 month	8.6	3.1	2.8	0.001
			SADS-D 1 year°	4.5	1.5	3.0	0.01
			SADS-PD 1 year°	8.9	3.1	2.9	0.001
			SADS-D lifetime°	5.5	3.6	1.5	NS
			SADS-PD lifetime°	9.9	6.6	1.5	NS
Meltzer	1995	Great Britain	CIS-R 1 week	1.4	0.7	2.0	NS
Filho	1992	Brasilia, Brazil	Checklist 1 year	17.2	6.0	2.9	
		Pôrto Alegre, Brazil	Checklist 1 year	6.6	7.6	0.9	
		São Paulo, Brazil	Checklist 1 year	7.2	2.8	2.6	
		Brasilia, Brazil	Checklist lifetime	22.7	10.8	2.1	
		Pôrto Alegre, Brazil	Checklist lifetime	10.4	4.9	2.1	
		São Paulo, Brazil	Checklist lifetime	20.5	7.7	2.6	

NS, not significant; SADS-PD, SADS-RDC Probable and Definite; SADS-D, SADS-RDC Definite.

°Unpublished data obtained from the author.

Table 13.16. Obsessive–compulsive disorder: Third-generation studies and gender

First author	Year	Site	Instrument & prevalence	Gender prevalence rate Female (%)	Male (%)	Ratio	p <
Regier	1993	ECA five sites	DIS 1 month[†]	1.5	1.1	1.3	NS
Karno	1988	ECA five sites	DIS 1 month[†]			1.1	NS
			DIS lifetime[†]			1.3	NS
Karno	1991	ECA five sites	DIS 1 month	1.5	1.1	1.4	
			DIS 1 year	1.9	1.4	1.4	
			DIS lifetime	3.0	2.0	1.5	
Blazer	1985	ECA Durham, NC	DIS 6 month			1.2	NS
Myers	1984	ECA New Haven	DIS 6 month	1.7	0.9	1.9	NS
		ECA Baltimore	DIS 6 month	2.2	1.9	1.2	NS
		ECA St. Louis	DIS 6 month	1.7	0.9	1.9	NS
Robins	1984	ECA New Haven	DIS lifetime	3.1	2.0	1.6	NS
		ECA Baltimore	DIS lifetime	3.3	2.6	1.3	NS
		ECA St. Louis	DIS lifetime	2.6	1.1	2.4	0.01
Bland	1988	Edmonton, Canada	DIS 6 month	1.6	1.6	1.0	NS
			DIS lifetime	3.1	2.8	1.1	NS
Canino	1987	Puerto Rico	DIS 6 month	2.3	1.3	1.8	NS
			DIS lifetime	3.1	3.3	0.9	NS
Wittchen et al.	1992	Munich, Germany	DIS lifetime	2.3	1.8	1.3	
Stefánsson	1994	Iceland	DIS 1 month	1.2	0.2	6.0	NS
			DIS 1 year	1.4	0.2	7.0	0.05
Stefánsson	1991	Iceland	DIS lifetime	2.1	1.8	1.2	NS
Oakley-Brown	1989	New Zealand	DIS 6 month	1.4	0.6	2.3	NS
Wells	1989	New Zealand	DIS lifetime	3.4	1.0	3.4	0.05
Hwu	1989	Taiwan — Taipei	DIS lifetime	1.1	0.8	1.4	NS
		Taiwan — towns	DIS lifetime	0.7	0.4	1.8	NS
		Taiwan — villages	DIS lifetime	0.2	0.4	0.5	NS
Lee	1990a,b	Korea — Seoul	DIS lifetime	2.4	2.2	1.1	NS
		Korea — rural	DIS lifetime	2.0	1.8	1.1	NS
Chen	1993	Hong Kong	DIS lifetime	1.2	0.9	1.3	0.05
Faravelli	1989	Florence, Italy	SADS unknown			1.0	
Levav	1993	Israel	SADS-D 6 month	0.7	0.9	0.8	NS
			SADS-PD 6 month	1.4	1.0	1.4	NS
			SADS-D 1 year°	0.7	0.9	0.8	NS
			SADS-PD 1 year°	1.4	0.9	1.6	NS
			SADS-D lifetime°	1.6	1.2	1.3	NS
			SADS-PD lifetime°	2.5	1.3	1.9	NS
Meltzer	1995	Great Britain	CIS-R 1 week	1.5	0.9	1.7	NS
Filho	1992	Brasilia, Brazil	Checklist 1 year	0.4	0.5	0.8	
		Pôrto Alegre, Brazil	Checklist 1 year	0.7	1.7	0.4	
		Brasilia, Brazil	Checklist lifetime	0.5	0.9	0.6	
		Pôrto Alegre, Brazil	Checklist lifetime	2.5	1.7	1.5	

NS, not significant; SADS-PD, SADS-RDC Probable and Definite; SADS-D, SADS-RDC Definite.

°Unpublished data obtained from the author.

[†]Adjusted for other sociodemographic covariates.

Table 13.17. Generalized anxiety disorder: Third-generation studies and gender

| First author | Year | Site | Instrument & prevalence | Gender prevalence rate | | | |
				Female (%)	Male (%)	Ratio	$p <$
Blazer	1991	ECA Durham, NC	DIS 1 month	1.4	1.1	1.3	NS
			DIS 1 year	4.0	3.1	1.3	NS
			DIS lifetime	7.3	5.7	1.3	NS
		ECA Los Angeles	DIS 1 month	2.3	0.5	4.6	0.001
			DIS 1 year	3.1	0.7	4.4	0.001
			DIS lifetime	5.5	2.6	2.1	0.05
		ECA St. Louis	DIS 1 month	1.2	1.4	0.9	NS
			DIS 1 year	3.3	2.3	1.4	NS
			DIS lifetime	7.8	5.2	1.5	0.05
Stefánsson	1994	Iceland	DIS 1 month	7.6	1.8	4.2	0.001
			DIS 1 year	11.6	3.9	3.0	0.001
Stefánsson	1991	Iceland	DIS lifetime	32.2	11.8	2.7	0.001
Oakley-Brown	1989	New Zealand	DIS 6 month	11.6	7.7	1.5	0.05
Wells	1989	New Zealand	DIS lifetime	35.1	27.1	1.3	0.01
Hwu	1989	Taiwan—Taipei	DIS lifetime	5.0	2.4	2.1	0.001
		Taiwan—towns	DIS lifetime	12.4	8.8	1.4	0.01
		Taiwan—villages	DIS lifetime	9.0	6.2	1.5	0.01
Lee	1990a,b	Korea—Seoul	DIS lifetime	4.3	2.4	1.8	NS
		Korea—rural	DIS lifetime	4.0	2.0	2.0	NS
Hollifield	1990	Lesotho	DIS 1 month	15.9	8.1	2.0	0.05
Chen	1993	Hong Kong	DIS lifetime	11.1	7.8	1.4	0.05
Lepine	1989	France (town)	DIS/CIDI 6 month	4.9	1.9	2.6	0.01
			DIS/CIDI lifetime	13.4	5.4	2.5	0.01
Wittchen	1994	USA	CIDI 1 month	2.1	1.0	1.9	0.05
Vicente	1992	Concepcíon, Chile	CIDI lifetime	1.4	1.6	1.1	NS
Kessler	1994	USA	CIDI 1 year	4.3	2.0	2.2	0.05
			CIDI lifetime	6.6	3.6	1.8	0.05
Vicente	1994	Santiago, Chile	CIDI 6 month	1.1	0.0		NS
Rioseco	1994	Santiago, Chile	CIDI lifetime	2.5	0.8	3.1	0.05
Offord	1996	Ontario, Canada	CIDI 1 year	1.2	0.9	1.3	
Faravelli	1989	Florence, Italy	SADS unknown			2.5	
Kinzie	1992	Indian village, USA	SADS lifetime	0.8	0.0		
Weissman	1980	New Haven	SADS-PD point	3.1	1.8	1.7	NS
Levav	1993	Israel	SADS-D 6 month	3.1	3.9	0.8	NS
			SADS-PD 6 month	6.3	6.8	0.9	NS
			SADS-D 1 year°	4.1	5.0	0.8	NS
			SADS-PD 1 year°	7.5	8.2	0.9	NS
			SADS-D lifetime°	11.6	13.3	0.9	NS
			SADS-PD lifetime°	17.1	19.6	0.9	NS
Meltzer	1995	Great Britain	CIS-R 1 week	3.4	2.8	1.3	0.05

NS, not significant; SADS-PD, SADS-RDC Probable and Definite; SADS-D, SADS-RDC Definite.

°Unpublished data obtained from the author.

Table 13.18. Post-traumatic stress disorder: Third-generation studies and gender

First author	Year	Site	Instrument & prevalence	Gender prevalence rate			
				Female (%)	Male (%)	Ratio	$p <$
Helzer	1987	ECA St. Louis	DIS 6 month	1.3	0.5	2.6	
Stefánsson	1994	Iceland	DIS 1 month	0.7	0.0		NS
			DIS 1 year	1.0	0.0		0.05
Stefánsson	1991	Iceland	DIS lifetime	0.5	0.0		0.05
Chen	1993	Hong Kong	DIS lifetime	0.7	0.6	1.2	NS
Vicente	1992	Concepcíon, Chile	CIDI lifetime	5.2	2.6	2.0	0.001
Kessler	1995	USA	CIDI lifetime[1]	10.4	5.0	4.9	0.05
Vicente	1994	Santiago, Chile	CIDI 6 month	1.9	1.2	1.6	NS
Rioseco	1994	Santiago, Chile	CIDI lifetime	5.1	2.7	1.9	0.05

[1]Adjusted for other sociodemographic covariates.

The median female-to-male ratio was 1.3 for both the prevalence period closest to 1 year and lifetime prevalence.

Table 13.17 lists the numerous studies examining the relationship of gender with generalized anxiety disorder. For the most part, women appeared to be at significant higher risk compared to men. The median female-to-male ratio was 2.0 for the prevalence period closest to 1 year and 1.8 for lifetime prevalence.

Only six community-based studies in general, as opposed to studies of special populations, have examined post-traumatic stress disorder (Chen et al., 1993; Helzer et al., 1987; Kessler et al., 1995; Stefánsson et al., 1991; Vicente, 1992, 1994). All of these studies found higher rates for women (Table 13.18), with a median female-to-male ratio of 2.6 for the prevalence period closest to 1 year and 2.0 for lifetime prevalence.

Personality Disorder

Each of the reports from third-generation studies suggested that the rates for antisocial personality disorder are elevated among men (Table 13.19). The median female-to-male ratio for lifetime prevalence was 0.2. Many of these studies reported significant female-to-male differences. This is consistent with true prevalence studies from 1950 to 1980 (Neugebauer et al., 1980), in which

10 of 14 studies had higher rates for men. That review found the female-to-male ratio on average to be 0.7. In their earlier review examining studies before 1950, Dohrenwend and Dohrenwend (1974) found three other studies that had information on gender; men again had higher rates. The increased preponderance for overall personality disorders in men, most likely attributable to antisocial personality disorder, has been noted in the 1981 community-based study conducted in Baltimore (Samuels et al., 1994), where men had twice the rate of women.

Relatively little is known, however, about the gender differences in other specific personality disorders. Schwartz et al. (1990) found borderline personality disorder to be significantly higher among women. Nestadt et al. (1991) found no significant differences between men and women for compulsive personality disorder, although the rates were higher among the men. Histrionic personality disorder (Nestadt et al., 1990), however, exhibited no gender differences.

Alcoholism

The most strikingly male-predominant disorder is alcohol abuse/dependence. All third-wave studies found marked gender differences, and virtually all have significantly higher rates among men (Table

Table 13.19. Personality disorders: Third-generation studies and gender

First author	Year	Site	Instrument & prevalence	Gender prevalence rate Female (%)	Male (%)	Ratio	$p <$
Antisocial personality							
Regier	1993	ECA five sites	DIS 1 month[†]	0.2	0.8	0.2	0.003
Robins	1991	ECA five sites	DIS 1 month	0.2	0.9	0.2	0.001
			DIS 1 year	0.4	2.1	0.2	0.001
			DIS lifetime	0.8	4.5	0.2	0.001
Blazer	1985	ECA Durham, NC	DIS 6 month[†]			0.2	0.01
Robins	1984	ECA New Haven	DIS lifetime	0.5	3.9	0.1	0.001
		ECA Baltimore	DIS lifetime	0.7	4.9	0.1	0.001
		ECA St. Louis	DIS lifetime	1.2	4.9	0.2	0.001
Bland	1988	Edmonton, Canada	DIS 6 month	0.2	3.3	0.1	0.001
			DIS lifetime	0.8	6.5	0.1	0.001
Stefánsson	1994	Iceland	DIS 1 month	0.0	0.0	0.0	NS
			DIS 1 year	0.0	0.2	0.0	NS
Stefánsson	1991	Iceland	DIS lifetime	0.0	1.4	0.0	0.05
Oakley-Brown	1989	New Zealand	DIS 6 month	0.5	1.3	0.4	NS
Wells	1989	New Zealand	DIS lifetime	1.9	4.2	0.5	NS
Hwu	1989	Taiwan — Taipei	DIS lifetime	0.1	0.2	0.5	NS
		Taiwan — towns	DIS lifetime	0.0	0.1	0.0	NS
		Taiwan — villages	DIS lifetime	0.0	0.1	0.0	NS
Lee	1990a,b	Korea — Seoul	DIS lifetime	0.8	3.5	0.2	0.001
		Korea — rural	DIS lifetime	0.3	1.6	0.2	0.01
Chen	1993	Hong Kong	DIS lifetime	0.5	2.8	0.2	0.05
Vicente	1992	Concepcíon, Chile	CIDI lifetime	0.5	3.4	0.1	0.001
Kessler	1994	USA	CIDI lifetime	1.2	5.8	0.2	0.05
Vicente	1994	Santiago, Chile	CIDI 6 month	0.3	1.2	0.3	NS
Rioseco	1994	Santiago, Chile	CIDI lifetime	0.3	1.9	0.2	0.05
Offord	1996	Ontario, Canada	CIDI lifetime	0.5	2.9	0.2	
Weissman	1980	New Haven	SADS-PD point	0.3	0.0		NS
Levav	1993	Israel	SADS-D lifetime	0.2	1.1	0.2	0.001
			SADS-PD lifetime	0.5	3.1	0.2	0.001
Borderline personality							
Swartz	1990	ECA Durham, NC	DIS/DIB			2.7	0.05
Compulsive personality							
Nestadt	1991	EBMHS Baltimore	SPE	0.6	3.0	0.2	NS
Histrionic personality							
Nestadt	1990	EBMHS Baltimore	SPE	2.1	2.2	1.0	NS

NS, not significant; SADS-PD, SADS-RDC Probable and Definite; SADS-D, SADS-RDC Definite.

[†]Adjusted for other sociodemographic covariates.

13.20). The median female-to-male ratio was 0.2 for the prevalence period closest to 1 year and for lifetime prevalence.

DISCUSSION

The sociodemographic correlates to psychopathology suggested in the first two generations of psychiatric epidemiology appear for the most part to have been confirmed when reinvestigated in third-generation studies. Descriptive epidemiological findings, such as differences in rates by SES or gender, permit formulation and testing of hypotheses about the etiology of mental illnesses.

Socioeconomic status appears to be inversely related with overall psychopathology, schizophrenia, panic disorder, phobic disorder, and antisocial personality disorder. An inverse relationship is also seen among men for alcoholism. The evidence is inconclusive for obsessive–compulsive and generalized anxiety disorders. The relationship of SES to major depression continues to require further investigation.

The increased risk for the lower socioeconomic strata to develop psychiatric disorders is highlighted by a study of healthy respondents followed longitudinally from the New Haven ECA. Rates of overall and specific psychiatric disorders were higher for individuals who were classified, according to federal guidelines, as living in poverty compared with those not living in poverty (Bruce et al., 1991).

The inverse relationship of psychiatric disorders to SES has long impressed epidemiologists. Jarvis (1971), for example, found that "insanity" was 64 times higher in the "pauper class" than in the "independent class" in data from 1855. These historical findings, as well as those of contemporary studies, have raised over the years the classic social causation–social selection issue (Dohrenwend, 1990). The social causation hypothesis suggests that rates of psychiatric disorders are higher in the lower socioeconomic strata because of greater environmental adversity. The selection theory argues that rates are higher in the lower strata because predisposed individuals drift down to or fail to rise out of the lower social strata. Methodological advances have allowed researchers to begin addressing this long-standing debate about the etiology of specific mental disorders. Using the relationship of ethnic status to SES, and knowing that ethnic status cannot be an effect of disorder, allowed Dohrenwend et al. (1992) to test the social causation–social selection issue for specific psychiatric diagnoses. Their results indicate that social selection may be more important in schizophrenia, but that social causation may be more important for depression in women and for antisocial personality and substance use disorders in men (see Chapter 14).

Of increasing interest is the relationship of pure compared with comorbid disorders and SES. For example, in major depression pure disorders do not appear to have as pronounced an inverse relationship with education, while the role of income is less clear (Blazer et al., 1994). In a comparison with healthy individuals and those with only one mental disorder, persons with two or more psychiatric diagnoses were more likely to be unemployed, be of lower income, receive public assistance, and not graduate from high school (Offord et al., 1994).

The third-generation psychiatric epidemiological studies do not support first- and second-generation findings regarding gender differences in rates of overall psychopathology. Apparently, men and women differ not in overall rates of disorders but in rates of specific disorders. Major depression and phobic disorders are predominantly more common in women. There is a trend toward female predominance for panic and generalized anxiety disorders. Alcoholism and antisocial personality disorder are male-predominant mental illnesses. Obsessive–compulsive disorder, schizophrenia, and overall rates of mental disorders show little evidence for any gender differences.

Still unanswered in the literature is what accounts for these gender differences in rates of specific disorders. Are these differ-

Table 13.20. Alcoholism: Third-generation studies and gender

First author	Year	Site	Instrument & prevalence	Female (%)	Male (%)	Ratio	p <
				Gender prevalence rate			
Helzer	1991	ECA five sites	DIS 1 month	1.1	5.7	0.2	0.05
			DIS 1 year	2.2	11.9	0.2	0.05
			DIS lifetime	4.6	23.8	0.2	0.05
Blazer	1985	ECA Durham, NC	DIS 6 month[1]			0.1	0.01
Myers	1984	ECA New Haven	DIS 6 month	1.9	8.2	0.2	0.05
		ECA Baltimore	DIS 6 month	1.7	10.4	0.2	0.05
		ECA St. Louis	DIS 6 month	1.0	8.5	0.1	0.05
Robins	1984	ECA New Haven	DIS lifetime	4.8	19.1	0.3	0.001
		ECA Baltimore	DIS lifetime	4.2	24.9	0.2	0.001
		ECA St. Louis	DIS lifetime	4.3	28.9	0.1	0.001
Bland	1988	Edmonton, Canada	DIS 6 month	1.6	9.2	0.2	0.001
			DIS lifetime	6.7	29.3	0.2	0.001
Canino	1987	Puerto Rico	DIS 6 month	0.5	10.0	0.1	NS
			DIS lifetime	2.0	24.6	0.1	0.01
Yamamoto	1993	Lima, Peru	DIS lifetime	2.5	34.8	0.1	0.001
Wittchen, Bronisch	1992	Munich, Germany	DIS 6 month	0.9	1.3	0.7	
		Munich, Germany	DIS lifetime	5.1	21.0	0.2	
Stefánsson	1994	Iceland	DIS 1 month	1.0	5.0	0.2	0.001
			DIS 1 year	1.4	11.3	0.1	0.001
Stefánsson	1991	Iceland	DIS lifetime	8.5	45.6	0.2	0.001
Oakley-Brown	1989	New Zealand	DIS 6 month	2.6	14.1	0.2	0.001
Wells	1989	New Zealand	DIS lifetime	6.1	32.0	0.2	0.001
Hwu	1989	Taiwan — Taipei	DIS lifetime	0.4	6.4	0.1	0.001
		Taiwain — towns	DIS lifetime	0.6	14.7	0.1	0.001
		Taiwain — villages	DIS lifetime	0.2	11.3	0.1	0.001
Lee	1990b	Korea — Seoul	DIS lifetime	1.6	25.6	0.1	0.001
		Korea — rural	DIS lifetime	0.9	20.5	0.1	0.001
Chen	1993	Hong Kong	DIS lifetime	0.6	8.9	0.1	0.05
Vincente	1992	Concepcíon, Chile	CIDI lifetime	1.9	10.6	0.2	0.001
Kessler	1994	USA	CIDI 1 year	3.7	10.7	0.3	0.05
			CIDI lifetime	8.2	20.1	0.4	0.05
Vincente	1994	Santiago, Chile	CIDI 6 month	1.0	6.5	0.2	NS
Rioseco	1994	Santiago, Chile	CIDI lifetime	2.1	8.3	0.3	0.05
Offord	1996	Ontario, Canada	CIDI 1 year	1.8	7.1	0.3	
Weissman	1980	New Haven	SADS-D current	1.0	1.8	0.6	
			SADS-PD current	1.7	3.6	0.5	NS
			SADS-D lifetime	3.8	9.6	0.4	
			SADS-PD lifetime	4.1	10.1	0.4	
Kinzie	1992	Indian village	SADS point	7.0	36.4	0.2	
			SADS lifetime	39.4	76.5	0.5	
Levav	1993	Israel	SADS-D 6 month	0.1	0.9	0.1	0.001
			SADS-PD 6 month	0.1	1.4	0.1	0.001
			SADS-D 1 year°	0.1	0.9	0.1	0.001
			SADS-PD 1 year°	0.2	1.5	0.1	0.001
			SADS-D lifetime°	0.1	0.9	0.1	0.001
			SADS-PD lifetime°	0.1	1.4	0.1	0.001

Table continued on next page

Table 13.20. *Continued*

First author	Year	Site	Instrument & prevalence	Gender prevalence rate			
				Female (%)	Male (%)	Ratio	*p* <
Meltzer	1995	Great Britain	CIS-R 1 year	2.1	7.5	0.3	0.01
Filho	1992	Brasilia, Brazil	Checklist 1 year	0.8	8.6	0.1	
		Pôrto Alegre, Brazil	Checklist 1 year	1.6	15.9	0.1	
		São Paulo, Brazil	Checklist 1 year	0.0	8.6	0.0	
		Brasilia, Brazil	Checklist lifetime	1.1	15.0	0.1	
		Pôrto Alegre, Brazil	Checklist lifetime	2.5	16.0	0.2	
		São Paulo, Brazil	Checklist lifetime	0.0	15.2	0.0	

NS, not significant; SADS-PD, SADS-RDC Probable and Definite; SADS-D, SADS-RDC Definite.

*Unpublished data obtained from the author.

†Adjusted for other sociodemographic covariates.

ences a result of biological or social–cultural factors, or perhaps a combination of the two? Research has focused primarily on two disorders, major depression and alcoholism. With regard to the former, there is evidence to suggest that social role diversity may have a larger effect than biological factors (Wilhem & Parker, 1989), that diagnostic criteria may determine the sex ratio (Angst & Dobler-Mikola, 1984), and that the cohort effect increases the rates for women disproportionately compared with men (Weissman et al., 1993). Studies have suggested that gender differences in major depression may be affected by the rates of alcoholism in a community. Egeland and Hostetter (1983) found no gender differences in rates of major depression among the Amish, a community with a practically nonexistent rate of alcoholism. Similarly, among American Jews, a population with low rates of alcoholism, men and women had nearly equal six months prevalence rates of major depression (Levav et al., 1997).

This chapter has attempted to present the current psychiatric epidemiological evidence regarding the association of SES and gender with overall psychopathology as well as with specific disorders. Although these third-generation studies are a major advancement, most are household surveys that still contain numerous potential biases. The most obvious is that errors in the numerator and denominator may occur using household samples. Psychiatric disorders reduce the chance that one lives at home; household surveys usually will undercount disorders related to institutionalization. In contrast, healthy young men and women may not live at home because they are enrolled in the military or attending college, resulting in an overrepresentation of emotionally ill individuals in the community for these groups (Robins, 1969). The next generation of psychiatric epidemiological studies should rely on (*1*) cohort designs (Levav et al., 1993) that overcome such problems and (*2*) on longitudinal outcomes.

Acknowledgments: The authors wish to thank Sheri Della Grotta for assisting with preparation of this manuscript, and Bruce G. Link, Ph.D., for reviewing an earlier version.

REFERENCES

Abas, M. A., & Broadhead, J. C. (1997). Depression and anxiety among women in an urban setting in Zimbabwe. *Psychological Medicine, 27*, 59–71.

American Psychiatric Association. (1980). *Diagnostic and statistical manual of mental disorders* (3rd ed.). Washington, DC: American Psychiatric Press.

American Psychiatric Association. (1987). *Diagnostic and statistical manual of mental disorders* (3rd ed., rev.). Washington, DC: American Psychiatric Press.

Andrews, G., Tennant, C., Hewson, D., et al. (1978). The relation of social factors to physical and psychiatric illness. *American Journal of Epidemiology, 108,* 27–35.

Aneshensel, C. S., Frerichs, R. R., Clark, V. A., et al. (1982). Measuring depression in the community: A comparison of telephone and personal interviews. *Public Opinion Quarterly, 46,* 110–121.

Angst, J. (1992). Epidemiology of depression. *Psychopharmacology, 106,* S71–S74.

Angst, J., & Dobler-Mikola, A. (1984). Do the diagnostic criteria determine the sex ratio in depression? *Journal of Affective Disorders, 7,* 189–198.

Angst, J., & Dobler-Mikola, A. (1985). The Zurich study: V. Anxiety and phobia in young adults. *European Archives of Psychiatry and Neurological Science, 235,* 171–178.

Anthony, J. C., Warner, L. A., & Kessler, R. C. (1994). Comparative epidemiology of dependence on tobacco, alcohol, controlled substances, and inhalents: Basic findings from the National Comorbidity Survey. *Experimental and Clinical Psychopharmacology, 2,* 224–268.

Bebbington, P., Hurry, J., Tennant, C., et al. (1981). Epidemiology of mental disorders in Camberwell. *Psychological Medicine, 11,* 561–579.

Berkman, L. F., Berkman, C. S., Kasl, S., et al. (1986). Depressive symptoms in relation to physical health and function in the elderly. *American Journal of Epidemiology, 124,* 372–388.

Bland, R. C., Stebelsky, G., Orn, H., et al. (1988). Psychiatric disorders and unemployment in Edmonton. *Acta Psychiatrica Scandinavica. Supplementum, 77,* 72–80.

Blazer D., Crowell, B. A., & George, L. K. (1987). Alcohol abuse and dependence in the rural South. *Archives of General Psychiatry, 44,* 736–740.

Blazer, D., George, L. K., Landerman, R., et al. (1985). Psychiatric disorders: A rural/urban comparison. *Archives of General Psychiatry, 42,* 651–656.

Blazer, D. G., Hughes, D., George, L. K., et al. (1991). Generalized anxiety disorder. In L. N. Robins, & D. A. Regier (Eds.), *Psychiatric disorders in America: The Epidemiologic Catchment Area study* (pp. 180–203). New York: The Free Press.

Blazer, D. G., Kessler, R. C., McGonagle, K. A., et al. (1994). The prevalence and distribution of major depression in a national community sample: The National Comorbidity Survey. *American Journal of Psychiatry, 151,* 979–986.

Boyd., J. H., Rae, D. S., Thompson, J. W., et al. (1990). Phobia: Prevalence and risk factors. *Social Psychiatry and Psychiatric Epidemiology, 25,* 314–323.

Boyd, J. H., & Weissman, M. M. (1981). Epidemiology of affective disorders: A reexamination and future directions. *Archives of General Psychiatry, 38,* 1039–1046.

Brown, G. W., Bhrolchain, M. N., & Harris, T. (1975). Social class and psychiatric disturbance among women in an urban population. *Sociology, 9,* 225–254.

Brown, G. W., & Harris, T. (1978). *Social origins of depression.* New York: The Free Press.

Brown, G. W., & Prudo, R. (1981). Psychiatric disorder in a rural and an urban population: I. Aetiology of depression. *Psychological Medicine, 11,* 581–599.

Bruce, M. L., Takeuchi, D. T., & Leaf, P. J. (1991). Poverty and psychiatric status: Longitudinal evidence from the New Haven Epidemiologic Catchment Area Study. *Archives of General Psychiatry, 48,* 470–474.

Cahalan, D. (1970). *Problem drinkers: A national Survey.* San Francisco: Jossey-Bass.

Canino, G. J., Bird, H. R., Shrout, P. E., et al. (1987). The prevalence of specific psychiatric disorders in Puerto Rico. *Archives of General Psychiatry, 44,* 727–735.

Caraveo-Anguaga, J. Medina-Mora, M. E., Rascón, M. L., Villatoro, J., Martínez-Vélez, A., & Gómez, M. (1996). La prevalencia de los trastornos psiquiátricos en la población urbana adulta en México. *Salud Mental, 19,* 14–21.

Carta, M. G., Carpiniello, B., Morosini, P. L., et al. (1991). Prevalence of mental disorders in Sardinia: A community study in an inland mining district. *Psychological Medicine, 21,* 1061–1071.

Chen, C. N., Wong, J., Lee, N., et al. (1993). The Shatin community mental health survey in Hong Kong: II. Major findings. *Archives of General Psychiatry, 50,* 125–133.

Clark, W., & Midanik, L. (1982). *Alcohol consumption and related problems* (Alcohol and Health Monograph No. 1). Rockville, MD: National Institute of Alcohol Abuse and Alcoholism.

Cochrane, R., & Stopes-Roe, M. (1980). Factors affecting the distribution of psychological symptoms in urban areas of England. *Acta Psychiatrica Scandinavica, 61*, 445–460.

Cochrane, R., & Stopes-Roe, M. (1981). Women, marriage, employment, and mental health. *British Journal of Psychiatry, 139*, 373–381.

Cockerham, W. C. (1990). A test of the relationship between race, socioeconomic status, and psychological distress. *Social Science and Medicine, 31*, 1321–1326.

Cooper, J. E., & Sartorius, N. (1996). *Mental disorders in China: Results of the National Epidemiological Survey in 12 areas.* Glasgow: Gaskell.

Derogatis, L. R. (1977). *SCL-90: Administration, scoring, and procedures manual for the revised version.* Baltimore: The Johns Hopkins University School of Medicine, Clinical Psychometrics Research Unit.

Dohrenwend, B. P. (1990). Socioeconomic status (SES) and psychiatric disorders: Are the issues still compelling? *Social Psychiatry and Psychiatric Epidemiology, 25*, 41–47

Dohrenwend, B. P., & Dohrenwend, B. S. (1969). *Social Status and Psychological Disorder.* New York: John Wiley & Sons.

Dohrenwend, B. P., & Dohrenwend, B. S. (1974). Social and cultural influences on psychopathology. *Annual Review of Psychology, 25*, 417–452.

Dohrenwend, B. P., & Dohrenwend, B. S. (1981). Perspective on the past and future of psychiatric epidemiology. *American Journal of Public Health, 72*, 1271–1279.

Dohrenwend, B. P., Levav, I., Shrout, P. E., et al. (1987). Life stress and psychopathology: Progress on research begun with Barbara Snell Dohrenwend. *American Journal of Community Psychology, 15*, 677–715.

Dohrenwend, B. P., Levav, I., Shrout, P. E., et al. (1992). Socioeconomic status and psychiatric disorders: The causation-selection issue. *Science, 255*, 946–952.

Dupuy, H. (1974). *Utility of the National Center for Health Statistics General Well-Being Schedule in the assessment of self-representations of subjective well-being and distress.* National Conference on Education in Alcohol, Drug Abuse, and Mental Health Programs. Washington, DC: Department of Health, Education, and Welfare.

Eaton, W. W., Dryman, A., & Weissman, M. M. (1991). Panic and phobia. In L. N. Robins & D. A. Regier (Eds.), *Psychiatric disorders in America: The Epidemiologic Catchment Area study* (pp. 155–179). New York: The Free Press.

Eaton, W. W., & Kessler, L. G. (1981). Rates of symptoms of depression in a national sample. *American Journal of Epidemiology, 114*, 528–537.

Eaton, W. W., Kessler, R. C., Wittchen, H.-U., et al. (1994). Panic and panic disorder in the United States. *American Journal of Psychiatry, 151*, 413–420.

Egeland, J. A., & Hostetter, A. M. (1983). Amish Study: I. Affective disorders among the Amish, 1976–1980. *American Journal of Psychiatry, 140*, 56–61.

Endicott, J., & Spitzer, R. L. (1978). A diagnostic interview: The Schedule for Affective Disorders and Schizophrenia. *Archives of General Psychiatry, 35*, 837–844.

Faravelli, C., Guerrini Degl' Innocenti, G., Aiazzi, L., et al. (1990). Epidemiology of mood disorders: A community survey in Florence. *Journal of Affective Disorders, 20*, 135–141.

Faravelli, C., Guerrini Degl' Innocenti, G., & Giardinelli, L. (1989). Epidemiology of anxiety disorders in Florence. *Acta Psychiatrica Scandinavica, 79*, 308–312.

Filho, N. A., Mari, J. J., Coutinho, E., et al. (1992). Estudo mulicêntrico de morbidade psiquiátrica em áreas urbanas brasileiras (Brasília, São Paulo, Porto Alegre). *Revista ABP-APAL, 14*, 93–104.

Frerichs, R. R., Aneshensel, C. S., & Clark, V. A. (1981). Prevalence of depression in Los Angeles County. *American Journal of Epidemiology, 113*, 691–699.

Fuhrer, R., Antonucci, T. C., Gagnon, M., et al. (1992). Depressive symptomatology and cognitive functioning: An epidemiological survey in an elderly community sample in France. *Psychological Medicine, 22*, 159–172.

Goering, P., Lin, E., Campbell, D., Boyle, M. H., & Offord, D. R. (1996). Psychiatric disability in Ontario. *Canadian Journal of Psychiatry, 41*, 564–571.

Goldberg, D. P. (1978). *The Manual of the General Health Questionnaire.* Windsor, Ontario, Canada: Nelson.

Goldthorpe, J., & Hope, K. (1974). *The social grading of occupations: A new approach and scale.* London: Oxford University Press.

Gove, W. R., & Tudor, J. F. (1973). Adult sex roles and mental illness. *American Journal of Sociology, 78*, 812–835.

Hay, D. I. (1988). Socioeconomic status and health status: A study of males in the Canada Health Survey. *Social Science and Medicine, 27*, 1317–1325.

Helzer, J. E., Burnam, A., & McEvoy, L. T. (1991). Alcohol abuse and dependence. In L. N. Robins & D. A. Regier (Eds.), *Psychiatric disorders in America: The Epidemiologic Catchment Area study.* (pp. 81–115). New York: The Free Press.

Helzer, J. E., & Canino, G. J. (Eds.). (1992). *Alcoholism in North America, Europe, and Asia.* New York: Oxford University Press.

Helzer, J. E., Robins, L. N., & McEvoy, L. (1987). Post-traumatic stress disorder in the general population: Findings of the Epidemiologic Catchment Area Survey. *New England Journal of Medicine, 317*, 1630–1634.

Henderson, S., Duncan-Jones, P., Byrne, D. G., et al. (1979). Psychiatric disorder in Canberra: A standardised study of prevalence. *Acta Psychiatrica Scandinavica, 60*, 355–374.

Hodiamont, P., Peer, N., & Syben, N. (1987). Epidemiological aspects of psychiatric disorder in a Dutch health area. *Psychological Medicine, 17*, 495–505.

Hollifield, M., Katon, W., Spain, D., & Pule, L. (1990). Anxiety and depression in village in Lesotho, Africa: A comparison with the United States. *British Journal of Psychiatry, 156*, 343–350.

Holzer, C. E., & Shea, B. M. (1990, July). *Ethnicity, social status, and psychiatric disorder in the Epidemiologic Catchment Area survey.* Paper presented at the XIIth World Congress of Sociology, Madrid.

Holzer, C. E., Shea, B. M., Swanson, J. W., et al. (1986). The increased risk for specific psychiatric disorders among persons of low socioeconomic status: Evidence from the Epidemiologic Catchment Area surveys. *American Journal of Social Psychiatry, 6*, 259–271.

Hwu, H. G., Chang, I. H., Yeh, E. K., Chang, C. J., & Yeh, L. L. (1996). Major depressive disorder in Taiwan defined by the Chinese Diagnostic Interview Schedule. *Journal of Nervous and Mental Disease, 184*, 497–502.

Hwu, H. G., Yeh, E. K., & Chang, L. Y. (1989). Prevalence of psychiatric disorders in Taiwan defined by the Chinese Diagnostic Interview Schedule. *Acta Psychiatrica Scandinavica, 79*, 136–147.

Jarvis, E. (1971). *Insanity and idiocy in Massachusetts: Report of the Commission of Lunacy (1855).* Cambridge, MA: Harvard University Press.

Karam, E. (1991, October 26). *War events and depression in Lebanon.* Paper presented at a seminar of the International Traumatic Society, Washington, DC.

Karno, M., & Golding, J. M. (1991). Obsessive compulsive disorder. In L. N. Robins & D. A. Regier (Eds.), *Psychiatric disorders in America: The Epidemiologic Catchment Area study* (pp. 204–219). New York: The Free Press.

Karno, M., Golding, J. M., Sorenson, S. B., et al. (1988). The epidemiology of obsessive-compulsive disorder in five US communities. *Archives of General Psychiatry, 45*, 1094–1099.

Keith, S. J., Regier, D. A., & Rae, D. S. (1991). Schizophrenic disorders. In L. N. Robins & D. A. Regier (Eds.), *Psychiatric disorders in America: The Epidemiologic Catchment Area study* (pp. 33–52). New York: The Free Press.

Kellner, R., & Sheffield, B. F. (1973). A self-rating scale of distress. *Psychological Medicine, 3*, 812–835.

Kendler, K. S., Gallagher, T. J., Abelson, J. M., & Kessler, R. C. (1996). Lifetime prevalence, demographic risk factors, and diagnostic validity of nonaffective psychosis as assessed in a US community sample: The National Comorbidity Survey. *Archives of General Psychiatry, 53*, 1022–1031

Kessler, R. C. (1982). A disaggregation of the relationship between socioeconomic status and psychological distress. *American Sociological Review, 47*, 752–764.

Kessler, R. C., McGonagle, K. A., Swartz, M., Blazer, D. G., & Nelson, C. B. (1993). Sex and depression in the National Comorbidity Survey: I. Lifetime prevalence, chronicity and recurrence. *Journal of Affective Disorders, 29*, 85–96.

Kessler, R. C., McGonagle, K. A., Zhao, S., et al. (1994). Lifetime and 12-month prevalence of DSM-III-R psychiatric disorders in the United States. *Archives of General Psychiatry, 51*, 8–19.

Kessler, R. C., Sonnega, A., & Bromet, E. (1995). Post-traumatic stress disorder in the National Comorbidity Survey. *Archives of General Psychiatry, 52*, 1048–1060.

Kinzie, J. D., Leung, P. K., Boehnlein, J., et al. (1992). Psychiatric epidemiology of an Indian village: A 19-year replication study. *Journal of Nervous and Mental Disease, 180*, 33–39.

Langner, T. S. (1962). A twenty-two item screening score of psychiatric symptoms indicating impairment. *Journal of Health and Human Behavior, 3*, 269–276.

Larraya, F. P., Casullo, M. M., & Viola, F. P. (1982). *Programa de investigaciones sobre epidemiologia psiquiátrica.* Buenos Aires: Cansejo Nacional de Investigaciones Cientificas y Tecnicas.

Leaf, P. J., Weissman, M. M., Myers, J. K., et al. (1984). Social factors related to psychiatric disorder: The Yale Epidemiologic Catchment Area study. *Social Psychiatry, 19,* 53–61.

Leaf, P. J., Weissman, M. M., Myers, J. K., et al. (1986). Psychosocial risks and correlates of major depression in one United States urban community. In J. Barrett & R. Rose (Eds.), *Mental disorders in the community: Findings from psychiatric epidemiology* (pp. 47–66). New York: The Guilford Press.

Lee, C. K., Han, J. H., & Choi, J. 0. (1987). The epidemiological study of mental disorders in Korea: IX. Alcoholism, anxiety, and depression. *Seoul Journal of Psychiatry, 12,* 183–191.

Lee, C. K., Kwak, Y. S., Yamamoto, J., et al. (1990a). Psychiatric epidemiology in Korea: I. Gender and age differences in Seoul. *Journal of Nervous and Mental Disease, 178,* 242–246.

Lee, C. K., Kwak, Y. S., Yamamoto, J., et al. (1990b). Psychiatric epidemiology in Korea: II. Urban and rural differences. *Journal of Nervous and Mental Disease, 178,* 247–252.

Lehtinen V., Lindholm, T., Veijola, J., et al. (1990). The prevalence of PSE-CATEGO disorders in a Finnish adult population cohort. *Social Psychiatry and Psychiatric Epidemiology, 25,* 187–192.

Leighton, D. C., Harding, J. S., Macklin, D. B., et al. (1963). *The character of danger.* New York: Basic Books.

Lepine, J. P., Lellouch, J., Lovell, A., et al. (1989). Anxiety and depressive disorders in a French population: Methodology and preliminary results. *Psychiatry and Psychobiology, 4,* 267–274.

Levav, I., Kohn, R., Dohrenwend, B. P., et al. (1993). An epidemiological study of mental disorders in a 10-year cohort of young adults in Israel. *Psychological Medicine, 23,* 691–707.

Levav, I., Kohn, R., Golding, J. M., & Weissman, M. M. (1997). Vulnerability of Jews to affective disorders. *American Journal of Psychiatry, 154,* 941–947.

Lin, T. (1953). A study of the incidence of mental disorder in Chinese and other cultures. *Psychiatry, 16,* 313–336.

Link, B. G., & Dohrenwend, B. P. (1980). Formulation of hypotheses about the true prevalence of demoralization in the United States. In B. P. Dohrenwend, B. S. Dohrenwend, M. S. Gould, et al. (Eds.), *Mental illness in the United States* (pp. 114–132). New York: Praeger.

Liu, J. S., & Cohen, P. (1994, March). *Parental socioeconomic status and child psychiatric disorders.* Paper presented at the 84th Annual Meeting of the American Psychopathological Association, New York.

MacMillan, A. M. (1957). The Health Opinion Survey: Technique for estimating prevalence of psychoneurotic and related types of disorder in communities. *Psychological Reports, 3,* 325–339.

Magee, W. J., Eaton, W. W., Wittchen, H. C., et al. (1996). Agoraphobia, simple phobia, and social phobia in the National Comorbidity Survey. *Archives of General Psychiatry, 53,* 159–168.

Mavreas, V. G., Beis, A., Mouyias, A., et al. (1986). Prevalence of psychiatric disorders in Athens. *Social Psychiatry, 21,* 172–181.

Meltzer, H., Gill, B., Petticrew, M., et al. (1995). *OPCS surveys of psychiatric morbidity in Great Britain, Report 1: The prevalence of psychiatric morbidity among adults living in private households.* London: Her Majesty's Stationery Office.

Mulford, H. A. (1968). Drinking and deviant drinking, USA, 1963. In S. P. Spitzer & N. K. Denzin (Eds.), *The mental patient: Studies in the sociology of deviance* (pp. 155–163). New York: McGraw-Hill.

Myers, J. K., Weissman, M. M., Tischler, G. L., et al. (1984). Six-month prevalence of psychiatric disorders in three communities. *Archives of General Psychiatry, 41,* 959–976.

Nam, C. B., & Power, M. B. (1965). Variations in socioeconomic structure by race, residence, and life cycle. *American Sociological Review, 30,* 97–103.

Neff, J. A., & Husaini, B. A. (1987). Urbanicity, race, and psychological distress. *Journal of Community Psychology, 15,* 520–536.

Nestadt, B., Romanoski, A. J., Brown, C. H., et al. (1990). An epidemiological study of histrionic personality disorder. *Psychological Medicine, 20,* 413–422.

Nestadt, B., Romanoski, A. J., Brown, C. H., et al. (1991). DSM-lII compulsive personality disorder: An epidemiological survey. *Psychological Medicine, 21,* 461–471.

Neugebauer, R., Dohrenwend, B. P., & Dohrenwend, B. S. (1980). Formulation of hypotheses about the true prevalence of functional psychiatric disorders among adults in the United States. In B. P. Dohrenwend, B. S. Dohrenwend, M. S. Gould, et al. (Eds.), *Mental illness in the United States* (pp. 45–94). New York: Praeger.

Noll, G. A., & Dubinsky, M. (1985). Prevalence and predictors of depression in a suburban county. *Journal of Community Psychology, 13*, 13–19.

Oakley-Brown, M. A., Joyce, P. R., Wells, E., et al. (1989). Christchurch psychiatric epidemiology study: II. Six month and other period prevalences of specific psychiatric disorders. *Australia and New Zealand Journal of Psychiatry, 23*, 327–340.

Offord, D., Boyle, M., Campbell, D., et al. (1994). *Mental health in Ontario: Selected findings from the Mental Health Supplement to the Ontario Health Survey.* Toronto, Ontario, Canada: Ministry of Health.

Offord, D. R., Boyle, M. H., Campbell, D., Goering, P., Lin, E., Wong, M., & Racine, Y. A. (1996). One-year prevalence of psychiatric disorder in Ontarians 15 to 64 years of age. *Canadian Journal of Psychiatry, 41*, 559–563.

Orley, J., Blitt, D. M., & Wing, J. K. (1979). Psychiatric disorders in two African villages. *Archives of General Psychiatry, 36*, 513–514.

Radloff, L. S. (1977). The CES-D scale: A self-report depression scale for research in the general population. *Applied Psychological Measurement, 1*, 385–401.

Radloff, L. S., & Locke, B. Z. (1986). The Community Mental Health Assessment Survey and the CES-D scale. In M. M. Weissman, J. K. Myers, & C. E. Ross (Eds.), *Community surveys of psychiatric disorders* (pp. 177–190). New Brunswick, NJ: Rutgers University Press.

Rajala, U., Uusimäki, A., Keinänen-Kiukaannieme, S., et al. (1994). Prevalence of depression in a 55-year-old Finnish population. *Social Psychiatry and Psychiatric Epidemiology, 29*, 126–130.

Regier, D. A., Boyd, J. H., Burke, J. D., et al. (1988). One-month prevalence of mental disorders in the United States. *Archives of General Psychiatry, 45*, 977–986.

Regier, D. A., Farmer, M. E., Rae, D. S., et al. (1993). One-month prevalence of mental disorders in the United States and sociodemographic characteristics: The Epidemiologic Catchment Area study. *Acata Psychiatrica Scandinavica, 88*, 35–47.

Regier, D. A., Narrow, W. E., & Rae, D. S. (1990). The epidemiology of anxiety disorders: The Epidemiologic Catchment Area (ECA) experience. *Journal of Psychiatric Research, 24*, 3–14.

Rioseco, P., Escobar, B., Vicente, B., Vielma, M., Saldivia, S., Cruzat, M., Medina, E., Cordero, M. L., & Vicente, M. (1994). Prevalencia de vida de algunos trastornos psiquiátricos en la Provencia de Santiago. *Revista de Psiquiatria, 11*, 186–193.

Robins, L. N. (1969). Social correlates of psychiatric disorders: Can we tell causes from consequences? *Journal of Health and Social Behavior, 10*, 95–104.

Robins, L. N., Helzer, J. E., Croughan, J., et al. (1981). National Institute of Mental Health Diagnostic Interview Schedule: Its history, characteristics, and validity. *Archives of General Psychiatry, 38*, 381–389.

Robins, L. N., Helzer, J. E., Weissman, M. M., et al. (1984). Lifetime prevalence of specific psychiatric disorders in three sites. *Archives of General Psychiatry, 41*, 949–958.

Robins, L. N., Locke, B. Z., & Regier, D. A. (1991a). An overview of psychiatric disorders in America. In L. N. Robins & D. A. Regier (Eds.), *Psychiatric disorders in America: The Epidemiologic Catchment Area study* (pp. 328–366). New York: The Free Press.

Robins, L. N., Tipp, J., & Przybeck, T. (1991b). Antisocial personality. In L. N. Robins & D. A. Regier (Eds.), *Psychiatric disorders in America: The Epidemiologic Catchment Area study* (pp. 258–290). New York: The Free Press.

Robins, L. N., Wing, J., Wittchen, H. U., et al. (1988). The Composite International Diagnostic Interview: An epidemiologic instrument suitable for use in conjunction with different diagnostic systems and in different cultures. *Archives of General Psychiatry, 45*, 1069–1077.

Rodgers, B. (1991). Socioeconomic status, employment and neurosis. *Social Psychiatry and Psychiatric Epidemiology, 26*, 104–114.

Romanoski, A. J., & Chahal, R. (1981). *The Standardized Psychiatric Examination.* Baltimore, MD: The Johns Hopkins University School of Medicine, Department of Psychiatry and Behavioral Sciences.

Romanoski A. J., Folstein, M. F., Nestadt, G., et al. (1992). The epidemiology of psychiatrist-ascertained depression and DSM-III depressive disorders: Results from the Eastern Baltimore Mental Health Survey Clinical Reappraisal. *Psychological Medicine, 22*, 629–655.

Romans-Clarkson, S. E., Walton, V. A., Herbison, G. P., et al. (1988). Marriage, motherhood, and psychiatric morbidity in New Zealand. *Psychological Medicine, 18,* 983–990.

Romans-Clarkson, S. E., Walton, V. A., Herbison, P., et al. (1990). Psychiatric morbidity among women in urban and rural New Zealand: Psycho-social correlates. *British Journal of Psychiatry, 156,* 84–91.

Samuels, J. F., Nestadt, G., Romanoski, A. J., et al. (1994). DSM-III personality disorders in the community. *American Journal of Psychiatry, 151,* 1055–1062.

Schneier, F. R., Johnson, J., Hornig, C. D., et al. (1992). Social phobia: Comorbidity and morbidity in an epidemiologic sample. *Archives of General Psychiatry, 49,* 282–288.

Spitzer, R. L., Endicott, J., & Robins, E. (1978). Research diagnostic criteria: Rationale and reliability. *Archives of General Psychiatry, 35,* 773–782.

Srole, L., Langner, T. S., Michael, S. T., et al. (1962). *Mental health in the metropolis.* New York: McGraw-Hill.

Stefánsson, J. G., Lindal, E., Björnsson, J. K., et al. (1991). Lifetime prevalence of specific mental disorders among people born in Iceland in 1931. *Acta Psychiatrica Scandinavica, 84,* 142–149.

Stefánsson, J. G., Lindal, E., Björnsson, J. K., et al. (1994). Periodic prevalence rates of specific mental disorders in an Icelandic cohort. *Social Psychiatry and Psychiatric Epidemiology, 29,* 119–125.

Surtees, P. G., Dean, C., Ingham, J. G., et al. (1983). Psychiatric disorder in women from an Edinburgh community: Associations with demographic factors. *British Journal of Psychiatry, 142,* 238–246.

Swartz, M., Blazer, D., George, L., et al. (1990). Estimating the prevalence of borderline personality disorder in the community. *Journal of Personality Disorders, 4,* 257–272.

Vázquez-Barquero, J. L., Díez-Manrique, J. F., Aldam, J., et al. (1987). A community mental health survey in Cantabria: A general description of morbidity. *Psychological Medicine, 17,* 227–241.

Vicente, B., Rioseco, P., Vielma, M., Uribe, M., Boggiano, G., & Torres, S. (1992). Prevalencia de vida de algunos trastornos psiquiátricos en la Provencia de Concepcion. *Revista de Psiquiatria, 9,* 1050–1060.

Vicente, B., Saldivia, S., Rioseco, P., Vielma, M., Escobar, B., Medina, E., Cordero, M. L., Cruzat, M., & Vicente, M. (1994). Trastornos psiquiátricos en diez comunas de Santiago: Prevalencia de seis meses. *Revista de Psiquiatria, 11,* 194–202.

Von Korff, M. R., Eaton, W. W., & Keyl, P. M. (1985). The epidemiology of panic attacks and panic disorder: Results of three community surveys. *American Journal of Epidemiology, 122,* 970–981.

Warheit, G. J., & Auth, J. B. (1995). Epidemiology of alcohol abuse in adulthood. In R. Michaels (Ed.), *Psychiatry.* Philadelphia: J. B. Lippincott.

Weissman, M. M., Bland, R. C., Canino, G. J., et al. (1994). The cross national epidemiology of obsessive compulsive disorder: The cross national collaborative group. *Journal of Clinical Psychiatry, 55* (3, Suppl.), 5–10.

Weissman, M. M., Bland, R., Joyce, P. R., et al. (1993). Sex differences in rates of depression: Cross-national perspectives. *Journal of Affective Disorders, 29,* 77–84.

Weissman, M. M., Bruce, M. L., Leaf, P. J., et al. (1991). Affective disorders. In L. N. Robins & D. A. Regier (Eds.), *Psychiatric disorders in America: The Epidemiologic Catchment Area study* (pp. 53–80). New York: The Free Press.

Weissman, M. M., & Klerman, G. L. (1977). Sex differences and the epidemiology of depression. *Archives of General Psychiatry, 34,* 98–111.

Weissman, M. M., Leaf, P. J., & Holzer, C. E. (1984). The epidemiology of depression: An update on sex differences in rates. *Journal of Affective Disorders, 7,* 179–188.

Weissman, M. M., & Myers, J. K. (1978). Affective disorders in a US urban community: The use of Research Diagnostic Criteria in an epidemiological survey. *Archives of General Psychiatry, 35,* 1304–1311.

Weissman, M. M., & Myers, J. K. (1980). Psychiatric disorders in a U.S.community: The application of Research Diagnostic Criteria to a resurveyed community sample. *Acta Psychiatrica Scandinavica, 62,* 99–111.

Weissman, M. M., Myers, J. K., & Harding, P. S. (1980). Prevalence and psychiatric heterogeneity of alcoholism in a United States urban community. *Journal of Studies on Alcohol, 41,* 672–681.

Wells, J. C., Tien, A. Y., Garrison, R., et al. (1994). Risk factors for the incidence of social phobia as determined by the Diagnostic Interview Schedule in a population-based study. *Acta Psychiatrica Scandinavica, 90,* 84–90.

Wells, J. E., Bushness, J. A., Hornblow, A. R., et al. (1989). Christchurch Psychiatric Epidemiology Study, part I: Methodology and lifetime prevalence for specific psychiatric disorders. *Australia and New Zealand Journal of Psychiatry, 23*, 315–326.

Wilhelm, K., & Parker, G. (1989). Is sex necessarily a risk factor to depression? *Psychological Medicine, 19*, 401–413.

Williams, D. R., Takeuchi, D. T., & Adair, R. K. (1992). Socioeconomic status and psychiatric disorder among blacks and whites. *Social Forces, 71*, 179–194.

Wing, J. H., Nixon, J., Mann, S. A., & Leff, J. P. (1977). Reliability of the PSE (ninth edition) used in a population survey. *Psychological Medicine, 7*, 505–516.

Wittchen, H. U., & Bronisch, T. (1992). Alcohol use, abuse, and dependency in West Germany: Lifetime and six-month prevalence in the Munich follow-up study. In J. E. Helzer & G. J. Canino (Eds.), *Alcoholism in North America, Europe, and Asia* (pp. 159–181). New York: Oxford University Press.

Wittchen, H. U., Essau, C. A., von Zerssen, D., Krieg, J. C., & Zaudig, M. (1992). Lifetime and six-month prevalence of mental disorders in the Munich follow-up study. *European Archives of Psychiatry and Clinical Neuroscience, 241*, 247–258.

Wittchen, H. U., Zhao, S., Kessler, R. C., et al. (1994). DSM-III-R generalized anxiety disorder in the National Comorbidity Survey. *Archives of General Psychiatry, 51*, 355–364.

World Health Organization. (1978). *Mental disorders: Glossary and guide to their classification in accordance with the ninth revision of the International Classification of Diseases.* Geneva: Author.

World Health Organization. (1992). *The ICD-10 classification of mental and behavioral disorders: Clinical descriptions and diagnostic guidelines.* Geneva.

Yamamoto, J., Silva, J. A., Sasao, T., et al. (1993). Alcoholism in Peru. *American Journal of Psychiatry, 150*, 1059–1062.

Yeh, E. K., & Hwu, H. G. (1992). Alcoholism in Taiwan Chinese communities. In J. E. Helzer & G. J. Canino (Eds.), *Alcoholism in North America, Europe, and Asia* (pp. 214–246). New York: Oxford University Press.

14

Ethnicity, Socioeconomic Status, and Psychiatric Disorders: A Test of the Social Causation–Social Selection Issue

Bruce P. Dohrenwend
Itzhak Levav
Patrick E. Shrout
Sharon Schwartz
Guedalia Naveh
Bruce G. Link
Andrew E. Skodol
Ann Stueve

STATEMENT OF THE PROBLEM

Since the turn of the century, no results from epidemiological research on psychiatric disorders have been more challenging than those centering on socioeconomic status (SES). Despite changes in concepts and measures of both psychiatric disorders and SES over the years, the highest overall prevalence rates of psychiatric disorders consistently have been found among persons of the lowest SES (see Dohrenwend et al., 1980a; Chapter 13, this volume). Our best evidence is that this relationship holds for a number of important subtypes of psychopathology: schizophrenia; major depression (at least in women); antisocial personality, alcoholism, and substance use disorders (at least in men) (Dohrenwend, 1990b; see also Chapter 13, this volume); and nonspecific distress or "demoralization" (Frank, 1973) as measured by self-report symptom scales with items on depressed mood, anxiety, and psychophysiological disturbance (Link & Dohrenwend, 1980; see also Chapter 13, this volume).

These findings have raised and re-raised over the years the classic social causation–social selection issue, as Kohn et al. (Chapter 13, this volume) point out. The social causation explanation, proposed by environmentally oriented theorists, holds that the rates of some types of psychiatric disorder are higher in lower SES groups because their members are exposed to greater environmental adversity and stress (e.g., Bebbington et al., 1981; Brown & Harris, 1978; Faris & Dunham, 1939; Hollingshead &

Redlich, 1958; Leighton et al., 1963; Srole et al., 1962). The social selection explanation, proposed by genetically oriented theorists, argues that the rates are higher in lower SES groups because persons with the disorder or with other personal characteristics predisposing to the disorder drift down into or fail to rise out of lower SES groups (e.g., Dunham, 1965; Häfner et al., 1995; Jarvis, 1971; Wender et al., 1973; see also Eaton, 1980).

Although genetic factors play a part in all of the disorders, the role is not so large as to rule out environmental factors (see review in Dohrenwend, Introduction, this volume). It is likely—even for schizophrenia, where the evidence of a substantial role for genetic factors is strongest—that both processes are operating (e.g., Dohrenwend & Dohrenwend, 1981; Kohn, 1972a; see also Link et al., Chapter 21, this volume). However, the goal of specifying the relative importance of these processes has proved elusive.

The most usual approach has been to conduct retrospective case–control studies of intergenerational social mobility. These investigations have focused mainly on schizophrenia. They have had the advantage of being able to compare the SES of each index case and control respondent with the clearly antecedent SES of his or her parents to test whether the cases, usually persons with histories of schizophrenia, have been downwardly mobile compared to the controls (e.g., Goldberg & Morrison, 1976). A finding from one of the best of these studies is that cases with low-SES parents are less likely to be upwardly mobile than controls with low-SES parents (Turner et al., 1967). This and other findings from these mobility studies are evidence of downward social mobility in the cases of schizophrenia compared with the controls.

The results raise the question, however, of whether transmission is environmental or genetic. The problem of interpretation arises from the fact that parental SES can influence the individual's SES through factors related to the disorder that are either genetic, environmental, or both (see Robins,

1969). None of the studies has data on family history of disorder that might help to clarify the etiological issue. This is a major reason, along with some inconsistencies in their results, that the findings from the case–control studies of social mobility have been inconclusive even for schizophrenia (Dohrenwend & Dohrenwend, 1969, pp. 41–48; Kohn, 1972b; Link et al., 1986; Mechanic, 1972). Prospective mobility and family history studies over several generations might clarify matters, but they are not practical (see Dohrenwend, 1975).

It is possible in the abstract to envision straightforward experimental approaches to the problem. Thoday and Gibson (1970), for example, have provided a model experiment showing not only how the causation–selection issue can be tested but also the larger environment–heredity issue it implies. Thoday and Gibson's subjects were flies, the characteristic to be explained was the number of bristles the flies developed, and the environmental variable was temperature. The experimental protocol involved

- Dividing the flies into two groups on the basis of the number of their bristles
- Raising the flies under different temperature conditions
- On the basis of the number of their bristles, retaining offspring in each group or transferring them to the other group
- Assessing the results over nine generations

The experiment is elegant, and the outcomes proved clear cut with regard to the relative roles of nature and nurture and their relation to each other—insofar as the development of bristles on flies is concerned. This choice of subjects allowed the investigators to solve all or most of the design problems—including that of history over succeeding generations—that have constituted insurmountable practical and ethical difficulties when the subjects of the research are human beings and the effects in which we are interested consist of various types of psychopathology.

It is against this background that one of us proposed a quasi-experimental strategy for testing the stress–selection issue that would make use of empirical facts that appeared to be more immediately available than would be the case with multigeneration prospective studies (Dohrenwend, 1966). The argument put forward at that time was that the issue would turn on the answer to a simple question of fact: With SES controlled, are rates of the disorders in question higher or lower in advantaged than in disadvantaged ethnic groups?

For a variety of reasons described in this chapter, these facts proved hard to come by. Between 1966 and the start of a later study in 1983, we were able to acquire some relevant but fragmentary data (Dohrenwend, 1975; Dohrenwend & Dohrenwend, 1969, 1974b, 1981). Some of those data, however, especially with regard to schizophrenia, were limited to patients in psychiatric treatment and hence likely to be affected by selective factors associated with treatment (Dohrenwend, 1975; Dohrenwend & Dohrenwend, 1981). Other data suffered from serious problems associated with a variety of approaches to identifying and classifying psychiatric disorders in contrasting SES and ethnic/racial groups independently of treatment status (Dohrenwend, 1975; Dohrenwend & Dohrenwend, 1969). We accordingly made a major investment of time and effort in developing and adapting procedures for dealing with the problem of how to identify and diagnose cases of various types of psychiatric disorders in contrasting SES and ethnic groups (Dohrenwend & Shrout, 1981). Toward the end of this period, we found a way to build on this foundation. We located a potential research setting that seemed ideal for the kind of investigation required, and we obtained a grant to conduct the research in this setting.

Our purposes in this chapter are to describe, more fully than was possible in the major report of this study to date (Dohrenwend et al., 1992), the theoretical formulation, the assumptions on which it is based, the analyses, and the results of this first systematic implementation of the strategy. The present report also includes some additional tests we have conducted and an expanded discussion of the implications of what we have found. We begin with the theoretical formulation of the strategy for testing the causation–selection issue and the assumptions on which it is based.

THEORETICAL FORMULATION OF A QUASI-EXPERIMENTAL STRATEGY FOR TESTING THE SOCIAL CAUSATION–SOCIAL SELECTION ISSUE

Where relations between SES and various types of psychopathology are concerned, social causation and social selection theories both make the same prediction about an inverse relationship. Our problem has been to find a set of circumstances in which the two contrasting theories lead to different predictions about why rates of various types of disorders are higher in lower SES groups. We have argued that such circumstances can be found in the assimilation of initially disadvantaged ethnic groups into the SES structures of relatively open-class, urban settings found in many modern, democratic societies—for example, blacks and Hispanics by contrast with non-Hispanic whites in New York, Indians and Pakistanis by contrast with whites in London, and North African Jews by contrast with European Jews in Israel (Dohrenwend, 1966, 1975; Dohrenwend & Dohrenwend, 1969, 1974a, 1974b, 1981; Dohrenwend et al., 1992). We hold that this situation provides a natural experiment in which birth into a disadvantaged ethnic group compared to birth into an advantaged ethnic group is analogous to random assignment to differentially adverse conditions.

Many years ago, Dunham (1955) described the aspects of an urban assimilation situation in U.S. society that illustrates why it is so important for our problem:

Let's consider for a moment the foreign born communities in our cities. Certainly, no one can seriously contend that these communities have been settled by people who have drifted into these areas because of personality instability. Rather have they represented the starting point for various immigrant groups as they have struggled for a better life and a more secure economic niche in our society. In these communities, like others, these people are born, grow up, and die, and the sons and daughters of these immigrant groups in many instances succeeded in getting out of these communities and assuming larger and more significant roles in the life of the community. This is so well known that it hardly bears repeating. (Dunham, 1955, p. 173)

Assimilation involves the adoption of the values, pursuits, and goals of the host society by members of the ethnic/racial minority, often at the expense of abandoning traditional ethnic values and goals (e.g., Dohrenwend & Smith, 1962). The usual endpoint of these processes for the ethnic/racial minority is achievement by most of its members of middle-class status in the larger society. The successful assimilation of ethnic/racial minorities to middle-class status that Dunham implies is a slow process in societies such as ours, usually taking several generations (see Glazer & Moynihan, 1963; Scribner, 1996). Sometimes for minorities with special histories of extraordinary adversity, such as that of African-Americans, the time is much longer.

Insofar as the implications for most health outcomes are concerned, and in the absence of evidence to the contrary, we assume that there are no specifically ethnic/racial differences in genetic vulnerability to the psychiatric disorders that are inversely related to SES (see Dohrenwend, 1975; Dohrenwend & Dohrenwend, 1969, 1974a; Dohrenwend et al., 1992, especially pp. 950–951). To increase the plausibility of this assumption, we focus on second-generation sons and daughters born of immigrants rather than the first-generation immigrants. This avoids possible problems of selective migration in which persons prone to poor adaptation (e.g., exports of criminals and mentally ill persons from Castro's Cuba) or, more usually, good adaptation (e.g., the "healthy worker" phenomenon wherein the most robust and en-

ergetic migrate to places of greater opportunity) are overrepresented in the ethnic/racial group to be studied (see Mortensen et al., 1997).

Moreover, by concentrating on the second generation, we can distinguish between adversity that may be associated with migration (e.g., the hardships of Vietnamese "boat people") and the very different types of adversity associated with acculturation and assimilation, which provide the contrasts that we require for our investigation of the reasons for the SES differences. For the second generation who are born and raised in the host society, only the latter types of adversity are present—and considerably more so than for the generally less acculturated members of the first generation. The reference groups for the first generation of immigrants and the native-born second generation are likely to differ. The immigrants are likely to see themselves as relatively advantaged in their new surroundings compared to the groups and circumstances they left behind; the second generation, however, born and raised in the new society, are likely to see themselves as relatively deprived compared to members of dominant ethnic groups. This is something they share with other native-born persons of low SES who compare themselves with those higher in SES.

Examples of the importance for our purposes of this distinction between first- and second-generation ethnic/racial minorities are evident in comparisons of more and less acculturated Mexican-Americans on such diverse matters as rates of low-birth-weight babies (Cobas et al., 1996), scores on symptom scales of psychological distress (e.g., Kaplan & Marks, 1990), and lifetime rates of diagnosable psychiatric disorders (Burnam et al., 1987). It is the more acculturated individuals, as indicated by ethnic identification and language preference, who show greater distress; more diagnosable psychiatric disorder, including major depression, alcohol abuse/dependence, and antisocial personality; and elevated rates of low-birth-weight babies. With these points about the nature of ethnic acculturation and assimilation in modern democratic societies as background, let us return to the social causation–social selection issue posed by inverse relations between SES and psychiatric disorders.

The opportunity to develop different predictions from the social causation position on the one hand and the social selection position on the other arises out of the similarities and contrasts between ethnic status and SES in urban assimilation situations. Like SES, ethnic status influences a person's chances of obtaining the valued goals of the society—for example, its goods and services, honors, and respect. However, there are important differences. An individual's SES depends not only on the SES of his or her parents, but also on his or her own educational and occupational achievements. Like one's parents' attainments, those of the individual can be affected by genetic predispositions.

By contrast, a person's ethnicity is determined at birth by immutable characteristics such as skin color, national background, and religious origin. Whether the person's ethnic status is advantaged or disadvantaged is determined by stage in the assimilation process of the ethnic group into which the person was born. As Dunham's (1955) description makes clear, none of these things can be effects of behaviors related to the presence of psychopathology or personal predispositions to psychopathology.

Because of these differences and similarities between ethnic status and SES, different predictions can be derived from social causation and social selection theories about inverse relations between SES and psychiatric disorders by introducing ethnic status into the equation. These contrasting predictions apply to an assimilation situation in a modern, democratic, urban society containing at least two ethnic groups: one relatively advantaged by virtue of having assimilated to middle-class status and dominant political power, and the other disadvantaged, mainly of lower SES, and in relatively early stages of acculturation and assimilation. We assume that the members of the disadvantaged ethnic group experience an increment

in adversity that is independent of SES. The main source of this additional adversity is assumed to be ethnic prejudice and discrimination. We also assume that the two ethnic groups do not differ in genetic inheritance in ways that predispose one more than the other to the disorders at issue on the basis of ethnic background per se. The social causation and social selection predictions for any disorder that is inversely related to SES follow from these assumptions.

The Social Causation Prediction

We draw on Merton's (1957) classic formulation to describe the basic ideas underlying the social causation prediction:

The central proposition is that ... aberrant behavior may be regarded ... as a symptom of dissociation between culturally prescribed aspirations and socially structured avenues for realizing these aspirations. (p. 134)

In our society, these aspirations or goals tend to center on monetary success and the goods, services, honor, and respect that so often come with wealth. These goals are widely shared and compelling. As Merton put it:

Thus the culture enjoins the acceptance of three cultural axioms: First, all should strive for the same lofty goals since those are open to all; second, present seeming failure is but a way-station to ultimate success; and third, genuine failure consists only in the lessening of withdrawal of ambition. (p. 139)

Of those located in the lower reaches of the social structure, the culture makes incompatible demands. On the one hand they are asked to orient their conduct toward the prospect of large wealth ... "Every man is king" ... and on the other, they are largely denied effective means to do so institutionally. The consequence of this structural inconsistency is a high rate of deviant behavior. (p. 145)

This formulation seems even more applicable with the advent of the "Age of Television" and the increasing dominance of free market concepts that television advertises

Social Causation Prediction:

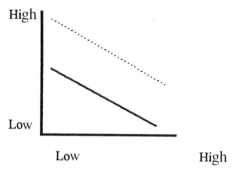

Social Selection Prediction:

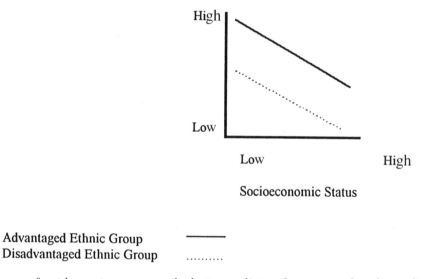

Figure 14.1. Summary of social causation versus social selection predictions for any type of psychiatric disorder that is inversely related to socioeconomic status in the general population.

than when Merton set it forth a few years after the end of World War II.

Because ethnic prejudice and discrimination restrict opportunities, disjunctions between means and goals are likely to be experienced more frequently by members of disadvantaged ethnic groups than by members of advantaged ethnic groups at every level of SES. The social causation prediction, therefore, is that this increment in

adversity and stress experienced by members of disadvantaged ethnic groups will lead to incrementally higher rates of psychopathology at every SES level, as shown in the top part of Figure 14.1.

The Social Selection Prediction

Under the social selection theory, the rate of psychopathology in a given SES stratum is assumed to be a function of sorting and sifting processes whereby the healthy and able tend to rise to or maintain high status and the unhealthy and disabled tend to drift down from high SES or fail to rise out of low SES (see Dunham, 1961; Gruenberg, 1961; Jarvis, 1971; see also Herrnstein & Murray, 1994, with regard to SES and IQ).

These selection processes are likely to affect individuals in an advantaged ethnic group very differently from individuals in a disadvantaged ethnic group. Because of prejudice and discrimination, healthy members of the disadvantaged ethnic group would be less likely to rise against great obstacles to higher SES positions and would be kept down in lower SES positions. This would dilute the rate of disorder among their lower SES members, with only the healthiest and most able members of the disadvantaged ethnic group rising against great obstacles to higher SES positions. With fewer obstacles to block them, the tendency of healthier members of the more advantaged ethnic group to rise would leave a relatively undiluted residue of disabled among their lower SES members. Moreover, the more advantaged the ethnic group, the more its members are able to support unhealthy individuals at higher SES levels. The resulting prediction of higher rates in advantaged ethnic groups (SES constant) is summarized in the bottom part of Figure 14.1.

Qualifications of the Predictions

Figure 14.1 has been drawn to portray one outcome in which social causation processes are clearly more important than social selection processes and one outcome in which the reverse holds true. To the extent that social causation processes and social selection processes are of equal strength in determining the inverse relation between SES and any particular type of psychopathology, we would expect the solid and dotted lines in Figure 14.1 to converge.

Note as well that there is no provision in Figure 14.1 for interactions between SES and ethnic status. However, such interactions may occur. For example, programs of

affirmative action in United States universities may alter differential pressures faced by blacks and other minorities. In such circumstances, the lines in Figure 14.1 might intersect at high levels of SES, especially when SES is measured by educational level. Unless the trace lines cross at the middle, however, an unlikely outcome if educational affirmative action programs are responsible, the interactions would not seriously compromise the test.

We also have made no distinction between men and women in formulating the social causation and social selection predictions above. This is another oversimplification in the interest of providing the most parsimonious presentation of the basic ideas. Gender, like ethnic status and unlike SES, is a status that is ascribed at birth. If psychopathology were a unitary phenomenon rather than a collection of distinct types of disorders, gender could be added to or substituted for ethnic status for purposes of investigating the social causation–social selection issue in urban, open-class societies that discriminate against women. However, as was pointed out by Kohn et al. (Chapter 13, this volume), some disorders, such as major depression, tend to show much higher rates in women; others, such as antisocial personality and alcoholism, show much higher rates in men. These disorders may be inversely related to SES only in the gender in which the disorder is more frequent; if so, the issue may be germane only or mainly within that gender.

As emphasized earlier, the predictions in Figure 14.1 are based on several key assumptions. For example, we focus on ethnic discrimination and the SES characteristics of low educational and occupational levels, and we assume that all of these factors are similar in that they limit opportunity. There may be other environmental factors, such as exposure to toxic substances in particular occupations, for which persons of lower SES in general but not persons of disadvantaged ethnic status specifically are at risk. Such factors would have to be considered separately, outside the framework of assumptions of this quasi-experimental strategy, if they were shown to be related to the type of psychopathology being investigated.

Moreover, we have assumed that there are no differences between the advantaged and disadvantaged ethnic groups in genetic vulnerability on the basis of ethnic background per se. This assumption is also essential for the predictions in Figure 14.1. Goldman (1994) has shown with simulated data, for example, that social selection outcomes can be indistinguishable from social causation outcomes as diagrammed in Figure 14.1 if the disadvantaged ethnic group is assumed to have a greater genetic predisposition to the disorder.

Choice of Research Setting for Tests of the Causation–Selection Issue

The setting chosen for the research is Israel, and the focus within this setting, is on a cohort of Israeli-born Jews of European background contrasted with Israeli-born Jews of North African background. Two main considerations guided this choice: First, the strategy requires a modern, urban democracy in which ethnic assimilation is an unachieved goal. Second, to secure unbiased estimates of rates of disorders in different gender, SES, and ethnic groups, it is important to be able to sample from a population register in which births, deaths, and migration into and out of the country are recorded and dated. Sampling from a population register makes it possible to identify persons who have died, migrated, or been institutionalized, so that something can be learned about their psychiatric status. Israel, probably uniquely, meets the requirements of both ethnic contrast and the presence of a population register. It also has the resource of a psychiatric register in which all psychiatric hospitalizations are reported by law.

In the years following Israel's establishment as a state in 1948, immigration from around the world more than trebled the Jewish population to approximately 3 million when the study was begun in 1982. For the most part, the migrants were seeking a haven from oppression in their countries of origin; self-selection related to psychiatric condition, therefore, has been at a minimum. At the same time, economic and industrial expansion led to increasingly complex differentiation of the occupational and social structure of this new country (Spilerman & Habib, 1976). One of the consequences of these simultaneous historical processes appears to students of Israeli society to be "partial institutionalization of congruence between economic and occupational classes and ethnic division" (Lissak, 1970, p. 152). At the grossest level, the "Ashkenazim," Jews of European background, who made up the majority of earlier immigrants, emerged as relatively advantaged, and the "Oriental" Jews from North African and Middle Eastern countries, who dominated later waves of migration, emerged as relatively disadvantaged. It has been argued that, as a consequence, "over and above the influence of socio-economic background, Oriental youth are exposed to an atmosphere of prejudice and to concrete unintended discrimination" (Yuchtman-Yaar & Semyonov, 1979). This describes precisely the conditions we require to test the social causation–social selection issue.

However, this portrayal is not without controversy among Israeli social scientists, and we have tested its accuracy in the present research. Moreover, two sets of special circumstances that could affect tests of the causation–selection issue in Israel must be considered. One is the fact that a large portion of the immigrants from European countries experienced the Shoa, the Hebrew term for the Holocaust in Europe. There is a controversy in the literature as to whether psychopathology generated in Shoa survivors (see Chapter 1, this volume) has been transmitted to their children (e.g., Sigal & Weinfeld, 1985).

The other special circumstance is related to Israel's history of war and exposure to terrorism. To take the most important example, about half the men in the cohort on which this study focuses were exposed to combat in one or more wars. If such exposure were greater for one than for another ethnic group, this also could affect the relative adversity faced by each and consequent rates of psychopathology. These matters also are investigated in the present study.

METHOD

The population with which we are concerned consists of Jews of European background and Jews of North African background who were born in Israel between 1949, just after it became a state, and 1958. This gives us a cohort of about 177,000 young Israeli adults ranging in age from 24 (when most have begun occupational careers even allowing for obligatory military service) through 33 (maximum age possible) at the time we began the study in 1982. By focusing on this cohort, we can maximize the central contrast, that between advantaged and disadvantaged ethnic status, while holding constant the social system, including its health care and educational, economic, and military institutions, to which the individuals have been exposed. We also avoid the problem of confounding the stress of migration with the stress of assimilation that would occur if we had included foreign-born Israelis in our study.

This cohort has two further advantages for our purpose. First, it has gone through much of the risk period for developing first episodes of the disorders with which we are centrally concerned: schizophrenia (see Cooper, 1978, p. 35), major depression (see Brown & Harris, 1978, pp. 223–227), antisocial personality (see Robins, 1966), alcohol abuse (see Cahalan & Room, 1972), and drug abuse (Kandel, 1980, p. 242). Second, as young adults, most of the cohort members have embarked on their own adult occupational careers. SES is therefore a more meaningful variable in this cohort than it would be if we had lowered the age to 18, when most Israelis begin 3 years of military service prior to undertaking further formal education or their first adult occupation.

Sample Design

Israel's population register makes feasible the sampling of specific birth cohorts of the Israeli-born population. In addition to gradations within the 10-year age range of the birth cohort, we wished to stratify the sample according to gender, education as an indicator of respondents' SES attainment, and advantaged/disadvantaged ethnic status as called for by our planned tests of the causation–selection predictions. We determined, on the basis of analyses of power considerations, that the total sample for the survey of psychiatric disorders needed to be about 5000 persons. To unconfound SES and ethnic advantage in the analyses, it was necessary to oversample higher SES members of the disadvantaged ethnic group and lower SES members of the advantaged ethnic group. This oversampling could not be done on the basis of information in the population register, which does not contain data on the SES indicators of educational level and occupation and does not provide complete information on parents' country of origin. For this reason, it was necessary to draw a much larger sample than we would eventually use, 19,000 in this case. Record checks and preliminary interviews were conducted to secure the necessary demographic information about these 19,000 persons; the relevant information was obtained for 97.7% of them.

Using information from the population register and from the demographic screening of the 19,000 member sample, the stratified sample was drawn. Six categories of education were employed in the stratification: (1) less than high school completion, (2) technical high school graduate, (3) academic high school (including Yeshiva or religious school) graduate, (4) some post–high school technical training, (5) some post–high school academic education, and (6) college or university degrees. Ethnic advantage was defined in terms of father's country of birth. Persons were considered to be from the disadvantaged ethnic group if their fathers were born in North Africa—more specifically, in Algeria, Libya, Morocco, Tangier, or Tunisia. Persons were considered to be from the advantaged ethnic group if their fathers were born in European U.S.S.R., Germany, Austria, Czechoslovakia, Hungary, Poland, or Romania.

The advantaged ethnic group of European background was further differentiated into those whose parents experienced Shoa and those whose parents did not. Because the possibility of exposure to Shoa is completely nested within the advantaged ethnic group, we incorporated the distinction into an "ethnic" variable with three categories (advantaged, not Shoa; advantaged, Shoa; disadvantaged). Although we did not include items on military history and exposure to combat and terrorism as sampling variables, we did include questions about these matters in subsequent interviews.

Excluded from the study population were first-generation Israelis whose fathers were born in countries other than those listed above. Also excluded by design were persons whose religious customs indicated that they were members of distinct enclaves outside the usual assimilation situation. Operationally, they were defined as follows: (1) highest level of education from a Yeshiva or religious school and (2) never worked or, if working, employed by a religious organization. On this basis, 141 persons were excluded from the sample.

Case Identification and Diagnosis

We used a two-phase procedure to identify and define cases of schizophrenia, major depression, substance use disorders (including alcoholism), antisocial personality, and several other disorders that, as explained later, might prove to be inversely related to SES (Dohrenwend, 1990a). The first phase consisted of relatively economical screening of the sample into screen positives (possible cases) and screen negatives; the second phase consisted of an intensive clinical follow-up interview with all screen positives and a subsample of screen negatives. We discuss each phase separately, indicating the checks on reliability and validity, comparisons of responders and nonresponders, and procedures for investigating possible bias that might affect ethnic differences in the results.

The First-Phase Screening Interview

Once the respondents were contacted and found eligible for the study (i.e., could be classified into either the advantaged or disadvantaged ethnic group as described above), they were asked anamnestic questions (e.g., mental hospitalizations, convictions for crimes [use of illicit drugs]) and questions about symptoms in seven screening scales from the Psychiatric Epidemiology Research Interview (PERI) originally developed and tested in New York (Dohrenwend et al., 1980b). These scales were Nonspecific Distress or "Demoralization," Enervation, Suicidal Ideation or Behavior, False Beliefs and Perceptions, Schizoid Tendencies, Drinking Problems, and Antisocial Behavior. Most of these self-report scales consist of items that have response categories such as "yes/no" or "very often/fairly often/sometimes/almost never/never" and refer to behavior in the preceding 12 months.

The screening scales had been tested for reliability and criterion validity and then were calibrated against known cases of psychiatric disorders in our pilot research in Israel (Shrout et al., 1986). This pilot research involved administering the seven scales and 11 other symptom scales to (1) known patient cases with the various types of disorder we are most interested in and (2) psychologically well persons sampled from the general population of the city of Jerusalem. Israelis of European and of North African background were overrepresented by design in both the patient and general population samples.

In calibrating the scales for screening purposes, tests were made to detect subcultural differences in reporting symptoms that would bias our results if the differences were not allowed for in the calibration. First, scales were checked for internal consistency and reliability within gender, SES, and ethnic groups, and the seven selected were found to be adequately reliable. We have re-checked these pilot study reliabilities in the present study for all symptom scales except Suicidal Ideation and Behavior, which was not composed of independent items. The reliabilities range from .91 (nonspecific distress) to .68 (schizoid) in the sample as a whole, and only one scale has a reliability of below .50 in any of the subgroups defined by ethnic group, gender, and educational level. This low alpha (.42) was for the scale of drinking problems among college graduates, where such problems are very rare.

Second, comparisons of the means of the seven screening scales revealed no consistent differences among the ethnic groups within either the well controls or the case groups in the pilot study. However, there was a tendency for North Africans to score higher than Europeans on the scale of false beliefs and perceptions in the well control group. To investigate the possible effect of this difference, we calculated the overall sensitivity and specificity of the screen for each ethnic group. The results indicated that North Africans were not more likely to be false positives, so no adjustment was made in the calibrations of this scale.

Although we found no indication in the pilot study of important subcultural differences, we have made provision for several additional checks on possible ethnic biases in the PERI screening scales in the main study. One is inclusion of measures of social desirability and acquiescence response styles by means of a subset of 15 alternately keyed items from the Need for Approval scale developed by Crowne and Marlowe (1960) and used previously in our work with the PERI symptom scales in New York (Dohrenwend et al., 1980b). The other is a provision for testing interviewer effects on the screening scales by assigning respondents to PERI interviewers without regard to the ethnic background of either. Although the large majority of the respondents of both European and North African backgrounds were interviewed by persons of European background, about a fifth of the respondents in each ethnic group were interviewed by individuals of North African background.

The PERI screening interview containing the symptom scales averaged an hour in length and was conducted by carefully trained and closely supervised mental health professionals, including mainly social workers but also nurses and psychologists. Most of the time, the PERI interviews were conducted in the respondents' homes. Our policy, however, was to locate and interview respondents wherever they were. For example, 12 interviews were conducted in prisons. Excluding the sample members who died or who were abroad, we obtained PERI screening data from 94.5% (4914/5200) of the demographically prescreened cohort sample, as Figure 14.2 shows.

Because identifying information was obtained in the demographic prescreening operation on the nonrespondents in the first-phase screening interview, it was possible to compare the gender, educational level, and ethnic status of the nonrespondents with those of the respondents. There was one difference, in educational level, that was statistically significant ($p < .02$). Among the nonrespondents, 37% did not graduate from high school, in contrast to 30% of the respondents.

We have also conducted checks on hospital admission and diagnostic information in the Israel Psychiatric Case Register, to which all psychiatric inpatient admissions are reported by law, for nonrespondents, emigrants, and dead members of the sample, and data have been obtained on causes of death for a subsample of the dead. The results of these checks are reported as they bear on the results of the tests of the causation–selection issue.

The Second-Phase Clinical Interview

More than 50% of the sample were screened positive in the first-phase interview. "Positive" was defined as (1) a score above empirically derived cut points of a discriminant function that had distinguished known cases from controls on the symptom scales in the preliminary calibration study (Shrout et al., 1986); and/or (2) a positive response on one or more anamnestic items such as psychiatric hospitalization, arrests, and use of illicit drugs; and/or (3) being unable to complete the PERI interview. All positives and a subsample of 18% of the negatives were designated for a follow-up clinical interview by one of 64 psychiatrists who participated in the research.

Figure 14.2 shows that diagnostic interviews were completed with 90.7% of the respondents designated for second-phase

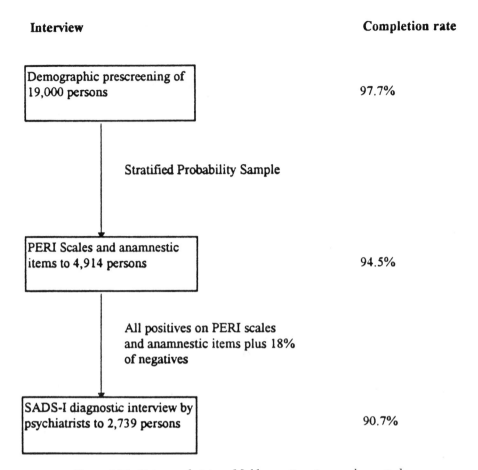

Figure 14.2. Nature and status of field operations in prevalence study.

follow-up. We compared the second-phase nonrespondents to second-phase respondents on demographic and screening variables in the first-phase interview. There was one statistically significant demographic difference: 42% of the second-phase nonrespondents did not graduate from high school, in contrast to 35% of the second-phase respondents. The main reason for this difference is the larger proportion of mentally retarded persons among the second-phase nonrespondents. There were no differences on any of the screening scales or in the proportions screened positive and negative.

The diagnostic interview administered by the psychiatrists in the second-phase oper-

ation is a modified lifetime version (SADS-L) of the Schedule for Affective Disorders and Schizophrenia (SADS) (Endicott & Spitzer, 1978). It is designed to make diagnoses according to Research Diagnostic Criteria (RDC) (Spitzer et al., 1978), a forerunner of the *Diagnostic and Statistical Manual of Mental Disorders (Third Edition)* (*DSM-III*) (American Psychiatric Association, 1980). Like the *DSM-III*, RDC observe hierarchies among diagnoses. If a person is diagnosed as meeting RDC criteria for schizophrenia at a particular time, for example, he or she cannot, according to the hierarchical rule, also be given a diagnosis of major depression. Similarly, to provide another example, depression takes precedence over generalized anxiety disorder. These hierarchies were observed in the present study.

Endicott and Spitzer (1978) described the SADS and SADS-L as follows:

The organization of the SADS and SADS-L is similar to that of a clinical interview focused on differential diagnosis. The schedule provides for a progression of questions, items, and criteria that systematically rule in and rule out specific RDC diagnoses . . . .

The most suitable personnel for administering the SADS and SADS-L, and for using the RDC, are individuals with experience in interviewing and making judgments about manifest psychopathology. (p. 838)

Some additions were made to the SADS-L for purposes of the present research. These included an introductory set of questions designed to elicit a developmental history of the respondent as an aid to recall and provisions for dating the onset of episodes of disorder. Because of these additions, we are calling the interview the SADS-I (for Israel) rather than the SADS-L. The psychiatrists involved in the research were intensively trained by one of us (Levav), who was himself trained at the New York State Psychiatric Institute, where the SADS was developed.

The SADS-I diagnostic interviews were tape recorded, permitting extensive quality and reliability checks. A preliminary reliability check involved independent reassessments of 64 taped interviews; the kappa between the interviewer's primary diagnosis and that of the reviewer was .68 (Cohen, 1960). Although adequate, it was evident that the reliability of the psychiatric examination could be improved. Reviews of the tapes indicated that inadequate information in the original interview sometimes reduced reliability. For this reason, all tape recordings were reviewed by Levav or one of the office-based clinical psychologists whom he trained. For about a fifth of the diagnostic interviews, it was deemed necessary to recontact the respondent to ask additional questions. The RDC diagnoses reported in this chapter incorporate changes made on the basis of this quality check of the tape-recorded clinical interviews.

Most past epidemiological studies reporting SES findings do so for "current" prevalence during the period of a few months to about a year prior to interview. To approximate this, and to ensure correspondence with the 1 year time set of the first-phase screening scales, we emphasized prevalence during the year prior to the SADS-I diagnostic interview for most disorders. An exception is antisocial personality; this is a "lifetime" diagnosis by definition, because it involves antisocial behavior in childhood that continues into adulthood. We have most confidence in these diagnoses of current prevalence because they are least dependent on the recall of the respondent. However, prevalence is a function of the rate at which the disorders occur and their duration; factors that contribute to occurrence may be quite different from those that contribute to recurrence or duration. Because of this limitation of current prevalence rates, we conducted supplementary analyses of lifetime rates for all the key disorders despite problems of recall that are involved (Anthony & Dryman, 1987; Bromet et al., 1986; Pulver & Carpenter, 1983). Lifetime rates are based on whether respondents have ever met criteria for the disorder regardless of number of episodes and their duration.

As with the SADS-L, RDC diagnoses based on the SADS-I can be made at either the "definite" or, where there is less confidence on the part of the diagnostician, the "probable" level. In most of the analyses, most details are provided for "definite-level" diagnoses. Although our emphasis has been on diagnoses made at the definite level, we have conducted additional analyses with definite and probable levels combined. The results of these additional analyses, like the results of the analyses of the lifetime diagnoses, are summarized as they support or contradict the analyses of current prevalence based on diagnoses made at the definite level.

Unfortunately, analyses of interviewer effects are not possible for the clinical interview because only one of the psychiatrists who participated in the study was of North African background, reflecting the scarcity of psychiatrists of North African background in Israel; this person conducted very few diagnostic interviews. However, we investigated the role of possible ethnic bias in the diagnoses in several ways:

1. By analyzing the ratios of probable to definite diagnoses made at each level of the screen (symptom scales plus anamnestic items; symptom scales alone; anamnestic items alone). We assume that diagnoses made at the probable level are nearer the cut point between case and noncase than diagnoses made at the definite level, and therefore more likely to reflect ethnic bias if it exists (Robins, 1985).
2. By investigating whether symptom scale scores are higher for definite-level diagnoses in one ethnic group than in the other.
3. By examining whether higher treatment rates in one ethnic group might have made it easier for psychiatrists to arrive at diagnoses in that ethnic group than the other.

Indicators of SES

In order to be able to control SES comprehensively in ethnic comparisons, we have constructed both continuous and categorical measures of each respondent's formal education and occupational status or, for married women, occupation of the respondent's spouse. The two measures of education are, first, level completed in the categories of low (not high school graduate), middle (high school graduate but not college graduate), and high (college graduate or more); and, second, number of years of formal education completed. The categorical occupation indicator consists of employed versus currently unemployed; if employed, the Kraus (1981) occupational prestige scores were used to group respondents into low (scores of 1–30), middle (31–66), and high (67–100) (V. Kraus, personal communication, 1989). We also investigated a continuous measure of occupational prestige that ran from 0 (never employed or currently unemployed) to 100 (highest occupational prestige possible on the Kraus scale); however, this measure did not show a statistically significant (p = .05 or better) relationship, independently of the other three indicators of SES, to any diagnostic rate and was therefore dropped as redundant. In each analysis, we added a dummy variable to represent people with an occupation for whom we had no prestige score; these totaled 439 respondents, the large majority of whom were in the military.

Measures of Prejudice

We used three approaches to assessing the extent of attitudinal prejudice. Details of these measures are presented elsewhere (Schwartz et al., 1991); only brief summaries are provided here. First, as an overall assessment, respondents were asked to evaluate the social standing of their own ethnic group using a 5 point Likert scale ranging from 1 ("very much favored") to 5 ("discriminated against to a great extent"). Second, in an experiment, vignettes describing an Israeli family with varying ethnic background and educational level were randomly allocated to the respondents, who then answered two sets of questions about (1) their own perceived social distance from the family described and (2) the social distance they judged "others" would be likely to express. Third, five situations were described that placed the respondent in hypothetical competition with another person who was dissimilar to him or her with respect to ethnic origin. The scenarios include competition for a job (qualifications equal), housing, fair adjudication of a court case, courtship, and acceptance at a university (qualifications equal). The respondents were requested to rate their competitors' chances of success in comparison to their own on a 5 point Likert scale. Possible responses ranged from 1 ("much worse than yours") to 5 ("much better than yours").

Statistical Analysis

Because SES and ethnic status are confounded in the population, the tests were conducted in a sample that was specially constructed to overrepresent ethnically disadvantaged persons who are high in SES and ethnically advantaged persons who are low in SES. Although the balance of SES between the two ethnic groups was improved, it remained far from complete. For example, only 14% (346) of the respondents of European background did not graduate from high school, compared with 45% (1135) of the respondents of North African background; only 3% (77) of the North African respondents were college graduates, compared with 20% (482) of the Europeans. The reason is that the SES difference between Israelis of North African compared with Israelis of European background is so great that we would have had to demographically prescreen a sample from the population register much larger than the 19,000 we drew to obtain equal proportions at the highest and lowest levels of SES in the two ethnic groups. Nevertheless, the improvement in balance that we achieved with this sampling plan has made it possible to gain considerable control of SES statistically in tests of ethnic differences.

Because only a minority of the negatives on the first-phase screening measures were sampled for inclusion in the second-phase diagnostic examination with the SADS-I, it was necessary in the analyses to weight the diagnostic results to represent the entire first-phase sample. Diagnostic interviews therefore were weighted by the inverse of the SADS-I sampling rates in each stratum. Regression analyses were done by computer software (Hidiroglou et al., 1980) that implements the methods of Fuller (1975).

To gain confidence in the robustness of the results to model specifications, both logistic regression and weighted least squares (WLS) multiple regression analyses were conducted. Except when the results are affected by the form of the regression model, we report the findings in terms of the logistic models. Separate analyses were done for men and women for disorders that typically have different rates in the two genders. For each set of analyses, we first tested main effects only and then included interactions between ethnic status and SES. When statistically significant interactions ($p = .05$ or better) were found, it is these rather than main effects that are interpreted.

For both symptom data (treated as continuous) and diagnostic data (treated as categorical), we present descriptive statistics and results from regression analyses. In the regression analyses, we add to the SES variables indicators of the additional stratification variables of gender, birth year, and Shoa versus non-Shoa parental background for respondents of European descent in order to produce results that are not an artifact of the sampling design (DuMouchel & Duncan, 1983). Although we do not employ sampling weights from these stratification variables in the regression analyses used to test the causation–selection hypotheses, we do use these demographic sampling weights for one purpose: to check whether the anticipated inverse relationship between SES and particular types of disorders in fact occurs in our cohort. Our presentation of results begins with theses checks on the relation of psychiatric disorders to SES in the cohort population.

RESULTS

Our tests of the social causation–social selection issue require a research setting in which relations between psychiatric disorders and SES are similar to those in the larger epidemiological literature that has generated the issue. In addition, the research setting must contain an assimilation situation in which members of the disadvantaged ethnic group do in fact face greater adversity attaching to their ethnic status. We begin, therefore, with an examination of relations between SES and various types of psychopathology in our cohort of young,

Israeli-born adults. We then turn to evidence that cohort members of North African background face greater adversity attaching to their ethnic background than cohort members of European background. Following this inquiry, we conduct tests of the social causation–social selection issue for the types of psychopathology that are inversely related to SES in this cohort of Israeli-born Jews of European and North African ethnic background.

Relationship between SES and Various Types of Psychopathology in the Israeli Cohort

On the basis of past research (see Kohn et al., Chapter 13, this volume), we chose overall disorder aggregated across diagnostic types (this consists of all RDC disorders plus the "other disorder" category for problems not covered by RDC); the specific RDC diagnoses of schizophrenia, major depression, antisocial personality, alcoholism, and other substance use disorders; and our symptom scale measure of high nonspecific distress or demoralization in persons with no history of diagnosable psychiatric disorder.

Table 14.1 shows that SES, as measured by educational levels, tends to be inversely related to the current prevalence of diagnosable disorder regardless of type and to each of the specific subtypes of disorder. These findings tend to hold whether diagnoses were made at the definite level of confidence or the probable and definite levels combined. Rates of high levels of nonspecific distress or demoralization also tend to be inversely related to educational level. As Table 14.1 also shows, the inverse relationships tend to hold for lifetime prevalence rates of the diagnosed disorders as well. It should be pointed out, however, that major depression does not show a statistically significant ($p < .05$) inverse relation among men when tested in further logistic regression analyses. Moreover, alcoholism, substance use disorders, and antisocial personality are extremely rare in women, and their relationship to SES for women is also not statistically significant.

We repeated the analysis shown in Table 14.1 with occupational prestige (grouped into the three categories described above in "Methods") substituted for the trichotomized educational variable shown in Table 14.1. The results are much the same as for educational level except that lifetime rates of major depression do not show an inverse relationship with occupational prestige.

We have also shown in Table 14.1 rates of diagnostic disorder according to gender and rates according to ethnic status. In general, the gender differences are consistent with the results of previous epidemiological research (see Kohn et al., Chapter 13, this volume). The tendency for North Africans to have higher rates than Europeans would be expected on the basis of the lower SES levels of the North African. These SES differences are strongly reflected in Table 14.1, where the rates have been weighted back to the distribution of SES indicators in the population from which the stratified samples were drawn. Note, however, the similarity in the rates of schizophrenia for the Europeans and North Africans despite the difference in SES between these two ethnic groups. We return to this point later on with reference to our assumption that there are no ethnically specific differences in genetic predisposition to the disorders of interest.

Some Evidence of Differences in Adversity Faced by Members of the Disadvantaged and Advantaged Ethnic Groups

Ethnic Prejudice

The results on ethnic prejudice are presented in detail elsewhere (Schwartz et al., 1991). In summary, both Europeans and North Africans within each social stratum perceived that others (i.e., members of society at large) desire greater social distance from North Africans than from Europeans. Additionally, the respondents of European background seem to desire greater personal social distance from North Africans. This desire is not reciprocated; the respondents of North African background do not indicate

Table 14.1. Base rates of diagnosable disorder by demographic characteristics of educational level, gender, and ethnic background[*]

Demographic characteristics	Any disorder		Schizophrenia		Major depression		Antisocial personality (lifetime only)[†]		Substance use disorders (including alcoholism)		High distress with no diagnosable disorder
	D	D&P	D	D&P	D	D&P	D	D&P	D	D&P	
Current											
Not high school graduate	37.63	50.52	1.36	1.54	4.43	7.01			4.01	5.60	2.37
High school graduate	23.87	38.61	0.52	0.52	4.24	5.63			0.35	0.96	1.46
College graduate	16.52	29.28	0.34	0.34	2.58	3.47			0.19	0.19	0.96
Female	27.41	40.48	0.35	0.42	4.90	6.39			0.33	0.56	1.21
Male	24.37	39.15	1.02	1.04	3.10	4.78			2.07	3.30	1.96
North African	32.97	47.26	0.57	0.60	6.58	9.12			2.85	4.31	2.65
European	22.21	35.96	0.75	0.80	2.65	3.80			0.36	0.72	1.04
Lifetime											
Not high school graduate	61.58	75.94	1.36	1.54	17.52	27.50	2.40	5.54	6.50	9.95	—
High school graduate	45.69	63.46	0.52	0.52	14.76	21.84	0.14	0.79	1.55	4.13	—
College graduate	41.26	56.09	0.84	0.84	11.91	15.69	0.00	0.00	0.49	1.60	—
Female	53.20	68.43	0.53	0.60	20.02	29.08	0.17	0.47	1.00	2.38	—
Male	44.22	61.94	1.02	1.04	9.92	15.28	1.13	3.09	4.04	7.73	—
North African	55.15	70.65	0.57	0.60	19.80	29.12	1.75	4.05	4.99	8.71	—
European	45.31	62.31	0.89	0.94	12.39	18.48	0.09	0.63	1.27	3.21	—

[*]"Current" (1 year before interview) and lifetime prevalence rates per hundred for disorders diagnosed at RDC definite (D) and RDC definite plus probable (D&P) levels of confidence are weighted to reflect the population from which the sample was drawn. Sample $n = 4914$ for first-phase screening interview; sample $n = 2741$ for second-phase diagnostic interview.

[†]Antisocial personality is by definition the same for lifetime as current prevalence.

Table 14.2.   Mean (standard error) occupational prestige by education, gender, and ethnic background[*]

Education	European		North African	
	Male	Female	Male	Female
Not high school graduate	29.76 (1.83)	31.19 (2.00)	22.10 (0.79)	24.40 (0.89)
High school graduate	48.18 (1.42)	53.13 (1.29)	33.05 (1.06)	38.22 (1.16)
College graduate	81.98 (2.22)	73.52 (2.59)	74.50 (4.72)	61.16 (5.29)

[*]Sample *n* = 4194, weighted to population.

a preference for social distance from the Europeans. There is also a perception by both groups that, to some extent, North Africans are at a disadvantage in the competition for socially desirable goals of obtaining a job, housing, and fair adjudication of a court case. Possibly reacting to policies of affirmative action, the Europeans as well as the North Africans tended to see themselves at a disadvantage in the competition for obtaining educational goals.

Status Attainment

Another way of assessing relative adversity has been through investigation of status attainment (i.e., Coleman et al., 1972; Duncan, 1968). Anticipating results of more detailed analyses being prepared for publication, Table 14.2 shows that, at every educational level and for both genders, re-

spondents of North African background tend to have lower prestige occupations than respondents of European background. The detailed analyses of status attainment by the respondents of North African by contrast with European background indicate that respondents of North African background experience considerably more downward pressure than do those of European background, and that this experience is associated with expectations of prejudice and discrimination on the part of the respondents of North African background.

Tests of the Issue for Diagnosed Disorders and Nonspecific Distress

Overall Rates of Diagnosed Disorders

For illustrative purposes, Table 14.3 presents the distribution of current and lifetime

Table 14.3.   Illustrative diagnostic results of second-phase clinical interviews for any disorder[*]

Education	Europe (1197)				North African (1544)			
	Male (602)		Female (595)		Male (852)		Female (692)	
	D	D&P	D	D&P	D	D&P	D	D&P
Current								
Not high school graduate	36.84	46.77	31.77	54.73	41.53	56.87	36.36	49.10
High school graduate	18.65	34.54	24.23	32.79	21.05	38.03	32.91	50.14
College graduate	18.67	25.13	13.45	32.74	15.69	27.45	34.69	52.36
Lifetime								
Not high school graduate	68.54	78.96	58.72	77.56	60.24	74.50	58.24	76.30
High school graduate	35.73	60.35	49.84	60.55	42.87	60.47	56.81	71.65
College graduate	35.54	45.17	43.27	67.56	34.31	50.00	59.73	74.38

[*]"Current" prevalence (1 year before interview) rates per hundred of RDC definite diagnoses by education, gender, and ethnic background (weighted to first-phase screen).

Table 14.4. Illustrative diagnostic results of second-phase clinical interviews for schizophrenia°

| Education | European (1197) | | | | North African (1544) | | | |
| | Male (602) | | Female (595) | | Male (852) | | Female (692) | |
	D	D&P	D	D&P	D	D&P	D	D&P
Current								
Not high school graduate	4.18	4.18	0.84	1.69	1.91	2.09	0.00	0.00
High school graduate	0.29	0.29	0.39	0.39	0.17	0.17	0.00	0.00
College graduate	0.00	0.00	0.39	0.39	0.00	0.00	0.00	0.00
Lifetime								
Not high school graduate	4.18	4.18	0.84	1.69	1.91	2.09	0.00	0.00
High school graduate	0.29	0.29	0.39	0.39	0.17	0.17	0.00	0.00
College graduate	0.00	0.00	0.78	0.78	0.00	0.00	0.00	0.00

°"Current" prevalence (1 year before interview) rates per hundred of RDC definite diagnoses by education, gender, and ethnic background (weighted to first-phase screen).

overall rates according to ethnic status with a control on one indicator of SES, the categorical groupings of educational level. These descriptive results suggest that ethnic differences shown in Table 14.1 between the Europeans and the North Africans in the four types of overall rate frequently tend to disappear when a control on educational level is introduced. This impression was tested with logistic regression analyses as described above under "Statistical Analysis." That is, each of the four types of overall rate in Table 14.3 was regressed on continuous and categorical measures of educational and occupational indicators of SES, ethnic background, date of birth, birth cohort used for sampling purposes, and gender. There were no statistically significant differences according to ethnic status for any of the rates with or without interactions among gender, ethnicity, and SES in the equation. The results of the tests are very different for individual diagnostic types.

Schizophrenia

Consistent with the social selection prediction, Table 14.4 suggests that rates of current, RDC-definite schizophrenia are higher among respondents of European background. According to the logistic regression analyses, this ethnic difference is statistically significant after comprehensive controls on SES and the other relevant variables (logistic regression results: adjusted odds ratio [OR] = 3.82; confidence interval [CI] = 1.46–11.22; $p < .05$). Additional analyses with current definite plus probable and with lifetime rates of both types give similar, slightly stronger results (e.g., adjusted OR = 4.30 for lifetime probable and definite combined; CI = 1.55–11.93; $p < .01$). Tests for interactions of ethnicity and the various indicators of SES were not statistically significant.

Additional regression analyses show that there is no significant difference in rates between respondents of European background whose parents were exposed to Shoa and respondents of European background whose parents were not exposed to Shoa. Thus the higher rates for respondents of European background are not a function of the Shoa experience of the parents of some of them. We also tested whether greater exposure of European men to combat could account for the results. Army service is negatively related to schizophrenia and, among those who did serve, there is no relation between exposure to combat and schizophrenia.

However, the regression analyses show, as the descriptive results in Table 14.4 suggest, that there is an unexpected gender difference: rates tend to be higher for men (e.g.,

Table 14.5. Illustrative diagnostic results of second-phase clinical interviews for major depression[°]

| | European (1197) | | | | North African (1544) | | | |
| | Male (602) | | Female (595) | | Male (852) | | Female (692) | |
Education	D	D&P	D	D&P	D	D&P	D	D&P
Current								
Not high school graduate	3.01	5.61	4.81	5.49	3.47	7.73	6.60	10.96
High school graduate	2.06	5.65	2.93	3.75	4.61	5.54	12.11	14.04
College graduate	0.67	1.18	1.68	4.80	2.94	2.94	10.70	19.54
Lifetime								
Not high school graduate	7.43	11.17	22.03	26.41	14.95	24.04	22.80	39.46
High school graduate	6.76	15.19	14.66	24.14	13.29	18.81	27.82	33.36
College graduate	6.10	8.87	11.97	16.54	9.80	9.80	27.13	46.36

[°]"Current" prevalence (1 year before interview) rates per hundred of RDC definite diagnoses by education, gender, and ethnic background (weighted to first-phase screen).

$p < .05$ for current definite). This may be due to the youthfulness of the sample and the well-established fact of gender differences in age of onset. This is discussed further later on.

Major Depression

By contrast with schizophrenia, the results for major depression are more consistent with the social causation prediction, as the illustrative descriptive findings in Table 14.5 suggest. Logistic regression analyses with full controls on SES show that, for all four types of rate, North African women are higher ($p < .01$), with ethnic contrast strongest for diagnoses at the current, definite level (adjusted OR = 3.22; CI = 1.79–5.80; $p < .001$). The main effects of ethnic status are not statistically significant ($p = .05$ or better) for men, and there are no significant ethnicity-by-SES interactions for men or women.

Note in Table 14.5 that depression is not inversely related to educational level among North Africans, especially women. In fact, when current probable and definite diagnoses are combined, we find an inverse relationship between depression and educational level for men but a direct relationship for North African women. The reasons may

be related to marital status and patterns of intermarriage and are discussed further later on.

Antisocial Personality

Table 14.6 shows that there were no cases of antisocial personality among college graduates. For this reason, college graduates from both ethnic groups were excluded from the regression analyses. The logistic regression analyses revealed no statistically significant ethnic differences in rates for women. For men, as the descriptive results in Table 14.6 suggest, there are significantly higher rates of RDC-definite antisocial personality among North Africans (adjusted OR = 5.09 for definite; CI = 1.00–25.97; $p = .05$; and adjusted OR = 3.51 for probable and definite combined; CI = 1.52–8.19; $p < .01$). There were no statistically significant interactions of SES indicators and ethnic status. As with major depression, these results are consistent with social causation prediction but for men rather than women.

Substance Use Disorders and Alcoholism

Substance use disorders and alcoholism have similarities with antisocial personality:

Table 14.6. Illustrative diagnostic results of second-phase clinical interviews for antisocial personality*

| | European (1197) | | | | North African (1544) | | | |
| | Male (602) | | Female (595) | | Male (852) | | Female (692) | |
Education	D	D&P	D	D&P	D	D&P	D	D&P
Not high school graduate	0.73	2.83	0.82	1.66	6.97	12.16	0.73	2.12
High school graduate	0.15	0.73	0.00	0.00	0.80	2.50	0.30	0.60
College graduate	0.00	0.00	0.00	0.00	0.00	0.00	0.00	0.00

*Lifetime rates per hundred of RDC definite diagnoses by education, gender, and ethnic background (weighted to first-phase screen).

they are more frequent among men, there are no statistically significant ethnic differences in their rates of among women, and these disorders are all but absent among college graduates. Because substance use disorders and alcoholism are rare in Israel, we have combined them in Table 14.7 and in the regression analyses.

With college graduates of both ethnic groups again omitted, regression analyses show significantly higher rates of substance use disorders, including alcoholism, diagnosed at the current, definite level among men of North African background (adjusted OR = 2.76; CI = 1.09–6.90; $p < .05$). There are significant main effects as well for definite lifetime diagnoses (adjusted OR = 1.77; CI = 1.00–3.12; $p = .05$). For neither of

these definite-level diagnoses is there a significant ethnicity-by-SES interaction. However, when probable cases are pooled with definite cases for both current and lifetime diagnoses, there are significant interactions of ethnic status and years of education, a quantitative indicator of SES ($p < .01$ for current; $p < .05$ for lifetime). These latter results imply, as the descriptive findings in Table 14.7 also suggest, that the social causation effects of disadvantaged ethnic status are strongest among men of lowest SES.

Because there is considerable comorbidity among alcoholism, other drug use disorders, and antisocial personality, we checked whether persons with only one of these disorders were distributed similarly to those with various combinations of the dis-

Table 14.7. Illustrative diagnostic results of second-phase clinical interviews for substance use disorders (including alcoholism)*

| | European (1197) | | | | North African (1544) | | | |
| | Male (602) | | Female (595) | | Male (852) | | Female (692) | |
Education	D	D&P	D	D&P	D	D&P	D	D&P
Current								
Not high school graduate	2.29	2.86	0.84	1.66	8.29	11.41	0.72	1.68
High school graduate	0.44	1.20	0.13	0.13	0.75	2.71	0.72	0.56
College graduate	0.49	0.49	0.00	0.00	0.00	0.00	0.00	0.00
Lifetime								
Not high school graduate	5.23	7.50	1.69	3.41	13.88	19.99	1.92	3.31
High school graduate	2.05	4.22	2.73	3.01	4.01	8.29	1.63	3.46
College graduate	1.04	1.48	0.00	1.68	0.00	0.00	0.00	0.00

*"Current" prevalence (1 year before interview) rates per hundred of RDC definite diagnoses by education, gender, and ethnic background (weighted to first-phase screen).

Table 14.8. Illustrative diagnostic results of first-phase screening interview for nonspecific distress°

| | European (1197) | | North African (1544) | |
Education	Male (602)	Female (595)	Male (852)	Female (692)
Not high school graduate	2.53	2.46	2.92	1.84
High school graduate	1.65	0.39	3.60	1.51
College graduate	1.53	0.51	2.94	4.65

°"Current" prevalence (1 year before interview) rates per hundred by education, gender, and ethnic background (weighted to first-phase screen).

orders. The highest rates of each type were consistently found among low-SES men of North African background.

Nonspecific Distress

Some respondents without any history of diagnosable psychiatric disorder scored in the top 20% of their respective gender samples on the symptom scale of nonspecific psychological distress that we have termed "demoralization." The descriptive results in Table 14.8 suggest that the inverse relation between such elevated distress and SES is more a function of social causation than social selection. Logistic regression analyses show that rates of high distress are significantly elevated in respondents of North African background with full controls on SES (adjusted OR = 2.87; CI = 1.57–5.30; $p <$ .01). Note in Table 14.8 that there is a tendency for rates to be elevated in North African women who graduated from college, as for rates of major depression in this subgroup.

Methodological Checks on the Results

As noted in the "Methods" section, we have built into the design of this study a number of opportunities to cross-check the results and to investigate the extent to which they might be artifacts of the data analysis procedures, diagnostic biases, or selective factors associated with inability to interview some members of the cohort because of refusal, death, or migration. We first take up the cross-checks on the methods of statistical analysis.

Comparisons Between Logistic and WLS Multiple Regression Analyses

The use of statistical adjustments in nonexperimental research to equate groups is problematic but necessary in fields such as psychiatric epidemiology. The confidence we have in the adjustments depends in part on the confidence we have in the specification of the statistical model. To determine whether our results are robust with respect to the choice of an analytical model, we used both logistic regression and WLS multiple regression methods. The former attempts to model the logarithm of the odds of disorder and the latter the simple risk of disorder.

The results for schizophrenia and major depression are entirely consistent for the two analyses. For substance use disorders and antisocial personality in men, the results are largely consistent, with the analysis of risk differences (WLS) suggesting that an SES by ethnic status interaction is more important. For substance use disorders, the logistic analyses revealed that the ethnic difference is strongest among less educated men for two of the four diagnostic outcomes, whereas the multiple regression of risks needed this interaction for all four outcomes (e.g., multiple regression interaction results for current definite: $b = $ .012; CI = .004–.020; $p <$ .01). For antisocial personality, the interactions were not statistically significant in the logistic regression but were significant in the risk regression (e.g., multiple regression for definite: $b = $ .011; CI = .003–.019; $p <$ .01). Regardless of the form of the analysis chosen, results for schizophrenia were consistent with the social se-lection prediction and results for major de-pression, substance use disorders, and antisocial personality with the social causa-tion prediction, at least in the lowest levels of SES.

Checks on Possible Bias in the Psychiatric Diagnoses

We have conducted three checks on whether the psychiatrists, almost all of whom were European, had a tendency to overdiagnose disorders in the respondents of North African background. First, we con-sidered the possibility that North Africans had higher psychiatric treatment rates, and that knowledge of treatment may have made it easier to give them a diagnosis. Slightly more of the North African respondents (4.3% of the men and 2.7% of the women) than of the European respondents (3.0% of the men and 2.0% of the women) reported ever having been in a psychiatric hospital. The percentages ever in outpatient treat-ment with a mental health professional (psy-chiatrist, psychologist, social worker) were slightly lower among North Africans (13% of the men and 15% of the women) in com-parison with Europeans (14% of the men and 19% of the women). It is unlikely that these ethnic differences in histories of psy-chiatric treatment could have biased our re-search diagnoses toward the ethnic differ-ences in rates that were obtained.

Second, probable diagnoses are likely to be nearer the cut point between cases and noncases than definite diagnoses. Probable diagnoses are more likely, therefore, to in-volve error (e.g., Robins, 1985), including error from ethnic bias if it exists. Thus, if bias operated, it would be likely to show up in a higher ratio of probable to definite di-agnoses for each type of psychiatric screen. As it turned out, the ratio of probable to definite diagnoses for the aggregated five subtypes of RDC diagnoses of greatest in-terest tends to be higher for the Europeans in relation to almost every type of screen. The only exception is in relation to the strongest screen, consisting of being positive

in the discriminant function and on the an-amnestic items. Here the ratios are almost identical in the two ethnic groups.

Finally, we would expect on the basis of similar reasoning that, if bias operated, North Africans would be diagnosed as cases with lower levels of symptomatology as mea-sured by the PERI symptom scales. This did not occur. Respondents of North African background with current diagnoses of the types we have been considering, made at the definite level, tend to score higher on five of the seven PERI screening scales than do Europeans with current, definite level di-agnoses of the same set of disorders.

Comparisons of Diagnostic and Symptom Scale Results

The seven psychometric symptom measures used in the first-phase screening consisted of demoralization, enervation, and suicidal ideation and behavior, each of which con-tains symptoms more characteristic of de-pression than of the other disorders; false beliefs and perceptions, and schizoid ten-dencies, both of which are more likely to be related to psychoses; antisocial history; and drinking problems. The descriptive findings are shown in Table 14.9.

Tests of ethnic differences on these scales were conducted that parallel those done with the diagnostic data, with the same com-prehensive controls on SES. Because the scales are quantitative, multiple regression was the method of analysis. By and large, the scale results are consistent with the di-agnostic findings. North African women have significantly higher scores on the De-moralization and Enervation scales than European women ($p < .001$), with no sig-nificant ethnicity-by-SES interactions. How-ever, there is no significant difference on the scale of suicidal ideation and behavior. Among men, there are statistically signifi-cant ethnicity-by–years of education inter-actions, indicating that scores on the scales of antisocial history ($p < .001$) and drinking problems ($p < .01$) are higher among North African than European men, with the

Table 14.9. Mean symptom scale scores (standard deviations) by education, gender, and ethnic background[*]

Symptom scale	European (2355)		North African (2468)	
	Male (1139)	Female (1216)	Male (1254)	Female (1214)
Demoralization				
Not high school graduate	0.92 (.57)	1.22 (.65)	1.12 (.61)	1.37 (.66)
High school graduate	0.77 (.39)	1.02 (.49)	0.94 (.48)	1.15 (.52)
College graduate	0.73 (.37)	0.94 (.46)	0.74 (.39)	1.19 (.45)
Antisocial behavior				
Not high school graduate	0.71 (.74)	0.24 (.47)	1.13 (.99)	0.31 (.43)
High school graduate	0.56 (.63)	0.21 (.28)	0.63 (.68)	0.22 (.31)
College graduate	0.47 (.56)	0.23 (.34)	0.50 (.48)	0.16 (.20)
Drinking problems				
Not high school graduate	0.05 (.23)	0.06 (.20)	0.15 (.44)	0.05 (.25)
High school graduate	0.02 (.11)	0.01 (.06)	0.07 (.31)	0.02 (.10)
College graduate	0.03 (.14)	0.01 (.06)	0.02 (.08)	0.02 (.10)
False beliefs and perceptions				
Not high school graduate	0.29 (.39)	0.32 (.38)	0.42 (.47)	0.43 (.52)
High school graduate	0.24 (.28)	0.26 (.32)	0.34 (.36)	0.35 (.40)
College graduate	0.18 (.24)	0.18 (.25)	0.24 (.30)	0.34 (.33)
Enervation				
Not high school graduate	0.94 (.71)	1.22 (.81)	1.15 (.82)	1.36 (.85)
High school graduate	0.84 (.54)	1.04 (.65)	0.98 (.63)	1.22 (.69)
College graduate	0.87 (.50)	1.03 (.64)	0.97 (.47)	1.50 (.72)
Schizoid tendencies				
Not high school graduate	0.95 (.62)	0.85 (.67)	1.09 (.72)	0.95 (.65)
High school graduate	1.01 (.58)	0.86 (.57)	0.99 (.59)	0.85 (.58)
College graduate	1.16 (.63)	0.96 (.63)	0.96 (.58)	1.00 (.60)
Suicidal ideation and behavior				
Not high school graduate	0.23 (.83)	0.43 (1.07)	0.27 (.90)	0.45 (1.18)
High school graduate	0.16 (.62)	0.16 (.63)	0.08 (.44)	0.23 (.81)
College graduate	0.16 (.56)	0.31 (.80)	0.00 (.00)	0.28 (.83)

[*]Sample n = 4823; 91 respondents are missing from these analyses. They were either mentally retarded or too disturbed to respond to the PERI items, but were screened positive and sent on for SADS interviews.

greatest differences occurring in persons of low SES.

The most striking exception occurs on the scale of false beliefs and perceptions. To be consistent with the diagnostic findings, Europeans should score higher on this scale. However, analyses reveal a significant interaction of ethnicity and years of education (p < .05), because North Africans with the fewest years of education tend to score the

highest. It is possible that there is ethnic bias in responses to this scale, as was hinted in our pilot research done to select and calibrate the screening scales (Shrout et al., 1986, p. 318). However, because this particular bias in a first-phase screening scale would lead, if anything, to overestimation of schizophrenia in respondents of North African background, eliminating the bias would not alter our finding of higher rates of schizophrenia in Europeans with SES controlled.

It was possible to conduct some tests of possible biases in these scales that could not be tested for the diagnoses. Because the results of these tests are reassuring, they enhance the value of the general concordance of the symptom scale results and the diagnostic results. These tests involve response styles and interviewer effects.

There were no differences on acquiescence response bias. There was, however, an ethnic difference in need for approval measured by the Crowne-Marlow items: the respondents of North African background showed higher need for approval. When this variable was entered into the regression analysis, tendencies for North Africans to score higher on the symptom scales actually increased.

With one exception, there were no effects of ethnicity of interviewer on the symptom differences between the respondents of North African and European background. The one interviewer effect occurred on the scale of false belief and perceptions. Male and female respondents of North African background and female respondents of European background tended to report more symptoms of false beliefs and perceptions to European interviewers, differences that are significant at the .01 level.

Diagnostic Base Rates According to Ethnic Status

The comparisons of population base rates for Europeans and North Africans in Table 14.1 provide useful additional information. There is no statistically significant ethnic difference in the base rates of schizophrenia (e.g., $z = .28$; $p > .50$ for the rates of 0.57% vs. 0.75% current, definite). By contrast, the current and lifetime base rates of major depression, substance use disorder (including alcoholism), and antisocial personality are significantly ($p < .001$) higher among persons of North African background. This is what would be expected if social causation processes were stronger than social selection processes for these disorders, with stress

from both ethnic prejudice and low SES contributing to their occurrence.

Possible Influence of Psychiatric Conditions of Nonrespondent, Migrant, and Dead Members of Cohort Sample on Ethnic Differences in Psychopathology

The resources of the population register and the Psychiatric Case Register provide the means of checking on possible biases in rates caused by selective factors related to death or migration of sampled members of the cohort, or to refusal to participate by sampled members living in Israel. As Figure 14.1 showed, we were unable to obtain PERI screening data from 5.5% (286/5200) of the cohort sample living in Israel; about nine out of ten of these were refusals after many attempts by PERI screening interviewers. A few persons were repeatedly unavailable after many attempts to make appointments; a few more could not be located. An additional 6.4% (334/5200) left Israel after age 15 (and hence were at risk of developing a psychiatric disorder for at least a brief period of time in Israel) and remained abroad during the several years of fieldwork. Finally, 160 potential members of the cohort sample died after age 15; we drew 59 of these into the cohort sample, and an estimated 65 (for a total of 2.4%) would have been drawn into the sample if we could have learned about their demographic characteristics.

It has been possible to trace these three groups through Israel's Psychiatric Case Register, with suitable aggregations into subgroups to preserve anonymity. We can thus compare the rates of persons ever hospitalized in the refusal, migrant, and dead samples with rates in the larger cohort sample of those interviewed in Israel according to gender and ethnic background. It is also possible to compare rates of persons with a last hospital diagnosis of schizophrenia with the rates of RDC schizophrenia in the cohort respondents, almost 90% of whom had been hospitalized at some time for their disorder. Such diagnostic comparisons are less informative for the other types of disorder with which we are concerned because only small minorities of those with the other disorders were ever hospitalized. Even for schizophrenia, there is the problem of imperfect correspondence between the hospital diagnoses and our research diagnoses according to RDC (Levav et al., 1987). The comparisons are useful, nevertheless, for what they tell us about the central questions with which we are concerned, questions about ethnic differences. The following is a summary of the findings from these checks.

As in the larger respondent sample, 48% of the 286 member *refusal sample* were of European background and 52% were of North African background. Israelis of European background in the refusal sample had higher rates of hospital diagnoses of schizophrenia than Israelis of North African background in the refusal sample (2.9% vs. 1.1%). It seems likely, therefore, that complete psychiatric data on the refusal sample would strengthen rather than contradict the ethnic difference for schizophrenia with SES controlled in the respondent sample, a result that was consistent with the social selection prediction.

Close to 60% of the 334 member *emigrant sample* were of European background. None of the hospitalizations in the emigrant sample (2.5% for emigrant Israelis of European background vs. 2.2% for emigrant Israelis of North African background) was associated with a diagnosis of schizophrenia. It is unlikely, therefore, that there was selective outmigration for schizophrenia on the part of either ethnic group, or that ethnic differences in rates of schizophrenia based on the respondent sample results would be much changed on the basis of full diagnostic data on the emigrant sample.

The psychiatric hospitalization rate in the 160 member *sample of those who died* after reaching age 15 was high, 5% versus 3% in the 4914 member respondent sample. We could find no evidence of ethnic differences in rates of hospital diagnoses of schizophrenia. However, our investigation was limited because we had data on the ethnic back-

ground of only 59 persons; none of them had a hospital diagnosis of schizophrenia.

We were able to analyze the reasons for the death of 41 of the estimated 160 sample members who died after reaching 15 years of age and whose ethnic background was known to us. From this information, we estimate that about three-quarters of the dead were men, and that the majority of these were combat casualties in Israel's wars. Moreover, the large majority of the combat casualties were among persons of European rather than North African background. For example, of the 16 men who died in the Yom Kippur war, 15 were of European background. Among the minority of male deaths for causes other than combat, those among Israelis of North African background tended to be associated with drugs, alcohol, or nonmilitary violence. This suggests that obtaining more detailed diagnostic data on the dead members of the cohort sample would strengthen the findings so far on ethnic differences in rates of antisocial personality and substance use disorders, including alcoholism. It also suggests that deaths were more likely to remove healthy members from the denominator in rate calculations for Israelis of European background than for Israelis of North African background because, in the Israel Army, those with the best physical and psychiatric profiles were most likely to be put into combat.

DISCUSSION

We argued at the outset that, within the framework of theory and assumptions that we set forth, the social causation–social selection issue could turn on a simple question of fact: Are rates or types of psychopathology that are inversely related to SES higher or lower in disadvantaged ethnic groups compared with advantaged ethnic groups when SES is controlled? How firm are the facts we have obtained in this study to answer this question, and how far do they take us in resolving the issue of the relative importance of social causation and social selection processes?

Firmness of the Facts

We consider each of the outcomes we obtained, starting with the "no difference" outcome for overall rates.

Social Causation and Social Selection of Equal Importance

This is the outcome we obtained for overall rates. With SES controlled, there was no statistically significant difference in overall rates between the advantaged and disadvantaged ethnic groups. In retrospect, this is not so surprising. Although the overall rates are inversely related to SES, they include subtypes, such as generalized anxiety disorder, that are not inversely related to SES in this cohort. Also, the overall rates include disorders that show causation outcomes (e.g., major depression), but they also include at least one disorder that shows a social selection outcome (e.g, schizophrenia) in the tests we reported for specific disorders. When aggregated, such contrasts would tend to cancel each other out. Moreover, some of the disorders included in the aggregate rate and not examined separately in the above analyses, even though they are inversely related to SES in this sample, show different outcomes when tested. For example, intermittent depression shows a social causation outcome, whereas minor depression shows no statistically significant difference according to ethnic status with SES controlled. The heterogeneity of the disorders in this aggregation is responsible for the "equal importance" outcome for the overall rate.

Social Causation More Important

Holding SES constant, rates of major depression in women and antisocial personality and substance use disorders, including alcoholism, in men were higher in the Israelis of North African background, as would be expected if an increment in adversity attaching to disadvantaged ethnic status produces an increment of psychopathology. The results for these three types of disorder, con-

sistent with the social causation prediction, are the strongest that we obtained, both empirically and theoretically. The reasons are as follows:

1. These diagnoses tend to show the same relationships to SES and ethnic status as do the relevant symptom scales of antisocial behavior and drinking problems (for diagnoses of antisocial personality and alcoholism) and the symptom scales of demoralization and enervation (for major depression).
2. It seems unlikely that these ethnic differences can be explained by diagnostic biases on the part of the psychiatrists or as artifacts of interviewer effects, response biases, or subcultural differences in modes of expressing distress on the symptom scales.
3. Analyses of data from the Psychiatric Case Register on nonrespondents, migrants, and dead members of the sample, supplemented by data from death records for the dead members, indicate that the ethnic differences in rates of antisocial personality and substance abuse are, if anything, underestimated from the findings on respondents living in Israel.
4. Where we have relevant comparisons with other ethnic groups in other settings, as we do with antisocial personality and substance use disorders, the patterns of present results are consistent with earlier findings (Dohrenwend, 1975; Dohrenwend & Dohrenwend 1981).
5. Results on major depression, substance use disorders (including alcoholism), and antisocial personality cannot be explained by greater exposure of respondents of North African background to combat in Israel's wars or to terrorism because it was the respondents of European background who tended to be more exposed.

Three factors must be examined, however, concerning results on major depression. First, with rates of diagnosed major depression and most of the relevant symptom scales higher among North Africans, it is surprising that the North Africans are not higher on the scale of suicidal ideation and behavior. A possible explanation may be found in the strong proscriptions against suicide in the Jewish religion and the fact that North Africans are generally more observant than Europeans (Levav & Aisenberg, 1989).

Second, rates of major depression were not inversely related to educational level among North African women, as we expected them to be. They tend, in fact to show a direct relationship to educational level among the women of North African background when probable- and definite-level diagnoses are combined. Moreover, rates of high nonspecific distress in the absence of diagnosable disorders are also sharply elevated in highly educated North African women. It is possible that the reasons are related to marital status and patterns of intermarriage among these highly educated women. Only 49% of the highly educated North African women have ever been married, and 70% of these are married to European men. This is in sharp contrast to North African women of lower educational levels, the large majority of whom (81%) are married and, except for small minorities, to North African men. It is possible that marginal status in the assimilation process involves an increment of stress for highly educated women of North African background compared not only with highly educated women of European background, but also with lower educated women of North African background.

Third, the ethnic differences in depression appear to be confined to women. This gender difference in depression, considered along with the opposite gender differences in antisocial personality and substance use disorders (including alcoholism), are consistent with the possibility that there are distinctively female and male modes of reacting to adversity (Dohrenwend & Dohrenwend, 1976). It will be important in further research to investigate the relation of depression to antisocial personality, alcoholism, and substance use disorders among

men in general and, especially, North African men. Nevertheless, these results provide strong support of the social causation hypothesis for these disorders.

We have used Jerome Frank's (1973) term *demoralization* to describe the type of nonspecific distress measured by most of the early screening scales in psychiatric epidemiology, scales composed of symptoms of depressed mood, anxiety, and physiological disturbance. We did so because we found that these types of symptoms were highly correlated with low self-esteem and feelings of helplessness and hopelessness that are the core components of Frank's concept (Dohrenwend et al., 1980b). Whether these measures are described as "demoralization" or as nonspecific distress or with some other term such as "neuroticism" or "negative affectivity" (Watson & Clark, 1984), we think these scales measure something analogous to temperature (Dohrenwend et al., 1980b) or, perhaps even better, blood pressure, with its more variable cut point between normal and abnormal. As with temperature and blood pressure, elevated scores indicate that something is wrong but do not indicate what the underlying problem is, whether it is chronic or acute, or even whether it is serious until more is learned about the sources of the elevation and the conditions that accompany it. In the measure used here, focus is on persons high on this measure of distress but with no history of psychiatric disorders. It may be, therefore, more acute than chronic and more reflective of transient stressful circumstances. If so, this would explain why we obtained a social causation outcome for otherwise psychiatrically well persons who reported many symptoms in this scale in the year prior to interview.

Social Selection More Important

Rates of schizophrenia were higher in the advantaged European ethnic group with SES controlled. This result would be expected if greater pressure from prejudice and discrimination on the disadvantaged North Africans functioned to hold down more healthy members of their group—as social selection theory would predict. The outcome for schizophrenia is not as empirically firm as the social causation outcomes for major depression, antisocial personality, and substance use disorders, including alcoholism, discussed above. It is, however, far from implausible.

One reason for caution is that the test may underestimate the role of environmental factors by our exclusive focus on the social environment (see Shrout & Link, Chapter 23, this volume). Physical environmental risks that may be related to low SES but not to disadvantaged ethnic status would have to be investigated separately. Some types of noxious conditions related to occupations, for example, could be such factors (see Link et al., Chapter 21, this volume).

There is also the problem that the symptom scale results on false beliefs and perceptions are not consistent with the diagnostic findings: North Africans score higher on this scale than Europeans. This appears to be due in part to an interviewer effect— North African respondents reported more symptoms on the scale of false beliefs and perceptions to European interviewers. However, there were no interviewer effects on the other symptoms scales, and this one seems counterintuitive. It was not predicted and may be a chance occurrence that does not replicate. In any case, as mentioned earlier, eliminating this possible bias on the scale of false beliefs and perceptions would not alter the social selection outcome because such a bias would have led, if anything, to an overestimation of rates of schizophrenia in the North Africans.

A second, more serious problem is the unexpected gender difference in schizophrenia, with men showing significantly higher rates than women. As mentioned earlier, this difference may be due to the fact that our respondents are all young adults. The onset of schizophrenia tends to be later in women than in men. The average difference appears to be 4–6 years (Hafner et al., 1989; Loranger, 1984). This indicates that our results for schizophrenia will be incomplete until we have been able to follow the cohort further through the age of risk.

Nevertheless, our findings for schizophrenia are consistent with those of Levav et al. (1987) based on their study of first hospital admission rates for all ages in the city of Jerusalem. Because the large majority of the schizophrenics in our sample were treated in psychiatric hospitals for their first episode of this disorder, the rates in the study by Levav and his colleagues were probably not seriously biased by selection factors in treatment, as is likely to have been the case with some earlier inconsistent findings that we obtained from studies in the United States (Dohrenwend & Dohrenwend, 1981). Moreover, results from case–control studies tend to show that adversity in the form of stressful life events is less important in schizophrenia than in depression (e.g., Stueve et al., Chapter 17, this volume), for which we obtained a social causation outcome.

We checked on whether the higher rates of schizophrenia in the Europeans could be explained by the exposure of many of their parents to the Shoa; we found no difference between respondents with such parents and respondents whose parents had not been exposed to Shoa. Nor could the greater exposure to combat of European as compared with North African men account for the difference. Finally, checks on refusals, emigrants, and dead members of the cohort sample through the Psychiatric Case Register did not reveal ethnic differences that would alter the general social selection outcome in the cohort sample.

CONCLUSION

There has long been controversy about social causation and social selection explanations of inverse relations between SES and psychiatric disorders. Although proponents of both theories have presented evidence and arguments to support their positions, no one has demonstrated previously that one position is more compelling. The present study offers a resolution, with findings strongly suggesting that the hypothesized processes differ in relative importance by diagnostic type.

These differences were masked when the quasi-experimental test was conducted for overall risks. Although overall rates are inversely related to SES, there were no statistically significant differences in overall rates according to ethnic status when SES was controlled. By contrast, there were sharp differences of considerable magnitude when individual types of psychopathology that are inversely related to SES were tested separately. For example, the adjusted odds ratios of disadvantaged compared with advantaged ethnic status ranged from 1.77 to 5.09, with most 3 or greater for the social causation outcomes.

We found that rates of schizophrenia are higher for respondents of European background with SES controlled, as would be expected if sorting and sifting processes function to hold down more healthy persons of disadvantaged North African background while leaving behind a residue of severely ill persons of advantaged European background. This outcome implies that social selection processes are more important than social causation processes in the relation between SES and schizophrenia. Could it be interpreted otherwise? It is difficult to think of an antecedent environmental adversity more common in high-status than in low-status ethnic or SES groups that would make a social causation interpretation of this outcome for schizophrenia plausible.

By contrast, holding SES constant, we found that rates of nonspecific distress or demoralization, of major depression in women, and of antisocial personality and substance use disorders, including alcoholism, in men are higher in Israelis of North African background, as would be expected if any increment in adversity attaching to disadvantaged ethnic status produces an increment in psychopathology. These results suggest that social causation processes are stronger than social selection processes in inverse relation between SES and these disorders. Is there a plausible social selection interpretation for this type of outcome? It

seems to us more reasonable, as argued earlier, that stage of assimilation process rather than genes accounts for disadvantaged ethnic status and, by extension, the low SES of most members of disadvantaged ethnic groups.

Although plausible, these outcomes are more complicated than the diagram of the social causation and social selection predictions shown in Figure 14.1. Most important, the ethnic difference in depression may be limited to women. This not wholly unexpected gender difference in depression, considered along with the opposite gender differences in antisocial personality and substance use disorders, is consistent with the possibility that there are gender-specific modes of reacting to adversity that affect the rates of different types of disorder that develop.

It will be recalled that the behavioral genetic strategies demonstrate the importance of heredity in most of the disorders we have been investigating. These strategies have not uncovered the modes of inheritance involved or located the genes that are responsible. The quasi-experimental tests we have conducted strongly suggest that environmental adversity related to low social status is important in the development of major types of psychopathology. Two lines of further investigation could test the firmness of these conclusions and pursue their implications. One would involve replications with different sets of advantaged and disadvantaged ethnic/racial groups in different assimilation settings; this would enable us to rule out idiosyncratic cultural/historical factors or idiosyncratic genetic factors that could affect results in a particular setting. The other would be intensive investigation of the specific stress and selection processes involved in relations among gender, ethic background, SES, and different types of psychiatric disorders. These matters are discussed further in the the two concluding chapters of this volume.

Acknowledgments: This research was supported by National Institute of Mental Health (NIMH) Research

Grant MH30710, NIMH Clinical Research Center Grant 30906, and NIMH Research Scientist Award MH14663. We acknowledge the invaluable collaboration with I. Rosenblum and others at the Public Opinion Research Institute of Israel (PORI) and with colleagues at the School of Public Health of the Hebrew University in Jerusalem and the Hadassah Medical Organization, especially E. Eisenberg, N. Turetsky, J. Magnes, and R. Lehrer. We also thank the following Israeli organizations and agencies for their generous cooperation: Israel Psychiatric Case Register, Israel Population Register, and Israel Defense Force. A number of Israeli researchers from outside the Hebrew University also provided valuable assistance and advice at various points in the research: Vered Kraus and Sammy Smooha, Department of Sociology, Haifa University; Yohanan Peres and Eli Ben Raphael, Department of Sociology, Tel Aviv University; S. Yavetz, Ministry of Police; Zahava Solomon, Israel Defense Force; and Israel's psychiatric institutions and social welfare agencies. We are grateful to L. Erlenmeyer-Kimling for consultation on genetic factors and to M. Reiff for computer assistance. A number of colleagues provided valuable criticisms of various drafts of this work: H. Hafner, D. Klein, N. Kreitman, D. Mechanic, and M. Rutter. The late Barbara Snell Dohrenwend had a major influence on this study; this chapter, like the book in general, is dedicated to her memory.

REFERENCES

American Psychiatric Association. (1980). *Diagnostic and statistical manual of mental disorders, 3rd Edition*. Washington, DC: American Psychiatric Press.

Anthony, J. C., & Dryman, A. (1987) *Analysis of discrepancy in lifetime diagnosis of mental disorders: Results from the NIMH Epidemiologic Catchment Area Program*. Paper presented at the September 1987 meeting of the World Psychiatric Association, Section on Epidemiology and Community Psychiatry, Reykjavik, Iceland.

Bebbington, P., Christopher, T., & Hurry, J. (1981). Adversity and the nature of psychiatric disorders in the community. *Journal of Affective Disorders, 3,* 345–366.

Bromet, E. J., Dunn, L., Connell, M. M., et al. (1986). Long-term reliability of lifetime major depression in a community sample. *Archives of General Psychiatry, 43,* 435–440.

Brown, G. W., & Harris, T. (1978). *Social origins of depression: A study of psychiatric disorder in women*. New York: The Free Press.

Burnam, A. M., Hough, R. L., Karno, M., et al. (1987). Acculturation and lifetime prevalence of psychiatric disorders among Mexican Americans in Los Angeles. *Journal of Health and Social Behavior, 28,* 89–102.

Cahalan, D., & Room, R. (1972). Problem drinking among American men aged 21–59. *American Journal of Public Health, 62,* 1474–1482.

Cobas, J. A., Balcazar, H., Benin, M. B., et al. (1996). Acculturation and low-birthweight infants among Latino women: A reanalysis of NHANES data with structural equation models. *American Journal of Public Health, 3,* 294.

Cohen, J. (1960). A coefficient of agreement for nominal scales. *Educational Psychological Measurement, 20,* 37–46.

Coleman, J. J., Blum, Z. D., Sorenson, A. B., et al. (1972). White and black careers during the first decade of labor force experience. Part I: Occupational status. *Social Science Research, 1,* 243–270.

Cooper, B. (1978). Epidemiology. In J. K. Wing (Ed.), *Schizophrenia: Toward a new synthesis* (pp. 31–51). New York: Grune & Stratton.

Crowne, D. P., & Marlow, D. (1960). A new scale of social desirability independent of psychopathology. *Journal of Consulting Psychology, 24,* 349–354.

Dohrenwend, B. P. (1966). Social status and psychological disorder: An issue of substance and an issue of method. *American Sociological Review, 31,* 13–35.

Dohrenwend, B. P. (1975). Sociocultural and social-psychological factors in the genesis of mental disorders. *Journal of Health and Social Behavior, 16,* 365–392.

Dohrenwend, B. P. (1990a). The problem of validity in field studies of psychological disorders revisited. *Psychological Medicine, 20,* 195–208.

Dohrenwend, B, P. (1990b). Socioeconomic status (SES) and psychiatric disorders: Are the issues still compelling? *Social Psychiatry/Psychiatric Epidemiology, 25,* 41–45.

Dohrenwend, B. P., & Dohrenwend, B. S. (1969). *Social status and psychological disorder: A causal inquiry*. New York: John Wiley & Sons.

Dohrenwend, B. P., & Dohrenwend, B. S. (1974a). Psychiatric disorders in urban settings. In G. Caplan (Ed.), *American handbook of psychiatry*. Vol. 2: *Child and adolescent psychiatry, sociocultural and community psychiatry* (2nd ed., pp. 424–447). New York: Basic Books.

Dohrenwend, B. P., & Dohrenwend, B. S. (1974b). Social and cultural influences on psychopathology. *Annual Review of Psychology, 25,* 417–452.

Dohrenwend, B. P., & Dohrenwend, B. S. (1976). Sex differences and psychiatric disorders. *American Journal of Sociology, 81,* 1447–1454.

Dohrenwend, B. P., & Dohrenwend, B. S. (1981). Socioenvironmental factors, stress, and psychopathology. Part 1: Quasi-experimental evidence on the social causation, social selection issue posed by class differences. *American Journal of Community Psychology, 2,* 129–146.

Dohrenwend, B. P., Dohrenwend, B. S., Gould, M. S., et al. (1980a). *Mental illness in the United States: Epidemiologic estimates.* New York: Praeger.

Dohrenwend, B. P., Levav, I., Shrout, P., et al., (1992). Socioeconomic status and psychiatric disorders: The causation-selection issue. *Science, 255,* 946–952.

Dohrenwend, B. P., & Shrout, P. E. (1981). Toward the development of a two-stage procedure for case identification and classification in psychiatric epidemiology. In R. G. Simmons (Ed.), *Research in community and mental health* (Vol. 2, pp. 295–323). Greenwich, CT: JAI Press.

Dohrenwend, B. P., Shrout, P. E., Egri, G., et al. (1980b). Measures of nonspecific psychological distress and other dimensions of psychopathology in the general population. *Archives of General Psychiatry, 37,* 1229–1236.

Dohrenwend, B. P., & Smith, R. J. (1962). Toward a theory of acculturation. *Southwestern Journal of Anthropology, 18,* 30–39.

DuMouchel, W. H., & Duncan, G. J. (1983). Using sample survey weights in multiple regression analyses of stratified samples. *Journal of the American Statistical Association, 78,* 535–543.

Duncan, O. D. (1968). Inheritance of poverty or inheritance of race?, In D. P. Moynihan (Ed.), *On understanding poverty, perspectives from the social sciences* (pp. 85–110). New York: Basic Books.

Dunham, H. W. (1955). Current status of ecological research in mental disorder. In A. M. Rose (Ed.), *Mental health and mental disorder* (pp. 168–179). New York: W. W. Norton.

Dunham, H. W. (1961). Social structures and mental disorders: Competing hypotheses of explanation. In *Causes of mental sisorders: A review of epidemiological knowledge* (pp. 227–265). New York: Millbank Memorial Fund.

Dunham, H. W. (1965). *Community and schizophrenia an epidemiological analysis.* Detroit: Wayne State University Press.

Eaton, W. W. (1980). A formal theory of selection for schizophrenia. *American Journal of Sociology, 86,* 149–158.

Endicott, J., & Spitzer, R. L. (1978). A diagnostic interview: The Schedule for Affective Disorders and Schizophrenia. *Archives of General Psychiatry, 35,* 837–844.

Faris, R. E. L., & Dunham, H. W. (1939). *Mental disorders in urban areas: An ecological study of schizophrenia and other psychoses.* Chicago: University of Chicago Press.

Frank, J. D. (1973). *Persuasion and Healing.* Baltimore: The Johns Hopkins University Press.

Fuller, W. (1975). Regression analysis for sample survey. *Sankhya O, 37,* 117–132.

Glazer, N., & Moynihan, D. P. (1963). *Beyond the melting pot.* Cambridge, MA: Massachusetts Institute of Technology.

Goldberg, E. M., & Morrison, S. L. (1976). Schizophrenia and social class. *British Journal of Psychiatry, 109,* 785–802.

Goldman, N. (1994). Social factors and health: The causation-selection issue revisited. *Proceedings of the National Academy of Sciences of the United States of America, 91,* 1251–1255.

Gruenberg, E. M. (1961). Comments on social structures and mental disorders: Competing hypotheses of explanation by H. Warren Dunham. In *Causes of mental disorders: A review of epidemiological knowledge* (pp. 266–270). New York: Millbank Memorial Fund.

Hafner, H., Nowotny, B., & Loffler, W. (1995). When and how does schizophrenia produce social deficits? *European Archives of Psychiatry and Clinical Neuroscience, 246,* 17–28.

Hafner, H., Riecher, A., Maurer, K., et al. (1989). How does gender influence age at first hospitalization for schizophrenia? *Psychological Medicine, 19,* 903–918.

Herrnstein, R. J., & Murray, C. (1994). *The bell curve: Intelligence and class structure in American life.* New York: The Free Press.

Hidiroglou, M. A., Fuller, W. A., & Hickman, R. D. (1980). *Supercarp.* Ames: Iowa State University Statistical Library.

Hollingshead, A. B., & Redlich, F. C. (1958). *Social class and mental illness.* New York: John Wiley & Sons.

Jarvis, E. (1971). *Insanity and idiocy in Massachusetts: Report of the Commission on Lunacy, 1855.* Cambridge, MA: Harvard University Press.

Kandel, D. B. (1980). Drug and drinking behavior among youth. *Annual Review of Sociology, 6,* 235–285.

Kaplan, M., & Marks, G. (1990). Adverse effects of acculturation: Psychological distress among Mexican-American young adults. *Social Science and Medicine, 12,* 1313–1319.

Kohn, M. L. (1972a). Class, family, and schizophrenia: A formulation. *Social Forces, 50,* 295–304.

Kohn, M. L. (1972b). Rejoinder to David Mechanic. *Social Forces, 50,* 310–313.

Kraus, V. (1981). Perception of the occupational structures in Israel. *Memagot, 26,* 283–294.

Leighton, D. C., Harding, J. S., Macklin, D. B., et al. (1963). *The character of danger.* New York: Basic Books.

Levav, I., & Aisenberg, E. (1989). Suicide in Israeli crossnational comparisons. *Acta Psychiatrica Scandinavica, 79,* 468–473.

Levav, I., Zilber, N., Danielovich, E., et al. (1987). The etiology of schizophrenia: A replication test of the social selection vs. the social causation hypotheses. *Acta Psychiatrica Scandinavica, 75,* 183–189.

Link, B. G., & Dohrenwend, B. P. (1980). Formulation of hypotheses about the true prevalence of demoralization in the United States. In B. P. Dohrenwend, B. S. Dohrenwend, M. S. Gould, B. Link, R. Neugebauer, & R. Wunsch-Hitzig (Eds.), *Mental illness in the United States: Epidemiological estimates* (pp. 114–132). New York: Praeger.

Link, B. G., Dohrenwend, B. P., & Skodol, A. E. (1986). Socio-economic status and schizophrenia: Noisome occupational characteristics as a risk factor. *American Sociological Review, 51,* 242–258.

Lissak, M. (1970). Pattern of change in ideology and class structure in Israel. In S. N. Eisenstadt, R. B. Yosef, & A. Adler (Eds.), *Integration and Development in Israel.* New York: Praeger–Pall Mall.

Loranger, A. W. (1984). Sex difference in age at onset of schizophrenia. *Archives of General Psychiatry, 41,* 157–161.

Mechanic, D. (1972). Social class and schizophrenia: Some requirements for a plausible theory of social influence. *Social Forces, 50,* 305–309.

Merton, R. K. (1957). Social structure and anomie. In R. K. Merton (Ed.), *Social theory and social structure* (pp. 131–160). Glencoe, IL: The Free Press.

Mortensen, P. B., Cantor-Graae, E., & McNeil, T. F. (1997). Increased rates of schizophrenia among immigrants: Some methodological concerns raised by Danish findings. *Psychological Medicine, 27,* 813–820.

Pulver, A. E., & Carpenter, W. T. (1983). Lifetime psychotic symptoms assessed with the DIS. *Schizophrenia Bulletin, 9,* 377–382.

Robins, L. N. (1966). *Deviant children grown up.* Baltimore: Williams & Wilkins.

Robins, L. N. (1969). Social correlates of psychiatric disorders: Can we tell causes from consequences? *Journal of Health and Social Behavior, 2,* 95–104.

Robins, L. N. (1985). Epidemiology: Reflections on testing the validity of psychiatric interviews. *Archives of General Psychiatry, 38,* 381–389.

Schwartz, S., Link, B. G., Dohrenwend, B. P., et al. (1991). Separating class and ethnic prejudice: A study of North African and European Jews in Israel. *Social Psychology Quarterly, 4,* 287–298.

Scribner, R. (1996). Editorial: Paradox as paradigm—the health outcomes of Mexican Americans. *American Journal of Public Health, 86,* 303–304.

Shrout, P. E., Dohrenwend, B. P., & Levav, I. (1986). A discriminant rule for screening cases of diverse diagnostic types: Preliminary results. *Journal of Consulting and Clinical Psychology, 54,* 314–319.

Sigal, J. J., & Weinfeld, M. (1985). Control of aggression in adult children of survivors of the Nazi persecution. *Journal of Abnormal Psychology, 94,* 556–564.

Spilerman, S., & Habib, J. (1976). Development towns in Israel: The role of community in creating ethnic disparities in labor force characteristics. *American Journal of Sociology, 81,* 781–812.

Spitzer, L., Endicott, J., & Robins, E. (1978). Research diagnostic criteria: Rationale and reliability. *Archives of General Psychiatry, 35,* 773–782.

Srole, L., Langner, T. S., Michael, S. T., et al. (1962). *Mental health in the metropolis: The midtown study* (Vol. I). New York: McGraw-Hill.

Thoday, J. M., & Gibson, J. B. (1970). Environmental and genetical contributions to class difference: A model experiment. *Science, 167,* 990–992.

Turner, R. J., Wagenfeld, M. O. (1967). Occupational mobility and schizophrenia: An assessment of the social causation and social se-lection hypotheses. *American Sociological Review, 32,* 104–113.

Watson, D., & Clark, L. A. (1984). Negative af-fectivity: The disposition to experience aver-sive emotional states. *Psychological Bulletin, 96,* 465–490.

Wender, P. H., Rosenthal, D., Kety, S. S., et al.

(1973). Social class and psychopathology in adoptees. *Archives of General Psychiatry, 28,* 318–325.

Yuchtman–Yaar, E., & Semyonov, M. (1979). Ethnic inequality in Israeli schools and sports: An expectation states approach. *American Journal of Sociology, 85,* 576–590.

15

Epidemiological Findings on Posttraumatic Stress Disorder and Co-morbid Disorders in the General Population

Naomi Breslau
Glenn Davis
Patricia Andreski
Belle Federman
James C. Anthony

Although there are numerous studies of posttraumatic stress disorder (PTSD) in special populations—primarily combat veterans but also rape victims and victims of other types of criminal violence and natural disasters (e.g., Alexander & Wells, 1991; Egendorf et al., 1981; Frank & Anderson 1987; Kilpatrick & Resnick, 1992; Shore et al., 1989) there are few studies on the PTSD sequelae of traumatic events in the general population. The prevalence of PTSD in the general population was estimated in two Epidemiologic Catchment Area (ECA) sites, one in St. Louis (Helzer et al., 1987) and the other in North Carolina (Davidson et al., 1991). The lifetime prevalence of PTSD as diagnosed by the criteria in the *Diagnostic and Statistical Manual of Mental Disorders (Third Edition)* (*DSM-III*; American Psychiatric Association, 1980), as measured by the National Institute of Mental Health

(NIMH) Diagnostic Interview Schedule (DIS), was approximately the same in these studies (1% and 1.3%, respectively) and was higher in women than in men.

Based on a survey of young adults conducted in 1989, we reported a lifetime prevalence of PTSD as diagnosed by the revised *DSM-III* (*DSM-III-R*; American Psychiatric Association, 1987), as measured by the NIMH Diagnostic Interview Schedule, Version III Revised (DIS-III-R; Robins et al., 1989), of 9.5%, 11.3% in women and 5.6% in men (Breslau et al., 1991). The higher prevalence we found might be due to the differences between the diagnostic criteria in *DSM-III* and *DSM-III-R*, or the difference in the age range between our sample of young adults and the ECA samples. It might also have resulted from a revision in the DIS approach to eliciting information on traumatic events and their PTSD sequelae. (A description of the revised version is presented in "Methods" below.)

By now, there is information as well on PTSD in the National Comorbidity Survey (NCS), a survey of a representative U.S. sample of 8098 persons, 15 to 54 years of age, conducted in 1991 (Kessler et al., 1994). The lifetime prevalence of PTSD in the NCS was 7.8%, 10.4% in women and 5.0% in men (Kessler et al., 1995). The similarity in the lifetime prevalence of PTSD between our study and the NCS is more coincidental than it might appear at first glance, because there were considerable differences between the two studies in the components that make up these estimates, namely, the lifetime prevalence of exposure to traumatic events and the prevalence of PTSD among exposed persons. Although the NCS found a higher prevalence of exposure than we did, it found a lower prevalence of PTSD among exposed persons.

All four general population studies reported that most persons with a lifetime history of PTSD had at least one other psychiatric disorder. On this count, they replicated reports from clinical samples, especially those of Veterans Administration (VA) patients (Green et al., 1989; Keane & Wolf, 1990; McFarlane & Papay, 1992; Sierles et al., 1983) and the report from the National Vietnam Veterans Readjustment Study (NVVRS; Kulka et al., 1990). In our study of young adults, 83% of persons with lifetime PTSD had at least one other disorder out of 11 specific affective, anxiety, and substance use disorders other than nicotine dependence (Breslau et al., 1991). The prevalence of one or more co-morbid disorders was the same in men and women with PTSD. The overall proportion of PTSD cases with co-morbidity in the NCS was about the same as in our study, although it was higher in men than in women (88% vs. 79%, respectively) (Kessler et al., 1995). The co-morbidity estimates from the two ECA studies were also above 80% (Davidson et al., 1991; Helzer et al., 1987). Studies in VA patients, as well as the NVVRS, have emphasized the high rate of substance use disorders in persons with PTSD. Studies of civilian samples of survivors of disasters and general population studies revealed a somewhat different pattern of co-morbidity, with depression and anxiety disorders predominating rather than substance use disorders.

The prevailing explanation for the high rates of co-morbidity in persons with PTSD is that substance use disorders, depression, and anxiety are complications of PTSD, caused by distressing PTSD symptoms. Alcohol and other psychoactive substances are believed to be used to self-medicate painful PTSD symptoms (Grady, 1990). It has also been suggested that PTSD symptoms may cause a reactive depression (Green et al., 1992). Little is known about the chronological order between the onset of PTSD and the onset of co-morbid disorders. One study (Davidson et al., 1990) reconstructed the chronology of disorders in two VA patient samples, using retrospective reports on the age of onset of lifetime disorders. Major depression, according to these data, occurred an average of 9 years after the onset of PTSD in World War II veterans and 4.8 years after the onset of PTSD in Vietnam veterans. Alcohol use disorder followed PTSD in World War II veterans but preceded PTSD in Vietnam veterans. There are no prospective studies on the risk for other disorders in persons with PTSD.

The top part of Figure 15.1 depicts the prevailing explanation of co-morbidity in PTSD, that is, that other psychiatric disorders are caused by, or are the sequelae of, PTSD. However, the lifetime association between PTSD and other psychiatric disorders might also reflect two other causal paths, depicted in the bottom of Figure 15.1: (1) the potential effect of preexisting disorders on the likelihood of PTSD following exposure; and (2) the potential effect of pre-existing disorders on the probability of experiencing traumatic events. Personal vulnerabilities, such as history of major depression, are recognized as factors that might predispose to PTSD, a notion reflected in the text of the *DSM-III* and *DSM-III-R* (American Psychiatric Association, 1980, 1987). However, it is generally assumed that PTSD-related events, such as violence, serious accidents,

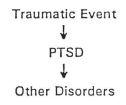

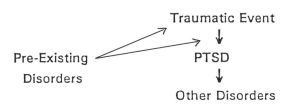

Figure 15.1. Alternative explanations of co-morbidity in PTSD.

or disaster, occur at random and are uninfluenced by individual differences.

In this chapter, we summarize results from our epidemiological study of young adults, which has been expanded into a longitudinal investigation with follow-up data gathered 3.5 years after baseline. The following three questions are addressed:

1. *Are persons with prior history of PTSD at increased risk for other psychiatric disorders?* Using our prospective data, we compare the incidence of major depression, any anxiety disorder, and alcohol and illicit drug use disorders during the 3.5 year follow-up in persons with and without history of PTSD at baseline. If we find no associations between PTSD and the subsequent onset of other disorders, then the plausibility that PTSD has caused these disorders will be severely diminished.

2. *Do pre-existing psychiatric disorders, specifically major depression and anxiety disorders, increase the vulnerability to PTSD following exposure to traumatic events?* This question could not be addressed in our prospective data because the number of new PTSD cases during the 3.5 years of follow-up was insufficient for yielding reliable answers. Therefore, we address the

question in the retrospective lifetime data, gathered at baseline, using survival analysis methods that take into account the age at which multiple disorders within individuals began.

3. *Do pre-existing psychiatric disorders, especially illicit drug use disorders, increase the risk for future exposure to traumatic events?* Evidence that history of psychiatric disorders increases the chances of exposure to traumatic events would account in part for the lifetime associations between PTSD and other disorders. Using our prospective data, we compare the incidence of traumatic events in persons with and without history of specific psychiatric disorders at baseline. We further calculate the odds ratios for traumatic events to self and to others, according to prior history of psychiatric disorders.

METHODS

A random sample of 1200 was drawn from all 21- to 30-year-old members of a 400,000 member health maintenance organization in southeast Michigan, which includes the city of Detroit and surrounding communities. A total of 1007 (84%) were interviewed in person in 1989. Follow-up interviews were con-

Table 15.1. Lifetime prevalence of traumatic events and PTSD in a sample of young adults (rate/100)

	Traumatic events ($n = 1007$)	PTSD in exposed ($n = 394$)	PTSD in sample ($n = 1007$)
Total	39.1	23.6	9.2
Sex			
Male	43.0	14.0	5.6
Female	36.7	30.7	11.3
Race			
White	38.5	24.3	9.5
Black	41.8	19.8	8.3
Education			
<HS	51.4	36.8	18.9
HS	43.4	23.9	10.4
>HS	40.3	24.7	10.0
College	32.8	18.6	6.1

ducted 3.5 years later, in 1992, with 979 persons (97% of the sample). At baseline, the median age was 26. Approximately 80% were white, and 62% were women. Psychiatric disorders, including PTSD, were measured by the DIS-III-R, which yields data on *DSM-III-R* disorders (Robins et al., 1989).

The PTSD section of the revised DIS opens with a question in which several typical PTSD events are mentioned, and respondents are asked whether any of these events has ever happened to them. The description of traumatic events follows closely the *DSM-III-R* text, using the examples it lists (e.g., "being attacked or raped," "being in a fire or flood or bad traffic accident," "being threatened with a weapon," or "watching someone being injured or killed"). A respondent's report of an event that does not fit the *DSM-III-R* stressor definition (e.g., severe illness, divorce, loss of job) is excluded from further inquiry, and the respondent is asked whether or not he or she has experienced another event of the sort described in the question. A report of a PTSD-type stressor is followed by questions about the occurrence of PTSD symptoms after the event. Up to three qualifying events are covered as to their PTSD se-

quelae. Information is elicited on age at exposure, the time of onset of symptoms, and symptom duration.

RESULTS

Traumatic Events and PTSD in Young Adults

The lifetime prevalence of exposure to traumatic events that qualify for the *DSM-III-R* stressor criterion in this sample of young adults was 39.1%. The lifetime prevalence of *DSM-III-R* PTSD was 9.2%. Table 15.1 presents information on the prevalence of traumatic events and PTSD by sex, race, and education. As can be seen, exposure to traumatic events was higher in men than in women and in persons with lower education than in college graduates. The lifetime prevalence of PTSD was higher in women than in men, reflecting the greater susceptibility of women to PTSD following exposure. Higher rates of PTSD were observed in persons with less than college education, especially those who did not complete high school, reflecting the combined trends for higher exposure and higher susceptibility to

Table 15.2. Lifetime co-morbidity of PTSD (% with other disorders) and sex-adjusted odds ratios

	PTSD (n = 93)	No PTSD (n = 914)	Odds ratio (95% CI°)
Major depression	36.6	11.0	4.4 (2.7–7.0)
Any anxiety	58.1	23.3	4.2 (2.7–6.6)
Alcohol abuse/dependence	31.2	20.5	2.2 (1.4–3.6)
Drug abuse/dependence	21.5	10.6	2.8 (1.6–4.8)
Any other disorder	82.8	44.3	6.2 (3.6–10.9)
Two other disorders	55.9	19.7	5.2 (3.3–8.10

°CI, confidence interval.

PTSD in persons with lower education (Breslau et al., 1991).

Lifetime Co-morbidity at Baseline

Table 15.2 summarizes the co-morbidity estimates ascertained at baseline. Percentages with lifetime history of specific disorders in persons with PTSD versus no PTSD are presented together with sex-adjusted odds ratios. The odds for all the disorders covered are increased in persons with history of PTSD, compared with persons with no history of PTSD. Major depression and anxiety disorders had stronger associations with PTSD than did substance use disorders. Of all persons with a lifetime history of PTSD, 83% had at least one other disorder, compared with 44% of those with no history of PTSD (Breslau et al., 1991). The prevalence of two or more additional disorders in persons with lifetime history of PTSD was 56%,

compared with 20% in persons with no history of PTSD.

Are Persons with PTSD at Increased Risk for Other Disorders?

Table 15.3 displays the 3.5 year incidence of specific disorders in persons with prior PTSD versus no PTSD. These results are calculated in six separate analyses, with each disorder considered alone. For each disorder, only those persons with no prior history were included in the analysis because our interest was in first-onset cases. PTSD was estimated to increase the risk for major depression 4.3 times. The odds for anxiety disorder and illicit drug use disorder were weaker and not significant, although in the direction of increased risk. The results for alcohol, which are not significant, suggest a protective effect of PTSD. If we consider anxiety disorders other than phobia, primar-

Table 15.3. The 3.5 year incidence of other disorders: Prospective data (n = 979)

New disorder	Prior PTSD	No PTSD	Odds ratio (95% CI°)
Major depression	21.0	5.4	4.3 (2.1–8.7)
Any anxiety	15.8	7.9	2.1 (0.8–5.3)
Alcohol abuse/dependence	3.2	5.4	0.7 (0.2–2.9)
Drug abuse/dependence	2.8	1.3	2.5 (0.5–11.8)
Generalized anxiety disorder	15.9	3.6	4.7 (2.2–9.9)
Nicotine dependence	26.2	8.7	3.6 (2.0–6.7)

°CI, confidence interval.

ily generalized anxiety disorder, the association with PTSD is similar in magnitude to the association with major depression. Nicotine dependence, a substance use disorder rarely examined, was found to be associated significantly with prior PTSD.

Is Exposure to Traumatic Events a Risk Factor for Other Disorders?

It has been suggested that it is not PTSD that is the cause of co-morbid disorders, but rather the exposure to the traumatic events that led to PTSD (McFarlane & Papay, 1992). We examined this possibility by comparing the incidence of disorders other than PTSD according to history of exposure. The results for major depression, any anxiety disorder, alcohol and illicit drug use disorders appear in Table 15.4. Persons who at baseline reported lifetime exposure to traumatic events but did not develop PTSD were only slightly different from those who reported that they had never been exposed, with respect to the incidence of other disorders during the follow-up period. The excess incidence of new disorders among persons exposed to traumatic events was concentrated in the subset with PTSD.

It might be argued that PTSD in exposed persons is a marker of more severe trauma and that those among the exposed persons who did not develop PTSD experienced less severe trauma, which is why they did not have a higher incidence of major depression or anxiety disorders. There is some evidence to suggest that the likelihood of developing PTSD varies by type and severity of stressors. General population studies suggest higher probability of PTSD associated with some types of trauma, primarily rape and childhood abuse (Breslau et al., 1991; Kessler et al., 1995). Among Vietnam veterans, those exposed to high war zone stress had considerably higher rates of PTSD than other Vietnam veterans (Kulka et al., 1990). The question remains of whether exposure to more severe stressors is associated with disorders other than PTSD. Data from the NVVRS on the prevalence of disorders other than PTSD are relevant to this ques-

tion. The prevalence of one or more disorders other than PTSD in all men exposed to high war zone stress, including a high proportion of persons who subsequently developed PTSD, was less than one-third higher than in all theater veterans (63.3% vs. 49%, respectively) (Kulka et al., 1990). The dramatic increase in the prevalence of one or more disorders other than PTSD among men exposed to high war zone stress was observed to be in the subset who developed PTSD (98.9%). A similar pattern was observed in women veterans (Kulka et al., 1990). Thus, in the NVVRS, as in our study, increased prevalence of other disorders was associated specifically with PTSD, rather than with exposure to the type of stressors that lead to PTSD.

These data suggest that other disorders might, in fact, be complications of PTSD because they are found primarily in those with PTSD, an interpretation that is plausible only if PTSD preceded the onset of other disorders. An alternative interpretation of the data is that PTSD, in addition to its association with the severity of stressors, serves to identify persons who are vulnerable to psychopathology.

Limitation of the Prospective Analysis Because of High Co-morbidity at Baseline

Although prospectively gathered data offer important advantages in risk estimates, their utility in this context is limited. The most important limitation is the already high comorbidity with PTSD at baseline (83%), a state of affairs that restricts our ability to estimate the risk for new disorders in persons with PTSD alone. Thus, for example, the estimated risk for major depression in persons with PTSD, displayed in Table 15.3, did not take into account the fact that persons with prior PTSD but with no history of major depression had higher rates of other co-morbidity, compared to persons with neither PTSD nor major depression, the reference group in that analysis. Although the increased risk for major depression during the follow-up might be due to pre-existing

Table 15.4. The 3.5 years incidence of other disorders by prior exposure: Prospective data

	Exposed, PTSD (%)	Exposed, no PTSD (%)	Not exposed (%)
Major depression	21.0	6.3	5.0
Any anxiety	15.8	9.8	7.1
Alcohol abuse/dependence	3.2	6.3	5.0
Drug abuse/dependence	2.8	0.8	1.5

PTSD, it also may have been influenced by history of coexisting anxiety or substance use disorders.

Although we are limited greatly by small numbers, we evaluated the incidence of other disorders in 15 persons with baseline history of "pure" PTSD, that is, PTSD with no other disorder. The incidence of each disorder during the follow-up period in the pure-PTSD group was not higher than in the reference group of persons with no history of prior PTSD. Of the 15 pure-PTSD cases, only 2 (13%) developed new disorders during the 3.5 years of follow-up.

Survival Analysis of Baseline Data

In light of the limitations of the prospective data, we took advantage of the retrospectively collected baseline data to examine the risk for other disorders associated with prior PTSD. Cox-proportional hazards models with time-dependent covariates allowed us to make use of the information on the age of onset of PTSD relative to that of other disorders. The results are presented in Table 15.5. Using models that included sex and race as fixed covariates and PTSD as a time-dependent covariate, we found significantly increased hazards ratios for major depression, any anxiety disorder, alcohol use disorder, and illicit drug use disorder following PTSD. Hazards ratios ranged from 1.8 for alcohol use disorder to 3.9 for any anxiety disorder. Thus, the results from the retrospective data provide stronger evidence than was found in the prospective data of an increased risk for other psychiatric disorders following the onset of PTSD.

Table 15.5. Hazards ratios (HR) for other disorders in persons with PTSD: Baseline retrospective data ($n = 1007$)

	Sex adjusted HR (p value)
Major depression	2.4 (.002)
Any anxiety	3.9 (.001)
Alcohol abuse/dependence	1.8 (.064)
Drug abuse/dependence	3.1 (.001)

Do Pre-existing Disorders Predispose to PTSD?

To examine the hypothesis that pre-existing disorders predispose to PTSD, we analyzed the baseline data on lifetime PTSD, using Cox-proportional hazards models with time-dependent covariates and sex and race as fixed covariates. The results appear in Table 15.6. As can be seen, pre-existing major depression and any anxiety disorder increased the risk for PTSD after exposure. The results for pre-existing substance use disorders are not significant, although they are in the direction of increased risk for PTSD. Other results of interest are that women were significantly more likely than men to develop PTSD (approximately 2 to 3 times), and that blacks were not different from whites with regard to the vulnerability for PTSD after exposure.

In additional analyses we estimated the relationship between major depression and PTSD, controlling for pre-existing anxiety disorder. This probe was necessitated by the frequent co-morbidity between major depression and anxiety disorders and the co-

Table 15.6. Hazards ratios (HR)° for PTSD following exposure by history of prior disorders (n = 394)

	Major depression	Any anxiety	Alcohol abuse/ dependence	Drug abuse/ dependence
Hazards ratio	3.3	1.9	1.6	1.2
p value	.001	.008	.133	.731

°Cox-proportional hazards, adjusted for sex and race, and with age of onset of disorder as a time-dependent covariate.

morbidity between PTSD and other anxiety disorders. In this analysis, history of anxiety was added to the model as a fixed covariate, dichotomized into prior anxiety versus no prior anxiety, in reference to age of onset of major depression. This approach was applied also to the analysis of any anxiety disorder as the independent variable, controlling for prior major depression. For the variable major depression, controlling for prior anxiety disorder yielded a slightly higher estimate of the hazards ratio for PTSD associated with pre-existing major depression. Controlling for prior major depression had no effect on the estimated risk for PTSD associated with pre-existing anxiety disorder.

Do Pre-existing Disorders Increase the Risk for Exposure?

Of the 979 persons on whom follow-up data are available, 187 (19%) reported exposure to traumatic events during the 3.5 years of follow-up. Using baseline data on lifetime history of psychiatric disorders and the prospectively gathered data on exposure, we estimated the risk for exposure associated with prior history of specific disorders. Table 15.7 presents the percentages with new exposure according to history of specific psychiatric disorders at baseline and shows higher rates of exposure associated with all but alcohol use disorder. Table 15.8 presents sex-adjusted odds ratios for new exposure associated with pre-existing disorders. Both major depression and any anxiety disorder significantly increased the risk for exposure. History of illicit drug use disorder was associated with a slight increase in the risk for exposure, but neither alcohol use disorder nor illicit drug use disorder was significantly related to future exposure.

Further analysis was performed to explore whether the effect of pre-existing psychopathology differed by *type of traumatic*

Table 15.7. New exposure by prior history of specific disorders: Prospective data

Prior history	n	% Exposed	p value
Major depression	133	27.1	.012
No major depression	846	17.8	
Any anxiety	260	23.1	.057
No anxiety	719	17.7	
Alcohol abuse/dependence	210	17.1	.415
No alcohol use	769	19.6	
Drug abuse/dependence	116	22.4	.334
No drug use	863	18.7	

Table 15.8. Sex-adjusted odds ratios for new exposure by prior disorders: Prospective data

	Odds ratio (95% CI[°])	p value
Major depression	1.7 (1.1–2.6)	.010
Any anxiety	1.4 (1.0–2.0)	.042
Alcohol abuse/dependence	0.8 (0.5–1.2)	.340
Drug abuse/dependence	1.2 (0.8–2.0)	.370

[°]CI, confidence interval.

event. Events were classified as events to self and events to others. Events to self included physical assault, rape, being threatened with a weapon, and a bad injury or accident. Events to others included witnessing someone being killed or injured and receiving news about a family member or close friend having been killed or badly injured. This classification overlaps with the distinction between personal and social network events used in previous research on stressful life events (Kendler et al., 1993). However, events to others in this analysis are not always network events, because they include witnessing violent injuries, accidents, or attacks to strangers.

Table 15.9 presents percentages with prior disorders in persons exposed to events to self and to others and Table 15.10 presents odds ratios for events to self and events to others associated with specific pre-existing disorders, controlling for coexisting disorders and sex. Exposure to events to self was significantly increased in persons with prior history of major depression. In contrast, exposure to events to others was un-

related to pre-existing major depression. The risk for exposure associated with prior anxiety disorder did not vary by type of event, and alcohol use disorder was unrelated to exposure. The event-specific analysis also suggested that prior history of illicit drug use disorder increased the risk for events to self, exposing a risk factor that the previous analysis on the combined events category had not revealed.

In a more elaborate model of exposure, in which social class indicators, personality traits, and prior history of exposure were included, both major depression and illicit drug use disorder were found to be associated with increased risk for exposure to events to self but not to events to others (Table 15.11).

DISCUSSION

The key findings of this study lead to several conclusions:

1. Persons with PTSD were at increased risk for first onset of other psychiatric disorders during 3.5 years of follow-up. The disorders with highest risk were major depression and generalized anxiety disorder. An increased risk for nicotine dependence was observed as well.
2. Based on lifetime data gathered at baseline, pre-existing major depression and any anxiety disorder signaled increased odds for PTSD following exposure to traumatic events.

Table 15.9. Prevalence of pre-existing disorders by type of exposure: Prospective data

Pre-existing disorders	Events to self (%) (n = 95)	Events to others (%) (n = 92)	Not exposed (%) (n = 792)
Major depression	27.4	10.9	12.2
Any anxiety	32.6	31.5	25.2
Alcohol abuse/dependence	22.1	16.3	22.0
Drug abuse/dependence	20.0	7.6	11.4

Table 15.10. Odds ratios for new exposure associated with specific psychiatric disorders, controlling for other disorders and sex

	Self vs. not exposed		Other vs. not exposed	
	Odds ratio	p value	Odds ratio	p value
Major depression	2.5	.001	0.8	.464
Any anxiety	1.1	.676	1.5	.093
Alcohol abuse/dependence	0.7	.196	0.7	.245
Drug abuse/dependence	1.8	.054	0.7	.477
Sex	1.3	.312	1.2	.478

3. The risks for direct personal exposure to traumatic events (events to self) during the 3.5 years of follow-up were increased in persons with prior history of major depression and prior history of illicit drug use disorder. In contrast, vicarious exposure (witnessing or receiving news about violent events to others) was not significantly associated with history of any prior psychiatric disorder.

The findings of this investigation can be generalized to the urban (inner-city and suburban) population of young adults in a midwestern region of the United States. Selected from the membership of a large health maintenance organization, the sample represents the socioeconomic range in the area, excluding the extremes of the distribution (primarily the uninsured poor). Differences in victimization rates across ge-

ographic areas, age, and income levels suggest that rates of exposure to typical PTSD events might also vary across different populations. National studies could further elucidate the effects of these social factors on exposure to traumatic events.

The results of this study shed some light on ways in which the lifetime associations of PTSD with major depression and any anxiety disorder, but primarily major depression, might come about. In contrast, they revealed little about the mechanisms that might have given rise to the lifetime association between PTSD and alcohol use disorder. A role for illicit drug use disorder in exposure to traumatic events was observed in the data as well, providing some insight into the lifetime association with PTSD.

The role of major depression in the PTSD–co-morbidity picture is multifaceted. First, prior history of PTSD increased the risk for subsequent major depression. Sec-

Table 15.11. Risk factors for new exposure: Odds ratios (95% confidence intervals)*

	Self (n = 95)	Other (n = 92)
Race (black)	2.9 (1.8–4.7)	1.7 (1.0–2.8)
Education (<college)	1.2 (0.7–4.7)	1.6 (1.0–2.8)
Extraversion†	1.2 (1.0–1.6)	1.1 (0.9–1.4)
Neuroticism†	1.3 (1.0–1.6)	1.2 (0.9–1.5)
History of drug abuse/dependence	1.8 (1.0–3.2)	0.6 (0.3–1.4)
History of major depression	1.9 (1.1–3.3)	0.7 (0.4–1.5)
History of exposure	2.1 (1.3–3.3)	1.6 (1.0–2.5)

*Results from two multivariable logistic regressions.

†Odds associated with a standard deviation increase in score.

ond, pre-existing major depression increased the vulnerability for PTSD following exposure to traumatic events. Third, history of prior major depression predisposed to exposure to traumatic events, specifically traumatic events to self. Major depression might have a direct effect on exposure to traumatic events by causing impairment in judgment, attention, or interpersonal relations. It should be noted that, although major depression is an episodic disorder, there is evidence that recovery from episodes of major depression is generally incomplete with respect to level of functioning. Even when symptoms remit, those with history of major depression manifest considerable personal and social impairment. History of major depression would be expected to predict events to self rather than events that occur to others and, as such, are less likely to be under one's control. Our results are consistent with this expectation. We found that major depression had an effect on exposure independent of other variables that predict exposure, including social class indicators, personality traits, and prior exposure. Furthermore, the prospective data allowed us to address an important concern, that is, that history of major depression might predispose to the reporting of traumatic events, rather than to actual exposure. By controlling for history of prior exposure to traumatic events, we controlled, at least in part, for the predisposition to report such events.

An effect of illicit drug use disorder on exposure to traumatic events was proposed at the outset of this analysis, based on the assumption that use of illicit drugs tends to be associated with a deviant lifestyle and involves risk-taking behaviors that extend beyond the periods during which the drug exerts its pharmacological effects. The results of this study support this proposition. The finding that alcohol use disorder was not associated with an increased risk for exposure might be explained by the sporadic nature of impairment resulting from intoxication. Behavioral tolerance to the adverse effects of alcohol might also minimize impaired function. Furthermore, in this sample of young adults, alcohol use disorder, as a rule, has not reached high levels of severity. It might be the case that among older adults, alcohol use disorder is associated with greater and more persistent impairment and consequently plays a role in exposure.

Our results suggest that personal vulnerability, such as personality traits or history of psychiatric disorders, does not exert its influence merely by increasing the odds for PTSD after exposure. The way in which it influences PTSD is in part by increasing the likelihood of exposure to traumatic experiences that lead to PTSD. Major depression appears to be one of several factors that influence exposure to trauma as well as to the psychopathological reactions that follow.

Acknowledgments: This research was supported in part by Research Scientist Development Award MH-00380 and by grant MH-48802 from the National Institute of Mental Health, Bethesda, MD (Dr. Breslau).

REFERENCES

Alexander, D. A., & Wells, A. (1991). Reactions of police officers to body-handling after a major disaster: A before-and-after comparison. *British Journal of Psychiatry*, *159*, 547–555.

American Psychiatric Association. (1980). *Diagnostic and statistical manual of mental disorders* (3rd ed.), Washington, DC: American Psychiatric Press.

American Psychiatric Association. (1987). *Diagnostic and statistical manual of mental disorders* (3rd ed., rev). Washington, DC: American Psychiatric Press.

Breslau, N., Davis, G., Andreski, P., et al. (1991). Traumatic events and posttraumatic stress disorder in an urban population of young adults. *Archives of General Psychiatry*, *48*, 216–222.

Davidson, J. R. T., Kudler, H. S., Saunders, W. B., & Smith, S. D. (1990). Symptom and morbidity patterns in World War II and Vietnam veterans with posttraumatic stress disorder. *Comprehensive Psychiatry*, *31*, 162–170.

Davidson, J. R. T., Hughes, D., & Blazer, D. G. (1991). Post-traumatic stress disorder in the community: An epidemiological study. *Psychology and Medicine*, *21*, 713–721.

Egendorf, A., Kashudin, C., Laufer, R. S., et al. (1981). *Legacy of Vietnam: Comparative adjustment of veterans and their peers* (Vol. V), New York: Center for Policy Research.

Frank, E., & Anderson, B. P. (1987). Psychiatric disorders in rape victims: Past history and current symptomatology. *Comprehensive Psychiatry, 28,* 77–82.

Grady, D. A. (1990). Epilogue: "A self-guide for Vietnam veterans." In R. Kulka, W. Schlenger, J. Fairbank, et al. (Eds.), *Trauma and the Vietnam war generation* (pp. 276–291). New York: Brunner/Mazel.

Green, B. L., Lindy, J. D., Grace, M. C. & Leonard, A. C. (1992). Chronic posttraumatic stress disorder and diagnostic comorbidity in a disaster sample. *Journal of Nervous and Mental Disorders, 180,* 760–766.

Helzer, J., Robins, L., & McEvoy, L. (1987). Post-traumatic stress disorder in the general population: Findings of the Epidemiologic Catchment Area Survey. *New England Journal of Medicine, 317,* 1630–1634.

Keane, T. M. & Wolfe, J. (1990). Comorbidity in post-traumatic stress disorder: An analysis of community and clinical studies. *Journal of Applied Social Psychology, 20,* 1776–1788.

Kendler, K. S., Neale, M., Kessler, R., Heath, A., & Eaves, L. (1993). A twin study of recent life events and difficulties. *Archives of General Psychiatry, 50,* 789–796.

Kessler, R. C., McGonagle, K. A., Zhao, S., Nelson, C. B., Hughes, M., Eshleman, S., Wittchen, H-U., & Kendler, K. S. (1994). Lifetime and 12-month prevalence of DSM-III-R psychiatric disorders in the United States. *Archives of General Psychiatry, 51,* 8–19.

Kessler, R. C., Sonnega, A., Bromet, E., Hughes, M., & Nelson, C. B. (1995). Posttraumatic stress disorder in the National Comorbidity Survey. *Archives of General Psychiatry, 52,* 1048–1060.

Kilpatrick, D. G., & Resnick, H. D. (1992). Posttraumatic stress disorder associated with exposure to criminal victimization in clinical and community populations. In J. R. T. Davidson, E. B. Foa (Eds.), *Posttraumatic stress disorder: DSM-IV and beyond.* Washington, DC: American Psychiatric Press.

Kulka, R., Schlenger, W., Fairbank, J., Hough, R. L., Jordan, B.K., Marmar, C. R., & Weiss, D. S. (1990). *Trauma and the Vietnam war generation.* New York: Brunner/Mazel.

McFarlane, A. C., & Papay, P. (1992). Multiple diagnoses in posttraumatic stress disorder in the victims of a natural disaster. *Journal of Nervous and Mental Disease, 180,* 498–504.

Robins, L. N., Helzer, J. E., Cottler, L., & Golding, E. (1989). *NIMH Diagnostic Interview Schedule, Version III Revised.* St. Louis: Washington University.

Shore, J. H., Vollmer, W. M., & Tahum, E. I. (1989). Community patterns of posttraumatic stress disorders. *Journal of Nervous and Mental Disease, 177,* 681–685.

Sierles, F. S., Chen, J. J., McFarland, R. E., & Taylor, M. A. (1983). Posttraumatic stress disorder and concurrent psychiatric illness: A preliminary report. *American Journal of Psychiatry, 140,* 1177–1179.

16

Exposure to "Fateful" Events: A Confounder in Assigning Causal Roles to Life Events

Lee N. Robins
Judith Robertson

ADVERSE LIFE EVENTS: THE SEQUENCING PROBLEM

Study of the relationships between life events and mental disorder is generally motivated by an interest in identifying adverse life events that serve as risk factors for mental disorders. Getting definitive evidence that life events are risk factors turns out to be difficult because, although it is easy to show that life events and mental disorders are related, it is difficult to decide which is cart and which is horse. The role of a life event as a consequence of disorder can be relatively clear when the employer who precipitated a job loss, the doctor who recommended hospitalization, or the spouse who sued for divorce directly states that his or her action was a response to behavior that is known to be a symptom of the mental disorder. The comparable claim by an affected person or his or her relative that an event precipitated the illness is viewed with more suspicion because people are known to be motivated to search for explanations of their misfortunes.

Recognizing the "cart versus horse" problem, some researchers have argued that only follow-up studies can definitively establish that adverse life events contribute to mental disorder. Follow-up studies can assess mental health at time 1 and consider as at risk of becoming mentally ill only those free of mental illness at the time 1 assessment. If more of those who experienced adverse events in the interval between times 1 and 2 are found to have a mental illness at time 2 than are those who did not, evidence for a causal role for life events is thought to have been provided. However, the follow-up design appears to have major limitations in resolving temporal sequences. First, mental disorders often have an insidious onset. Thus someone considered to be at risk because criteria were not met at time 1 may nonetheless have had a partial expression of the disorder at that time. When this was the case and an association between life events and disorder is discovered at follow-up, there are three viable alternatives to perceiving the life event as a risk factor for the disorder: (1) the life event was the result of

331

the incipient disorder, (2) the life event hastened the full expression of the incipient disorder without causing it, or (3) both the life event and the disorder were the result of some unidentified third variable. One could avoid including those with an incipient disorder from the group declared as at risk by requiring that no symptom of the disorder be present at time 1, but a second problem would remain—dating the independent variable. As Harris et al. (1986) have shown, some events have a lasting impact only if an equilibrium cannot be restored rapidly. Although the event itself, such as a parent's departure, may be easily datable, if its impact depends on how the remaining parent goes about reconstituting the household, is it the parent's departure that we want to date? Or is it the child's becoming convinced that the parent will not return, or the child's being moved to a relative's home?

Even if one knew how to define onset of disorder and the stage in the cascade of consequences following an event that marks it as having a long-term impact, follow-up studies would face a third problem: If disorder and event are correlated at follow-up, there may be no way to determine whether the event or the disorder came first during the interval other than through retrospection by the affected person or some observer of the follow-up interval. Retrospection at follow-up has the same cart versus horse problem that it has in cross-sectional studies, except that the period of recall is shorter.

It has been suggested that adding a second follow-up contact would avoid the problem of errors in recall. If the three contacts produced the pattern "Time 1: Well, no event; Time 2: Well, event; Time 3: Ill," the event would unequivocally precede the disorder, but that pattern will be rare. It can occur only when the time 2 contact is so close to the event that there has not been time for the event's effects to appear. Because many life events occur at variable times, and reactions to them are typically rapid, it would be pure luck to have the first

follow-up fall within that narrow window between the event's occurrence and the symptoms it caused. Thus longitudinal designs are no panacea; they often leave the sequencing problem unsolved.

A suggestion by Dohrenwend and Dohrenwend (1981) would seem to make solving the sequence problem unnecessary. They argued that the most defensible candidates for risk factors are events that by their very nature could not be caused by the individual's pre-existing mental illness, what they called "fateful negative events." Life events that fit this category would include most negative events occurring in early childhood, when the child still has little control over his or her experiences (e.g., departure of a parent). They also include those occurring later but that are beyond the individual's control (e.g., human-made and natural disasters, assaults or thefts inflicted by strangers, deaths and illnesses of loved ones, unemployment resulting from plant closings that eliminate all jobs regardless of worker performance, and exposure to combat). If these events are found to be associated with increased risk of mental illness, the mental disorder certainly cannot have caused the event to occur.

The issue this chapter addresses is whether the fact that the disorder cannot cause the event means that an association between the two indicates that the event is a risk factor for the mental illness. The possibility that must be considered is that, even if psychiatric disorder cannot cause the event, it may influence whether or not the individual is exposed to the event.

This possibility was underscored in our study of Vietnam veterans who had been enlisted men in the American army in 1970–1971. We studied the relation between combat experience and depression at 10 months and again at 3 years after their return from Vietnam (Helzer, 1981). Initially, finding an association between combat and subsequent depression seemed a perfect example of a life event over which individuals had no control leading to mental disorder. Not only was there a draft lottery operating at the time we studied Vietnam veterans, but the Vietnam war was spoken of as the war without a front, implying that every soldier was at risk of being fired on. However, the association between depression and combat almost disappeared when we controlled for the veterans' preservice deviant behavior, measured with many of the criteria for conduct disorder—school dropout, juvenile arrest, fighting, and substance use. We discovered that, despite news stories to the contrary, risk of exposure to combat was not an equal opportunity event for Vietnam soldiers. Infantrymen had the greatest exposure, while some Army enlisted men saw no combat at all. Soldiers in the infantry were often high school dropouts who had enlisted voluntarily rather than waiting to be drafted, presumably because, being unskilled, they could not find a civilian job. If they had stayed in school and learned a trade of use to the Army, they would have been back at the base camp serving as cooks, medical aides, typists, and the like instead of being in combat.

We learned again that exposure to events beyond an individual's control is associated with psychiatric history when we looked at psychiatric symptoms following exposure to natural and human-made disasters in an area of rural Missouri that suffered severe flooding and where dioxin was discovered in the soil in the winter of 1982–1983. Residents whose homes had been flooded reported more symptoms than those whose homes had escaped, but this difference was greatly reduced when we controlled for pre-disaster symptoms (Smith et al., 1986). We found an explanation: those exposed to the disaster were younger, poorer, less well educated, and more often separated or divorced, characteristics repeatedly found to be associated with psychiatric disorder. Presumably these individuals had greater exposure to floods because they more often lived on the flood plain, where homes were cheap. Thus exposure to both combat and natural disaster, two events that psychiatric illness cannot cause, was more likely among those with pre-existing psychiatric disorder.

FATEFUL EVENTS AND PSYCHIATRIC DISORDERS IN AN URBAN POPULATION

The study described in this chapter provides further evidence that "independent" or "fateful" events are not immune from concern about whether they precede or follow mental disorders when considering their plausibility as risk factors. We examined the association of a variety of life events with substance abuse and with the adult symptoms of antisocial personality, dividing these events into those thought to be consequences of these disorders and those thought to be independent. The disorders we studied almost always have their first symptoms in the late teens or early twenties, and the events we examined occurred *after* the age of risk of onset, and therefore cannot be the causes of the disorders. These particular disorders are well known to lead to experiencing adverse life events engendered by the poor occupational functioning and illegal behaviors that are the essence of antisocial personality and the consequences of excessive use of psychoactive substances. These disorders are also associated with poor interpersonal relationships, and therefore with marital failure.

If fateful events occur after a psychiatric disorder is already present, they are clearly not its cause and they cannot be its consequences, because, by definition, they are events unaffected by the individual experiencing them. Therefore, we have no reason to expect an association between *postonset* independent events and disorder. Yet the experience in the previous studies of Vietnam combat and disaster exposure suggests that associations *may* exist between disorders and "independent" events that follow them.

If such associations exist, we also must ask whether they continue once the disorder remits. Events that are not caused by a mental disorder should be as likely to occur when the disorder is in remission as when it is active, whereas events caused by the disorder should diminish when the disorder remits. To answer this question, we investigated the relationship between events occurring in the previous year and disorders present in the past but for which there were no symptoms in the current year.

METHODS

Source

The data come from Wave 1 and Wave 2 interviews with the St. Louis Epidemiologic Catchment Area (ECA) sample. They are restricted to a single site because many of the questions about life events were not uniform across sites. The methods used to obtain these interviews are detailed in Eaton and Kessler (1985).

Sample

The St. Louis ECA sample of 3500 adults was interviewed in 1981 and again in 1982. Subjects were representative of adults (over 18) in three mental health catchment areas. Because life events are more abundant at younger ages, and because forgetting might be a confounding factor in older subjects, we restricted the sample to the 1826 persons under 45, the cohort in whom antisocial personality and substance abuse and dependence disorders are more common. The age span is broad enough to include both active cases and a substantial number in remission. The St. Louis study oversampled blacks and those in institutions (predominantly jails and prisons in this age group). In most reports from the ECA, the oversamples are appropriately weighted to make the population representative of the areas surveyed. We did not weight respondents in this study because we were not interested in estimating the prevalence of either disorder or events but only their interrelationships. However, we did include the principal weighting elements in our multivariate analyses.

Variables

Disorders

We created a measure of the severity of substance abuse by counting the number of types of substances a subject had abused or was dependent on, according to criteria of the *Diagnostic and Statistical Manual of Mental Disorders (Third Edition)*. (*DSM-III*; American Psychiatric Association, 1980), among four categories: (*1*) alcohol, (*2*) marijuana, (*3*) heroin or cocaine, and (*4*) all other illicit drugs. We created a measure of severity of adult antisocial behavior by counting how many of the 35 questions asking about adult antisocial acts were answered positively. In order to be able to compare the two disorder scales with respect to their association with outcomes, we chose cut points for "absent," "mild," and "severe" in such a way that the two scales had nearly identical proportions in the three categories both for the total sample and for subgroups by age and sex (Table 16.1). This was achieved by dividing the substance abuse scale into "none" (70%), "one or two types" (26%), and "three or four types" (4%) and the count of antisocial behaviors into "fewer than 4" (72%), "4–9" (24%), and "10 or more" (4%).

We also created a combination of the two types of disorder (Table 16.1,C), and divided the combined disorders into active and remitted categories. Those in remission are defined as having had one or both of these disorders in the past but no symptom of either in the last year (Table 16.1,D).

Life Events

We examined both Wave 1 and Wave 2 interviews for items that could be considered to be life events and classified each event as plausibly having occurred because of the behaviors characterizing persons with antisocial personality or substance abuse or as independent of these behaviors. Events were then classified as "recent," that is, present at the time of interview or having occurred within the past year, or "not known to be recent." The data analysis is limited to re-

Table 16.1. Percentage of substance abuse and adult antisocial behavior in Wave 1 or 2 for 1826 St. Louis ECA subjects ages 18–44

Diagnosis	Total	Men	Women	Age <30	Age 30–44
A: Abused substances: number of types among four categories (see text)					
Absent: none	70	52	83	68	72
Mild: 1 or 2	26	40	15	27	26
Severe: 3 or 4	4	8	1	5	3
B: Number of adult antisocial behaviors (out of 35)					
Absent: <4	72	57	77	70	67
Mild: 4–9	24	34	21	26	28
Severe: 10+	4	9	1	4	5

C: Abused substances and adult antisocial behavior combined

	Total
Neither: both absent	57
Both: both severe	2
Others: either or both mild; one absent and the other severe	41

D: Current vs. past abuse of substances and antisocial behavior combined

Absent: never enough antisocial symptoms or substance abuse to trigger recency question	68
Previous: last symptom for both more than 1 year ago	7
Current: symptoms of either within the year	25

cent events when investigating whether relationships decline more for affected than independent events when the disorders remit.

Analysis

We first determined which life events are related to substance abuse or antisocial behavior. For those significantly related, we performed logistic regressions, including as independent variables four factors that could be confounders because they are associated with both life events and disorder and predate both. That is, they might be a cause of both disorders and events and thus responsible for a statistical association between them even if neither causes the other. These possible confounders are year of birth (age 18–30 vs. 30–44 in 1981), sex, race (black vs. others), and parent's occupation when the respondent was 16 [parent with an occupational score of 700 or better vs. below 700 on the *Alphabetical Index of Occupations and Industries* (U.S. Bureau of the Census, 1960)].

Next we examined whether the associations between substance abuse and antisocial behavior and life events cease when the disorders remit. For this purpose we selected that subset of persons with the disorders who had had no symptoms in the current year and compared the rate of recent life events experienced by those who previously had a disorder with rates for persons who had never had either disorder.

RESULTS

The substance abuse and antisocial personality scales' separate and combined associations with each life event initially were calculated by dividing the proportion of those with severe disorder who experienced the event by the proportion without disorder who experienced the event (Table 16.2). Persons with mild disorder were omitted. The fact that the relative risks are often higher for the combined disorders than for either substance abuse or antisocial behaviors shows that the disorders have independent effects on most life events.

The notable finding is that all adverse life events but one, whether from the "affected" or "fateful" list, were statistically significantly associated with severe adult antisocial behaviors and substance abuse, both singly and combined. The one exception, being on welfare, was an event from the "affected" list.

To be certain that these relationships were not spuriously created by the fact that both disorders and events were associated with the same demographic characteristics, we entered the count first of substances abused and then of adult antisocial behaviors into a logistic regression, along with age, sex, race, and parental occupation as independent variables, with each event as the dependent variable. (The "mild" disorder categories were included in these analyses.) *All* of the relationships between disorders and adverse events remained statistically significant, as shown in Table 16.2. Even receiving welfare was now positively associated with both types of disorder. Its previous inverse relationship with substance abuse and lack of relationship with antisocial behavior is explained by the fact that women are much more likely to be on welfare than men, and substance abuse and antisocial behaviors are predominantly male disorders. Once sex was controlled, there was a strong positive relationship between receiving welfare and both substance abuse and antisocial behavior.

Not only were all "fateful" events positively correlated with disorder, but their average level of significance and their risk ratio averages were only slightly lower than those of events known often to be consequences of these disorders (Table 16.3).

Although subsequent "fateful" events were associated with disorders in the same way and to approximately the same extent as events known to be consequences of the disorders, even when controlled for demographic variables that might have made the relationships spurious, it was still possible that other sources of spuriousness had been overlooked. One test remained that could make the association convincing. If the association between disorder and subsequent fateful events *were* spurious (i.e., could be explained by disorders and events sharing a common cause), then the association should not be affected by the *course* of the disorder. The relationship should not diminish when recovery from disorder occurred. Conversely, if the association was causal, and the disorder led to the "fateful" event, the relationship should diminish or disappear with recovery, as would be expected for events known to be consequences of the disorder.

To explore whether events known to be "consequences" were more sensitive to recovery than were "independent" events, we limited the analysis to persons without symptoms of either disorder in the past year. We then compared life events experienced within the past year by those who had had either disorder in the past with life events experienced by those who never had had either disorder. It was necessary to limit the events studied to those that had been dated as present at interview or as occurring within the year prior to interview to be sure that they occurred when disorders were *not* active. We had to require that *neither* disorder be active because, if we examined one disorder at a time, persons who had recovered from one disorder might have experienced the event because of the presence of symptoms of the other disorder.

The relative risks (calculated as before) were lower for persons in remission than they had been for those ever affected *both* for events considered "fateful" and for events known to be affected by disorder, although the drop was less dramatic for fateful events (Table 16.4).

Table 16.2. Relative risks of adverse life events in severe vs. absent disorder

	Relative risks		
	Substance abuse[†,‡] (*n* severe = 74) (*n* absent = 1270)	Antisocial[†,‡] (*n* severe = 90) (*n* absent = 1235)	Combined[†] (*n* severe = 32) (*n* absent = 1092)
A: Events Likely Affected by Disorder			
Occupation			
Fired more than once	9.0[a]	8.4[a]	10.0°
Unemployed 6 months in 5 years	1.4[a]	1.6[a]	1.9°
Lost job in last 6 months	2.2[a]	2.8[a]	2.6
Not full time	1.4[c]	1.6[a]	1.6
Residence			
Ever homeless	8.4[a]	13.8[a]	18.3°
3+ addresses in 5 years	4.7[a]	6.1[a]	6.4°
Moved last 6 months	2.7[a]	2.7[a]	3.1°
Finances			
Problems from overspending	7.4[a]	9.5[a]	18.7°
No medical insurance currently	2.5[a]	3.1[a]	3.7°
Sued, repossession in last 6 months	3.0[b]	6.0[a]	6.5
On welfare currently	0.5[b]	1.0[a]	0.7
Health			
Ever unable to work for weeks	2.2[a]	1.7[a]	2.0
Amnesia	8.4[a]	5.6[a]	13.7°
Marital status			
Breakup in last 6 months	3.0[a]	3.8[a]	4.7°
Currently divorced/separated	1.3[c]	1.9[a]	1.8
Legal status			
Incarcerated for 1 month or longer	16.3[a]	64.0[a]	78.0°
Arrested in last 6 months	11.3[a]	16.7[a]	29.5°
B: Events Considered Independent			
Health			
Hospitalized in last year	1.8[c]	1.4[a]	1.9°
Physical illness in last 6 months	2.6[a]	2.0[a]	2.2
Death and illness			
Household member sick/died in last 6 months	1.9[a]	2.2[a]	6.5°
Traumatic experiences			
Plotted against	7.8[a]	9.8[a]	12.5°
Robbed in last 6 months	1.9[a]	2.3[a]	2.4
Mugged in last 6 months	6.0[a]	12.0[a]	16.0°
PTS symptoms from			
Accident	4.0[d]	3.0[c]	4.0
Attack	5.5[a]	11.0[a]	17.0°
Threat	5.0[d]	6.0[d]	13.0°

°Substance abuse and antisocial symptoms additive or interactive, as shown by combination higher than either alone.

[†]As detailed in Table 16.1.

[‡]Significance of differences calculated by logistic regression, controlling for sex, age, race, and parent's occupation when respondent was age 16: [a]*p* < .0001; [b]*p* < .001; [c]*p* < .01; [d]*p* < .05.

Table 16.3. Disorders' average relative risks and percentage of events predicted at different levels of significance: Affected events vs. independent events—1815 St. Louis ECA respondents ages 18–44

	17 Affected events	9 Independent events
Average relative risks (severe vs. none or low)		
Substance abuse	5.0	4.1
Adult antisocial	8.8	5.5
Combined	12.0	8.4
Logistic regression, controlling for age, sex, race, childhood socioeconomic status		
Substance abuse (%)		
$p < .05$	100	100
$p < .0001$	76	67
Antisocial behavior (%)		
$p < .05$	100	100
$p < .0001$	100	82

Table 16.4. Does past disorder forecast recent fateful events?

Recent events	Past disorder[a,b] ($n = 123$) (%)	No disorder ($n = 1184$) (%)	Relative risk
Likely affected by disorder			
No health insurance	19	19	1.0
On welfare currently	10	10	1.0
Lost job in last 6 months	29[d]	21	1.4
Moved in last 6 months	28	24	1.2
Breakup with spouse/lover in last 6 months	20[d]	13	1.5
Arrested in last 6 months	5	2	2.5
Currently divorced/separated	25[d]	20	1.3
Sued, repossession in 6 months	5	2	2.5
Not currently full time	30	37	0.8
Considered to be independent of disorder			
Household member sick/died in last 6 months	12	10	1.2
Robbed in last 6 months	26[d]	19	1.4
Mugged in last 6 months	2	2	1.0
Hospitalized this year	19	20	1.0
Serious illness in last 6 months	11[d]	6	1.8

[a] Last symptom more than 1 year ago.

[b] Significance of differences vs. no disorder calculated by logistic regression, controlling for sex and age: [d] $p < .05$.

Table 16.5. Recent life events in 123 subjects whose substance abuse or adult antisocial behaviors had remitted vs. unaffected persons ($n = 1184$)—St. Louis ECA respondents ages 18–44

	9 Affected events	5 Independent events
Average relative risks (severe vs. absent)	1.5	1.3
Logistic regression, controlling for age, sex (%)		
$p < .05$	44	40
$p < .0001$	11	0

We then tested these differences with logistic regression, controlling for sex and age (we omitted race and parent's occupational status because they had been weak variables in the prior regressions, and the small numbers made it unwise to use many variables). Fewer than half the recent "affected" events and two of five recent "fateful" events showed a significant relationship with past disorder, and only one of these associations was strong (Table 16.5). Thus the two types of events appeared to be similarly affected by remission; when the symptoms remitted, the risk for both types of events dropped to a level only slightly higher than that found in persons who had never had the disorder.

DISCUSSION

We divided events measured in the St. Louis ECA into (*1*) those that would generally be considered to be possible consequences of the early-appearing disorders of substance abuse and antisocial personality—events such as poverty, marital disruption, poor employment history, arrest, being sued, and moving frequently or having no home—and (*2*) events that are commonly thought unlikely to be the consequences of disorder because the individual has no control over them—events such as being mugged, robbed, attacked, plotted against, or threatened; having a family member die or get seriously ill; and developing a serious illness or a need for hospitalization. This distinction between events the individual can or cannot affect has been offered as grounds for regarding the latter group as plausible causes of disorder, while the role of the former group is ambiguous and can be resolved only when temporal order is known.

Controlling for possible demographic confounders, we found that both categories of events strongly and almost equally correlated with psychiatric disorder. We also found that there was a marked decline in those correlations for both categories of events after the disorder went into remission. These findings for "fateful" events occurring after the disorder has begun are counterintuitive. The only plausible explanation would seem to be that, even when the disorder cannot have *caused* the event, it may have increased chances of *exposure* to the event.

With hindsight, it is not difficult to imagine why that could be so. If there is a genetic contribution to a psychiatric disorder, or if the disorder is associated with assortative mating, the chances that other household members will have the same disorder are increased. This in turn will increase chances that those household members experience events caused by their disorders. The affected index case will then be exposed to these events by virtue of living with these relatives or spouses, although his or her disorder did not cause the events. Another mechanism also can operate: mental disorders frequently affect capacity to work. Work disability leads to lower income, which in turn means living in worse neighborhoods than one's healthy peers. This puts the affected person at risk of a series of "fateful" events, including being a victim of crime. If the affected person is the head of the household, his or her inability to earn much also will make other family members poor, thus increasing their risk of illness and premature death. The affected person will thereby experience more deaths of family members.

Because mental disorder affects exposure to adverse events through these and other indirect routes, life events that cannot be *caused* by disorder may still not be entirely "independent" of disorder. Therefore, as attractive as was the idea that associated "fateful" events *had* to be causes because they could not be consequences, it does not solve the troubling problem of attempting to determine which came first—the disorder or the life event—when searching for etiological explanations of psychiatric disorder. There probably are events to which exposure is truly random, but each case must be considered on its merits. The fact that an association exists between disorder and events not under the victim's control is clearly not sufficient to guarantee a causal relationship.

Perhaps there is no sure way to distinguish life events that act as causes from those that are either consequences or to which exposure is facilitated by disorder in nonexperimental studies. The experiment with random assignment still serves as the benchmark for avoiding misinterpretation of correlations. It has rarely been used to demonstrate a causal relationship between life events and mental disorder because intentionally exposing persons to life events suspected of causing disorder is clearly unethical. The search for the etiology of mental illness remains a bootstrap operation of approximations and rethinking questions of plausibility with each association discovered.

REFERENCES

American Psychiatric Association. (1980). *Diagnostic and statistical manual of mental disorders* (3rd ed.). Washington, DC: American Psychiatric Press.

Dohrenwend, B. S., & Dohrenwend, B. P. (1981). Life stress and illness: Formulation of the issues. In B. S. Dohrenwend & B. P. Dohrenwend (Eds.), *Stressful life events and their context* (Monographs in psychosocial epidemiology, Vol. 2, pp. 1–27). New York: Prodist.

Eaton, W. W., & Kessler, L. G. (1985). *Epidemiologic field methods in psychiatry: The NIMH Epidemiologic Catchment Area program.* Orlando, FL: Academic Press.

Harris, T. O., Brown, G. W., & Bifulco, A. (1986). Loss of parent in childhood and adult psychiatric disorder: The role of lack of adequate parental care. *Psychological Medicine, 16*, 641–659.

Helzer, J. E. (1981). Methodological issues in the interpretations of the consequences of extreme situations. In B. Z. Locke, A. E. Slaby (Eds.), *Stressful life events and their context* (Monographs in psychosocial epidemiology, Vol. 2, pp. 108–129). New York: Prodist.

Smith, E. M., Robins, L. N., Przybeck, T. R., Goldring, E., & Solomon, S. D. (1986). Psychological consequences of a disaster. In J. H. Shore (Ed.), *Disaster stress studies: New methods and findings* (pp. 49–76). Washington, DC: American Psychiatric Press.

U.S. Bureau of the Census. (1960). *1960 census of population, Alphabetical index of occupations and industries* (rev. ed.). Washington, DC: U.S. Government Printing Office.

17

Relationships between Stressful Life Events and Episodes of Major Depression and Nonaffective Psychotic Disorders: Selected Results from a New York Risk Factor Study

Ann Stueve
Bruce P. Dohrenwend
Andrew E. Skodol

The notion that stressful life experiences contribute to psychopathology is hardly novel. Clinicians are routinely taught to inquire about recent events and interpersonal difficulties when treating new patients, and people readily explain their distress in terms of stressful experiences and circumstances. So it is not surprising that researchers, too, have focused on life events as a possible risk factor for psychiatric disorders and as a vehicle for understanding the social distribution of psychopathology. Yet despite the seeming obviousness of a relationship between stressful events and psychopathology, and despite more than two decades of research on this relationship, controversy persists about whether and to what extent life events play a causal role. Some conclude that life events play a substantial causal role in the development or recurrence of at least

some disorders (e.g., Brown & Birley, 1968; Brown & Harris, 1978); others argue that the evidence is too weak, limited, or problematic to warrant such a strong conclusion (e.g., Guze, 1989; Heston, 1988). Of course, the focus of discussion varies by disorder and the availability of evidence. In schizophrenia research, for example, debate focuses on whether there is any association between recent life events and the occurrence of psychotic episodes; in research on depression, where there is ample evidence of some association (e.g., Brown & Harris, 1978; Brown et al., 1986; Costello, 1982; Kendler et al., 1993a; Lewinsohn, 1988; Paykel et al., 1969; Surtees et al., 1986), debate focuses on the nature and importance of the relationship.

This chapter focuses on relationships between stressful life events and two categories of psychiatric disorders, major depression and nonaffective psychotic disorders. We present results from a case–control study carried out by Dohrenwend and colleagues in New York City (Dohrenwend et al., 1995; Shrout et al., 1989) and discuss these results in the context of other research. In doing so, we also review important methodological issues that have hampered understanding of event–disorder relationships and discuss our response to these issues.

Before describing our study and approach, however, we address a commonly heard critique of life events research. The importance of life events as a possible risk factor for disorder is sometimes minimized, if not dismissed, because [to paraphrase Paykel (1974), Guze (1989), and others] the kinds of events that predate onset typically are not catastrophic but fall in the range of usual human experiences—deaths of loved ones, loss of employment, marital separations, and the like—that most people negotiate without becoming ill. At first glance such an observation seems reasonable— until the same standard is applied to other relatively common risk factors and relatively rare outcomes. Take, for example, the still all-too-common behavior of smoking and a disorder such as lung cancer. Most people who use tobacco do not develop lung cancer, yet few would dismiss smoking as an inconsequential risk factor for this disease. Similarly, although most women who drink alcoholic beverages while pregnant do not deliver infants with birth defects, few would encourage such behavior. Stressful life events may never elicit a warning label from the Surgeon General, but the fact that most people weather adversity without developing a psychiatric disorder does not in and of itself rule out the possible importance of life events as a risk factor. With this in mind, we turn to our study and evidence regarding the relationship between stressful life events and two forms of psychopathology.

STUDY DESCRIPTION AND RATIONALE

The data come from personal interviews with 96 patients with recent episodes of ma-

jor depression, 65 patients with recent episodes of schizophrenia or other nonaffective psychotic disorder, and 404 community controls. Half ($n = 48$) of the depressed cases were in treatment for their first episode of major depression, as were one-third ($n = 21$) of those diagnosed with a nonaffective psychotic disorder. Patients were primarily recruited from inpatient and outpatient units of the Columbia–Presbyterian Medical Center and the New York State Psychiatric Institute (NYSPI). The control group was sampled from residents living in the geographic area where the treatment settings are located.

To be selected, cases had to have onsets of episodes within the year prior to admission to treatment. Diagnoses were made by psychiatric residents using criteria from the *Diagnostic and Statistical Manual of Mental Disorders* (*DSM-III*; American Psychiatric Association, 1980) and were systematically reviewed by members of the Biometrics Department of the NYSPI. The depressed cases met *DSM-III* criteria for major depression. The second case group met criteria for various *DSM-III* nonaffective psychotic disorders. The majority (30/44) of the repeat-episode cases met *DSM-III* criteria for schizophrenia; only a minority (6/21) of the first-episode cases were diagnosed with *DSM-III* schizophrenia, probably because of the criterion of 6-month duration of symptoms. Episodes were dated to their month of occurrence using clinical data and patient reports. Onset was conservatively defined by the earliest significant change in the respondent's usual behavior or functioning that could be attributed to the disorder. It is not possible to give completion rates for the patient cases because diagnoses and their date of onset were ascertained only after patients were recruited; we thus have no denominator within each diagnostic type. In general, very few refusals by patients were encountered.

Members of the control group were randomly sampled from households with telephone listings in the Washington Heights area of New York City. Households were screened to determine the presence of an adult between 19 and 60 years of age.

Table 17.1. Demographic composition of case and control groups: New York risk factor study

	Nonaffective psychotic disorders (NAPD) n = 65	Major depression (MD) n = 96	Community controls (CC) n = 404	NAPD vs. CC°	MD vs. CC°	NAPD vs. MD°
Gender (%)						
Female	52.3	74.0	56.2	n.s.	p < .01	p < .01
Ethnicity (%)						
Black	44.6	34.4	30.2			
Latino	16.9	26.0	27.2	p < .05	n.s	n.s
Non-Latino white	38.5	39.6	42.6			
Education (%)						
<High school	38.5	27.1	25.7			
High school graduates	49.2	50.0	46.0	p < .01	n.s.	n.s.
College graduates	12.3	22.9	28.2			
Marital status (%)						
Married	9.2	31.3	52.5			
Separated, divorced	38.5	37.5	22.5	p < .00001	p < .001	p < .01
Never married, widowed	52.3	31.3	25			
Mean age (yr)	34.2	37.0	39.2	p < .01	n.s.	n.s.
Mean father's prestige[†]	37.1	41.9	41.1	p < .05	n.s.	p < .05

[†]Prestige scores were assigned to fathers usual (or last) occupation.

°p level from chi square test for categorical variables; from *t*-test for continuous variables.

Ninety-three percent of the households provided screening information; 68% of the households contained an eligible member. Of the 943 eligible members, 57% (n = 541) were interviewed between 1980 and 1982. These respondents (like the cases) initially participated in a methodological study of psychiatric symptom inventories; they were subsequently recontacted and asked to participate in the "risk factor" study presented below. Of the original participants, 429 (i.e., 79%) were successfully reinterviewed. Community respondents found to have a current or recent (within a year) episode of a nonaffective psychotic disorder or major depression were removed from the control group, yielding a final sample of 404 persons (see Dohrenwend et al., 1986, for further details.)

We have conducted two checks on the representativeness of the community control sample: we compared the demographic characteristics of the sample with data from the 1980 U.S. Census for Washington Heights, and we compared reports of life events from the 33 respondents who were most difficult to recruit into the study with reports from the rest of the community sample. The results of these checks are reassuring. First, the demographic characteristics of our community sample are quite similar to those reported in the census when our procedures for ethnic stratification are taken into account. Second, the 33 hard-to-recruit respondents do not appear to differ in their reports of life events from those who were easier to interview. We assume that these hard-to-recruit respondents have much in common with respondents we were unable to interview and, therefore, that our obtained community sample is not seriously biased with regard to rates of life events.

Table 17.1 shows the demographic composition of case and control groups. Because case and control groups differed in a number of respects, the odds ratios reported later are adjusted for these demographic characteristics.

Although the study is not without limitations (see next section), two strengths of the sample should be highlighted. First, having two case groups lets us test the specificity of the events–disorder relationship and, in the case of positive evidence for one disorder and negative for the other, helps rule out poor measurement as the explanation of the negative result. Second, having first-episode cases is a distinct advantage because it lets us speak more directly to the question of etiology. In most studies repeat-episode cases almost certainly outnumber first-onset cases, unless a concerted effort has been made to recruit the latter. This may weaken the association between life events and episode occurrence if, as some have argued (e.g., Post, 1992, for depression), previous episodes increase the likelihood of subsequent episodes without environmental provocation.

Measurement of Life Events

Methodological Issues

Cases and controls were interviewed about a wide range of possible risk factors, including recent life events. Because the measurement of life events is critical to our analyses and to the conclusions that can be drawn, we describe the alternatives considered and the procedures implemented in detail.

The earliest and still most common procedure for measuring life events is the checklist method, in which respondents are presented with a list of event categories and asked which they have experienced during a designated time interval. As we and others have noted (e.g., Brown, 1974, 1989; Dohrenwend, 1974; Dohrenwend et al., 1987, 1993; Rabkin & Struening, 1976; Shrout et al., 1989), measurement problems associated with this procedure not only distort (and often attenuate) the association be-

tween life events and disorder but also cloud the interpretation when an association is found.

Two problems are particularly troublesome. First, the checklist method does not differentiate events of different magnitudes (Brown, 1989; Dohrenwend et al., 1987, 1993). Events recorded for a single category (e.g., death of a close friend, personal injury or illness) can range from trivial (e.g., death of a childhood friend not heard from in years, a bout of the flu) to severe (e.g., death of a confidant, diagnosis of a life-threatening disease). Insofar as there is a dose–response relationship between event magnitude and disorder, and insofar as small events are more common than large ones, such mixing of magnitudes both dilutes the association between events and psychopathology and reinforces the criticism (mentioned earlier) that precipitating events are only ordinary troubles tripping up highly vulnerable individuals.

The checklist approach also does not differentiate events in terms of their independence from the personal dispositions and behaviors of respondents; this, in turn, limits interpretations about the causal role of events (Dohrenwend et al., 1993; Rutter, 1986). The strongest evidence that environmental stress plays a causal role in the onset of psychopathology comes from events that are severe and whose occurrence is clearly outside the control of respondents—events that are highly unlikely to have been brought about either by the prodromal phase or insidious onset of the episode or by personal dispositions (e.g., genetic, psychological) that may also predispose to disease. Events that are at least partly the consequence of respondents' behaviors may still be part of the causal pathway, but they do not provide clear evidence that social conditions outside the individual contribute to psychopathology.

Three strategies have been developed to deal with these problems. One entails relying on the subjective assessments of respondents (e.g., Grant et al., 1976; Rahe, 1981; Sarason et al., 1978). For example, respondents are asked to rate such aspects as the stressfulness of the events they experienced and their control over the events. Unfortunately such assessments, although easy to obtain, are likely to be influenced by respondents' personal dispositions and psychopathology, thus confounding the measurement of stress with that of the disorder of interest.

A second strategy, the Life Events and Difficulties Schedule, was developed by Brown & Harris (1978, 1989). It entails collecting extensive information from respondents about the events they have experienced and then having these event narratives rated for their likely impact and independence by a team of researchers. Impact (i.e., magnitude) is rated in terms of "contextual threat," defined as the likely threat imposed by the event given respondents' personal histories and current situations. In making this determination, raters are instructed to disregard the actual distress reported by respondents.

Although the Brown and Harris strategy is a clear advance over both the checklist approach and reliance on respondent assessments, problems have been pointed out regarding both the rating of contextual threat and independence. As noted by Tennant, et al. (1981), the measure of contextual threat "combines events with other antecedent variables" (e.g., employment status, number of children at home, quality of the marital relationship) and consequently potentially "overestimate[s] the causal role of life events in illness" (p. 380). In addition, the definition of independence is usually limited to independence from disorder or its insidious onset; it does not include independence from the behaviors of individuals. However, the new 12-point scale developed by Brown and Harris does distinguish events that are, or are likely to have been, beyond the control of the individual.

The third strategy for measuring life events, the Structured Event Probe and Narrative Rating method (SEPRATE), was developed by Dohrenwend and colleagues (1993). An early version of this method was used in the study reported here.

SEPRATE Method of Measuring Life Events

The SEPRATE method of measuring life events is similar to the method used by Brown and Harris in that event narratives are rated by a team of researchers who are blind to the case status of respondents reporting the events. We differ, however, on how the events are elicited and on how magnitude and independence are defined and measured.

Both cases and controls were first asked about the occurrence of positive and negative events using a checklist containing 88 content categories plus a category for "other." Cases were asked about events that happened during the year prior to episode onset, controls about the year prior to interview. Like episode onsets, events were dated to their month of occurrence. As a result, there is slippage in our measurement of the temporal proximity of events to episode onset for cases and date of interview for controls. For example, an individual experiencing an onset in late September and an event in early August, and an individual experiencing an onset in early September and an event in late August are both coded as reporting an event during the month prior to episode.

Once events were elicited and dated, respondents were asked for more detail about negative events. Priority was given to events for which the respondent was the central figure; negative events occurring to significant others and positive events were probed only if the respondent reported fewer than six events. We took the event descriptions provided by respondents, stripped them of information that might reveal their case status or social characteristics (other than gender), and had our research team rate each event narrative on several dimensions.

Three ratings were used to measure the construct of independence, or what we refer to as the *fatefulness* of the event. Events were rated for the extent to which respondents' behaviors influenced either the sequence of transactions leading to the event or the event's actual occurrence. In addition, an overall judgment was made of the like- lihood that personal dispositions influenced the occurrence of the event. Events were defined as "fateful" if both the sequence of transactions leading to the event and its ac- tual occurrence were rated as mostly or completely outside the control of the re- spondent and as almost certainly indepen- dent of his or her personal dispositions.

The *magnitude* of events was evaluated in terms of the amount of change in usual ac- tivities entailed by the event. For fateful events we used a normative rating; specifi- cally, we rated "the amount of change in usual activities the average person encoun- tering such an event would be likely to ex- perience." We used the normative rating to avoid confounding the assessment of event magnitude with differences in coping ability that could affect the actual amount of change reported. For nonfateful events we used a less ideal measure: we rated the ac- tual amount of change reported in the nar- rative. For events involving physical illness or injury to the respondent, we substituted physicians' ratings of seriousness for the change ratings. These illness severity ratings were modeled after procedures developed by Wyler et al. (1968).

We divided negative events into three cat- egories of magnitude: (*1*) *major* negative events involving more than moderate change (i.e., mean score > 2 on a scale of 0 to 4 points); (*2*) *minor* negative events in- volving no change or less than a little change (i.e., mean score < 1); and (*3*) *moderate* neg- ative events that are intermediate. Physical illnesses and injuries with ratings above 334, the median, on the modified Wyler index were included as major negative events; those rated 334 or below were included in the moderate category.

Recall and Reporting Issues

Although the SEPRATE procedures go far toward increasing our confidence in the measurement of event exposure, there is still the possibility of recall and reporting bi- ases. Even in longitudinal studies, the re- ports of life events are retrospective, with

time intervals ranging from a week to more than a year. The retrospective nature of re- porting is important because it can lead to either underreporting or overreporting of events by cases relative to controls (see Norman & Malla, 1993).

On the one hand, both cognitive impair- ments (e.g., active psychotic symptoms) and, in case–control studies such as ours, the longer recall period for cases (i.e., year prior to episode onset rather than year prior to interview) potentially lead to an underre- porting of events on the part of cases. On the other hand, cases may be more likely to overreport events either because they are more likely than controls to be demoralized at the time of interview [negative material tends to be recalled more frequently by those in negative moods (Blaney, 1986; Cohen et al., 1988)] or because cases are more likely to engage in "effort after mean- ing" (see Brown, 1974), that is, to be ac- tively searching for explanations for their episode, onset, or both. Processes leading to overreporting by cases are more problem- atic than those leading to underreporting because overreporting biases in favor of the event–disorder hypothesis.

To address the possibility of differential recall by respondents in the case and com- parison groups, we controlled for negative affect at the time of interview, using the 27- item Demoralization Scale from the Psychi- atric Epidemiology Research Interview (Dohrenwend et al., 1980). Items in this scale ask about demoralized mood during the prior 6 months and thus tap negative affect at or close to the time of the inter- view. We could not directly address the problem of "effort after meaning"; however, we examined case–control differences in the temporal patterning of reported events for evidence that cases are pulling events forward in time.

Measurement of Other Risk Factors

Many other facets of the stress process, in- cluding respondents' location in the social structure, ongoing situation, and personal dispositions, were included in the study

(Dohrenwend et al., 1995). In addition to the demographic variables listed in Table 17.1, we included family history of psychiatric disorder, presence of a confidant, and mastery orientation in some of the analyses reported here. Each is a hypothesized risk factor for major depression, nonaffective psychotic disorders, or both and thus serves as a possible benchmark for assessing the relative importance of life events. Also, there is evidence that genetic factors influence the occurrence of some types of events as well as psychiatric disorders (Kendler et al., 1993b; Plomin et al., 1990; see also Chapter 26, this volume). We included family history of disorder to provide some control for this potentially confounding effect. Although family history of disorder can indicate environmental as well as genetic transmission, it is our best measure of genetic vulnerability.

Our measures of family history of psychiatric disorder are based on reports given by respondents about the psychiatric problems of their first-degree relatives. Respondents were asked to list their first-degree relatives and to indicate whether any had ever had "serious mental or emotional problems such as problems with depression, suicide attempts, odd or violent behavior, or difficulties with drugs or alcohol." For each positive answer, respondents were asked to name "the specific mental or emotional problem(s) that the relative(s) had" and whether the relative was "ever in a hospital" for the specific problem. Two psychiatrists rated these reports on each relative for the likely presence of a psychiatric disorder (kappa = .71) (Dohrenwend et al., 1986). Five dichotomous measures were constructed: a global measure indicating the presence of one or more (versus no) first-degree relatives with a history of psychiatric disorder, and four more specific measures indicating the presence of one or more first-degree relatives with a psychiatric disorder involving psychotic symptoms, affective symptoms, alcoholism, or antisocial behavior.

Mastery orientation was assessed using a subset of items from the Personal Attributes Questionnaire developed by Spence and Helmreich (1978). In our sample, the internal consistency reliability is .82 for patients diagnosed with a nonaffective psychotic disorder, .73 for patients with a diagnosis of major depression, and .68 for the control group.

Finally, our measure of confidant status is modeled after work by Brown and colleagues (Brown & Harris, 1978; Brown et al., 1986). Married respondents are defined as having a confidant if they report turning to their mates to discuss personal worries or important decisions and also name their mates as the people they felt closest to last year. Unmarried respondents are defined as having a confidant if they live with or speak with someone weekly who meets the same criteria.

RESULTS: MAJOR DEPRESSION

The Role of Fateful Negative Life Events

As mentioned above, the strongest test of whether recent life events play an important role as environmental risk factors for psychopathology centers on major fateful negative events. These events occur independently of the individual's behavior and would likely entail substantial disruptions in the lives of most individuals who experience them. However, before investigating whether such events are associated with the onset of major depression, we addressed a prior question: What is the relevant risk period? Whereas most studies have focused on a time interval ranging from 6 to 12 months as the period of interest (see review in Brown & Harris, 1989), there is evidence that events tend to cluster in the few weeks prior to onset (Brown & Harris, 1989; Emmerson et al., 1989; Surtees et al., 1986). Consistent with the literature, we began with a 1 year period and then look for evidence of greater temporal proximity.

As Table 17.2 shows, individuals diagnosed with recent episodes of major depression were significantly more likely than controls to report one or more major fateful

Table 17.2. Depression–control differences in exposure to one or more fateful negative events (1 year approx.): percentages and adjusted exposure odds ratios[†]

Event magnitude	% Reporting one or more events		Major depression vs. community controls	
	Major depression (n = 96)	Community controls (n = 404)	Adjusted odds ratio	95% confidence interval
Major	25.0	10.4	3.04°°°	1.66, 5.56
Major & moderate	49.0	29.0	2.38°°°	1.48, 3.83
Major & moderate & minor	56.3	44.3	1.66°	1.03, 2.66

[†]Adjusted for age, sex, ethnicity, education, marital status, father's prestige, and father's prestige × ethnicity (Hispanic).

°$p < .05$; °°°$p < .001$.

negative events during the 1 year risk period (adjusted odds ratio = 3.04). The odds ratios decreased when moderate fateful events were added to major fateful and decreased again when major, moderate, and minor events were combined. When we look at the three categories of magnitude separately (results not shown), only major fateful events have an effect (adjusted odds ratio = 3.07, $p < .001$). The pattern of results remains unchanged when negative affect at time of interview is controlled, although the odds ratios decrease. The same pattern holds when first-episode cases are compared with controls (not shown), providing stronger evidence for an etiological effect.

A 1 year risk period may be excessively long, however. In order to examine the temporal relationship between stressful events and the onset of depressive episodes, we broke the 1 year risk period into several segments—1 month before onset/interview, 2–3 months, 4–6 months, 7–9 months, and 10–12 months—and ran a logistic regression with case–control status as the outcome and with exposure to one or more major fateful negative events during each temporal segment as predictors. As Table 17.3 indicates, there appears to be an excess of major fateful negative events during the 3 months prior to episode onset and especially during the most proximate month. We

Table 17.3. Temporal proximity of major fateful negative events and episode onset—depression–control differences in event exposures throughout the year prior to episode onset (cases)/interview (controls): percentages and adjusted odds ratios[†]

Proximity of event to episode onset or interview	% Reporting 1 or more major fateful negative events		Major depression vs. community controls	
	Major depression (n = 96)	Community controls (n = 404)	Adjusted odds ratio	95% confidence interval
Within ~1 month	11.5	0.7	22.21°°°	5.50, 89.62
~2–3 Months	4.2	1.0	6.99°	1.56, 31.29
~4–6 Months	0	2.2	0	0.00, >1 mil
~7–9 Months	4.2	4.2	0.78	0.23, 2.69
~10–12 Months	7.3	2.5	3.21°	1.72, 9.84

[†]Adjusted for age, sex, ethnicity, education, marital status, father's prestige, and father's prestige × ethnicity (Hispanic).

°$p < .05$; °°°$p < .001$.

see the same pattern when first- and repeat-episode cases are separately compared with controls; that is, at least with our sample of treated cases, the risk period is similar for first-onset and recurrent depressive episodes (results not shown).

Next we considered whether the association between recent major fateful negative events and depressive episodes is spurious. Are there personal attributes or dispositions that both increase one's risk for major depressive episodes and make one more prone to encounter stressful life events? Although we tried to diminish this possibility by applying a stringent definition of fatefulness, we also introduced four potential confounders into the analysis: presence of one or more family members with a history of affective disorder, presence of one or more family members with a history of other psychiatric disorders (i.e., psychotic symptoms, antisocial behavior, or alcoholism), the personality attribute of mastery, and our measure of negative affect (a large component of which we believe is trait neuroticism).

Adding these variables does not explain the greater tendency of individuals diagnosed with major depression to report one or more major fateful negative events during the 3 months prior to episode. Controlling for family history of affective and other psychiatric disorders, mastery, negative affect, and a host of demographic characteristics, patients were almost 14 times (adjusted odds ratio = 13.8) more likely to report a major fateful negative event during the 3 months prior to episode than were community controls to report such an event during the 3 months prior to interview. We repeated this analysis with first- and repeat-episode cases separately with similar results.

Finally, we considered the relative importance of major fateful negative life events as a risk factor for depression. That is, how does the effect size for stressful events compare with other risk factors? Here we ran a series of logistic regression analyses in which we pitted major fateful events against other risk factors, including family history of affective disorder, low mastery orientation, and absence of a confidant. Whereas re-

spondents reporting a recent (within 3 months) major fateful event were about 14 times more likely to be a depressed patient in our sample, the comparable odds ratio was 3.5 for having any first-degree relative with a history of affective disorder ($p < .0001$), about 1.8 for absence of a confidant ($p < .05$), and about 7 for low mastery (comparing those in the bottom vs. top quartile on the mastery index using the community sample to define the cut points). Although we acknowledge that the association between these other risk factors and depression might have been higher had we had equally good measures of our competing risk factors, nonetheless, like Kendler et al. (1993a), we find recent stressful life events to be a strong predictor of liability to episodes of major depression, and we do so using a far more convincing measure of environmental adversity.

Role of Nonfateful Negative Life Events

We repeated the above analyses for nonfateful negative events. These events were clearly or possibly influenced by the personality and behavior of our study participants, and as a result provide less clear-cut evidence for a causal relationship between adversity and psychopathology.

Our results largely parallel those for fateful events. As Table 17.4 shows, cases were more likely than controls to report exposure to one or more major nonfateful negative events during the 1 year risk period, with and without the control for negative affectivity (latter results not shown). There was also a dose−response relationship with respect to event magnitude. The odds ratios decreased when moderate nonfateful events were added to major nonfateful and decreased again when major, moderate, and minor events were combined. As with fateful events, the pattern holds when first-episode cases are compared with controls.

Table 17.5 shows the temporal relationship between exposure to major nonfateful negative events and the occurrence of depressive episodes. Again, we found an excess

Table 17.4. Depression–control differences in exposure to one or more nonfateful negative events (1 year approx.): percentages and adjusted exposure odds ratios[†]

Event magnitude	% Reporting 1 or more events		Major depression vs. community controls	
	Major depression (n = 96)	Community controls (n = 404)	Adjusted odds ratio	95% confidence interval
Major	36.5	12.4	4.67°°°	2.68, 8.14
Major & moderate	65.6	37.9	3.25°°°	1.95, 5.44
Major & moderate & minor	68.8	47.0	2.49°°°	1.48, 4.21

[†]Adjusted for age, sex, ethnicity, education, marital status, father's prestige, and father's prestige × ethnicity (Hispanic).

°°°$p < .001$.

of events during the month prior to episode for cases but no excess of events reported by cases during the 2–3 months prior to episode. In general, there was a stronger relationship between recent major fateful negative events and episodes of depression than between recent major nonfateful negative events and this form of psychopathology (see Tables 17.3 and 17.5). Again, the temporal relationship between exposure to major nonfateful events and episode onset is repeated when first-episode cases are compared with community residents (results not shown).

Finally, the relationship between exposure to recent (within 3 months) major nonfateful events and case status is not explained by self-reported family history of affective disorders, family history of other psychiatric disorders, mastery orientation, or demoralization at the time of interview. Also, as with exposure to recent major fateful events, the effect size for recent major nonfateful events generally equals or exceeds that for family history of psychiatric disorder, lack of a confidant, and low mastery.

Summary

Both the case group as a whole and the subset of cases experiencing their first episode of major depression were more likely than members of the control group to have ex-

Table 17.5. Temporal proximity of major nonfateful negative events and episode onset—depression–control differences in event exposures throughout the year prior to episode onset (cases)/interview (controls): percentages and adjusted odds ratios[†]

Proximity of event to episode onset or interview	% Reporting 1 or more major nonfateful negative events		Major depression vs. community controls	
	Major depression (n = 96)	Community controls (n = 404)	Adjusted odds ratio	95% confidence interval
Within ~1 month	10.4	1.0	10.22°°°	2.89, 36.11
~2–3 Months	5.2	2.5	2.39	0.64, 8.98
~4–6 Months	9.4	4.2	1.30	0.48, 3.53
~7–9 Months	9.4	3.5	2.45	0.90, 6.61
~10–12 Months	12.5	3.7	4.14°°	1.71, 10.01

[†]Adjusted for age, sex, ethnicity, education, marital status, father's prestige, and father's prestige × ethnicity (Hispanic).

°°$p < .01$; °°°$p < .001$.

perienced major fateful events during the 1 year and 3 month risk periods. Insofar as environmental adversity is measured by major fateful negative events, our results are consistent with the hypothesis that environmental adversity contributes to the development and recurrence of major depressive episodes. Our results also indicate that other highly disruptive negative events, although less pure indicators of environmental adversity, are associated with severe depressive symptomatology.

OVERVIEW AND RESULTS: NONAFFECTIVE PSYCHOTIC DISORDERS

Overview of the Issues

Although clinical observations suggest that stressful events may precipitate episodes of schizophrenia, epidemiological evidence for this event–disorder association is limited. In the late 1960s, Brown and Birley (1968; Birley & Brown, 1970) presented results suggesting that stressful life events may contribute to the development and recurrence of schizophrenic disorder, based on data from 50 patients and a control group of 325 employees of six local firms. Specifically, they found that cases were more likely to have experienced an independent event during the 3 weeks prior to onset than were control group members during the 3 weeks prior to interview. Moreover, they reported that episode status made no difference; the result held for first- and repeat-episode cases. They also found that rates of nonindependent events tended to be higher among cases throughout the 13 week period investigated.

Since this early and pivotal study, there have been several attempts at replication and extension. We located six case–control studies that compare patients with samples of nonpatient controls (Al Khani et al., 1986; Bebbington et al., 1993; Chung et al., 1986; Gureje & Adewunmi, 1988; Jacobs & Myers, 1976; Malzacher et al., 1981) and eight other studies that, although lacking nonpatient control groups, either compare relapsing with nonrelapsing patients or compare patients with themselves at different periods of time (Day et al., 1987; Hardesty et al., 1985; Hirsch et al., 1993; Leff et al., 1973, 1983; Malla et al., 1990; Ventura et al., 1989, 1993). These studies by and large have not replicated the results reported by Brown and Birley. Although most report statistically significant elevations of at least some types of events in at least some subgroups for some risk period (although typically with no adjustments for multiple comparisons), it is rarely clear that severe events, much less severe events that are independent of personal dispositions, play an etiological role. Only three studies report results for first-episode cases, and none finds evidence for a causal relationship. Two (Malzacher et al., 1981; Gureje & Adewunmi, 1988) report no differences in event exposure between first-episode cases and the control group; the third (Al Khani et al., 1986) reports that repeat-episode cases, not first-onset cases, experienced significantly higher rates of life events than controls.

By contrast, there is some evidence that exposure to stressful life events plays a role in psychotic relapse or exacerbation, at least among patients on medication (Hirsch et al., 1993; Leff et al., 1973, 1983; Ventura et al., 1989). However, there is no consistent evidence of increased exposure to life events (large or small) during the month prior to episode occurrence; some studies show temporal proximity (e.g., Day et al., 1987) and others do not (e.g., Hirsch et al., 1993). Thus, despite numerous attempts to locate an association between life events and the onset of psychotic episodes, as Day and colleagues (1987) point out, the original Brown and Birley study remains the primary source of evidence that stressful life events play a causal role in schizophrenic episodes.

Results from the New York Risk Factor Study

In our own study we also found little evidence that major fateful negative events

Table 17.6. Nonaffective psychotic disorders–control differences in exposure to one or more fateful negative events (3 months approx.): percentages and adjusted exposure odds ratios°

| Event magnitude | % Reporting 1 or more events | | Nonaffective psychotic disorders vs. community controls | |
	Nonaffective psychotic disorders (n = 65)	Community controls (n = 404)	Adjusted odds ratio	95% confidence interval
Major	3.1	1.7	2.24	0.34, 14,89
Major & moderate	9.2	8.2	0.86	0.32, 2.29
Major & moderate & minor	10.8	17.3	0.47	0.20, 1.14

°Adjusted for age, sex, ethnicity, education, marital status, father's prestige, and father's prestige × ethnicity (Hispanic).

play a role in the occurrence of psychotic episodes, whether we look at a 1 month, 3 month (see Table 17.6), 6 month, or 12 month risk period. Nor was there evidence that moderate or minor fateful negative events are associated with disorder; to the contrary, the odds ratios decreased when smaller events are combined with major disruptions.

Major nonfateful negative events, by contrast, may be risk factors for psychotic episodes, although their causal role as representative of adversity is much less clear. As Table 17.7 shows, respondents with diagnoses of nonaffective psychotic disorders were more likely to report exposure to one or more major nonfateful negative events

during the 3 month risk period than were respondents in the control group. Note, however, that the adjusted odds ratio is smaller than that found for major depression (4.12 vs. 6.23). The case–control difference was not statistically significant when negative affect at the time of interview is added to the equation, nor was the rate of events significantly elevated during the most proximal 1 month period (results not shown).

We also investigated the possibility of subgroup differences. The stress–diathesis hypothesis as developed by Zubin and Spring (1977), among others, suggests that the greater the individual's vulnerability to schizophrenia, the less the role for stressful

Table 17.7. Nonaffective psychotic disorders–control differences in exposure to one or more nonfateful negative events (3 months approx.): percentages and adjusted exposure odds ratios[†]

| Event magnitude | % Reporting 1 or more events | | Nonaffective psychotic disorders vs. community controls | |
	Nonaffective psychotic disorders (n = 65)	Community controls (n = 404)	Adjusted odds ratio	95% confidence interval
Major	9.2	3.2	4.12°	1.16, 14.70
Major & moderate	23.1	13.4	1.60	0.76, 2.09
Major & moderate & minor	32.3	18.3	1.87	0.96, 3.65

[†]Adjusted for age, sex, ethnicity, education, marital status, father's prestige, and father's prestige × ethnicity (Hispanic).

°$p < .05$.

life events. We divided our case group into high- and low-vulnerability subsets (e.g., repeat- vs. first-episode cases, insidious vs. acute-onset cases, those meeting *DSM-III* criteria for schizophrenia vs. others) and investigated whether rates of major fateful events during the full 1 year risk period were higher within the low vulnerability groups. There were no significant differences in rates by these indicators of vulnerability, and patterns were not consistent with the hypothesis. In part this may be because our so-called low-vulnerability cases did not differ appreciably from our high-vulnerability cases on other possible risk factors (e.g., family history of psychiatric disorders).

The seven major fateful negative events reported by cases were clustered, however, in the group where we least expected them: repeat-episode cases meeting *DSM-III* criteria for schizophrenia. We cannot fully account for this clustering; it is quite possibly a chance occurrence. However, if people with a history of psychosis meeting *DSM-III* criteria for schizophrenia are more likely to have been prescribed and be taking medication, then our results are consistent with the longitudinal results by Leff and Ventura and their colleagues (see above) and with the early speculation by Birley and Brown (1970) that stress plays a role in precipitating relapse among patients protected by medication. Where possible, we reviewed the medical charts of selected patients in our sample for evidence of medication prescription and compliance; the results are consistent with, although not confirming of, this view.

DISCUSSION AND CONCLUSION

Our purpose in this chapter was to examine relationships between recent stressful life events and two forms of psychopathology using data from a case–control study of major depression and nonaffective psychotic disorders. We focused on major fateful events because this event category provides the clearest evidence regarding the role of environmental adversity in the initial devel-

opment and recurrence of psychiatric episodes.

Our analyses suggest, first, that the association between stressful life events and psychopathology is disorder specific. Major stressful life events, both fateful and nonfateful, are consistently associated with the onset of major depressive episodes but not consistently associated with the onset of nonaffective psychotic episodes. Depressed cases were more likely than community controls to report exposure to one or more major fateful negative events at the 1 year, 3 month, and 1 month risk intervals; they were more likely to report major nonfateful negative events as well. These results hold when controlling for demographic differences between case and control groups, demoralized mood at the time of interview, and other measured risk factors. In addition, the effect size for major fateful life events is not inconsequential; it equals or exceeds that for family history of affective disorder and other risk factors in our study. More important, parallel results are obtained when we restrict the case group to individuals experiencing their first episode of major depression, thus providing stronger evidence for an etiological effect.

The event–disorder association is strikingly different for nonaffective psychotic disorders. Cases, including first-episode cases, were no more likely than controls to have experienced a major fateful negative event during the 3 month risk period or during the most proximal 1 month interval. Reports of major fateful events were clustered among patients with a diagnosed history of schizophrenic episodes, however, suggesting that such events may play some role in precipitating relapse among patients protected by antipsychotic medication. There is also some evidence of increased exposure to recent major nonfateful events among patients compared with the control group, but this association is not statistically significant when controlling for demoralization at the time of interview. Taken together, these results are consistent with the bulk of the research literature: Major negative events, both fateful and nonfateful, play a much larger role in episodes of major depression than in episodes of nonaffective psychotic disorders.

Also consistent with other research, our results indicate that the event–depression relationship is temporally bounded. Cases reported increased exposure to major fateful and nonfateful events during the month prior to onset and to major fateful events during the most proximal 3 month period as well. Depressed cases and controls did not differ significantly in their event reports for the more distal periods, with the exception of the most remote interval inquired about (10 to 12 months prior to onset/interview). This may reflect a greater tendency toward telescoping on the part of respondents diagnosed with major depression; that is, cases may have pulled distant major events closer to onset than they actually were. We found no comparable "critical period" for nonaffective psychotic disorders, even where we found some evidence of an events–disorder relationship.

Finally, our work suggests that the events–disorder association is limited to stressful events of considerable magnitude. Events rated as moderate or minor show little relationship with episode onset for either major depression or nonaffective psychotic disorders. It is possible, of course, that the longer recall period for cases than controls led to greater forgetting of smaller events on the part of cases, thus obscuring an effect for negative events of lesser magnitude. However, our findings highlight the importance of employing a measurement strategy that differentiates events according to magnitude. Insofar as small to moderate events dominate life experiences, failing to discriminate on the basis of magnitude risks attenuating the event–disorder relationship.

Several caveats to our study should be noted. First, the participation rate in the control group is low by contemporary standards, in large part because their initial recruitment was for a measurement study where high completion rates were less critical. Insofar as we disproportionately lost residents who had recently experienced adversity, we overestimate case–control differences in exposure to stress. We examined this possibility by comparing hard-to-recruit community residents with other members of the control group and found no differences in reported event exposure. We also compared demographic characteristics of the control group with census data for the recruitment area and again found few differences. Thus, although selection effects cannot be ruled out entirely, these checks provide evidence for the representativeness of the community control group.

Second, both case groups were drawn from patient populations, which raises the possibility of other selection processes that could inflate or depress the observed event–disorder relationships. If patients are more likely than untreated persons to have experienced, or to recall and report, stressful events, then our results overestimate the effects of life events. Although some investigators have reported a weaker relationship between life events and disorder for patients than for community cases (e.g., Bebbington et al., 1981), it is certainly plausible both that the coupling of distressing experiences and depressive symptoms motivates treatment seeking and that therapy itself trains patients to recall adverse events and link their symptoms with them.

Finally, our reliance on a treated sample also raises the possibility that our cases do not represent the full range of individuals who are vulnerable to the disorders of interest. With respect to nonaffective psychotic disorders, our sample of first-episode cases not only is small but may also overrepresent individuals most vulnerable to psychotic episodes. Insofar as we (and other investigators of these disorders) tend to undersample those first-episode cases who are less vulnerable to psychosis, we may have missed those whose psychotic episodes were most likely to be precipitated by major fateful events. Our sample of cases with recent episodes of major depression may be biased in the opposite direction. The age of onset for patients in their first episodes is substantially older than that reported for general population samples. To the extent that vulnerability varies inversely with age, such a treated sample may be biased toward less vulnerable cases. Unfortunately, studies such as ours of relations between stressful life events and patient cases of major depression are rare, and published studies of life events and first-episode cases in the general population are nonexistent (Kessler, 1997). Most research on this topic is about relationships between life events and recurrence rather than first onset of major depression. In the course of our large-scale epidemiological research in Israel (e.g., Dohrenwend et al., 1992), we are conducting extensive studies of subsamples of cases and controls drawn from the larger sample. Data from this research will examine the extent to which the substantial role of major fateful events found in the New York sample of first- and repeat-episode cases of major depression is replicated in a sample of first- and repeat-episode cases drawn from a general population sample of young adults who tend to have earlier ages of onset.

Acknowledgments: This research was supported by a New Investigator Award from the Ann P. Lederer Institute and the National Alliance for Research on Schizophrenia and Depression (NARSAD) to Ann Stueve and by research grant MH36208 and Research Scientist Award K05-MH14663 from the National Institute of Mental Health to Bruce Dohrenwend. An earlier version of this work was presented at the annual meeting of the American Psychopathological Association, New York City, March 3–5, 1994. We acknowledge the many and diverse contributions of other members of the research team, including Michael Flory, Bruce Link, and Patrick Shrout, and the insightful criticisms and suggestions of Sharon Schwartz.

REFERENCES

Al Khani, M. A. I., Bebbington, P. E., Watson, J. P., & House, F. (1986). Life events and schizophrenia: A Saudi Arabian study. *British Journal of Psychiatry*, *148*, 12–22.

American Psychiatric Association. (1980). *Diagnostic and statistical manual of mental disorders* (3rd ed.). Washington, DC: American Psychiatric Association.

Bebbington, P., Tennant, C., & Hurry, J. (1981). Adversity and the nature of psychiatric disorder in the community. *Journal of Affective Disorders*, *3*, 345–366.

Bebbington, P., Wilkins, S., Jones, P., Foerster, A., Murray, R., Toone, B., & Lewis, S. (1993). Life events and psychosis: Initial results from the Camberwell Collaborative Psychosis Study. *British Journal of Psychiatry*, *162*, 72–79.

Birley, J. L. T., & Brown, G. W. (1970). Crises and life changes preceding the onset or relapse of acute schizophrenia: Clinical aspects. *British Journal of Psychiatry*, *116*, 327–333.

Blaney, P. H. (1986). Affect and memory: A review. *Psychological Bulletin*, *99*, 229–246.

Brown, G. W. (1974). Meaning, measurement, and stress of life events. In B. S. Dohrenwend & B. P. Dohrenwend (Eds.), *Stressful life events: Their nature and effects* (pp. 214–243). New York: John Wiley & Sons.

Brown, G. W. (1989). Life events and measurement. In G. W. Brown & T. O. Harris (Eds.), *Life events and illness* (pp. 3–45). New York: The Guilford Press.

Brown, G. W., Andrews, B., Harris, T. O., Adler, Z., & Bridge, L. (1986). Social support, self-esteem, and depression. *Psychological Medicine*, *16*, 813–831.

Brown, G. W., & Birley, J. L. T. (1968). Crises and life changes and the onset of schizophrenia. *Journal of Health and Social Behavior*, *9*, 203–214.

Brown, G. W., & Harris, T. (1978). *Social origins of depression*. New York: The Free Press.

Brown, G. W., & Harris, T. (1989). Depression. In G. W. Brown and T. O. Harris (Eds.), *Life events and illness* (pp. 49–93). New York: The Guilford Press.

Chung, R. K., Langeluddecke, P., & Tennant, C. (1986). Threatening life events in the onset of schizophrenia, schizophreniform psychosis, and hypomania. *British Journal of Psychiatry*, *148*, 680–685.

Cohen, L. H., Towbes, L. C., Flocco, R. (1988). Effects of induced mood on self-reported life events and perceived and received social support. *Journal of Personality and Social Psychology*, *55*, 669–674.

Costello, C. G. (1982). Social factors associated with depression: A retrospective community study. *Psychological Medicine*, *12*, 329–339.

Day, R., Nielsen, J. A., Korten, A., Ernberg, G., Dube, K. C., Gebhart, J., Jablensky, A., Leon, C., Marsella, A., Olatawura, M., Sartorius, N., Stromgren, E., Takahashi, R., Wig, N., & Wynne, L. C. (1987). Stressful life events preceding the acute onset of schizophrenia: A cross-national study from the World Health Organization. *Culture, Medicine, and Psychiatry, 11*, 123–205.

Dohrenwend, B. P. (1974). Problems in defining and sampling the relevant population of stressful life events. In B. S. Dohrenwend & B. P. Dohrenwend (Eds.), *Stressful life events: Their nature and effects* (pp. 275–310). New York: John Wiley & Sons.

Dohrenwend, B. P., Levav, I., Shrout, P. E., Schwartz, S., Naveh, G., Link, B. G., Skodol, A. E., & Stueve A. (1992). Socioeconomic status and psychiatric disorders: The causation-selection issue. *Science, 255*, 946–952.

Dohrenwend, B. P., Link, B. G., Kern, R., Shrout, P. E., & Markowitz, J. (1987). Measuring life events: The problem of variability within event categories. In B. Cooper (Ed.), *Psychiatric epidemiology: Progress and prospects* (pp. 103–119). London: Croom Helm.

Dohrenwend, B. P., Raphael, K. G., Schwartz, S., Stueve, A., & Skodol, A. E. (1993). The Structured Event Probe and Narrative Rating method (SEPRATE) for measuring stressful life events. In L. Goldberger & S. Bresnitz (Eds.), *Handbook of stress: Theoretical and clinical aspects* (2nd ed.), (pp. 174–199). New York: The Free Press.

Dohrenwend, B. P., Shrout, P. E., Egri, G., & Mendelsohn, F. S. (1980). Measures of nonspecific psychological distress and other dimensions of psychopathology in the general population. *Archives of General Psychiatry, 37*, 1229–1236.

Dohrenwend, B. P., Shrout, P. E., Link, B. G., Martin, J. L., & Skodol, A. E. (1986). Overview and initial results from a risk factor study of depression and schizophrenia. In J. E. Barrett & R. M. Rose (Eds.), *Mental disorders in the community: Progress and challenge* (pp. 184–215). New York: The Guilford Press.

Dohrenwend, B. P., Shrout, P. E., Link, B. G., Skodol, A. E., Stueve, A. (1995). Life events and other possible psychosocial risk factors for episodes of schizophrenia and major depression: A case-control study. In C. M. Mazure (Ed.), *Does stress cause psychiatric illness?* (pp. 43–65). Washington, DC: American Psychiatric Press.

Emmerson, J. P., Burvill, P. W., Finlay-Jones, R., & Hall, W. (1989). Life events, life difficulties, and confiding relationships in the depressed elderly. *British Journal of Psychiatry, 155*, 787–792.

Grant, I., Gerst, M., & Yager, J. (1976). Scaling of life events by psychiatric patients and normals. *Journal of Psychosomatic Research, 20*, 141–149.

Gureje, O., Adewunmi, A. (1988). Life events and schizophrenia in Nigerians: A controlled investigation. *British Journal of Psychiatry, 153*, 367–375.

Guze, S. B. (1989). Biological psychiatry: Is there any other kind? *Psychological Medicine, 19*, 315–323.

Hardesty, J. P., Fallon, I. R. H., & Shirin, K. (1985). The impact of life events, stress, and coping on the morbidity of schizophrenia. In I. R. H. Fallon (Ed.), *Family management of schizophrenia* (pp. 137–152). Baltimore: The Johns Hopkins University Press.

Heston, L. L. (1988). What about environment? In L. Dunner, E. S. Gershon, & J. P. Barrett (Eds.), *Relatives at risk for mental disorder* (pp. 205–213). New York: Raven Press.

Hirsch, S., Bowen, J., Emami, J., Crammer, P., Jolley, A., Haw, C., & Dickinson, M. (1996). A one year study of the effect of life events and medication in the aetiology of schizophrenic relapse. *British Journal of Psychiatry, 168*, 49–56.

Jacobs, S. C., & Myers, J. K. (1976). Recent life events and acute schizophrenic psychosis: A controlled study. *Journal of Nervous and Mental Diseases, 162*, 75–87.

Kendler, K. S., Kessler, R. C., Neale, M. C., Heath, A. C., & Eaves, L. J. (1993a). The prediction of major depression in women: Toward an integrated etiologic model. *American Journal of Psychiatry, 150*, 1139–1148.

Kendler, K. S., Neale, M., Kessler, R., Heath, A., & Eaves, L. (1993b). A twin study of recent life events and difficulties. *Archives of General Psychiatry, 50*, 789–796.

Kessler, R. C. (1997). The effects of stressful life events on depression. *Annual Review of Psychology, 48*, 191–214.

Leff, J. P., Hirsch, S. R., Gaind, R., Rohde, P. D., & Stevens, B. C. (1973). Life events and maintenance therapy in schizophrenic relapse. *British Journal of Psychiatry, 123*, 659–660.

Leff, J., Kuipers, L., Berkowitz, R., Vaughn, C., & Sturgeon, D. (1983). Life events, relatives' expressed emotion, and maintenance neuroleptics in schizophrenic relapse. *Psychological Medicine, 13*, 799–806.

Lewinsohn, P. M., Hoberman, H. M., & Rosenbaum, M. (1988). A prospective study of risk factors for unipolar depression. *Journal of Abnormal Psychology, 97*, 251–264.

Malla, A. K., Cortese, L., Shaw, T. S., & Ginsberg, B. (1990). Life events and relapse in schizophrenia: A one-year prospective study. *Social Psychiatry and Psychiatric Epidemiology, 25,* 221–224.

Malzacher, M., Merz, J., & Ebnother, D. (1981). Einschneidende lebensereignisse im vorfeld akuter schizophrener episoden: Erstmals erkrankte patienten im vergleiich mit einer normalstichprobe. *Archiv fur Psychiatrie und Nervenkrankeiten, 230,* 227–242.

Norman, R. M. G., & Malla, A. K. (1993). Stressful life events and schizophrenia II: Conceptual and methodological issues. *British Journal of Psychiatry, 162,* 167–174.

Paykel, E. S. (1974). Life stress and psychiatric disorder: Applications of the clinical approach. In B. S. Dohrenwend & B. P. Dohrenwend (Eds.), *Stressful life events: Their nature and effects* (pp. 135–149). New York: John Wiley & Sons.

Paykel, E. S., Myers, J. K., Dienelt, M. N., Klerman, G. L., Lindenthal, J. J., & Pepper, M. P. (1969). Life events and depression: A controlled study. *Archives of General Psychiatry, 21,* 753–760.

Plomin, R., Lichtenstein, P., Pedersen, N. L., McClearn, G. E., & Nesselroade, J. R. (1990). Genetic influence on life events during the last half of the life span. *Psychology and Aging, 5,* 25–30.

Post, R. M. (1992). Transduction of psychosocial stress into the neurobiology of recurrent affective disorder. *American Journal of Psychiatry, 149,* 999–1010.

Rabkin, J. G., & Struening, E. L. (1976). Life events, stress, and illness. *Science, 194,* 1013–1020.

Rahe, R. H. (1981). Developments in life change measurement: Subjective life change unit scaling. In B. S. Dohrenwend & B. P. Dohrenwend (Eds.), *Stressful life events and their contexts* (pp. 48–62). New York: Prodist.

Rutter, M. (1986). Meyerian psychobiology, personality development, and the role of life experiences. *American Journal of Psychiatry, 143,* 1077–1087.

Sarason, I. G., Johnson, J. H., & Siegel, J. M. (1978). Assessing the impact of life changes: Development of the life experiences survey. *Journal of Consulting Clinical Psychology, 46,* 932–946.

Shrout, P. E., Link, B. G., Dohrenwend, B. P., Skodol, A. E., Stueve, A., & Mirotznik, G. (1989). Characterizing life events as risk factors for depression: The role of fateful loss events. *Journal of Abnormal Psychology, 98,* 460–467.

Spence, J. T., & Helmreich, R. (1978). *Masculinity and feminity: Their psychological dimensions, correlates, and antecedents.* Austin: University of Texas Press.

Surtees, P. G., Miller, P. McC., Ingham, J. G., Kreitman, N. B., Rennie, D., & Sashidharan, S. P. (1986). Life events and the onset of affective disorder: A longitudinal general population study. *Journal of Affective Disorders, 10,* 37–50.

Tennant, C., Bebbington, P., & Hurry, J. (1981). The role of life events in depressive illness: Is there a substantial causal relation? *Psychological Medicine, 11,* 379–389.

Ventura, J., Neuchterlein, K. H., Hardesty, J. P., & Gitlin, M. (1992). *Life events and schizophrenic relapse after medication withdrawal: A prospective study.* British Journal of Psychiatry, 161, 615–620.

Ventura, J., Nuechterlein, K. H., Lukoff, D., & Hardesty, J. P. (1989). A prospective study of stressful life events and schizophrenic relapse. *Journal of Abnormal Psychology, 98,* 407–411.

Wyler, A. R., Masuda, M., & Holmes, T. H. (1968). Seriousness of illness rating scale. *Journal of Psychosomatic Research, 11,* 363–374.

Zubin, J., & Spring, B. (1977). Vulnerability: A new view of schizophrenia. *Journal of Abnormal Psychology, 86,* 103–126.

18

Loss and Depressive Disorders

George W. Brown

This chapter focuses on one issue—the degree to which life events provoking depressive disorders do so because of loss. This narrow focus perhaps needs no apology, because effective conceptualization of this proximal link undoubtedly enables broader questions to be tackled more effectively—cross-cultural comparisons, macrolevel social influences, life-span processes, vulnerability, biological contributions, and so on.

I deal here with clinically relevant depression at a "caseness" level of the order defined by the *Diagnostic and Statistical Manual of Mental Disorders (Third Edition, Revised)* (*DSM-III-R*; American Psychiatric Association, 1987) as major depression (Finlay-Jones et al., 1980). I also deal only with studies of women. A convincing etiological model for men is only beginning to emerge, but it is already clear that it is unlikely to differ a great deal from that for women (Bolton & Oatley, 1987; Eales, 1985). However, Nazroo et al. (1997) have suggested that the well-recognized gender difference in the experience of depression may be due to women being particularly susceptible to threatening events (defined objectively) involving the household arena—more specifically, severely threatening events concerning procreation, children, and housing. If this result is replicated, it

would underline the relevance of my overall thesis: that it is not improbable that most cases of depressive disorder result from a failure to meet goals derived from evolutionary-based needs such as being admired, forming friendships, having a core adult attachment figure, having children, and so on. These goals are almost entirely social in nature, and in this sense rates of depression are likely to be largely the result of psychosocial processes. However, one may also argue that the gap between what is wanted and what is not forthcoming must on the whole have special qualities for clinical depression to emerge.

It is difficult to conceive of an alternative explanation other than a broadly social one for the large differences in rates of depression that can occur in population terms. For example, two studies have revealed a 1 year prevalence of major depression of 3% among women in a Basque-speaking rural community (Gaminde, et al., 1993) and of 30% in a black urban setting in Zimbabwe (Broadhead & Abas, 1997), a tenfold difference. Both studies used the same instruments, including the Present State Examination (PSE) employed by Maudsley-trained psychiatrists, and the differences in rate were parallelled by differences in the frequency of adverse life events. Studies of western urban populations have rates falling roughly between these extremes. There are, of course, bound to be biological risk factors of importance, but they can be seen as contributing to variability in risk within populations, with differences across populations largely driven by psychosocial factors (Brown, 1996).

THE ROLE OF LIFE EVENTS IN ONSET OF CLINICAL DEPRESSION

The study of life events has been critical in developing such a radical social perspective. This chapter does not deal with the methodological issues that have tended to dominate the life events literature. The instrument used in the research described here, the Life Events and Difficulties Schedule (LEDS), has been good enough to establish that certain kinds of adverse events do occur not long before onset in the majority of depressive disorders, and that they are of etiological significance (Brown & Harris, 1986, 1989).

The LEDS has now been used in some 20 studies covering depressed patients and nonpatients. It requires skilled interviewing focused on the broad context of the event and its timing *vis-à-vis* other events and any onset of psychiatric disorder (Brown & Harris, 1989). Findings concerning the onset of depression have been broadly comparable—in adult samples between two-thirds and 90% of episodes have at least one severely threatening life event occurring not long before onset. It is important to emphasize that long-term threat is involved—that is, such events must have long-term threatening implications at a point in time some 10 days after their occurrence. Events with short-term threat, however adverse—say a child admitted to the hospital apparently dangerously ill, but on the mend within a few days—do not provoke depression (Brown & Harris, 1978).

Table 18.1 summarizes the findings of one study in terms of onsets of depression in a 12 month period. This longitudinal study was carried out in Islington, an inner-city

Table 18.1. Depression onset rate among 303 women in terms of provoking agent status

Provoking agent status	No. of onsets	% Onset rate
No provoking agent	2/153	1
Provoking agent		
Major difficulty only	1/20	5
Severe event	29/130	22
Total onset rate	32/303	11

area in North London, with 400 women with a child living at home (Brown et al., 1987). The women were largely working class; approximately one-fourth were single mothers. They were followed up at 12 month intervals. The data in Table 18.1 represent the results for 303 women at risk of an onset in the sense that, at the time of first contact, they did not have depression at a clinical level. These results are fairly typical for such studies.

Two findings from the Islington study are relevant. First, as many as 29 of the 32 women developing a depressive disorder had experienced a severely threatening life event in the 6 months before onset—most within a matter of weeks. Second, only about one-fifth of the women experiencing a severe event in the year went on to develop depression. This second result raises the issue of vulnerability, a topic discussed later in the chapter, after a discussion of the nature of the provoking life events. Before proceeding, however, I must comment on one obvious objection to a radical psychosocial perspective.

THE QUESTION OF ENDOGENOUS DEPRESSION

There can be little doubt of the existence of genuine "endogenous" depressive disorders, but one of the puzzling findings of life event research is that, except in cases of the comparatively rare bipolar conditions, life events appear to play a significant role in all forms of depression (e.g., Brown & Harris, 1978; Paykel et al., 1971). Studies of patient pop-

Table 18.2. Ordinal number of adult episodes of depression in north London patients by melancholic/psychotic score and presence of a severe life event within 6 months of onset

Melancholic/psychotic score	% Severe event by adult episode number					
	1st	2nd	3rd	4th	5th	Total
Low	71 (25/35)*	70 (21/30)	83 (10/12)	60 (3/5)	80 (8/10)	73 (67/92)
			74 (42/57)[†]			
High	59 (10/17)*	15 (2/13)	33 (1/3)	100 (1/1)	0 (0/1)	40 (14/35)
			22 (4/18)[†]			
Total	67 (35/52)	53 (23/43)	73 (11/15)	67 (4/6)	73 (8/11)	64 (81/127)

*Not significant.

[†]$\chi^2 = 13.18$, 1 df, $p < .001$.

ulations have consistently failed to show that endogenous and nonendogenous conditions, when defined in clinical terms, are notably different, although there has been a fair amount of variability in results (Bebbington & McGuffin, 1989; Katschnig et al., 1986).

The findings in a depressed patient series (Brown et al., 1994a) in North London may shed some light on this impasse. This study distinguished between melancholic/psychotic and non–melancholic/psychotic depressive conditions based on a score derived from the presence and severity of the following PSE symptoms: diurnal variation, guilty ideas of reference, pathological guilt, delusions of guilt, hypochondriacal delusions, delusions of catastrophe, depressive hallucinations, delusions of reference, delusions of misinterpretation, delusions of persecution, appetite/weight loss, early waking, retardation, loss of libido, perceptual distortion, auditory hallucinations, visual hallucinations, distinct quality, lack of reactivity, and constipation coinciding with episode. (The psychotic symptoms in this list were mood congruent.) One point was allotted for each symptom. However, it was decided beforehand on theoretical grounds that important information might be lost if degree (rather than simple presence) of vegetative disturbance was ignored. Thus in three instances (weight loss, early waking, and retardation) a score of 2 was given if the PSE score was severe (i.e., 2). The term *psychotic* added to that of *melancholic* conveys that more than traditional melancholic

symptoms have been included. A score of 6 or more, based loosely on earlier results from a survey of patients living in Camberwell, was used to define a melancholic/psychotic condition (Brown & Harris, 1978).

Among depressed psychiatric inpatients and outpatients, the presence of a severely threatening life event in the 6 months before onset was common among those with non–melancholic/psychotic conditions whether or not it was a first episode (Table 18.2). However, among patients with conditions that would be expected to be endogenous—that is, the contrasting melancholic/psychotic group defined by a score of 6 or more—the proportion with a severe event was just as high among those with a first onset but much lower among those who had had a prior episode. The number of patients with a high melancholic/psychotic score is small but, given that the findings held when two other patient series were taken into account, the results are probably reasonably accurate (Brown et al., 1994a). The fact that only those who had a melancholic/psychotic diagnosis *and* a prior episode differed in their experience of severe events may well go a long way toward explaining the puzzling inconsistencies in published results, because the proportion of patients with both these characteristics is bound to vary by type of treatment center, and studies have often been carried out in tertiary treatment centers. The results would also appear to be worth pursuing in biological terms. It is possible that first onset in the melancholic/psychotic group results in some kind of "scarring," that increases the chance of a spontaneous episode (Post et al., 1986), and the accurate delineation of a truly endogenous group (albeit fairly small) would probably help in the search for relevant brain mechanisms.

A key point of my argument, however, is that melancholic/psychotic depressive conditions as a whole are unlikely to form more than one-tenth of the total range of clinically relevant depression—that is, when psychiatric patients and nonpatients with conditions of at least "major depression" severity in *DSM-III-R* terms are considered. If we turn our attention to this much larger group, there is little doubt that the majority of cases of clinically relevant depression, whether a first episode or not, are provoked by a severely threatening life event occurring in the 6 months, and in most instances in a matter of weeks before onset (Brown & Harris, 1989).

THE ROLE OF LOSS

The most obvious starting point in considering the nature of provoking severely threatening life events is with the experience of loss. Few would be likely to reject this. In a curious fashion this is reflected in the exclusion criteria of the *DSM-III-R*, which rule out, except under special circumstances, a diagnosis of major depression following bereavement (American Psychiatric Association, 1987). But why just death? What about a miscarriage? What about a broken love affair or marital separation? Such a criterion must be viewed as scientifically misjudged while the nature of the role of loss in depression remains unsettled.

To proceed requires a confrontation with the question of meaning. The LEDS has made a start by relying on investigator-based judgments along the lines of the notion of *verstehen*—that is, of the likely response of a particular individual to a particular event once his or her biography and immediate circumstances have been taken into account (Brown, 1989). The LEDS ratings take ac-

count of an event's impact on likely central goals, plans, and concerns. This contextual approach is used to delineate the severely threatening life events mentioned earlier. For example, a young university student finding out she was pregnant 8 weeks after her boyfriend, who had planned to marry her, had suddenly left her would be judged to have suffered a severely threatening life event, irrespective of anything she might say about her actual reaction. This, it should be noted, is a typical example of a severe life event—by and large there is not much doubt about their essential unpleasantness.

The LEDS approach is without doubt crude, but it has been successful in the sense that very few events of etiological significance where depression is concerned appear to be missed. No evidence has emerged that any other class of event is of importance for depression. This is so despite the fact that severe events form only a relatively small proportion of the total events covered by the LEDS.

However, research has not relied entirely on contextual ratings. In the longitudinal Islington research it has been possible to take into account "soft" material concerning feelings expressed in a lengthy interview carried out 1 year before the interview collecting life-event material. One set of ratings recorded a woman's *commitment* to six domains of her life—marriage, motherhood, employment, and the like—on the basis of not only what was said but how it was said. High commitment was defined in terms of the top scale point of a 4 point scale and only occurred on average in 1.5 of the 6 domains (Brown et al., 1987). When a severe life event in the following year matched such an area of high commitment, risk of a depressive onset trebled in contrast with that of other severe events (Table 18.3).

The result suggests that the methodological criticism that contextual ratings soak up too much extraneous information is misplaced (Dohrendwend et al., 1987). The trebling of the size of the association between severe life event and onset of depression makes clear just how much is left out by the approximate assessment of goals

Table 18.3. Onset of depression among the 130 women in Islington with severe life event in terms of matching commitment

At least one severe event matching a prior marked commitment	% Onset
Yes	40 (16/40)
No	14 (13/90)
Total	22 (29/130)°

°$p < .01$.

Table 18.4. Onset of depression among 130 women in Islington with severe life event in terms of matching ongoing difficulty

	% Onset
A: At least one severe event matching a prior marked difficulty	
Yes	46 (16/35)
No	14 (13/95)
Total	22 (19/130)°
B: Any matching severe event (difficulty or commitment)	
Yes	37 (24/65)
No	8 (5/65)
Total	22 (29/130)†

°$p < .01$.
†$p < .001$.

and concerns utilized in making such contextual ratings. As I noted earlier, the importance of the ratings has been their ability to isolate events of *potential* etiological significance.

So far the kind of evidence I have touched on suggests that depressogenic events are typically highly unpleasant and that a core identity is likely to be involved. Each severe event has in addition been considered in terms of the presence of loss, extending the concept to cover not only loss of a person but that of a role or cherished idea. In the Islington study, we have taken the top two points of a 4 point scale to represent a clear loss (i.e., "marked" or "moderate" contrasted with "some" or "little or none"). Put another way, losses in LEDS terms are intended to reflect the likelihood of being cut off from a key source of self-value or the development of a grave impediment to carrying out a core activity. A woman told that nothing could be done for her crippling arthritis or one finding out that her new husband is a compulsive gambler would be considered to have experienced a loss. However, like the severity ratings, the Islington measure attempts to reflect only what is *likely* to have been experienced. As in all the ratings of events discussed in this chapter, any report of what was felt as a result of the event is ignored in making contextual-type ratings.

Loss has been contrasted with danger— that is, the threat of future loss—although a particular event may reflect both. Several studies have shown that at least three-

quarters of severely threatening life events leading to depression involve a definite loss (Brown, 1993; Finlay-Jones, 1989; Finlay-Jones & Brown, 1981). Despite this, there are reasons for questioning the centrality of loss for clinical depression. That something more is likely to be involved can be seen in another result concerning matching: A severe event matching a marked ongoing difficulty present at the time of first interview increased the risk of onset of depression in exactly the same way as an event matching high commitment (Table 18.4A). (Table 18.4B gives results in terms of either a matching-commitment or matching-difficulty event.)

A critical point for my argument is that loss is by no means always involved in such matching-difficulty events. One woman with such event had had a serious problem for 2 years with the hyperactivity of her 8-year old child. The event that led to onset of depression was a teacher complaining about the child in front of many other mothers. It is doubtful if anything had been "lost" at this particular point in time. She had been long aware of her son's difficulties and had received complaints from the school well over a year before—albeit not in public.

Table 18.5. Depression onset rate by type of severe life event over a 2 year period in Islington community series

Event type	Rate	% Onset
A: Humiliation/trapped	41/131	31
1. Humiliation: separation	12/34	35
2. Humiliation: other's delinquincy	7/36	19
3. Humiliation: put down	12/32	38
4. Trapped	10/29	34
B: Loss alone	14/157	9
5. Death	7/24	29
6. Separation: subject initiated	2/18	11
7. Other key loss	4/58	7
8. Lesser loss	1/57	2
C: Danger alone	3/89	3
D: Total	58/367	15

THE ROLE OF HUMILIATION/ENTRAPMENT

There is a second perspective on depression that is more able to deal with such exceptions, one that underlines situations leading to powerlessness, defeat, and the lack of any means of escape from one's circumstances. I find particularly interesting in this context arguments concerning ranking derived from ethological observations of evolutionary-based response tendencies—that is, a biological system of the same order as those involving, say, attachment or anxiety. Responses to the experience of defeat have been viewed by commentators such as John Price as critical for human depression, and as originating in an evolutionary sense from either the activity of defending territory, or submission following being "outranked" in a group-living species (e.g., Price et al., 1994). Paul Gilbert (1992), with this perspective in mind, outlined a number of depressogenic situations that closely parallel those identified by LEDS life-event research:

- Direct attacks on persons' self-esteem and forcing them into a subordinate position.

- Events undermining persons' sense of rank, attractiveness, and value, particularly via the consequences of the event for core roles.
- Blocked escape.

Such ideas go beyond the concept of loss. In discussing human despair, Unger (1984), for example, also underlined the key importance of what he calls the experience of imprisonment. This can occur in the "blocked escape" described by Gilbert when we are unable to free ourselves from an unrewarding setting, but also in grief when despair arises from a disbelief in our ability to re-affirm an identity in the absence of the relationship.

In order to reflect these ideas, my colleagues and I have used material collected about events in the Islington general population sample within a 2 year period rather than the 1 year period used earlier (see Brown et al., 1995). A *hierarchical* scheme has been used, again based on contextual ratings of likely response to the events, (see Table 18.5). I must emphasize that only severe events are considered. Events were placed together where they had been part of some developmental sequence—say, learning of a husband's cancer and a major operation 3 weeks later. The overall risk of onset from a severe event, or sequence, was approximately 1:6 in the 6 months following the event (Table 18.5D). (Where an onset had occurred, only the event temporally *nearest* onset was considered to play a role in provoking onset. However, a more complex alternative approach that allowed all events with 6 months of onset to be considered as provoking arrived at essentially the same set of conclusions.)

The first three categories in the hierarchical scheme concern possible humiliation. The ratings assume that one consequence of the event was likely to be either a sense of being put down or a marked devaluation of self. The first category, for example, includes any separation from a partner or lover where the other person either took the initiative or where the woman was "forced" to leave or break off a relationship because of violence or discovery of infidelity. Finding out that her 12-year-old daughter had been stealing from her and playing truant from school would have been placed in category 2, and a woman criticized by a judge in public for failing to pay her son's fine and warned she could go to prison, or one learning of a husband's infidelity, placed in category 3.

Given the hierarchical rules, events associated with entrapment, the fourth category, must have failed to meet criteria for the three humiliation categories. Such events had to involve difficulty-matching and in addition were also judged to underline the fact the woman was trapped in a punishing situation that had gone on for some time— the woman mentioned earlier with severe arthritis would be placed here.

Loss alone has four component categories. That for "death" had to have reached "1—marked" or "2—moderate" on the Islington measure. "Separation–subject initiated" involved a separation (typically from a partner or lover) where the women either clearly took the initiative or in a few instances separated by mutual argument. Category 7, other key loss, involved important losses such as that of a job held for some

Table 18.6. Percent onset of depression resulting from separation or rift in a core tie by degree of control on woman's part—Islington series

Other's initiative	Woman "forced" to act	Woman's initiative
53 (9/17)	25 (4/16)	11 (2/18)

years or a close friend or confident leaving to live abroad. The eighth category, lesser loss, involved events rated only "3—some" on loss—for example, going to the funeral of a mother in the West Indies who had not been seen for several years. Only the "death" category had an obviously high risk of onset of depression. The final group of events, involving danger alone (without humiliation, entrapment, or loss), had a rate of onset of only 3% (Table 18.5C).

Table 18.5 as a whole shows that there were large differences in risk of depression by current category. If those entrapped are combined with the humiliated (Table 18.5A), risk of depression is three times more likely than those with a loss alone (Table 18.5B)—31% versus 9%. The relatively low risk associated with a "loss alone" event, except the category of "death," and the fact that a third of the humiliating and entrapping events did not involve loss, suggests that something more than loss is usually necessary to bring about a depressive onset.

The likely importance of humiliation and devaluation of self and entrapment is apparent in the results shown in Table 18.6. Separations associated with humiliation were further divided into whether the woman took *some* initiative (forced to act) after learning of an infidelity or marked violence. When the category of woman who clearly took the initiative (category 6) is taken into account, a clear gradient in depressive onset emerges, with the greatest rate of onset among those women whose partners or lovers left them and the least among those who left on their own initiative. Hammen (1988) has made the point that the one finding that has clearly emerged from the extensive research on the reformulated learned helplessness model involves the importance of lack of control.

Very similar results concerning the role of humiliation/entrapment events have been obtained in a patient series (Brown et al., 1995) and in the study of women in a township in Harare in Zimbabwe (Broadhead & Abas, 1998).

To recapitulate, severely threatening life events provoking onset of depression will tend to have many, but not all, of the following characteristics:

- high commitment in the role area involved in the event
- loss—defined in a broad sense
- devaluation in one's own or others' eyes
- experience of defeat
- entrapment
- lack of a sense of control

It should be added that almost all such events involved some kind of interpersonal crisis.

PSYCHOSOCIAL VULNERABILITY

I mentioned earlier the way in which work on life events opens up many other avenues of enquiry. This general conclusion concerning types of depressogenic life events fits well into current findings concerning vulnerability to depression seen in psychosocial terms. Two background factors measured at the time of the first interview in Islington have proved highly predictive of onset of depression in the following 12 months: (*1*) *negative psychological* (negative evaluation of self or chronic subclinical symptoms); and (*2*) *negative environmental* (negative interaction with a partner or child in the home, or lack of a close confidant in the case of single mothers). The order of prediction can be judged by the fact that, although only 23% of the 303 women at risk for developing a depressogenic disorder had both risk factors, three-quarters of all onsets occurring in the 12-month follow-up period occurred among them (Brown et al., 1990b).

I do not need to spell out the conceptual similarity of humiliation and entrapment events and these two risk factors. It is clear, for example, with low self-esteem, a key component of the negative psychological factor. However, I must emphasize that I do not view low self-esteem as essential for the development of depression. The depressed women in Islington fairly often had high self-esteem when seen during the episode (Brown et al., 1990b). It would appear quite possible following, say, an entrapment event to retain high self-esteem and in no way blame oneself for the event, and yet still develop depression. [Gilbert (1992) argues this point with some force.] It is, however, obviously likely that low self-esteem prior to the experience of a severe life event will raise the chances of responding to it in terms of defeat and general hopelessness.

Figure 18.1 puts the type of provoking event and vulnerability results together. (It deals only with the 1 year follow-up period because we only rated negative evaluation of self at the time of first interview.) It shows that a severe life event (or sequence), however adverse, was never enough to produce depression; nor, for that matter, was vulnerability on its own. The size of the interactive effects of vulnerability and a provoking event are impressive. For example, for loss without humiliation/entrapment, onset was almost absent without the presence of both risk factors. The results as a whole underline the groundlessness of the fear that has sometimes been expressed that contextual-type ratings of events encompass too much detail. The basic Islington findings have been replicated in a 1 year follow up of high-risk women (based on vulnerability measures) when seen on three separate occasions at 4 month intervals (Bifulco et al., 1998). However, it is also clear that the finding in the earlier Islington series concerning a total lack of onset among those with a severe event but without vulnerability (Fig. 18.1) is likely to have been an extreme result, and that on occasions onsets do occur under these circumstances. However, the main thrust of the earlier results remain (see also Edwards et al., 1998). One other im-

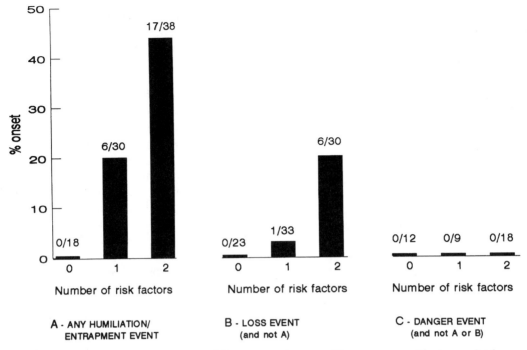

Figure 18.1. Rates of onset of depression in follow-up year by severe life event type and background risk among 130 Islington women. All onsets and severe events (or sequences) noted; only those nearest onset considered provoking.

plication is that, if risk of onset is considered in terms of traditional event-type categories such as loss of job, move of house, illness, and divorce, only a very small proportion of most types are likely to lead to depression.

Research has also made a case that psychosocial factors are equally involved in determining *course* of a depressive disorder. Fortunately, the findings are entirely consistent with what I have so far presented. The research on the role of "fresh start" or "relief" events in recovery can be seen in terms of relieving a sense of entrapment and powerlessness (Brown et al., 1992). Studies concerning determinants of chronicity underline the importance of "negative" predictors such as an interpersonal difficulty (but no other kind) at point of onset and childhood neglect and abuse (Brown & Moran, 1994; Brown et al., 1994b).

SOME FINAL COMMENTS

Much remains to be explained concerning the role of adverse life events in the onset

of depression. I finish by mentioning briefly three of many issues that are still unresolved.

First, why should an adverse life event usually be necessary to provoke depression? In terms of Frijda's Laws of Emotion, that of Habituation reads: "Continued pleasures wear off; continued hardships lose their poignancy" (Frijda, 1988). For whatever reason, we humans have an uncanny tendency to adapt to adversity and deprivation —not in the sense of ruling out suffering, but apparently enough to ward off any onset of clinical depression.

An adverse life event is typically required to overcome this habituation. In an extraordinary story, *Alfred Nobbs*, George Moore tells of the experiences of a woman who spent much of her life in a Dublin hotel disguised as a male waiter. A crisis occurred when she was found out. In telling her story, she says: "I thought nobody would ever hear [my story], and I thought I would never cry again. . . . it is much sadder than I thought it was, and if I had known how sad it was I shouldn't have been able to live through it." (p.121). Life events can, as here, tell us what we already know but, because of the event, we now "know" in a different, more disturbing, way. I believe that a depressive onset might well follow under these circumstances if there is also a realization that the discovery of her real sex would make it impossible in her judgment (however arrived at) to continue this sad way of life—particularly if this realization were coupled with an inability to conceive of an alternative.

I suspect adverse life events also are usually necessary to provoke onset of depression, even when levels of background deprivation and adversity are great, because we do not always recognize the degree of our dependence on a particular social arrangement until that arrangement goes wrong. In Proust's *Albertine Disparue*, Marcel's servant tells him simply "Mademoiselle Albertine has gone." (This constitutes a "humiliation: separation" event in the scheme described earlier.) Marcel had over the previous months come to believe that this was just what he wanted. He had recognized his boredom and had entertained fantasies of her leaving, thereby enabling him to indulge in new sexual adventures on a visit to Venice. Yet, within a few seconds, he realizes otherwise: "And so, what I had believed to mean nothing to me was quite simply my whole life" (Proust, 1989). Frijda (1988) writes of the *reality* an event can bring— the iron of the world. He emphasizes how events can make situations real for us via the emotion they provoke. In Marcel's words, "the idea of Albertine's departure on her own initiative might have occurred to my mind a thousand times over, in the clearest, the most sharply defined form, without my suspecting any the more what, in relation to myself, that is to say in reality, that departure would be, what an unprecedented, appalling, unknown thing, how entirely novel a calamity" (Proust, 1989).

Second, it may also be asked why psychosocial vulnerability factors typically also must be present for clinical depression to emerge. I suspect this is because the sense of defeat and hopelessness brought about by the event must be matched by inability to contemplate dealing with its implications for depression to occur.

Two broad processes are likely to prove critical. The first is a cognitive–emotional process in which interpretations of hopelessness and helplessness are brought to the situation. Psychological research on depression has tended to place particular emphasis on the inappropriateness of negative cognitive sets. By contrast, I would emphasize their appropriateness and how such cognitions may be fully understandable in the light of the person's current milieu. The Islington research has made clear, for example, the predictive importance of low self-esteem (defined on the basis of negative comments) as a vulnerability factor; and furthermore how such negative evaluation of self is highly related to difficulties in the women's current environment (Brown et al., 1990a, 1990b, 1990c). Although complex transactional processes involving personal characteristics and environment are undoubtedly involved, it would be foolhardy to rule out on current evidence the idea that doubts about ability to deal effectively with the consequences and implications of an event typically have a realistic basis. [I leave undiscussed the likely importance of social support (Brown, 1992; Harris, 1992) and the reawakening of memories of childhood (and subsequent) adverse experiences (Bifulco et al., 1994).] The second process is one of biological vulnerability stemming from ongoing stressors. Depletion of serotonin in the brain is one possibility, and this, indeed, may be one way in which self-esteem is lowered (Deakin, 1990).

Finally, as a third point, there is an urgent need to relate such findings to broader cultural and societal issues. Large differences, for example, in the frequency of severe life events by type of population have been documented (Gaminde et al., 1993), and this doubtless also holds for the experience of humiliation and entrapment events (Broadhead & Abas, 1994). In this context the reason for the surprising success of the LEDS in cross-cultural research must be considered. Basic findings concerning the role of

severe life events so far have been replicated almost exactly. I suspect that this success relates in large part to the fact that
changes in the *delivery* system serving central goals are typically reflected in life-event
ratings of severity—and such changes can
occur only in a limited number of ways. As
long as the fact that such a change has taken
place is established, it is probably not vital
in the current contextual ratings to be especially accurate about the nuances of the
particular concerns and goals that are involved. The presence of a husband, or a
healthy body for oneself, doubtless tends to
serve somewhat different goals in London
and in Zimbabwe—or, for that matter,
within these populations. A LEDS severity
rating places weight on the disruption of
broad goals following loss of a husband or
debilitating illness, rather than considering
any exact delineation of the concerns
affected.

It is not possible to feel the same degree
of confidence in dealing cross-culturally
with ongoing difficulties that are more directly concerned with *level* of deprivation.
For example, the notion of what constitutes
"good" housing differs dramatically in Zimbabwe and in London; such factors must be
accommodated in rating LEDS difficulties.
By contrast, the actual loss of a place to live
as an event may well be associated with a
broadly similar range of emotional reactions
in the two populations. In terms of themes
such as humiliation, shame, and defeat, depressogenic events therefore may have surprisingly universal characteristics. Because
depression appears to be provoked by a
change from an ongoing state (which may
be highly satisfactory or highly unsatisfac-
tory), assessment of the exact nature of what
is involved in the change is not necessarily
crucial for establishing etiological links.

CONCLUSION

I have reviewed some representative findings concerning life events based on a measure that is without doubt crude in terms of
what is ideally required. However, it has

been good enough to get research underway
and has led to a considerable amount of
replicable findings. For me the excitement
of such results is the impetus they give to
explore other issues: cross-cultural comparisons, gender differences, the contribution
of childhood experience, the role of adult
attachment style in both creating life events
and influencing how they are dealt with, biological correlates, and so on.

I need not point out that life events are
the very phenomenon that our brains have
evolved to deal with, and that what happens
in the outside world can have profound biological implications. This has been implicit
in all the research results I have presented.
I believe that life events are important to
study for two further reasons. First, they are
a marvellous way of finding out just what
living in a particular society means for individuals within it. I have mentioned the use
of the LEDS in other cultures. In practice
this requires putting an event such as an accusation of witchcraft into context. In real
life, culturally recognized practices tend to
serve purposes that are not necessarily obvious in the sense of strictly being a part of
the practices as such. Thus someone accused of being a witch will find that those
individuals involved in the accusation are
likely to be important within the social
group in a practical and an emotional sense.
Because of this the accusation is likely to
have highly idiosyncratic consequences. It
may, for example, be made in the context of
a husband blaming his wife for the illness of
a co-wife's child, and so perhaps suggest an
initial move in a divorce in which the
women will lose her spouse and her children
(Broadhead & Abas, 1998). A witchcraft example may seem extreme—albeit not uncommon in Zimbabwe—but such wider
consequences hold to some degree for most
life events rated severe by the LEDS.

Second, the study of life events, at least
when collected by semistructured instruments such as the LEDS, inevitably leads to
a concern with needs, plans, and goals that
are easily overlooked in our current emphasis on cognitive and biological processes.
The human experience is centrally about

wanting, about goals, about meaning—and in a way not necessarily easily put into words. I have come to believe that, without this grounding, social science contributions to psychiatry will often find themselves searching, if not badly stumbling, in the dark.

REFERENCES

American Psychiatric Association. (1987). *Diagnostic and statistical manual of mental disorders* (3rd ed., rev.). Washington, DC: American Psychiatric Press.

Bebbington, P., & McGuffin, P. (1989). Interactive models of depression. In E. Paykel & K. Herbst (Eds.), *Depression: An integrative approach* (pp. 65–80). London: Heinemann Medical Books.

Bifulco, A., Brown, G. W., & Harris, T. O. (1994). Childhood experience of care and abuse (CECA): A retrospective interview. *Child Psychology and Psychiatry, 35,* 1419–1435.

Bifulco, A., Brown, G. W., Moran, P., Ball, C., & Campbell, C. (1998). Predicting depression in women: The role of past and present vulnerability. *Psychological Medicine, 28,* 39–50.

Bolton, W., & Oatley, K. (1987). A longitudinal study of social support and depression in unemployed men. *Psychological Medicine, 17,* 453–460.

Broadhead, J., & Abas, M. (1998). Life events, difficulties and depression among women in an urban setting in Zimbabwe. *Psychological Medicine, 28,* 29–38.

Broadhead, J., & Abas, M. (1997). Depression and anxiety among women in an urban setting in Zimbabwe. *Psychological Medicine, 27,* 59–71.

Brown, G. W. (1989). Life events and measurement. In G. W. Brown & T. O. Harris (Eds.), *Life events and illness* (pp. 49–94). New York: The Guilford Press.

Brown, G. W. (1992). Social support: An investigator-based approach. In H. O. F. Veiel & U. Baumann (Eds.), *The meaning and measurement of social support* (pp. 235–257). Washington, DC: Hemisphere.

Brown, G. W. (1993). Life events and affective disorders: Replications and limitations. *Psychomatic Medicine, 55,* 248–259.

Brown, G. W. (1996). Genetics of depression: A social science perspective. *International Review of Psychiatry, 8,* 387–401.

Brown, G. W., Andrews, B., Bifulco, A., & Veiel, H. (1990a). Self-esteem and depression: 1. Measurement issues and prediction of onset. *Social Psychiatry and Psychiatric Epidemiology, 25,* 200–209.

Brown, G. W., Bifulco, A., & Andrews, B. (1990b). Sefl-esteem and depression: 3. Aetiological issues. *Social Psychiatry and Psychiatric Epidemiology, 25,* 235–243.

Brown, G. W., Bifulco, A., & Harris, T. O. (1987). Life events, vulnerability and onset of depression: Some refinements. *British Journal of Psychiatry, 150,* 30–42.

Brown, G. W., Bifulco, A., Veiel, H., & Andrews, B. (1990b). Self-esteem and depression: 2. Social correlations and self-esteem. *Social Psychiatry and Psychiatric Epidemiology, 25,* 225–234.

Brown, G. W., & Harris, T. O. (1978). *Social origins of depression: A study of psychiatric disorder in women.* New York: The Free Press.

Brown, G. W., & Harris, T. O. (1986). Establishing causal links: The Bedford College Studies of Depression. In H. Katschnig (Ed.), *Life events and psychiatric disorders: Controversial issues* (pp. 107–187). Cambridge, England: Cambridge University Press.

Brown, G. W., & Harris, T. O. (1989a). Depression. In G. W. Brown & T. O. Harris (Eds.), *Life events and illness* (pp.49–94). New York: The Guilford Press.

Brown, G. W., & Harris, T. O. (Eds.). (1989b). *Life events and illness.* New York: The Guilford Press.

Brown, G. W., Harris, T. O., & Eales, M. J. (1993). Aetiology of anxiety and depressive disorders in an inner city population. 2. Comorbidity and adversity. *Psychological Medicine, 23,* 155–165.

Brown, G. W., Harris, T. O., & Hepworth, C. (1994a). Life events and endogenous depression: A puzzle reexamined. *Archives of General Psychiatry, 51,* 525–534.

Brown, G. W., Harris, T. O., & Hepworth, C. (1995). Loss, humiliation and entrapment among women developing depression: A patient and non-patient comparison. *Psychological Medicine, 25,* 7–21.

Brown, G. W., Harris, T. O., Hepworth, C., & Robinson, R. (1994b). Clinical and psychosocial origins of chronic depressive episodes. II. A patient enquiry. *British Journal of Psychiatry, 165,* 457–465.

Brown, G. W., Lemyre, L., & Bifulco, A. (1992). Social factors and recovery from anxiety and depressive disorders: A test of the specificity. *British Journal of Psychiatry, 161,* 44–54.

Brown, G. W., & Moran, P. (1994). Clinical and psychosocial origins of chronic depressive episodes. I. A community survey. *British Journal of Psychiatry, 165,* 447–456.

Deakin, J. W. (1990). Serotonin subtypes and affective disorder. In C. Idzidwoski & P. Cowen (Eds.), *Serotonin—sleep and mental disorder.* Oxford, England: Blackwell Scientific Publishers.

Dohrenwend, B. P., Link, B. G., Kern, R., Shrout, P. E., & Markowitz, J. (1987). Measuring life events: The problem of variability within event categories. In B. Cooper (Ed.), *Psychiatric epidemiology—progress and prospects* (pp. 103–119). London: Croom Helm.

Eales, M. J. (1988). Depression and anxiety in unemployed men. *Psychological Medicine, 18,* 935–945.

Eales, M. J. (1985). *Social factors in the occurrence of depression, and allied disorders, in unemployed men.* Ph.D. thesis, Royal Holloway & Bedford New College (University of London).

Edwards, A. C., Nazroo, J., & Brown, G. W. (1998). Gender differences in marital support following a shared life event. *Social Science and Medicine, 46,* 1077–1085.

Finlay-Jones, R. (1989). Anxiety. In G. W. Brown & T. O. Harris (Eds.), *Life events and illness* (pp. 95–112). New York: The Guilford Press.

Finlay-Jones, R., & Brown, G. W. (1981). Types of stressful life event and the onset of anxiety and depressive disorders. *Psychological Medicine, 11,* 803–815.

Finlay-Jones, R., Brown, G. W., Duncan-Jones, P., Harris, T. O., Murphy, E., & Prudo, R. (1980). Depression and anxiety in the community. *Psychological Medicine, 10,* 445–454.

Frijda, N. H. (1988). The laws of emotion. *American Psychologist, 43,* 349–358.

Gaminde, I., Uria, M., Padro, D., Querejeta, I., & Ozamiz, A. (1993). Depression in three populations in the Basque country—a comparison with Britain. *Social Psychiatry and Psychiatric Epidemiology, 28,* 243–251.

Gilbert, P. (1992). *Depression: The evolution of powerlessness.* Hillsdale, NJ: Lawrence Erlbaum Associates.

Hammen C, (1988). Depression and cognition about personal stressful life events. In L. B. Alloy (Ed.), *Cognitive processes in depression.* New York: The Guilford Press.

Harris, T. O. (1992). Some reflections on the process of social support; and nature of unsupportive behaviors. In H. O. F. Veiel & U. Baumann (Eds.), *The meaning and measurement of social support* (pp. 171–189). Washington, DC: Hemisphere.

Katschnig, H., Pakesch, G., & Egger-Zeidner, E. (1986). Life stress and depressive subtypes: A review of present diagnostic criteria and recent research results. In H. Katschnig (Ed.), *Life events and psychiatric disorders: Controversial issues* (pp. 201–245). Cambridge, England: Cambridge University Press.

Moore, G. (1985). Alfred Nobbs. In minor keys—The uncollected short stories of George Moore. Syracuse, NY: Syracuse University Press.

Nazroo, J. Y., Edwards, A. C., & Brown, G. W., (1997). Gender differences in the onset of depression: A study of couples. *Psychological Medicine, 27,* 9–19.

Paykel, E. S., Prusoff, B. A., & Klerman, G. L. (1971). The endogenous-neurotic continuum in depression: Rater independence and factor distribution. *Journal of Psychiatric Research, 8,* 73–90.

Post, R. M., Rubinow, D. R., & Ballenger, J. C. (1986). Conditioning and sensitization in the longitudinal course of affective illness. *British Journal of Psychiatry, 149,* 191–201.

Price, J., Sloman, L., Gardner, R., Jr., Gilbert, P., & Rohde, P. (1994). The social competition hypothesis of depression. *British Journal of Psychiatry, 164,* 309–315.

Proust, M. (1989). *Albertine disparue.* Paris: Éditions Grasset & Fasquelle.

Unger, R. M. (1984). *Passion: An essay on personality.* New York: The Free Press.

IV

STRESS-MODERATING AND -AMPLIFYING FACTORS

David Mechanic

Variants of the stress–coping model have been major organizing frames of reference for more than 30 years (Lazarus, 1966; Mechanic, 1962). In the earlier years, attention was focused on stressful life events, and there was a tendency to seek simple associations between the magnitude of life stressors and adverse outcomes (Holmes & Masuda, 1974). Attention now has shifted to the various mediators between the occurrence of such events and response, focusing particularly on mediators that reflect personality characteristics, coping, and social support. The four chapters in this section are helpful in moving the field ahead not only because they provide new and interesting data but also because they help point the way for needed amplifications and new directions.

Personality, coping, and social support, which are the foci of this section, are useful integrative concepts, but they are all too general and vaguely defined to capture the extraordinary complexity of causal processes affecting adaptation. Adaptation is an iterative process in which earlier events and interactions influence subsequent adaptive pathways. Few studies capture these inter-

linked processes. Also, most analyses of stress and coping are highly individualistic, ignoring important structural aspects. This poses no problem for personality analyses, but coping and social support could and should be studied in terms of their structural dimensions as well as personal ones. People's abilities to deal with adversities depend as much on the organization of everyday life, on the stratification of social groups, and on the networks in which they are embedded as on individual characteristics (Mechanic, 1974). It is also clear that stress and coping processes, and important mediators, vary depending on the particular health challenges under consideration (Brown & Harris, 1989). There is need for specificity and differentiation among the many health, disease, and functioning outcomes possible. It is also essential that we keep constantly in mind that coping is a process, not a static situation. Thus the same coping strategy, such as denial, may be helpful or counterproductive, depending on the dimensions of the challenge and needs of the person at a specific time. Denial may be helpful if it protects the person for a time from being overwhelmed. It may be dysfunctional if it interferes with acquiring the information and resources needed to engage challenging situations.

In an important paper in *Science*, House and his colleagues (1988) concluded that "the evidence regarding social relationships and health increasingly approximates the evidence in the 1964 Surgeon General's report that established cigarette smoking as a cause or risk factor for mortality and morbidity from a range of diseases" (p. 543). There have been impressive findings on social support in varying studies (Cohen & Syme, 1985), but the concept remains ambiguous. There are different proxies for social support, including friendships, intimacy, confidants, networks of association, participation in voluntary groups, and the like. Many studies use a number of these indicators, which are not necessarily highly intercorrelated, and find effects for some and not others. As one considers results across studies, there are substantial inconsistencies. Such inconsistencies relate not only to the predictiveness of varying support measures but also to whether support acts directly on outcome variables or only buffers or mediates stressors when they occur. In some studies intimacy seems the key, whereas in others embeddedness in social networks seems more important. Treating results using these varying concepts as equivalent discourages needed exploration that might bring order to the inconsistencies that are now common.

It may be that these findings could be sorted by carefully distinguishing outcome measures, the specific challenges associated with various stressors, and the stage of stressful events, but I am not aware that this has been done successfully or even attempted. Intimacy may be most important for affective disorders where emotional support in the face of a humiliating severe difficulty may be a primary issue, while instrumental assistance may be more crucial in coping with events that overload the person and that pose risks for cardiovascular disease or other disease outcomes. In these latter instances, embeddedness in a network of stable associations that offer the availability of instrumental assistance may help give regularity to daily routines, encourage positive health behaviors, and influence behavior in other health-promoting ways.

The selection of positive findings and discounting of results affecting measures that fail may be one aspect of a more general problem. Social support measures are used commonly in psychosocial studies, and it is likely that the published literature exaggerates their influence because negative studies probably are much less likely to be submitted for publication or published. My informal observation is that such publication selection occurs and may be substantial.

The issue of social selection, of course, goes well beyond differential publication. As Henderson's important chapter in this section indicates, it remains unclear how much of the social support effect reflects the characteristics of individuals who can attract and mobilize such support and how much it reflects the product of social support itself. In his longitudinal study, Henderson suggests that the effect is due primarily to personality. In this vein, Werner and Smith's (1992) study in Hawaii of a cohort followed from birth found that some children at risk have a temperamental capacity to elicit interest and support from teachers, neighbors, and others in a manner that is protective. Fortunately, social support is an area of research where carefully designed experimental interventions can help resolve issues suggested by the literature. I believe we have gone beyond the point where further multivariate statistical studies of social support will yield large gains. We now must move to theoretically based, carefully designed controlled trials in which we provide various types of social support interventions and assess their utility. I have no illusions about the difficulties of doing this well, or about the barriers to implementation, but such efforts are needed if we are to move forward.

Some years ago, I suggested that social scientists should give more attention to social selection as a useful theoretical framework (Mechanic, 1975) and not simply treat social selection as an annoyance that makes it difficult to identify "real effects." People are active in structuring their environments and opportunities in seeking certain friends, jobs, and activities: they also make choices affecting almost every other aspect of their lives, ranging from schooling to mating. Thinking about such selection effects systematically may contribute importantly to our ultimate understanding of the stress–coping process. As chapters in this volume demonstrate, even some of the most seemingly independent events are to some degree influenced by selection processes. Henderson's findings may or may not ultimately be sustained by other investigations, but his chapter is important because it affirms that social support and coping are not randomly assigned resources but also involve important selective processes.

The chapters by Link and his colleagues and by Lennon are important in needed efforts to "deconstruct" highly complex environments to identify the aspects of situations that contribute to varying important outcomes. Too much of the work on stressful life events treats statuses and roles as "black boxes," thus limiting our understanding of what aspects of these social locations are noxious or protective. Work on "expressed emotion" represents one successful area of research where identification of particular aspects of family interaction has proved useful in developing successful psychoeducational programs (Hogarty et al., 1991). People, including those with serious mental illness, spend much of their time in contexts other than the family, including work, clubhouse programs, and the like. Learning about the emotional climate of these programs is also important. The research by Link and his colleagues nicely shows how noisome work conditions and having direction and control over one's work have differential effects for schizophrenia and affective disorder. Lennon's study, informed by a relevant theoretical orientation, shows how the characteristics of varying types of labor, whether housework or job, affect relevant outcomes. Both studies have the advantage of using theory mean-

ingfully to enhance understanding of psychopathology.

As Skodal's chapter shows, it has been difficult to identify consistent and reliable dispositional and coping effects. Coping, in particular, has been a major theoretical construct used to explain differential outcomes under common stressors, but measurement of coping repertoires has not advanced significantly. Despite large advances in rigor and quality of longitudinal data, intervals between interviews are too long to capture meaningfully the problem-solving activities that people apply to life challenges. Most longitudinal studies consist of linked static "snapshots" that fail to capture the variety and iterative quality of how people cope. The quality of coping and its dynamic character are often better represented through naturalistic observations and aids such as diaries. These observations provide more substance for theorizing about the coping process and its complex contingencies. We need efforts that combine the large samples and rigor of population research with smaller naturalistic studies that better identify the specific processes involved within the time intervals covered by the larger studies. Combining the advantages of both types of studies within an integrative framework offers opportunities to push the field forward.

My earlier comments on the importance of specifying which measures of social support are expected to affect which outcomes also applies to socioeconomic status (SES), discussed extensively in this volume. Although education, income, and occupation are intercorrelated, they each often have independent effects on health outcomes (Kessler, 1982). Each aspect of SES is also a complex proxy. Education, for example, captures in more or less efficient ways such varied concepts as knowledge acquisition and retention, coping, sense of mastery, lifestyles, preferences, and the like (Mechanic, 1989). It also represents, with other indicators, the amount of disposable income, quality of housing and neighborhood, and occupational risks. We need to develop and test more specifically hypotheses explaining the associations between the components of SES and varying outcomes.

We also need to give attention to identifying appropriate measures beyond American Psychiatric Association diagnoses. As the Medical Outcomes Study (Wells et al., 1989) has demonstrated, depressive symptoms short of a clinical diagnosis are often as disabling as the clinical diagnosis itself, and diagnosis is a poor predictor of need or resource use. As we proceed, more attention must be focused on the disability dimension, with the understanding that the risk factors for disorder might be quite different from those for disability.

The study of moderating factors depends on the quality of the survey questions we ask that seek to capture the theoretical dimensions of the stress–coping process. Many of the common questions we ask are inefficient in eliciting the desired information, and respondents often fail to understand our questions as we intend them. Increasing efforts have been made to apply findings from cognitive science to survey methodology, a process that may be helpful in refining some of our frequently used measures. It is also extremely useful to develop independent criteria for rating environments or life events, as Link and his colleagues skillfully did in their chapter.

We still have much to learn about what people have in mind when they answer conventional health questions. A number of longitudinal studies, some covering periods as long as 17 years, have found that individuals' assessments of their health are more predictive of future mortality than other indicators, including physician assessment, risk factors, and medical history (Idler, 1992). No one has been fully successful in identifying the mediating factors, although a wide range of objective and subjective indicators has been examined. Interviews with respondents who report varying levels of health make clear that respondents consider a large range of dimensions in making these assessments. Why health assessments have such predictive power still remains a puzzle.

In sum, it is reasonable to conclude that, in our quest to understand moderating and amplifying processes, our cup is both half full and half empty. On the positive side, the quality of the questions, the rigor of our methodologies, and the sophistication of our concepts have improved a great deal over the past few decades. However, we have made less progress than we hoped in elucidating underlying processes and in measuring more subtle aspects of coping, support, and other features of the adaptational process. The chapters in this section reflect the increasing sophistication of our questions and methods. They also make clear that a larger agenda remains.

REFERENCES

Brown, G. W., & Harris, T. O. (Eds.). (1989). *Life events and illness*. New York: The Guilford Press.

Cohen, S., & Syme, L. (Eds.). (1985). *Social Support and Health*. New York: Academic Press.

Hogarty, G. E., Anderson, C. M., Reiss, D. J., et al. (1991). Family psychoeducation, social skills training, and maintenance chemotherapy in the aftercare treatment of schizophrenia. *Archives of General Psychiatry*, *48*, 340–347.

Holmes, T. H., & Masuda, M. (1974). Life change and illness susceptibility. In B. S. Dohrenwend & B. P. Dohrenwend (Eds.), *Stressful life events: Their nature and effects* (pp. 45–72). New York: Wiley-Interscience.

House, J. S., Landis K. L., & Umberson, D. (1988). Social relationships and health. *Science 241*, 540–546.

Idler, E. (1992). Self-assessed health and mortality: a review of studies. In S. Maes, H. Leventhal, & M. Johnston (Eds.), *International review of health psychology* (Vol. 1). New York: John Wiley & Sons.

Kessler, R. C. (1982). A disaggregation of the relationship between socioeconomic status and psychological distress. *American Sociological Review*, *47*, 752–764.

Lazarus, R. S. (1966). *Psychological stress and the coping process*. New York: McGraw-Hill.

Mechanic, D. (1962). *Students under stress: A study in the social psychology of adaptation*. New York: The Free Press.

Mechanic, D. (1974). Social structure and personal adaptation: Some neglected dimensions. In G. Coelho, D. Hamburg, & J. Adams (Eds.), *Stress and adaptation* (pp. 32–44). New York: Basic Books.

Mechanic, D. (1975). Sociocultural and social-psychological factors affecting personal responses to psychological disorder. *Journal of Health and Social Behavior, 16,* 393–404.

Mechanic, D. (1989). Socioeconomic status and health: An examination of underlying processes. In J. P. Bunker, D. S. Gomby, & B. H. Kehrer (Eds.), *Pathways to health: The role of social factors* (pp. 9–26). Menlo Park, CA: Henry J. Kaiser Family Foundation.

Wells, K. B., Stewart, A., Hays, R. D., et al. (1989). The functioning and well-being of depressed patients: Results from the Medical Outcomes Study. *JAMA, 262,* 914–919.

Werner, E. E., & Smith, R. S. (1992). *Overcoming the odds: High risk children from birth to adulthood.* Ithaca, NY: Cornell University Press.

19

Personality and Coping as Stress-Attenuating or -Amplifying Factors

Andrew E. Skodol

The effects of life events and chronic stressors on people experiencing them are far from uniform. Many studies reveal a relatively weak effect of psychosocial stressors on production of psychopathology (Rabkin & Struening, 1976), and some studies suggest that stressors may lead to personal growth and improved functioning (Baltes, 1987; Masten et al., 1991; Schaefer & Moos, 1992). These observations have prompted examination of individual differences among people experiencing stress, in an attempt to understand why some experience distress or disability and others exhibit resiliency in the face of adversity (Rutter, 1985).

The two types of individual differences that are the focus of this chapter are personality and coping processes. Personality refers to constellations of traits or attributes that determine how people perceive, think about, and relate to themselves and the environment (American Psychiatric Association, 1994). Personality includes both fundamental behavioral predispositions such as emotionality, activity, and sociability, commonly referred to as temperament (Buss & Plomin, 1986), and more complex organizing and integrative systems that include cognitive and motivational components (Rutter,

1987). Personality traits are assumed to be relatively stable over time and to be relatively consistent across situations.

Coping refers to specific processes that a person engages in expressly for the purpose of dealing with stress (Lazarus & Folkman, 1984; Pearlin & Schooler, 1978). Coping involves cognitive, behavioral, and emotional responses. In contrast to personality, coping strategies may or may not be characteristic of a person or consistent across stressful situations or functional roles. Personality and coping should be related in that certain traits or dispositions should predispose to, or be associated with, the use of certain coping strategies and not others. Personality traits, coping processes, or a combination of both are likely to either ameliorate or aggravate the impact of stressful experiences.

Personality traits and coping styles are part of a larger set of personal attributes that include intelligence, genetic predispositions, abilities and disabilities, motivation, and values. Together, these are sometimes referred to as *personal dispositions* in life stress research. Along with external resources, such as social support, these characteristics of a person may interact with stressful events and situations in a number of ways to contribute to the development of psychopathology or to help to protect against it.

MAJOR MODELS OF PERSONALITY

Although hundreds, perhaps thousands, of trait scales have been developed by personality researchers, the lack of a coherent theory integrating single dimensions of personality (Rorer & Widiger, 1983) has led many personality psychologists toward multidimensional models of personality. Nonetheless, research involving single traits such as self-esteem and particularly locus of control as potential buffers against stress has accumulated. Self-esteem is a sense of self-worth, self-respect, and self-acceptance that is usually linked to an expectation of success in life (Rosenberg, 1979). Locus of control is a generalized belief concerning personal control over important outcomes (Rotter, 1966).

In addition, two personality types have appeared repeatedly in the stress literature: hardiness and type A behavior pattern. Hardiness is a personality construct consisting of control (i.e., a tendency to feel and act as if one is influential rather than helpless, in the face of external forces); commitment (i.e., a tendency to be involved and find purpose and meaning in, rather than feel alienated from, life's activities and encounters); and challenge (i.e., a belief that change is normal in life and that the anticipation of change is an opportunity for growth rather than a threat to security) (Kobasa et al., 1982). The type A behavior pattern (Friedman & Rosenman, 1959) or personality is characterized by excessive competitive drive, impatience, hostility, and accelerated speech and motor movements (Matthews, 1982).

Multitrait models of personality are theories about the number and kind of personality traits most important in describing an individual; they involve simultaneous assessment on many (usually 10–20) different personality dimensions. Instruments based on these models are designed to provide a comprehensive assessment of personality.

An example is the Jackson Personality Inventory (Jackson, 1976), which measures anxiety, breadth of interest, complexity, conformity, energy level, innovation, interpersonal affect, organization, responsibility, risk taking, self-esteem, social adroitness, social participation, tolerance, and value orthodoxy. Another well-known example is the Sixteen Personality Factor Questionnaire (Cattell et al., 1980), which measures apprehensiveness, assertiveness, contentiousness, conservativism, control, emotional instability, forthrightness, imaginativeness, intelligence, self-sufficiency, surgency, tender-mindedness, tension, trust, venturesomeness, and warmheartedness.

Although these and other omnibus personality inventories contain some synonymous or closely related terms, and several opposites, there is very little overlap in the content of the traits across questionnaires (Watson et al., 1994). Furthermore, these instruments in their entirety have not been used in life stress research, although several of their component traits (e.g., self-esteem, control) have been studied.

Some multitrait models have been derived using quantitative techniques in order to identify a basic structure of personality indicated by the covariation of personality traits together, or apart from, one another (Watson et al., 1994). Work on personality structure has produced several *three-factor models*, represented by Eysenck's, Tellegen's, or Watson and Clark's systems, and a *five-factor model* originated by Fiske (1949), developed by Norman (1963), but now most commonly associated with Costa and McCrae (1992) and McCrae and Costa (1987).

The three factors in Eysenck's model are called neuroticism (vs. emotional stability), extraversion (vs. introversion), and psychoticism (Eysenck & Eysenck, 1975). Tellegen's (1985) model includes negative emotionality, positive emotionality, and constraint. Watson and Clark (1993) have a very similar model with factors named negative temperament, positive temperament, and disinhibition (vs. constraint). The five-factor model includes neuroticism, extraversion, conscientiousness, agreeableness, and openness to experience or intellect (Digman, 1990; Goldberg, 1990).

The three- and five-factor models can be integrated (Watson et al., 1994): neuroticism (negative emotionality, negative temperament) and extraversion (positive emotionality, positive temperament) are common to both; the third three-factor dimension, psychoticism or disinhibition vs. constraint, may correspond to five-factor dimensions of conscientiousness and agreeableness. Conscientiousness and agreeableness, however, appear to be broader domains than psychoticism that can at times be in opposition and thus may be better represented by separate factors than as facets of a single "superfactor" (Costa & McCrae, 1995). The final "Big Five" factor, openness or intellect, appears to be unrelated to any "Big Three" dimension.

The neuroticism or negative emotionality factor represents a tendency to see and react to the world as threatening, problematic, and distressing. People with such a personality trait would be prone to make negative cognitive appraisals of situations demanding coping efforts. The extraversion or positive emotionality factor represents a tendency to engage and confront the world. People with such a personality trait would be expected to be action oriented in their approach to problems. The third factor, conscientiousness or constraint, reflects impulse control. People with such a personality trait would be likely to plan rather than act in problem-solving situations. Agreeableness represents sociability. Openness reflects flexibility of mind and emotion.

The five-factor model of personality structure has also been shown to be complementary to interpersonal models of personality as represented by the interpersonal circumplex (Kiesler, 1983; Wiggins, 1979), a circular arrangement of interpersonal dispositions arrayed around the orthogonal dimensions of dominance (vs. submission) and nurturance (vs. hostility). According to this synthesis, extraversion is related to dominance and agreeableness to nurturance (McCrae & Costa, 1989). The five-factor model has also been related (Costa & Widiger, 1994; Widiger & Costa, 1994) to personality disorders as described in the *Diagnostic and Statistical Manual of Mental Disorders*, (*Third Edition, Revised*) (*DSM-III-R*, American Psychiatric Association, 1987). Most personality disorders studied reveal strong associations with neuroticism. Borderline personality disorder also shows consistently negative correlations with agreeableness, suggesting a significant facet of antagonism in the diagnosis. Avoidant personality disorder appears to be a combination of high neuroticism and low extraversion.

Personality factors of the five-factor model are stable over time (Costa & McCrae, 1994) and can be used to describe gender-related individual differences in personality (Lippa, 1995). Masculinity has been linked to extraversion, openness, and neuroticism. Femininity has been linked to agreeableness and, to a lesser degree, to conscientiousness. The factor structure of the five-factor model in six highly diverse cultures and languages (German, Portuguese, Hebrew, Chinese, Korean, and Japanese) has been found to be highly congruent with the American normative factor structure (McCrae & Costa, 1997). These data suggest that personality trait structure may be universal.

An alternative approach to delineating the basic structure of personality is Cloninger's (1987) biosocial theory, which includes dimensions of novelty seeking, harm avoidance, and reward dependence, based on three postulated brain systems concerned with behavioral activation, inhibition, and maintenance. Cloninger has revised his system to include seven personality dimensions: four of temperament (adding persistence) and three of character, including self-directedness, cooperativeness, and self-transcendence (Cloninger et al., 1993). The four temperamental dimensions are hypothesized to be more biologically based and genetically determined, whereas the later developing character dimensions involve conceptual learning.

The factor structure of the Cloninger dimensions has been difficult to establish empirically using conventional methods, and the relationship of these dimensions to factor models is unclear (Cannon et al., 1993; Waller et al., 1991). However, Cloninger's four-dimensional structure of temperament was confirmed by genetic and environmental analyses in female twins (Stallings et al., 1996). Male twins had a three-factor genetic structure, not including persistence; for men, variance in persistence appeared to be environmental. Low self-directedness and low cooperativeness have been shown to indicate the presence of a *DSM-III-R* personality disorder of some type, and clusters A (odd, eccentric), B (dramatic, emotional, erratic), and C (anxious, fearful) are characterized by low reward dependence, high novelty seeking, and high harm avoidance, respectively (Goldman et al., 1994; Svrakic et al., 1993).

The boundaries between personality characteristics and other characteristics of the person and of his or her social situation are not always clear. Nor can personality and psychopathology always readily be cleaved apart. Finally, not all personality characteristics have been investigated as buffers or stress-aggravating factors in life stress studies. This brief review of personality models and measures focused primarily on personality characteristics that are most clearly traits of the person, not his or her social situation, that are commonly accepted as distinct from the signs and symptoms of mental disorders, and that have played a role in the literature on factors affecting the life stress process.

MAJOR MODELS OF COPING

The prevailing models of coping have been those of Pearlin and Schooler and of Lazarus and Folkman. As conceptualized by Pearlin and Schooler (1978), coping refers to behavior that protects people from being psychologically harmed by adverse experiences. This protective function can take three forms. A person can (*1*) modify or change problematic conditions, (*2*) control the meaning of an experience to neutralize its problematic character, or (*3*) manage the emotional consequences of the experience.

According to the model of Lazarus and Folkman (1984), initially, a person makes a cognitive appraisal of harm, threat, or challenge embodied by a stressor. Harm refers to damage already done—a loss; threat is the anticipation of harm; and challenge represents demands that can be met. Next, there is a secondary appraisal of the extent to which a stressful situation might be changed or must be accepted. These appraisals are followed by either *problem-focused coping, emotion-focused coping*, or both.

Problem-focused coping refers to efforts to resolve the threatening problem or to diminish its impact by taking direct action. Emotion-focused coping refers to efforts to reduce the negative emotions aroused in response to a threat by changing the way the threat is attended to or interpreted. These two types of coping often co-occur and may interact with one another; for example, emotion-focused coping may reduce distress to an extent that facilitates problem-focused coping, and problem-focused coping may reduce threat to an extent that also relieves emotional distress.

One model of coping differentiates cognitive from behavioral coping, either approach or avoidance (Moos & Schaefer, 1993); another emphasizes the distinction between dispositional coping styles and situational coping strategies (Silver & Wortman, 1980). Some aspects of the coping process may not be totally deliberate or conscious, as represented by the psychoanalytical concept of defense mechanism (Vaillant, 1977) and the social cognition concept of controlled versus automatic processing (Bargh, 1994).

Coping has been assessed by a variety of measures, including the Coping Responses Inventory (Moos, 1992), the Ways of Coping Questionnaire (Folkman & Lazarus, 1988), and the COPE Inventory (Carver et al., 1989), among others. The most commonly studied types of coping, however, have been variants of these six: planful problem solving, seeking support, focusing on the positive, distancing or distraction, wishful thinking or escape, and accepting responsibility or self-blame.

MODELS OF STRESS AND COPING

According to the model of the life stress process proposed by Dohrenwend and Dohrenwend (1981), maladaptive personal dispositions may exert a direct additive effect on adverse mental health outcomes along with stressful events (the so-called additive burden hypothesis), or an indirect effect, by increasing a person's vulnerability to stressors for a negative outcome (the "vulnerability" hypothesis). Alternatively, or in addition, maladaptive predispositions may lead to the occurrence of stressors by a mechanism that is referred to as "proneness." Adaptive personal biological or psychological characteristics would operate in the opposite direction, that is, to reduce the occurrence of, vulnerability to, or burden from life's stressors, so that the risk for psychopathology would be diminished.

In considering ways in which personality characteristics might interact with coping, Cohen and Edwards (1989) proposed two alternatives. Personality traits might either increase or decrease a person's appraisal of an experience as stressful or influence his or her actual coping response. In the former case, a perception that the person has the necessary resources to handle a situation should reduce the threat perceived in the situation or increase the perceived efficacy of his or her coping efforts. A negative perception would have the opposite effect. In the latter case, more adaptive coping behaviors and emotional responses to a stressor should directly counteract its pathogenic impact; less adaptive coping responses would aggravate the situation.

PROBLEMS IN PERSONALITY, COPING, AND LIFE STRESS RESEARCH

The literature on the relationship of coping processes to the outcomes of life stress has been reviewed by others (e.g., Coyne & Downey, 1991; Kessler et al., 1985). In general, these reviews suggest that studies of the effect of personality and coping on the outcome of stressful experiences have suffered from many of the problems that have plagued life events research in general, as well as from some problems specific to these variables. These problems can be summarized as follows:

1. Most studies have been retrospective, thus potentially confounding the measurement of the outcome of psychological distress with the measurement of the personality or coping factor presumed to attenuate or amplify the effect of the stressor on outcome.

2. Few studies take into account symptom status prior to the stressor or past history of depressive symptoms or disorder (for example), thus ignoring the crucial question of the direction of causality between personality attribute or coping mechanism and psychopathology. The chronic nature of many mental disorders raises the question of whether stress initiates a disorder or exacerbates or maintains it.

3. Studies have often allowed respondents to identify the most significant stressor over a given time period or have investigated coping with life stress in general, thus introducing heterogeneity of the stressor itself into the equation. Even seemingly similar stressors have been shown to vary considerably on factors such as desirability, fatefulness, or magnitude of normative change that is induced.

4. Studies have often used college students as subjects and simple symptom measures of psychological distress as outcomes, thus casting doubt on the generalizability of the findings and their relevance to clinical psychopathology. Most studies have used simple self-report scales for measuring distress; very few have used a semistructured interview to assess diagnoses of mental disorders.

5. Studies are most often cross-sectional, giving the potentially misleading impression that coping is a static as opposed to a dynamic process.

6. Few studies have attempted to measure stable personality dispositions and situational coping attempts independently and to determine the relative contributions of each to outcome.

7. Studies that have investigated personality factors have been limited for the most part to traits related to neuroticism, not a full array of personality dimensions, or have introduced new constructs such as hardiness, not clearly related to prevailing personality models.

8. Most studies on coping have not considered the relationship of other potentially mediating variables, such as availability of social support, on coping efforts. For example, whether someone seeks social support or engages in wishful thinking or fantasy may be determined by the availability of a support system.

9. Most studies on coping have not investigated characteristics of the stressful situation itself that might make certain coping strategies potentially more adaptive and others less so.

RESEARCH ON PERSONALITY, COPING, AND LIFE STRESS

The Question of Independent Effects

Do dispositional coping styles or personality traits and situational coping strategies have independent effects on the pathogenic aspects of stress? McCrae and Costa (1986) found in a community sample that both neuroticism and coping were related to distress. Coping, however, showed no relationship to distress when neuroticism was statistically controlled. The authors concluded that reports of coping efforts may be "epiphenomena of personality" and have no independent effects on reactions to stress.

Their study, however, asked subjects to recall how they coped with an event that occurred from 10 to 21 months earlier. This time lapse would be consistent with subjects reporting their typical, dispositional coping styles, more consistent with their personality traits, rather than the specific situational coping strategies they employed at the time of the event's occurrence.

In a longitudinal study by Bolger (1990) of college students taking the Medical College Admissions Test, the personality trait of neuroticism was related to increases in anxiety, controlling for initial levels of anxiety. Ineffective coping mechanisms, specifically wishful thinking and self-blame, as measured by the Ways of Coping Scale, mediated over half of the effect of neuroticism on anxiety. This suggests that neuroticism leads people to cope ineffectively, and that ineffective coping, in turn, leads to increases in distress. The focus on a specific stressor (an examination) and a particular population (premedical students) was both a strength and a weakness in this study. Although the narrow focus limited the potential generalizability of the results to other stressors and other populations, it also afforded methodological leverage in allowing for a prospective design and in studying a uniform event.

In a longitudinal study of breast cancer patients, Carver et al. (1993) found that the personality trait of optimism (vs. pessimism), a variable reflecting aspects of the Big Five dimensions of extraversion and neuroticism, was inversely related to measures of anxiety, depression, and anger at diagnosis and at five points in time covering a 1 year postsurgical follow-up period, controlling for prior distress. Evidence was found for mediating effects of coping strategies of acceptance, denial, and behavioral disengagement on levels of distress. This study did not specifically measure neuroticism, which consists partly of pessimism and could account for the study's findings. However, controls for previous distress, a tentative proxy for neuroticism, did not eliminate the effects of pessimism on subsequent distress.

In a subsequent study, Scheier et al. (1994) demonstrated that dispositional optimism continued to be significantly correlated with aspects of coping, including planning, active coping, positive reinterpretation, and seeking instrumental support, and with symptoms of depression, even when other personality traits, such as mastery, trait anxiety, self-esteem, and neuroticism, were controlled. The authors argue that the broad factor of neuroticism, although related to optimism (i.e., pessimism), may create problems of interpretation in coping research because it may be difficult to determine which components of neuroticism would be responsible for a given effect.

These three studies suggest independent roles for personality traits, especially neuroticism and its lower order component trait pessimism, and for coping behaviors on the outcome of stressful events.

The Question of Consistency in Coping

Is there consistency in coping behaviors over time or across situations, suggesting a particular coping style, or does coping change based on the demands of a particular situation or the outcome of previous coping efforts? If coping is consistent, how much of the consistency is related to personality traits, and what patterns are evident?

Some evidence supports the notion of stable coping styles or dispositions. Several investigators have demonstrated significant correlations between coping measured at time intervals of up to 7 years (Carver et al., 1989; Holahan & Moos, 1987; McCrae, 1989). These correlations may be inflated, however, by the similarity of the stressful situations encountered at the two times, which would be expected also to increase coping consistency. Terry (1994) demonstrated that much of the stability in coping over a relatively short (10 week) period in response to a variety of different life events was dependent on the extent of cross-situational consistency in the type of event and levels of appraised stress. These findings echo earlier

results of Folkman and Lazarus (1980), who found that people were more variable than consistent in their coping with different kinds of stressful events. Work contexts favored problem-focused coping, while health contexts favored emotion-focused coping. Situations in which a person believed that something could be done elicited more problem-focused coping, whereas those that had to be accepted elicited more emotion-focused coping.

Personality traits might also exert a stable influence on coping (Carver et al., 1989). Persons high on internal locus of control or self-esteem are more likely to use problem-focused coping than emotion-focused coping because they believe they can influence the outcome of a stressful situation for the better (Fleishman, 1984; Holahan & Moos, 1987). People high on neuroticism rely more on emotion-focused coping (Bolger, 1990; Carver et al., 1989). Carver et al. (1989) found that the coping efforts of Type A individuals were characterized by planning, active confrontation, and persistence. Terry (1994) found that high self-esteem and Type A behavior were related to problem-focused coping, especially for work-related problems that were appraised as controllable. Personality traits of denial and external locus of control were related in her study to emotion-focused strategies, such as minimization and seeking meaning. When stable influences on coping were controlled, Terry found that situational factors, such as situation type and situation appraisal, influenced the type of coping used.

In studies that have followed people sequentially through a stressful experience, such as a major college exam (Bolger, 1990; Carver & Scheier, 1994; Folkman & Lazarus, 1985) or surgical treatment for breast cancer (Carver et al., 1993), there is evidence that cognitive appraisals and coping strategies employed change in anticipation of, during, and following the stressor. People appear to respond to different demands at different stages. Furthermore, not only do cognitive appraisals of, for example, threat or challenge influence coping strategy, but coping strategy and its outcome affects subsequent cognitive appraisal, in a feedback loop pattern.

The Question of Attenuating Versus Amplifying Effects

What are beneficial personality traits or coping styles, and which are maladaptive? In their 1985 review, Kessler et al. conclude, "Although it is widely assumed that the choice of coping strategies can ameliorate the impact of stressful experiences, there is surprisingly little sound, empirical research bearing on this assumption." This situation is essentially unchanged today.

Examples of maladaptive coping include escapism (e.g., fantasizing, daydreaming, use of drugs or alcohol), self-blame (e.g., taking full responsibility for the problem in a self-punitive manner), overt denial, and behavioral disengagement (e.g., thoughts of giving up). These strategies are related to elevated symptoms of anxiety and depression and diagnoses of depression in response to diverse stressors such as college exams, diagnosis of breast cancer, in vitro fertilization failure, chronic illness, and general life stressors, both large and small (Bolger, 1990; Carver & Scheier, 1994; Carver et al., 1993; Felton & Revenson, 1984; Litt et al., 1992; Rohde et al., 1990; Stanton & Snider, 1993).

In general, the effects of coping depend somewhat on the characteristics of the stressful situation, that is, whether steps can be taken to diminish the stressor's impact or whether there must be accommodation to the stressor for successful adaptation. Therefore, personality traits or coping mechanisms that involve mental withdrawal or disengagement from a situation in which there is potential for control are detrimental. This may even be true in circumstances such as chronic physical illness, where the course of the illness may not be controllable but some of the consequences, such as daily physical symptoms or emotional reactions, may be (Thompson et al., 1993).

Self-perception of coping successfully with loss of a spouse by older adults (Zautra & Wrabetz, 1991), with an elective abortion by young women (Cozzarelli, 1993), and

with stressful events in general by a community sample of respondents (Aldwin & Revenson, 1987) has been associated with lower levels of psychological distress. Self-efficacy has been shown to mediate some of the effects of personality traits such as feelings of control and optimism on poststressor adjustment. These studies could not definitively separate cause and effect in the analyses of relationships between coping efficacy and mental health, but contained longitudinal assessments and controlled for initial symptom levels and neuroticism.

Three studies have found that some aspect of problem-focused coping exerted a positive effect on emotional distress following a stressor (Aldwin & Revenson, 1987; Aspinwall & Taylor, 1992; Glyshaw, et al., 1989). A fourth study indicated that positive reappraisal had a beneficial effect on dealing with problems in the workplace (Menaghan & Merves, 1984). Although these studies had the advantage of being prospective and thus able to deal with issues of confounding and, to some extent, the direction of causality, none studied a particular stressor, focusing instead on nominated stressors occurring over a particular time period.

Only one study, by Carver et al. (1993), demonstrated prospectively beneficial effects of acceptance and use of humor in coping with the diagnosis of breast cancer and subsequent surgery. However, the beneficial effects of both active coping (Bolger, 1990; Carver & Scheier, 1994; Mattlin et al., 1990) and acceptance (Carver & Scheier, 1994) have been contradicted by the results of studies of other stressful situations. These contradictions again suggest that characteristics of a stressful situation—possibly whether the situation realistically represents challenge and should be dealt with actively or is one that must be endured and accommodated to—may determine which coping strategies are most beneficial (Vitaliano et al., 1990).

The Question of Direction of Effects

Does personality lead people into stressful situations by increasing their exposure to stressful events? In a prospective longitudinal study by Magnus et al. (1993), extraversion was found to predispose young adults to experience more positive objective life events, whereas neuroticism predisposed them to experience more negative objective life events. Similarly, Breslau et al. (1995) found that neuroticism and extraversion increased the likelihood of being exposed to an extreme stressor, as well as the likelihood of developing post-traumatic stress disorder following exposure. Genetic variance in personality (primarily extraversion and openness) has been found to mediate genetic variance on controllable, desirable, and undesirable life events (Saudino et al., 1997). Genetic influences have been demonstrated for situation-specific components of behavior (more akin to coping) as well as cross-situational consistency (more akin to personality) (Phillips & Matheny, 1997). Bolger and Schilling (1991) found that exposure to daily stressors was only half as important as reactivity to daily stressors, however, in explaining how neuroticism leads to distress in daily life. People high in neuroticism had both higher exposure to interpersonal conflicts and greater emotional reactivity (e.g., anger and depression); the latter may have been due to the differential choice of coping mechanisms and the reduced effectiveness of those efforts (Bolger & Zuckerman, 1995).

CONCLUSIONS

On the basis of both early and more recent research on the effects of personality or coping on the pathogenic aspects of stress, the following conclusions may be drawn:

1. Both dispositional coping styles or personality traits and situational coping strategies appear to exert an effect on the emotional impact of stress.
2. People may be relatively consistent in the coping strategies used to deal with similar problems at different times, but they show little consistency in dealing with stressors across life situations or across role domains, such as work, health, or marriage.
3. Coping is a dynamic process that involves changing appraisals and coping efforts in relationship to outcomes over time, in phases of a stressful encounter.
4. A large majority of studies that show coping effects indicate that maladaptive coping contributes to adverse outcomes rather than adaptive coping buffering against stress. There continue to be surprisingly few sound empirical studies documenting the assumption that adaptive coping strategies can ameliorate the effects of stressful experiences.
5. Personality traits or coping mechanisms that involve mental withdrawal or disengagement from a stressful situation in which there is potential for control are detrimental.
6. Perceived self-efficacy in coping may be the most emotionally protective factor in a stressful situation.
7. Additional studies are needed on the relationship of personality traits as measured by the prevailing three- and five-factor models of personality to coping styles. Axis II personality disorders should also be integrated theoretically and empirically into models of the personality/coping/life stress equation. Additional studies are also needed to assess the effects of personality traits and disorders or coping styles on the *occurrence* of stressful life events and on recovery from adverse mental health outcomes.

Acknowledgments: The author gratefully acknowledges Peggy E. Gallaher, Ph.D., for her helpful comments and suggestions.

REFERENCES

Aldwin, C. M., & Revenson T. A. (1987). Does coping help? A reexamination of the relation between coping and mental health. *Journal* of *Personality and Social Psychology*, 53, 337–348.

American Psychiatric Association. (1987). *Diagnostic and statistical manual of mental disorders* (3rd ed., rev.). Washington, DC: American Psychiatric Press.

American Psychiatric Association. (1994). *Diagnostic and statistical manual of mental disorders* (4th ed.). Washington, DC: American Psychiatric Press.

Aspinwall, L. G., & Taylor, S. E. (1992). Modeling cognitive adaptation: A longitudinal investigation of the impact of individual differences and coping on college adjustment and performance. *Journal of Personality and Social Psychology*, 63, 989–1003.

Baltes, P. B. (1987). Theoretical propositions of life-span developmental psychology: On the dynamics between growth and decline. *Developmental Psychology*, 23, 611–626.

Bargh, J. A. (1994). The four horsemen of automaticity: Awareness, intention, efficiency, and control in social cognition. In R. S. Wyer & T. K. Srull (Eds.), *Handbook of social cognition, Vol. 1, Basic Processes*, (pp. 1–40). Hillsdale, NJ: Lawrence Erlbaum Associates.

Bolger, N. (1990). Coping as a personality process: A prospective study. *Journal of Personality and Social Psychology*, 59, 525–537.

Bolger, N., & Schilling, E. A. (1991). Personality and the problems of everyday life: The role of neuroticism in exposure and reactivity to daily stressors. *Journal of Personality*, 59, 355–386.

Bolger, N., & Zuckerman, A. (1995). A framework for studying personality in the stress process. *Journal of Personality and Social Psychology*, 69, 890–902.

Breslau, N., Davis, G. C., & Andreski, P. (1995). Risk factors for PTSD-related traumatic events: A prospective analysis. *American Journal of Psychiatry*, 152, 529–535.

Buss, A. H., & Plomin, R. (1986). The EAS approach to temperament. In R. Plomin & J. Dunn (Eds.), *The study of temperament: Changes, continuities and challenges*, (pp. 67–79). Hillsdale, NJ: Lawrence Erlbaum Associates.

Cannon, D. S., Clark, L. A., Leeka, J. K., et al. (1993). A reanalysis of the Tridemensional Personality Questionnaire (TPQ) and its relationship to Cloninger's type 2 alcoholism. *Psychological Assessment*, 5, 62–66.

Carver, C. S., Pozo, C., Harris, S. D., et al. (1993). How coping mediates the effect of optimism on distress: A study of women with early stage breast cancer. *Journal of Personality and Social Psychology*, 65, 375–390.

Carver, C. S., & Scheier, M. F. (1994). Situational coping and coping dispositions in a stressful transaction. *Journal of Personality and Social Psychology*, 66, 184–195.

Carver, C. S., Scheier, M. F., & Weintraub, J. K. (1989). Assessing coping strategies: A theoretically based approach. *Journal of Personality and Social Psychology*, 56, 267–283.

Cattell, R. B., Eber, H. W., & Tatsuoka, M. M. (1980). *Handbook for the Sixteen Personality Factor Questionnaire (16PF)*. Champaign, IL: Institute for Personality and Ability Testing.

Cloninger, C. R. (1987). A systematic method for clinical description and classification of personality variants: A proposal. *Archives of General Psychiatry*, 44, 573–538.

Cloninger, C. R., Svrakic, D. M., & Przybeck, T. R. (1993). A psychobiological model of temperament and character. *Archives of General Psychiatry*, 50, 975–990.

Cohen, S., & Edwards, J. R. (1989). Personality characteristics as moderators of the relationship between stress and disorder. In R. W. J. Neufeld (Ed.), *Advances in the investigation of psychological stress*, (pp. 235–283). New York: John Wiley & Sons.

Costa, P. T., Jr., & McCrae, R. R. (1992). *Revised NEO Personality Inventory (NEO-PI-R) and NEO Five-Factor Inventory (NEO-FFI) professional manual*. Odessa, FL: Psychological Assessment Resources.

Costa, P. T., Jr., & McCrae, R. R. (1994). Set like plaster? Evidence for the stability of adult personality. In T. F. Heatherington & J. L. Wemberger (Eds.), *Can personality change?* (pp. 21–40). Washington, DC: American Psychological Association.

Costa, P. T., Jr., & McCrae R. R. (1995). Primary traits of Eysenck's P-E-N system: Three- and five-factor solutions. *Journal of Personality and Social Psychology*, 69, 308–317.

Costa, P. T., Jr., & Widiger, T. A. (1994). *Personality disorders and the five-factor model of personality*. Washington, DC: American Psychiatric Press.

Coyne, J. C., & Downey, G. (1991). Social factors and psychopathology: Stress, social support, and coping processes. *Annual Review of Psychology*, 42, 401–425.

Cozzarelli, C. (1993). Personality and self-efficacy as predictors of coping with abortion. *Journal of Personality and Social Psychology*, 65, 1224–1236.

Digman, J. M. (1990). Personality structure: Emergence of the five-factor model. *Annual Review of Psychology, 41*, 417–440.

Dohrenwend, B. S., & Dohrenwend, B. P. (1981). Life stress and psychopathology. In D. A. Regier & G. Allen (Eds.), *Risk factor research in the major mental disorders* (National Institute of Mental Health, DHHS Publ. No. ADM 81-1086) (pp. 131–141). Washington, DC: National Institute of Mental Health.

Eysenck, H. J., & Eysenck, S. B. G. (1975). *Manual of the Eysenck Personality Questionnaire.* San Diego, CA: Educational and Industrial Testing Service.

Felton, B. J., & Revenson, T. A. (1984). Coping with chronic illness: A study of illness controllability and the influence of coping strategies on psychological adjustment. *Journal of Consulting and Clinical Psychology, 52*, 343–353.

Fiske, D. W. (1949). Consistency of the factorial structures of personality ratings from different sources. *Journal of Abnormal and Social Psychology, 44*, 329–344.

Fleishman, J. A. (1984). Personality characteristics and coping patterns. *Journal of Health and Social Behavior, 25*, 229–244.

Folkman, S., & Lazarus, R. S. (1980). An analysis of coping in a middle-aged community sample. *Journal of Health and Social Behavior, 21*, 219–239.

Folkman, S., & Lazarus, R. S. (1985). If it changes it must be a process: A study of emotion and coping during three stages of a college examination. *Journal of Personality and Social Psychology, 48*, 150–170.

Folkman, S., & Lazarus, R. S. (1988). *Manual for the Ways of Coping Questionnaire.* Palo Alto, CA: Consulting Psychologists Press.

Friedman, M., & Rosenman, R. H. (1959). Association of specific overt behavior pattern with increases in blood cholesterol, blood clotting time, incidence of arcus senilis, and coronary artery disease. *JAMA, 169*, 1286–1296.

Glyshaw, K., Cohen, L. H., & Towbes, L. C. (1989). Coping strategies and psychological distress: Prospective analyses of early and middle adolescents. *American Journal of Community Psychology, 17*, 607–623.

Goldberg, L. R. (1990). An alternative "description of personality": The big-five factor structure. *Journal of Personality and Social Psychology, 59*, 1216–1229.

Goldman, R. G., Skodol, A. E., McGrath, P. J., et al. (1994). Relationship between the Tridimensional Personality Questionnaire and DSM-III-R personality traits. *American Journal of Psychiatry, 151*, 274–276.

Holahan, C. J., & Moos, R. H. (1987). Personal and contextual determinants of coping strategies. *Journal of Personality and Social Psychology, 52*, 946–955.

Jackson, D. N. (1976). *Jackson Personality Inventory manual.* Port Huron, MI: Research Psychologists Press.

Kessler, R. C., Price, R. H., & Wortman, C. B. (1985). Social factors in psychopathology: Stress, social support, and coping processes. *Annual Review of Psychology, 36*, 531–572.

Kiesler, D. J. (1983). The 1982 Interpersonal Circle: A taxonomy for complementarity in human transactions. *Psychological Reviews, 90*, 185–214.

Kobasa, S. C., Maddi, S. R., & Kahn, S. (1982). Hardiness and health: A prospective study. *Journal of Personality and Social Pscyhology, 42*, 168–177.

Lazarus, R. S., & Folkman, S. (1984). *Stress, appraisal, and coping.* New York: Springer-Verlag.

Lippa, R. (1995). Gender-related individual differences and psychological adjustment in terms of the big five and circumplex models. *Journal of Personality and Social Psychology, 69*, 1184–1202.

Litt, M. D., Tennen, H., Affleck, G., et al. (1992). Coping and cognitive factors in adaptation to in-vitro fertilization failure. *Journal of Behavioral Medicine, 15*, 171–187.

Magnus, K., Diener, E., Fujita, F., et al. (1993). Extraversion and neuroticism as predictors of objective life events: A longitudinal analysis. *Journal of Personality and Social Psychology, 65*, 1046–1053.

Masten, A. S., Best, K. M., & Garmezy, N. (1991). Resilience and development: Contributions from the study of children who overcome adversity. *Development and Psychopathology, 2*, 425–444.

Matthews, K. S. (1982). Psychological perspectives on the type-A behavior pattern. *Psychological Bulletin, 91*, 293–333.

Mattlin, J. A., Wethington, E., & Kessler, R. C. (1990). Situational determinants of coping and coping effectiveness. *Journal of Health and Social Behavior, 31*, 103–122.

McCrae, R. R. (1989). Age differences and changes in the use of coping mechanisms. *Journal of Gerontology, 44*, 161–169.

McCrae, R. R., & Costa, P. T., Jr. (1986). Personality, coping, and coping effectiveness in an adult sample. *Journal of Personality, 54,* 385–405.

McCrae, R. R., & Costa, P. T., Jr. (1987). Validation of a five-factor model of personality across instruments and observers. *Journal of Personality and Social Psychology, 52,* 81–90.

McCrae, R. R., & Costa, P. T., Jr. (1989). The structure of interpersonal traits: Wiggins's circumplex and the five-factor model. *Journal of Personality and Social Psychology, 56,* 586–595.

McCrae, R. R., & Costa, P. T., Jr. (1997). Personality trait structure as a human universal. *American Psychologist, 52,* 509–516.

Menaghan, E., & Merves, E. (1984). Coping with occupational problems: The limits of individual efforts. *Journal of Health and Social Behavior, 25,* 406–423.

Moos, R. (1992). *Coping responses inventory manual.* Palo Alto, CA: Center for Health Care Evaluation, Department of Veterans Affairs and Stanford University Medical Centers.

Moos, R. H., & Schaefer, J. A. (1993). Coping resources and processes: Current concepts and measures. In L. Goldberger & S. Bresnitz (Eds.), *Handbook of stress: Theoretical and clinical aspects* (2nd ed., pp. 234–257). New York: The Free Press.

Norman, W. T. (1963). Toward an adequate taxonomy of personality attributes: Replicated factor structure in peer nomination personality ratings. *Journal of Abnormal Social Psychology, 66,* 574–583.

Pearlin, L. I., & Schooler, C. (1978). The structure of coping. *Journal of Health and Social Behavior, 19,* 2–21.

Phillips, K., & Matheny, A. P. (1997). Evidence for genetic influence on both cross-situation and situation-specific components of behavior. *Journal of Personality and Social Psychology, 73,* 129–138.

Rabkin, J. G., & Struening, E. L. (1976). Life events, stress, and illness. *Science, 194,* 1013–1020.

Rohde, P., Lewinsohn, P. M., Tilson, M., et al. (1990). Dimensionality of coping and its relation to depression. *Journal of Personality and Social Psychology, 58,* 499–511.

Rorer, L. G., & Widiger, T. A. (1983). Personality structure and assessment. *Annual Review of Psychology, 34,* 431–463.

Rosenberg, M. (1979). *Conceiving the self.* New York: Basic Books.

Rotter, J. B. (1966). Generalized expectancies for internal versus external control of reinforcement. *Psychological Monographs: General and Applied, 80* (No. 609).

Rutter, M. (1985). Resilience in the face of adversity: Protective factors and resistance to psychiatric disorder. *British Journal of Psychiatry, 147,* 598–611.

Rutter, M. (1987). Temperament, personality and personality disorder. *British Journal of Psychiatry, 150,* 443–458.

Saudino, K. J., Pedersen, N. L., Lichtenstein, P., McClearn, G. E., & Plomin, R. (1997). Can personality explain genetic influences on life events? *Journal of Personality and Social Psychology, 72,* 196–206.

Schaefer, J., & Moos, R. (1992). Life crises and personal growth. In B. N. Carpenter (Ed.), *Personal coping: Theory, research, and applications* (pp. 149–170). New York: Praeger.

Scheier, M. F., Carver, C. S., & Bridges, M. W. (1994). Distinguishing optimism from neuroticism (and trait anxiety, self-mastery, and self-esteem): A reevaluation of the Life Orientation Test. *Journal of Personality and Social Psychology, 67,* 1063–1078.

Silver, R. L., & Wortman, C. B. (1980). Coping with undesirable life events. In J. Garber & M. E. P. Seligman (Eds.), *Human helplessness: Theory and applications* (pp. 279–340). San Diego, CA: Academic Press.

Stallings, M. C., Hewitt, J. K., Cloninger, C. R., Heath, A. C., & Eaves, L. J. (1996). Genetic and environmental structure of the Tridimensional Personality Questionnaire: Three or four temperamental dimensions? *Journal of Personality and Social Psychology, 70,* 127–140.

Stanton, A. L., & Snider, P. R. (1993). Coping with a breast cancer diagnosis: A prospective study. *Health Psychology, 12,* 16–23.

Svrakic, D. M., Whitehead, C., Przybeck, T. R., et al. (1993). Differential diagnosis of personality disorders by the seven-factor model of temperament and character. *Archives of General Psychiatry, 50,* 991–999.

Tellegen, A. (1985). Structures of mood and personality and their relevance to assessing anxiety, with an emphasis on self-report. In A. H. Tuma, & J. D. Maser (Eds.), *Anxiety and the anxiety disorders* (pp. 681–706). Hillsdale, NJ: Lawrence Erlbaum Associates.

Terry, D. J. (1994). Determinants of coping: The role of stable and situational factors. *Journal of Personality and Social Psychology, 66,* 895–910.

Thompson, S. C., Sobolew-Shubin, A., Galbraith, M. E., et al. (1993). Maintaining perceptions of control: Finding perceived control in low-control circumstances. *Journal of Personality and Social Psychology, 64,* 293–304.

Vaillant, G. E. (1977). *Adaptation to life*. Boston: Little, Brown.

Vitaliano, P. P., DeWolfe, D. J., Maiuro, R. D., Russo, J., Katon, W. (1990). Appraised changeability of a stressor as a modifier of the relationship between coping and depression: A test of the hypothesis of fit. *Journal of Personality and Social Psychology, 59,* 582–592.

Waller, N. G., Lilienfeld, S. O., Tellegen, A., et al. (1991). The Tridimensional Personality Questionnaire: Structural validity and comparison with the Multidimensional Personality Questionnaire. *Multivariate Behavioral Research, 26,* 1–23.

Watson, D., & Clark, L. A. (1993). Behavior disinhibition versus constraint: A dispositional perspective. In D. M. Wegner & J. W. Pennebaker (Eds.), *Handbook of mental control* (pp. 506–527). Englewood Cliffs, NJ: Prentice-Hall.

Watson, D., Clark, L. A., & Harkness, A. R. (1994). Structures of personality and their relevance to psychopathology. *Journal of Abnormal Psychology, 103,* 18–31.

Widiger, T. A., & Costa, P. T., Jr. (1994). Personality and personality disorders. *Journal of Abnormal Psychology, 103,* 78–91.

Wiggins, J. S. (1979). A psychological taxonomy of trait-descriptive terms: The interpersonal domain. *Journal of Personality and Social Psychology, 37,* 395–412.

Zautra, A. J., & Wrabetz, A. B. (1991). Coping success and its relationship to psychological distress for older adults. *Journal of Personality and Social Psychology, 61,* 801–810.

20

Social Support: Its Present Significance for Psychiatric Epidemiology

A. Scott Henderson

The aim of this chapter is to examine the present state of knowledge about social support as a determinant of mental health. Evidence is presented that what has been measured in most studies is probably not a valid estimate of the actual social environment; it is instead the subject's personal perception of this. It may be that it is the internal representation of the social environment rather than its true state that has a protective effect on mental health. The significance of such a conclusion is not trivial for psychiatric epidemiology, which traditionally has expected the social environment to play a major role in etiology.

FORMULATION OF HYPOTHESES ON SOCIAL SUPPORT

After some two decades of research on adverse life events, attention began to be accorded not only to malignant forces in the environment but also to the possibility that the environment may contain positive or health-promoting elements. It should be noted that such a hypothesis had been central to the work of Alexander Leighton and his collaborators in the Stirling County

Study, with their concept of sociocultural integration and disintegration (Leighton et al., 1963). Five bodies of information pointed to the possible relevance of social support for mental health. These were the role of social relationships in higher primate and human evolution, attachment theory, observations from clinical practice, and both medical and psychiatric epidemiology. In each of these five fields of information, there is the common component that individuals receive from others something that is beneficial.

Social Bonds in Human Evolution

In 1920, Emile Kraepelin wrote

It will be necessary to search for the roots and the manifestations of our inner lives everywhere—in the souls of children, of primitive men, of animals. Furthermore, it will be necessary to establish to what degree lost emotions of the individual and of the phylogenetic past are reborn in illness. (pp. 1–29)

By saying this, Kraepelin revealed that he was aware of the relevance of primate and human evolution in understanding some abnormal mental conditions. To think in evolutionary terms can be heuristically useful not only in biology but also in medicine and in the behavioral sciences.

This is the approach adopted by Boyden (1980) in considering the effect of civilization on human biology. He has introduced the term *evodeviations* for situations where there is a mismatch between contemporary human conditions and those to which our species has adapted over some 2 million years. The capacity to form and maintain social bonds during adulthood has been an important acquisition during higher primate evolution. It has carried selective advantage since the Middle Pleistocene period. The questions one now must ask are whether the contemporary social environment is different from the primeval conditions of hunters and gatherers, and, if so, whether this could have consequences for mental health. Clinicians usually presume that social relationships are somehow related to the maintenance of normal mood. Although the disruption of such relationships is invariably associated with transient dysphoria, it may also be that individual environments that are conspicuously deficient in social relationships contribute to the onset of common psychological symptoms.

Attachment Theory

The next pointer to the hypothesis comes from theory about affectionally close relationships between adults. Although the work of Bowlby on attachment referred to the relationship of the infant to its mother, it has become apparent that attachment also occurs in adults. Bowlby (1973, p. 359) wrote that "human beings of all ages are found to be at their happiest and to be able to deploy their talents to best advantage when . . . there are one or more trusted persons who will come to their aid should difficulties arise." Attachment theory is certainly consistent with an expectation that affectionally close relationships make some contribution to mental health.

Clinical Practice

There are occasions in epidemiological research when an impression based on clinical work with patients can be a valuable stimulus. Our group noted that patients with what Goldberg and Huxley (1992) usefully term *common mental disorders* often described being deficient in the amount of care or affection they obtained from others (Henderson et al., 1978, 1981). It was not clear if the deficiency we were being told about existed in the objective world of patients' social environments or if it was largely a consequence of how they construed it. Our concept of caring behavior includes the following: affording comfort through one's physical presence, demonstration of affection by physical contact, genuine interest in the other's well-being, showing concern and giving encouragement in the presence of distress, the expression of liking the other or of esteeming him or her highly, and affording opportunities for the unburdening of painful affect.

We went on to propose that both psychological symptoms and abnormal illness behavior (Pilowsky, 1997) could often be viewed as a communication of affective discomfort, and that the symptoms or behavior carried a corrective effect by bringing about an increase in the caring behavior shown by others to the patient. It is not a new idea that psychiatric symptoms or behaviours can act as operants and are reinforced by the responses they elicit in others. Freud (1946), in the *Fragment of an Analysis of a Case of Hysteria*, describes a woman for whom "ill health will be her one weapon for maintaining her position. It will procure for her the care she longs for . . . it will compel him [her husband] to treat her with solicitude if she recovers, for otherwise a relapse will threaten" (Vol. 3, pp. 55–56). This statement makes it clear that Freud was aware not only of the social impact of neurotic symptoms but also of the possibility that the need for care was part of the reason they developed.

Formulated in this way, some of the phenomenology of common mental disorders can be construed as morbid variants of an ethological category of behavior called *care eliciting*, as discussed by Henderson (1974). The propositions were that some common mental disorders arise in persons who are deficient or have a perceived deficiency in what is supplied to them by their social environment, and that the symptoms or behavior have a care-eliciting effect on the person's primary group.

A further lead from clinical practice is the possible role of personality factors. Traits such as neuroticism may confer vulnerability to development of psychological symptoms, particularly anxiety and depression (Fergusson et al., 1989; Ormel & Wohlfarth, 1991). At the same time, it must be borne in mind that some personality traits, possibly including neuroticism, may influence the formation and maintenance of supportive social relationships, thereby having a possible effect on mental health through this additional pathway. A study of social support therefore must include personality attributes in the etiological model.

Psychiatric Epidemiology

Early encouragement for looking more closely at the social environment came from the work of Brown and his colleagues. In looking for factors that would increase vulnerability to developing depression in the face of adversity, they had identified the lack of a close, confiding relationship as one such attribute (Brown & Harris, 1978; Brown et al., 1975). This work was conducted on community samples of women, first in the London borough of Camberwell, then on the Hebridean island of North Uist (Brown et al., 1977), and subsequently in Islington (Brown et al., 1986).

Medical Epidemiology

Within medical epidemiology, there have been a number of reports suggesting a possible causal link between deficiencies in social ties and increased rates for some types of physical morbidity. Cassel (1976) reviewed these in an important paper in which he brought together observations relating the absence of social ties to increased rates for hypertension and stroke. To this, there is now added the interesting work on social

support and reduced *mortality* in the elderly, as reviewed by House et al. (1988).

THE HYPOTHESES

There are at least five distinct hypotheses on the association that may exist between the construct of social support and health. These are (*1*) that a deficiency in social support is an independent determinant of common mental disorders, including anxiety and depression; (*2*) that the relationship holds only in the presence of adversity (i.e., there is an interaction effect); (*3*) that social support promotes well-being; (*4*) that social support contributes to restitution of mental health, not to its destabilization, in the language of Goldberg and Huxley (1992), so that, rather than contributing to the onset of common mental disorders, it favorably influences the course and outcome of psychopathological states that are already established; and (*5*) that a deficiency in social support is associated with increased physical morbidity, mortality, or both.

In the work my colleagues and I have undertaken, only the etiological hypotheses have been considered. That is, a therapeutic or health-promoting effect is specifically set aside here because it is of a different conceptual order and requires a different design to test it.

MEASUREMENT

To make further progress with social support as a new class of variable for epidemiological research, it was necessary to be able to measure it. Remarkably, when we began our work in this field in 1975, humankind had been able to land on the moon, but there was at that time no research interview to measure social support as an aspect of human relationships.

Greatly assisted conceptually by the work of Robert Weiss (1974), who has attempted to delineate the major "provisions of social relationships," we developed the Interview Schedule for Social Interaction (ISSI)

(Henderson et al., 1980, 1981). This structured interview assesses four principal indicators: the availability of affectionally close relationships and of more diffuse interaction with others, and the perceived adequacy of these two types of relationship. A number of other instruments subsequently have been developed that provide information on a person's primary group or personal network and that measure in different ways what the person receives and gives in the course of interaction with these others. Examples are the instruments by Sarason et al. (1983) and by Brown et al. (1986), the Duke Social Support Index by Landerman et al. (1989), and the Mannheim instrument by Veiel (1990).

FINDINGS

I report our own experience here, and then contrast it with some others. The Canberra Longitudinal Study has been fully reported elsewhere (Henderson et al., 1981). A general population sample was examined on four occasions over 12 months. Respondents who had psychological symptoms at Wave 1 were, perhaps unwisely, excluded from the analysis, leaving a cohort of 169 persons on whom there were measures of symptoms, life events, and social support at 3 month intervals. Contrary to expectation, the finding was that only a weak association could be established between a deficiency in the availability of diffuse social relationships and the subsequent onset of symptoms. The lack of close affectional ties was not associated with an increased risk of morbidity. The adequacy indices for both close and diffuse ties had a substantial predictive power, but only when there was coexistent adversity. The ISSI indices at Wave 1 collectively accounted for 30.0% of the variance in the symptom score at Wave 2 in the high-adversity group (n = 62) but for only 4.1% in those with low adversity (n = 115). Neuroticism explained 40.5% of the variance in symptoms among those exposed to high adversity over the 12 months but only 7.5% in those with low adversity.

A contrasting methodology is to be found in the Bedford College studies by Brown and his colleagues (Brown, 1992). They have used an investigator-based approach to measuring social support rather than an unprocessed acceptance of respondents' replies to questionnaire or interview items. Their work suggests that, in women, a close confiding relationship is protective in the face of adversity. Their second important observation is that there is a high incidence of symptoms in those women who have been "let down" in the face of adversity, in that they received no support from those with whom they had believed that they had an affectionally close and confiding relationship.

There are now a large number of other studies of psychological symptoms and social support, varying greatly in the quality of the measures used and in whether they were cross-sectional or longitudinal. In a meta-analysis of 80 studies, Schwarzer and Leppin (1992) found an effect size of -0.07 for morbidity and the same for mortality. This is a very weak association. By contrast, at the same Bad Homburg Symposium on Social Support, convened by Veiel and Baumann (1992), I presented a conspectus of 35 studies of social support and depression (Henderson, 1992). This set out the type of sample, its size, the gender, the measures of social support and of depression, and the finding on whether there was no effect, a direct effect, or a buffering effect. The conclusion was that across this *mélange* of studies, two findings emerged with remarkable consistency: there is an inverse association between perceived support and affective symptoms, and there is a buffering effect in the presence of severe stressors. One study had the interesting finding that support from relatives and friends, in the presence of adverse events, was directly associated with *higher* levels of symptoms.

In prospective longitudinal studies of the elderly, there is consistent evidence that lack of perceived social support predicts subsequent depression. This holds even when baseline symptoms have been controlled (Krause et al., 1989; Oxman et al., 1992; Russell & Cutrona 1991; Wallace & O'Hara

1992). In his review of this work, Jorm (1995) noted that low social support predicted depression even after controlling for impaired physical health. He also noted the evidence that social support affects both destabilization from a state of mental health (Phifer & Murrell 1986) and restitution (George et al. 1989; Kivelä & Pahkala, 1989), although not all studies have found an effect on restitution (Burvill et al., 1991; Murphy, 1983).

One finding from genetic epidemiology must be embraced in any attempt to understand this field. Kessler et al. (1992) have conducted genetic analyses of the measures of social support on an adult twin sample of woman in the Virginia Twin Registry. Regrettably, these measures were only brief items in a questionnaire. When social support was examined in relation to a genetic factor, a shared environment common to both twins, and a unique environment for each, there was a significant genetic influence in five of the eight measures of social support. This finding suggests that there may be a genetic basis, at least in part, either for the capacity to establish and maintain supportive relationships or to perceive that these exist and to report this at a research interview. The evidence for a genetic contribution is further extended by the important work of Kendler and Karkowski-Shuman (1997), who found that genes may cause individuals "to select themselves into high-risk environments" (p. 539).

DISCUSSION

In the interpretation of the data from social support studies, the following issues must be considered. First is the validity of the measures of social support. These typically have been only self-report, without using collateral informants and certainly not using direct observation. The measures must therefore be open to information bias. If the rigor with which case–control studies are conducted elsewhere in epidemiology were applied to the published data on social support, the conclusions of the majority of studies would have to be rejected.

Next, Sarason et al. (1987, 1992) have undertaken an assessment of methods for measuring social support. They conclude that measures of received support are not strongly related to perceived support; that the measure of perceived support is a factor common to many instruments, and represents a feeling that one is valued and esteemed by one's primary group; and that it is this variable that is protective. In short, they note that "It is the perception of support, rather than the receipt of support, that is most indicative of good adjustment" (p. 830). This conclusion must have considerable significance for research on social support and on interpretation of the available data.

Most of the measures of social support are, on close inspection, of perceived and not received support. An exception is the effort made by the Bedford College group to reconstruct what actually happened and to have a research team rate this, rather than accept the respondent's unprocessed account of the event. However, in longitudinal studies elsewhere (e.g., George et al., 1989), it is perceived support that has the stronger association with symptom onset. In contrast, measures of received support typically have a weaker contribution. It has been suggested (Kessler, 1992) that the association between perceived support and symptoms could be due to the support variable serving as a measure of personality, including appraisal and coping processes, or of social competence (Heller & Swindle, 1983). We suggested years ago that persons who are lacking in social support may be less competent in establishing personal relationships and maintaining these over time; that is, people are to some extent the architects of their own social environment (Henderson et al., 1981, p. 133).

A third issue is that investigators have usually considered at most three sets of variables: symptoms, adversity, and social support. Previous psychiatric history or family history of mental disorders has rarely been incorporated in the explanatory model. A fourth issue is that the studies have usually been conducted on community samples or even on student groups. Insofar as research on social support may have relevance to services for the mentally ill, this could be misleading. Among persons with mental disorders, the level of symptoms, the personal network, and personality variables all will have base rates very different from those in general population samples. This may influence the associations that can be observed.

CONCLUSIONS

In light of the findings set forth above, three conclusions can be offered:

1. [Perceived social support]protects against destabilization of mental health.
2. What people describe as the social support available to them, or received by them, may not always be a valid measure of the support they actually received. As expressed by Kessler (1992), "the effect of perceived support on adjustment to stress seems not to be mediated by actual supportive behaviors"(p. 268). The conclusion is that, for etiological research, there may be important differences between perceived social support and the individual's actual social environment.
3. A hypothesis that deals with the support actually obtained from the social environment at the time when psychological symptoms emerged has yet to be tested in a design that overcomes the problem of information bias.

The available data on social support suggest that it is not the social environment per se that matters but rather its internal representation in people's minds. This means that the external world and the people in it are not so important as how these elements are construed. Our excursion into social psychiatry has led us, unexpectedly, to recognize the value of the statement by psychoanalyst Harry Guntrip (1974):

Thus by projection and introjection, human beings live in two worlds at once, the inner mental world and the external material world, and constantly confuse the two together. (p. 830)

Our own research on the social environment makes this most clear. If our conclusions are correct, the implication for psychiatric epidemiology is that the actual social environment is not the source of some protective factor for mental health; instead, what may be more important is how that environment is perceived. The active component seems to be intrapsychic, not really social. It is puzzling that the social environment can be the source of toxic factors, in the form of adverse life events, but not of protective factors. This asymmetry seems wrong. The explanation may be that the measures of social support used so far have lacked validity, or that it is technically very difficult to disentangle a person's actual social environment from how he or she construes it and then reports it to a research interviewer.

In conclusion, there are at least three questions that remain to be resolved in future research:

1. If it is indeed true that perceived and received support have only a weak correlation, why is this so?
2. Is perceived support determined largely by personality variables rather than by the actual social environment? Is there a substantial genetic basis for personality, exposure to adversity, and competence in personal relationships?
3. For common mental disorders, is it possible to estimate the etiological contribution attributable to poor social support after accounting for the contribution of personality variables?

These three questions alone provide a demanding agenda for further efforts in this field. Most of all, however, this line of work has led to exciting new opportunities for psychiatric epidemiology; these come from bringing molecular genetics into population-based research on etiology (Henderson, et al., 1997).

REFERENCES

Bowlby, J. (1973). *Attachment and Loss. Vol. 2. Separation: Anxiety and anger*. London: Hogarth Press.

Boyden, S. (1980). The need for a holistic approach to human health and well-being. In N. F. Stanley & R. A. Joske (Eds.), *Changing disease patterns and human behaviour* (pp. 621–644). Sydney: Academic Press.

Brown, G. W. (1992). Social support: An investigator-based approach. In H. O. F. Viel & U. Baumann (Eds.), *The meaning and measurement of social support*. New York: Hemisphere.

Brown, G. W., Andrews, B., Harris, T., et al. (1986). Social support, self-esteem and depression. *Psychological Medicine, 16*, 813–831.

Brown, G. W., Davidson, S., Harris, T., et al. (1977). Psychiatric disorder in London and North Uist. *Social Science and Medicine, 11*, 367–377.

Brown, G. W., & Harris, T. O. (1978). *Social origins of depression: A study of psychiatric disorder in women*. London: Tavistock.

Brown, G. W., Ní Bhrolcháin, M. N., & Harris, T. (1975). Social class and psychiatric disturbance among women in an urban population. *Sociology, 9*, 225–254.

Burvill, P. W., Hall, W. D., Stampfer, H. G., et al. (1991). The prognosis of depression in old age. *British Journal of Psychiatry, 158*, 64–71.

Cassel, J. (1976). The contribution of the social environment to host resistance. *American Journal of Epidemiology, 104*, 107–123.

Fergusson, D. M., Horwood, L. J., & Lawton, J. M. (1989). The relationships between neuroticism and depressive symptoms. *Social Psychiatry and Psychiatric Epidemiology, 24*, 275–281.

Freud, S. (1946). *The complete psychological works*. London: Hogarth Press.

George, L. K., Blazer, D. G., Hughes, D. C., et al. (1989). Social support and the outcome of major depression. *British Journal of Psychiatry, 154*, 478–485.

Goldberg, D. P., and Huxley, P. (1992). *Common mental disorders: A bio-social model*. London & New York: Tavistock/Routledge.

Guntrip, H. (1974). Psychoanalytic object theory. In S. Arieti (Ed.), *American handbook of psychiatry* (Vol. I). New York: Basic Books.

Heller, K., and Swindle, R. V. (1983). The effects of social support: Prevention and treatment implications. In A. P. Goldstein & F. H. Kanfer (Eds.), *Maximizing treatment gains: Transfer enhancement in psychotherapy*. New York: Academic Press.

Henderson, A. S. (1974). Care-eliciting behavior in man. *Journal of Nervous and Mental Disorders, 159*, 172–181.

Henderson, A. S. (1992). Social support and depression. In H. O. F. Veiel & U. Baumann (Eds.), *The meaning and measurement of social support*. New York: Hemisphere.

Henderson, A. S., Byrne, D. G., & Duncan-Jones, P. (1981). *Neurosis and the social environment*. Sydney: Academic Press.

Henderson, S., Duncan-Jones, P., McAuley, H., et al. (1978). The patient's primary group. *British Journal of Psychiatry, 132*, 74–86.

Henderson, S., Duncan-Jones, P., Byrne, D. G., et al. (1980). Measuring social relationships: The Interview Schedule for Social Interaction. *Psychological Medicine, 10*, 723–734.

Henderson, S., Jorm, A., Jacomb, P., Korten, A., & Easteal, S. (1997). Molecular genetics and the epidemiology of common mental disorders: New opportunities. *Epidemiologia e Psychiatria Sociale, 6*, 167–171.

House, J. S., Landis, K. R., & Umberson, D. (1988). Social relationships and health. *Science, 241*, 540–545.

Jorm, A. F. (1995). The epidemiology of depressive states in the elderly: Implications for recognition, intervention and prevention. *Social Psychiatry and Psychiatric Epidemiology, 30*, 53–59.

Kendler, K. S., & Karkowski-Shuman, L. (1997). Stressful life events and genetic liability to major depression: Genetic control of exposure to the environment? *Psychological Medicine, 27*, 539–547.

Kessler, R. C. (1992). Perceived support and adjustment to stress: Methodological consideration. In H. O. F. Veiel & U. Baumann (Eds.), *The meaning and measurement of social support*. New York: Hemisphere.

Kessler, R. C., Kendler, K. S., Heath, A., et al. (1992). Social support, depressed mood, and adjustment to stress: A genetic epidemiologic investigation. *Journal of Personality and Social Psychology, 62*, 257–272.

Kivelä, S.-L., and Pahkala, K. (1989). The prognosis of depression in old age. *International Psychogeriatrics, 1*, 119–133.

Kraepelin, E. (1920). Die Erscheinungsformen des Irreseins. *Zeitschrift für die Gesamte Neurologie und Psychiatrie, 62*, 1–29.

Krause, N., Liang, J., & Yatomi, N. (1989). Satisfaction with social support and depressive symptoms: A panel analysis. *Psychology and Aging, 4*, 88–97.

Landerman, R., George, L. K., Campbell, R. T., et al. (1989). Alternative models of the stress buffering hypothesis. *American Journal of Common Psychology, 17*, 625–642.

Leighton, D. C., Harding, J. S., Macklin, D. B., et al. (1963). Psychiatric findings of the Stirling County Study. *American Journal of Psychiatry, 119*, 1021–1026.

Murphy, E. (1983). The prognosis of depression in old age. *British Journal of Psychiatry, 142*, 111–119.

Ormel, J., & Wohlfarth, T. (1991). How neuroticism, long-term difficulties, and life-situation change influence psychological distress: A longitudinal model. *Journal of Personality and Social Psychology, 60*, 744–755.

Oxman, T. E., Berkman, L. F., Kasl, S., et al. (1992). Social support and depressive symptoms in the elderly. *American Journal of Epidemiology, 135*, 356–368l.

Phifer, J. F., and Murrell, S. A. (1986). Etiologic factors in the onset of depressive symptoms in older adults. *Journal of Abnormal Psychology, 95*, 282–291.

Pilowsky, I. (1997). *Abnormal illness behaviour.* Chichester, England: John Wiley & Sons.

Russell, D. W., & Cutrona, C. E. (1991). Social support, stress, and depressive symptoms among the elderly: Test of process model. *Psychology and Aging, 6*, 190–201.

Sarason, B. R., Shearin, E. N., and Pierce, G. R. (1987). Interrelations of social support measures: Theoretical and practical implications. *Journal of Personality and Social Psychology, 52*, 813–832.

Sarason, I. G., Sarason, B. R., & Pierce, G. R. (1983). Assessing social support: The Social Support Questionnaire. *Journal of Personality and Social Psychology, 44*, 127–139.

Sarason, I. G., Sarason, B. R., and Pierce, G. R. (1992). Three contexts of social support. In H. O. F. Veiel & U. Baumann (Eds.), *The meaning and measurement of social support.* New York: Hemisphere.

Schwarzer R., & Leppin, A. (1992). Possible impact of social ties and support on morbidity and mortality. In H. O. F. Veiel & U. Baumann (Eds.), *The meaning and measurement of social support.* New York: Hemisphere.

Veiel, H. O. F. (1990). The Mannheim Interview on Social Support: Reliability and validity data from three samples. *Social Psychiatry and Psychiatric Epidemiology, 25*, 250–259.

Veiel, H. O. F., and Baumann, U. (1992). Comments on concepts and methods. In H. O. F. Veiel & U. Baumann (Eds.), *The meaning and measurement of social support.* New York: Hemisphere.

Wallace, J., & O'Hara, M. W. (1992). Increases in depressive symptomatology in the rural elderly: Results from a cross-sectional and longitudinal study. *Journal of Abnormal Psychology, 101*, 398–404.

Weiss, R. S. (1974). The provisions of social relationships. In Z. Rubin (Ed.), *'Doing Unto Others'* (pp. 17–26). Englewood Cliffs, NJ: Prentice-Hall.

21

Some Characteristics of Occupations as Risk or Protective Factors for Episodes of Major Depression and Nonaffective Psychotic Disorder

Bruce G. Link
Mary Clare Lennon
Bruce P. Dohrenwend

Perhaps the most important legacy of the descriptive epidemiological studies of mental disorder is the consistency with which such studies show associations between sociodemographic factors such as gender and socioeconomic status (SES) and the prevalence of various types of mental disorders (Dohrenwend & Dohrenwend, 1974; 1980; Link & Dohrenwend, 1989; 1994; Neugebauer et al., 1980; see also Kohn et al., Chapter 13, this volume). A full etiological explanation of the major mental disorders must somehow account for these consistent patterns. If accumulating knowledge cannot explain these associations, this is an indicator that the knowledge is incomplete. In short, even if a group of investigators wish to ignore temporarily the relevance of their findings for these consistent associations, in the end they will have to return to them. We think it is appropriate to start with them.

The consistent relationship we have chosen as the starting point for our inquiry into the effects of occupational conditions is the association between SES and mental disorder. This association suggests the possibility that adversity associated with lower SES plays a role in the onset and course of major mental disorders (Dohrenwend, 1990; Dohrenwend et al., 1992). We use results from a case–control study of major depression and nonaffective psychosis–the New York Risk Factor Study (Dohrenwend et al., 1986)—to examine the role of occupational conditions in explaining why we find an association between SES and these two disorders. The results we report have been described in more detail in two earlier publications, one focused on nonaffective psychosis (Link et al., 1986) and another on major depression (Link et al., 1993). In this chapter, we expand on the research strategy that is common to these investigations, recount the results of the two analyses, and then assess their implications for understanding the association between SES and each of the two disorders.

DESCRIPTIVE EPIDEMIOLOGY

The association between SES and schizophrenia was documented in what Bruce and Barbara Dohrenwend called the first- and second-generation studies in psychiatric epidemiology (Dohrenwend & Dohrenwend, 1974, 1982). It is also found in the Epidemiological Catchment Area (ECA) studies (Robins & Regier, 1990) and in the study conducted by Dohrenwend et al. (1992) in Israel. The review by Kohn et al. in this volume suggests that the median prevalence ratio of highest to lowest class for 1 year prevalence is 3.4.

The association between major depression and SES has been somewhat more controversial, in part because it was not particularly strong in the ECA study. Still, when Holzer and colleagues (1986) aggregated results across the five ECA sites and used a composite measure of SES, they found an almost twofold difference between people in the two lowest SES quartiles and those in the top quartile. Moreover, other major studies have documented the association. The study conducted by Dohrenwend et al. (1992) in Israel found an inverse association between SES and major depression, and a co-morbidity study by Kessler and colleagues (1994) found an inverse association between SES and affective disorders most of which were major depressions. Moreover, the review in this volume by Kohn et al. documents a median prevalence ratio of 1.6 comparing the lowest socioeconomic group to the highest across the studies reviewed. Only one of the third-generation studies found a higher rate in the highest class than in the lowest. In fact, the 1.6 prevalence ratio is only slightly smaller than the median prevalence ratio reported by Kohn et al. (1.9) for the widely accepted gender difference in depression (see Chapter 13, this volume).

Such results posed the classic social selection–social causation question about the association between SES and mental disorder (Kohn, 1972; Mechanic, 1972). Dohrenwend et al. (1992) published the results of a quasi experiment that was designed to assess whether social selection or social causation processes predominate in accounting for the SES relationship with various disorders. With respect to schizophrenia, this study indicated that social selection predominated in explaining the association, whereas for major depression social causation was more important, particularly for women.

For the Dohrenwend's, the quasi experiment was one major part of a multipart inquiry (Dohrenwend & Dohrenwend, 1969). In the original statement of their research plan, they also laid out a series of studies that would reflect on the mechanisms that might be involved in accounting for the relationship between SES and mental disorder. The two analyses presented in this chapter are of this latter sort. They are designed to examine mechanisms that may explain why SES is related to each of these disorders. Moreover, because the quasi experiment is designed to assess which predominates in explaining the association, such further studies can reflect on the relative magnitude of processes associated with each of these major explanations.

RESEARCH STRATEGY

The basic research strategy underlying our inquiry into the association between SES and major mental disorders is as follows. The two broad explanations for the association—social causation and social selection—imply very different intervening mechanisms. If the SES–disorder association is due to selection, we should find factors such as genetic endowments or early environmental risk factors (with parental class held constant) that determine both the onset of disorder and low SES. Also consistent with selection would be evidence showing that disorder-produced disability ac-

Social Causation

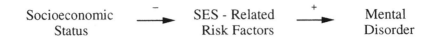

Social Selection

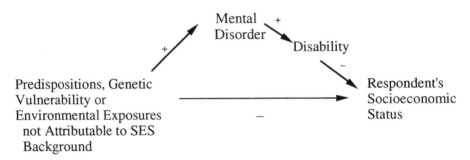

Figure 21.1. Social causation–social selection models.

counts for the association between SES and mental disorder. Alternatively, from a social causation point of view, we should find risk factors that are a consequence of SES and are in turn related to major depression or nonaffective psychosis. The idea is that we can learn a great deal about what accounts for the SES–disorder association by the success or failure of attempts to explain the association according to processes implied by the social causation and social selection perspectives.

Figure 21.1 presents this reasoning in diagrammatic form. Both the social causation and the social selection models in this diagram depict an inverse association between SES and mental disorder. What is different about the models is the processes through which the association is presumed to arise. The idea is to develop designs and measures that allow us to assess which set of processes best explains the association between SES and mental disorder. Thus, social selection would be supported to the extent that mea-

sures of genetic vulnerability and disability caused by mental disorder account for the association between SES and disorder. In contrast, social causation would be supported to the extent that SES-related risk factors explain the association.

IMPLEMENTING THE STRATEGY

Social Causation

The approach we adopted for addressing the social causation aspect of this strategy was to evaluate the impact of occupational conditions as one plausible mechanism linking SES to mental disorder. Thus occupational conditions are, in terms of Figure 21.1, the SES-related risk factor we have chosen to evaluate. The rationale for this is that aspects of socioeconomic status determine one's position in the occupational structure, thereby exposing people to very different conditions while at work. In keeping with this idea, sociological analyses have shown strong associations between father's SES, respondent's education and job prestige, and occupational conditions such as job complexity, routinization, and closeness of supervision (Kohn & Schooler, 1983).

Our analysis of episodes of non-affective psychosis focused on noisome occupational conditions (e.g., excessive noise, hazards), while our analysis of episodes of depression focused on whether or not occupations allowed direction, control, and planning as measured in the U.S. Department of Labor's *Dictionary of Occupational Titles* (DOT, 1977). Noisome conditions are particularly important for schizophrenia spectrum disorders such as the cases of nonaffective psychosis we studied based on the idea that people with schizophrenia may be vulnerable to overstimulation (Leff & Vaughn, 1985). The effectiveness of interventions based on the psychoeducational model and its variants have been impressive (Falloon et al., 1982; Hogarty et al., 1986). These interventions seek to decrease stimulation of a particular type and appear to reduce dramatically the occurrence of subsequent relapse. These studies have tended to focus on the nature of the home environment—but what about the work context? Perhaps noxious stimulation is harmful to people vulnerable to episodes of schizophrenia spectrum disorders in this context as well.

Our analysis of occupational control and depression is motivated by research showing that (1) occupational control is related to sense of personal control or mastery (Langer, 1976; Kohn, 1983), and (2) that a sense of personal control protects against depression (Mirowsky & Ross, 1986; Rosenfield, 1989).

Social Selection

The approach we adopted for addressing the social selection aspect of the strategy involved both design and analysis issues. To assess the potential impact of genetic vulnerability and environmental exposures not attributable to socioeconomic background, we included measures of these concepts in our analysis. We knew from a previous analysis (Dohrenwend et al., 1986) and from the research literature that these variables were strongly related to nonaffective psychosis and major depression. Therefore, they might explain the association between SES and mental disorder and thereby support a social selection interpretation of the SES–disorder association. We addressed the potential impact of disability caused by disorder through our study design. For major depression, we included people experiencing their first episode of depression and identified the occupational conditions they were exposed to before the onset of that first episode. Because the occupational conditions predated the onset of disorder, disability resulting from the disorder cannot account for the occupational conditions or the socioeconomic standing of the occupation in question. For nonaffective psychosis we chose to examine the first full-time occupations of our cases and controls, occupations that arguably predate the onset of nonaffective psychosis.

METHODS

Samples

The two analyses are based on a case–control study of major depression and nonaffective psychotic disorders in the Washington Heights section of New York City (Dohrenwend et al., 1986). Most cases were selected from inpatient and outpatient facilities in this general area of New York City and were diagnosed according to criteria in the *Diagnostic and Statistical Manual of Mental Disorders (Third Edition) (DSM-III*; American Psychiatric Association, 1980), under the supervision of members of the biometrics department at the New York State Psychiatric Institute. Special efforts were made to locate people experiencing their first episode of these disorders.

Altogether, 65 people with nonaffective psychotic disorder were recruited. Only 21 people experiencing a first episode of nonaffective psychotic disorder were located despite extensive efforts. Of 122 people with major depression who were interviewed, 50 were in treatment for a first episode of major depression. The sample also included 24 people from the community who had experienced an episode of major depression in the 12 month period before we interviewed them.

Finally, the 404 controls are a sample of community residents living in the Washington Heights section of New York City. The community respondents initially were recruited to participate in a methodological study of symptom scales. They were interviewed again approximately 6 months later for the present research. In the original community sample, households were enumerated and contacted to determine whether an eligible respondent between 19 and 59 years of age lived there. Information about ethnic background was obtained to permit the selection of roughly equal proportions of blacks, Hispanics, and non-Hispanic whites from this urban neighborhood, in which most residents are Hispanic. In 93% of the households, screening information was provided; 68% of these contained one eligible respondent or more ($N = 943$). Of these 57% (541) were interviewed successfully.

The original methodological study involved random assignment of respondents to 1 month or 1 year recall of symptoms from the Psychiatric Epidemiology Research Interview. Given the methodological focus, no intensive efforts were made to interview hard-to-schedule respondents or to covert refusals. When the case–control study was conceived and implemented near the end of the methodological study, and when questions of generalizability became more compelling, special efforts were made to interview a subsample of hard-to-schedule subjects ($N = 48$). An attempt also was made to ensure an adequate re-interview rate in the second wave of data collection. As a result, 79% ($N = 404$) of the initial sample was located and re-interviewed and used as the controls for this research.

The representativeness of the sample was assessed by comparing it to census data and by comparing the hard-to-schedule respondents with those who were easily obtained. The details of these comparisons can be found in Link et al. (1993). Neither comparison suggested severe sample selection bias.

Measures

We used the *DOT* to measure occupational conditions in this study. The *DOT* includes 44 ratings derived from on-site assessments by occupational analysts at the U.S. Department of Labor. In all, the *DOT* includes 12,099 distinct occupations, each of which is associated with a nine-digit code. We located the occupations of our respondents in the *DOT* and then used the nine-digit codes to append data regarding the 44 ratings of occupational conditions to our data file.

A shortcoming of the *DOT* ratings is that they miss variability within occupations. Therefore our *DOT* measure is restricted to between-occupation variance. At the same time, this drawback is offset by the objective nature of the *DOT* ratings. In retrospective studies such as ours, in which people are asked to recall conditions of their lives before their episode of mental disorder, one must be extremely careful in interpreting self-reports. Because the *DOT* ratings of occupational conditions are made by objective observers, biases that arise from self-report data in a case–control study are minimized.

Noisome Occupations

Six ratings from the *DOT* clustered empirically in our data and fit the concept of a noisome occupation—excessive noise, hazardous conditions, extreme heat, extreme cold, excessive humidity, and aversive atmospheric conditions. We scored our measure as a dichotomy, assigning "1" to a person who was exposed to one or more of the six potentially noisome conditions and "0" to a person who was exposed to none of them.

These conditions are almost entirely restricted to blue-collar occupations. In fact, 95% of the noisome occupations are blue-collar occupations in our community sample. This means that exposure to such conditions is strongly influenced by SES. Examples of occupations involving noisome features that were held by people who later developed a nonaffective psychosis are machinist, flatwork finisher, pest control worker, and crane operator.

Occupations Involving Direction, Control, and Planning

An occupation involves direction, control, and planning when the "worker is in a position to negotiate, organize, direct, supervise, formulate practices, or make final decisions." Examples of these occupations are civil engineer, manager of an industrial cafeteria, and high school principal. Only a minority (25.1%) of the occupations in our community sample were rated as involving direction, control, and planning. Most important, being in such an occupation is strongly related to SES. In fact, 90% of such occupations in our full community sample are white-collar occupations. In the *DOT*, the rating of direction, control, and planning is a dichotomy; in our analysis, it is scored "1" for those who have the occupation and "0" for those who do not.

Sociodemographics and SES Indicators

When appropriate, we control for age, gender, ethnicity (black, Hispanic, and other), and education measured in years. We assess socioeconomic origin by asking respondents about their fathers' usual occupations. If a respondent had no knowledge of his or her father or was raised by his or her mother only, we used the occupation of the major caregiver. We defined first occupation as the first full-time job held for 6 months or more in order to exclude summer jobs and part-time jobs held while in school. We assigned Treiman (1977) prestige scores to father's occupation, respondent's first occupation, and respondent's most recent occupation.

Social Selection Variables

These are antecedent factors indicating possible genetic vulnerability or early stressful experience (with SES held constant) that might limit the ability to obtain high-status jobs and also predispose to depression or nonaffective psychosis. These would include family history of mental disorder, being raised in a household where only the mother was present and there was no knowledge of the father, and remote life-threatening illnesses and injuries. Although this is not a comprehensive list of all possible confounding variables, previous research with this sample has shown that these variables are strongly related to depression and nonaffective psychosis (Dohrenwend et al., 1986).

We generated the family history measure (Dohrenwend et al., 1986) by asking each respondent whether his or her first-degree relatives had ever had "serious mental or emotional problems such as problems with depression, suicide attempts, odd or violent behavior, or difficulties with drugs or alcohol." Using responses to this query and information about family members' psychiatric treatment, we made a dichotomous rating of "family history present/absent" based on the consensus rating of two psychiatrists.

Being raised in a mother-headed household with no knowledge of one's father is indexed by a dichotomy with "1" for yes and "0" for no. As McLanahan (1985) pointed out, such circumstances involve the likely loss of the father's contribution to family income, the lack of a male role model, and exposure to stressful circumstances associated with family discord or disruption.

The measure of remote life-threatening illnesses and injuries is created from a question that asks respondents to list the three most serious illnesses or injuries they ever had. They also were asked whether these illnesses still bothered them (if they did so, we excluded the conditions as not being "remote") and whether the health problems were "life-threatening." Respondents with at least one remote life-threatening illness or injury were scored "1," whereas all other respondents were scored "0."

RESULTS

Nonaffective Psychosis

We focused our attention on the first full-time occupations of cases with nonaffective psychosis and compared them to the first full-time occupations of controls. The reason for this focus on first jobs was that several studies had shown that much of the downward mobility experienced by people with nonaffective psychosis occurred between the attainment of education and the occupation held before admission to treatment (Dunham et al., 1966; Goldberg & Morrison, 1963; Turner, 1968; Wiersma et al., 1983). However, there is a gap in our knowledge about what actually happens in the transition period between completion of education and occupation at the time of first admission—a considerable period of time in the lives of people who develop nonaffective psychosis.

With this as background, we addressed four major questions in our analysis. Our first question was whether the findings of other studies would be replicated in our sample. Specifically, we assessed whether first-episode cases of nonaffective psychosis were downwardly mobile into the jobs they held before their first admission to treatment by comparing them with controls who did not develop nonaffective psychosis. The dependent variable in the multiple regression analysis was the prestige level of the current or last occupation held by cases and controls. We held constant age, sex, ethnicity, respondent's years of education, and father's occupational prestige.

We found that the occupations held by people with nonaffective psychosis before their first treatment contact were about one-half standard deviation lower in prestige than the occupations of controls. The magnitude of this effect is roughly comparable to the difference in prestige attributable to an additional 4 years of education—a sub-

stantial difference. Although less relevant to our question about downward mobility at the time of first admission, the repeat-episode cases also showed evidence of downward mobility into the jobs held before their readmission. Thus our results were consistent with what other studies had found. But what about the gap between educational attainment and the jobs held before first admission. What about first full-time occupations?

Our second question focused on whether people who develop nonaffective psychosis were downwardly mobile into these first full-time occupations. In this analysis, we used the prestige level of the first full-time occupation as the dependent variable. In a multiple regression analysis, we held constant age at the time of first full-time occupation, ethnicity, sex, years of education, and father's occupational prestige. There was no significant difference between cases and controls. Thus we found no evidence to suggest that people who develop nonaffective psychosis are downwardly mobile into their first full-time occupations.

Our third question focused on possible case–control differences in exposure to noisome occupations in these first full-time occupations. We found that cases were far more likely to have been exposed to noisome occupational condition than controls. Thirty-five percent of nonaffective psychosis cases (21 of 60) had noisome first full-time occupations compared to 13.5% of controls. The findings held for both first- and repeat-episode cases and for the 31 cases that met *DSM-III* criteria for schizophrenia. We used logistic regression to control for sex, ethnicity, age at first job, years of education, being raised by a mother alone, prestige of respondent's first job, father's occupational prestige, and respondent's report of family history of mental disorder. As Table 21.1 shows, the effect remains. In fact, the adjusted odds ratio is remarkably similar in magnitude to the unadjusted odds ratio, and both are quite strong. Exposure to noisome occupational conditions more than triples one's odds of developing nonaffective psychosis.

Table 21.1. Association between occupations involving noisome features and nonaffective psychosis before and after controls

	Regression coefficient (standard error)	Odds ratio (95% confidence interval)
Before controls	1.238*** (.306)	3.45 (1.89, 6.28)
After controls[a]	1.294*** (.345)	3.65 (1.85, 7.17)

***$p < .001$.

[a]Adjusted for age at first job, sex, ethnicity (African-American, Latino, other), father's occupational prestige, prestige of respondent's first occupation, years of education, family history of mental disorder, remote life-threatening illness or injury, and being raised in a single-parent household.

Our fourth question focused on whether the association of noisome occupations was specific to nonaffective psychosis. We found no association between noisome occupational conditions and depression either in bivariate associations or when controls for other variables were entered in a logistic regression. This led us to interpret the association of noisome occupational conditions and nonaffective psychosis in a vulnerability model because noisome conditions did not appear to be a general stress factor causing several types of disorder.

In sum, we found evidence consistent with a social causation model—SES leads to noisome occupational conditions, and those occupational conditions appeared to be risk factors for nonaffective psychosis.

What about social selection explanations? To begin, we note that results showing substantial downward mobility into occupations held at the time of illness onset are consistent with a social selection explanation. They suggest that some part of the association between SES and nonaffective psychosis occurs because of downward mobility. At the same time, our analysis suggests that social selection processes cannot account for the pattern of results we presented concerning first full-time jobs. Our focus on first full-time jobs that were held before the on-set of psychosis means that disability caused by disorder cannot explain selection into noisome jobs. In addition, there was no evidence of downward mobility into first full-time jobs. This finding suggests that any pre-existing vulnerabilities that might predispose people to develop nonaffective psychosis (e.g., genetic vulnerabilities) had no discernible effect on the SES of their first jobs. Together, these results indicate that social selection processes cannot account for the association between noisome conditions and nonaffective psychosis.

Major Depression

In this analysis, we focus on the occupations that people with major depression held before the onset of their most recent episode and the occupations that controls held in the period before they were interviewed. Our analysis is concerned with three main questions regarding these occupations.

Our first question focused on the issue of whether SES was related to case–control status in our sample as the descriptive epidemiology of major depression would lead us to expect. Consistent with previous research, we found that cases had significantly lower levels of education and lower occupational prestige than controls.

Our second question focused on the association between occupations involving direction, control, and planning and depression. We formed three groups—people who were highly distressed on a demoralization screening scale but who did not meet criteria for major depression, cases of major depression, and controls. Community controls were almost twice as likely (27.8%) as people with major depression (14.9%) or people with high demoralization (15.4%) to have occupations involving direction, control, and planning. Moreover, when we break down the case groups into first-episode cases, repeat-episode cases, and cases of major depression identified in the community, we found remarkably similar results. The consistency of the results in these subgroups is important because it shows that the finding concerning direction, control, and planning cannot be explained by selection of cases into treatment—it appears to hold for cases randomly selected from the community. Even more important is the fact that the difference holds for first-episode cases. Because the occupations assessed were those held before the onset of major depression, it means that disability caused by major depression per se cannot explain why first-episode cases are less likely to hold occupations involving direction, control, and planning.

Our third question focused on whether the association between direction, control, and planning and depression could be explained by factors related to social selection processes. One factor we wanted to control was an individual's tendency to achieve a higher or a lower prestige occupation than one might expect based on background factors. It may be that people who develop major depression achieve lower-than-expected occupational prestige and, as a result, rarely are found in the comparatively high-status occupations that involve direction, control, and planning. To address this possibility, we included controls for years of education, prestige of the respondent's first job and father's job, and prestige of the respondent's current job. When partialled for education and prestige of first job and father's job, the current job can be considered a measure of the tendency to do better or worse than expected. Thus it represents a control for unmeasured dispositional factors that affect status attainment above and beyond the variables included in the model.

We also controlled for variables that were clearly related to depression and might also affect status attainment—potential confounding variables that would be consistent with a social selection explanation. Thus we entered controls for self-reported family history of mental disorder, being raised by a mother alone, and remote life-threatening illnesses and injuries. Table 21.2 shows the unadjusted odds ratio and the adjusted odds ratio when variables consistent with a social selection explanation are controlled. As Table 21.2 shows, the protective effect of occupations involving direction, control, and planning remains despite controls for variables consistent with social selection.

Table 21.2. Association between occupations involving direction, control, and planning and depression before and after controls

	Regression coefficient (standard error)	Odds ratio (95% confidence interval)
Before controls	−.822*** (.301)	.44 (.24, .79)
After controls[a]	−.922*** (.364)	.40 (.22, .90)

***$p < .001$.

[a]Adjusted for age, sex, ethnicity (African-American, Latino, other) father's occupational prestige, respondent's first occupational prestige, respondent's current occupational prestige, years of education, family history of mental disorder, remote life-threatening illness or injury, and being raised in a single-parent household.

These results are consistent with a social causation model, which says that high SES leads to occupations that allow direction, control, and planning of one's own and others' activities, and that this experience is then protective with respect to depression. Social selection processes cannot entirely explain these findings. Disability caused by major depression is not a parsimonious explanation for the results because of the finding of an association between direction, control, and planning and depression in first-episode cases. In addition, our strategy of controlling for less-than-expected levels of occupational prestige as a means of assessing unmeasured variables that influence status attainment did not explain the association between direction, control, and planning and depression. Finally, direct measures of potential social selection processes such as family history of mental illness and other vulnerability factors had no discernible effect on the association between direction, control, and planning and depression.

DISCUSSION

At the outset of this chapter, we noted that the Dohrenwend's conceived of a multifaceted approach to addressing the impact of adversity on psychopathology. One part consisted of a quasi experiment that was designed to assess the extent to which social selection or social causation processes predominated in determining the inverse association between SES and major mental disorders. Another part consisted of investigations like those described above that were designed to understand the mechanisms involved. We now consider the implications of these analyses in the context of the results from the quasi experiment.

Noisome Occupations and the Quasi Experiment

The study of noisome occupations suggests a possible role for social causation in the SES–schizophrenia association, whereas the quasi experiment leads to the conclusion that social selection is a stronger determinant of the SES–schizophrenia association than social causation. The two sets of findings are not necessarily incompatible, however. First, as noted above, the analysis of noisome occupations and nonaffective psychosis does not deny the importance of selection processes. Indeed, one aspect of the analysis—the finding that people who develop nonaffective psychosis are downwardly mobile into occupations held at the time of first onset—is consistent with a selection explanation. Moreover, the quasi experiment tests whether selection or causation predominates in explaining the association between SES and mental disorder. Thus, even in the context of a selection outcome such as the one obtained by Dohrenwend et al. (1992), it still may be that social causation factors play some role. The finding of a role for noisome occupations supports this possibility.

Occupations Involving Direction, Control, and Planning and the Quasi Experiment

In this instance, the quasi experiment and the results from the New York Risk Factor Study cohere in suggesting a role for social factors in explaining the SES–depression association. The quasi experiment suggests that social causation predominates, and the results of direction, control, and planning suggest one mechanism through which this may occur.

CONCLUSION

Taken in the context of the quasi experiment, these studies are consistent with the possibility that exposure to varying occupational conditions explains some part of the association between SES and major mental disorders. To the extent they do so, they support, but do not fully confirm, a social causation explanation for at least a part of this association. At the very least, these studies represent empirical tests that did not fail. They could have. Their survivor status increases our confidence in them and poses a challenge to those who believe that SES and its consequences play no causal role in the onset and course of major mental disorders.

Acknowledgments: This research was supported by National Institute of Mental Health grants MH38773 (Link), MH42974 (Lennon), and MH36208 (Dohrenwend).

REFERENCES

American Psychiatric Association. (1980). *Diagnostic and statistical manual of mental disorders* (3rd ed.). Washington, DC: American Psychiatric Press.

Dohrenwend, B. P. (1990). Socioeconomic status (SES) and psychiatric disorders: Are the issues still compelling? *Social Psychiatry and Psychiatric Epidemiology*, 25, 41–47.

Dohrenwend, B. P., & Dohrenwend, B. S. (1969). *Social status and psychological disorder*. New York: John Wiley & Sons.

Dohrenwend, B. P., & Dohrenwend B. S. (1974). Social and cultural influences on psychopathology. *Annual Review of Psychology*, 25, 417–452.

Dohrenwend, B. P., & Dohrewend, B. S. (1982). Perspectives on the past and future of psychiatric epidemiology. *American Journal of Public Health*, 72, 1271–1279.

Dohrenwend, B. P., Levav, I., Shrout, P., et al. (1992). Socioeconomic status and psychiatric disorders: The causation-selection issue. *Science, 255*, 946–952.

Dohrenwend, B. P., Shrout, P., & Link, B. (1986). Overview and initial results from a risk-factor study of depression and schizophrenia. In J. E. Barret & R. M. Rose (Eds.), *Mental disorders in the community* (pp. 184–215). New York: The Guilford Press.

Dunham, W., Phillips, P., & Shrinivasan, B. (1966). A research note on diagnosed mental illness and social class. *American Sociological Review, 31*, 223–227.

Falloon, I., Boyd, J., McGill, J. R., et al. (1982). Family management in the prevention of exacerbations of schizophrenia. *New England Journal of Medicine, 306*, 1437–1440.

Goldberg, E. M., & Morrison, S. L. (1963). Schizophrenia and social class. *British Journal of Psychiatry, 109*, 785–802.

Hogarty, G., Anderson, C., Reiss, D., et al. (1986). Family psychoeducation, social skills training and maintenance chemotherapy in the aftercare treatment of schizophrenia. *Archives of General Psychiatry, 43*, 633–642.

Holzer, C., Shea, B., Swanson, J., et al. (1986). The increased risk for specific psychiatric disorders among persons of low socioeconomic status. *American Journal of Social Psychiatry, 6*, 259–271.

Kessler, R. C., McGonagle, K. A., Zhao, S., et al. (1994). Lifetime and 12-month prevalence of DSM-IIIR psychiatric disorders in the United States. *Archives of General Psychiatry, 51*, 8–19.

Kohn, M. (1972). Class, family and schizophrenia: A reformulation. *Social Forces, 50*, 295–304.

Kohn, M., Schooler, C. (1983). *Work and personality: An inquiry into the impact of social stratification*. Norwood, NJ: Ablex.

Langer, E., & Benevento, A. (1976). Self-induced dependence. *Journal of Personality and Social Psychiatry, 36*, 886–893.

Leff, J., & Vaughn, C. (1985). *Expressed emotions in families*. New York: The Guilford Press.

Link, B. G., & Dohrenwend, B. P. (1989). The epidemiology of mental disorders. In H. Freeman & S. Levine (Eds.), *The handbook of medial sociology* (pp. 102–127). Englewood Cliffs, NJ: Prentice-Hall.

Link, B. G., Dohrenwend, B. P., & Skodol, A. E. (1986). Socioeconomic status and schizophrenia: Noisome occupational characteristics as a risk factor. *American Sociological Review, 51*, 242–258.

Link, B. G., Lennon, M. C., & Dohrenwend, B. P. (1993). Socioeconomic status and depression: The role of occupations involving direction, control and planning. *American Sociological Review, 98*, 1351–1387.

McLanahan, S. (1985). Family structure and the reproduction of poverty. *American Journal of Sociology, 90*, 873–901.

Mechanic, D. (1972). Social class and schizophrenia: Some requirements for a plausible theory of social influence. *Social Forces, 50*, 305–309.

Mirowsky, J., & Ross, C. E. (1986). Social patterns of distress. *Annual Review of Sociology, 12*, 23–45.

Neugebauer, R., Dohrenwend, B. P., & Dohrenwend, B. S. (1980). Formulation of hypotheses about the true prevalence of functional psychiatric disorders among adults in the United States. In B. P. Dohrenwend, B. S. Dohrenwend, M. Gould, et al. (Eds.), *Mental illness in the United States: Epidemiological estimates* (pp. 45–94). New York: Praeger.

Robins, L., & Regier, D. (1990). *Psychiatric disorders in America*. New York: The Free Press.

Rosenfield, S. (1989). The effects of women's employment: Personal control and sex differences in mental health. *Journal of Health and Social Behavior, 30*, 77–91.

Treiman, D. (1977). *Occupational prestige in comparative perspective*. New York: Academic Press.

Turner, R. J. (1968). Social mobility and schizophrenia. *Journal of Health and Human Behavior, 9*, 194–203.

Wiersma, D., Giel, R., DeJond, A., & Sloof, C. (1983). Social class and schizophrenia in a Dutch cohort. *Psychological Medicine, 13*, 141–150.

U.S. Department of Labor. (1977). *Dictionary of occupational titles*. Washington, DC: Author.

22

Domestic Arrangements and Depressive Symptoms: An Examination of Housework Conditions

Mary Clare Lennon

One of the most consistent findings in psychiatric epidemiology is the greater prevalence of depressive disorders and symptoms of nonspecific psychological distress in women than in men (Dohrenwend & Dohrenwend, 1976; Kessler et al., 1994; McGrath et al., 1990; Pearlin, 1975; Robins & Regier, 1991; Weissman & Klerman, 1977, 1987). Gender differences are found on measures of anxiety, depressed mood, and psychophysiological complaints—what Dohrenwend and colleagues (1980) call demoralization (see Dohrenwend & Dohrenwend, 1976, and McGrath et al., 1990, for reviews)—and on measures designed to yield a psychiatric diagnosis of major depressive disorder and dysthymia according to criteria set forth by the *Diagnostic and Statistical Manual of Mental Disorders* of the American Psychiatric Association (1987, 1994; for example, see Kessler et al., 1994; Robins & Regier, 1991). Although the rates of disorder vary widely according to how the disorders are defined, women have, on average, about twice as many depressive disorders as men (McGrath et al., 1990; Paykel, 1991; Weissman & Klerman, 1977).

In seeking to explain these gender differences, a number of investigators have examined the social roles that women and men typically occupy. This literature assumes that women's family and work roles are more stressful than men's and that this greater stress accounts for women's increased psychological distress. Support for this general idea exists in studies that find higher rates of depression and demoralization among married women compared with married men (Gove & Geerken, 1977; Radloff, 1975); among mothers of young children compared with mothers of older children or nonmothers (Gore & Mangione, 1983; McLanahan & Adams, 1987; Radloff, 1975, 1980); and among housewives compared with employed women and with men (Horwitz, 1982; Radloff, 1975; Rosenfield, 1980). However, there are a sufficient number of studies that fail to document these effects, leading many investigators to examine factors that may mediate the association between occupancy of a social role and distress.

Within this area of study, attention has focused on domestic arrangements, that is, the structure of households and the allocation of domestic work. Although this domain incorporates a wide range of living arrangements and domestic responsibilities, I focus in this chapter on just one aspect of domestic arrangements: the structure of household chores. This is an increasingly relevant area of research, given the changes in work and family life that have occurred during the twentieth century. Primary among these changes is the increased participation of women in the labor force. The most dramatic shift in employment is seen among married women with young children. In 1960, 20% of married women with children younger than 6 were employed; by 1990, this had tripled to 60% (Gibson, 1993). This is in stark contrast with the division of labor inside the home, which has remained largely unchanged. Studies estimate that employed married women perform about two-thirds of the household chores, such as cooking, cleaning, repairs, and laundry. This is approximately twice as much as employed married men (Lennon & Rosenfield, 1994; Pleck, 1985; Ross, 1987).

Hochschild (1989) refers to this situation as a "stalled revolution": while women's social roles have changed to accommodate paid work, men's domestic roles have not changed to accommodate housework. Several studies suggest that husbands of employed wives are somewhat more involved in housework and child care than are husbands of unemployed wives (see, e.g., Barnett & Baruch, 1987; Pleck, 1985). Nevertheless, men's participation generally involves tasks that are more pleasant and autonomous, such as playing with children, whereas women generally assume the more time-pressured and essential tasks, such as preparing meals and bringing children to the doctor (Thompson & Walker, 1989).

Studies of the consequences of this situation for employed wives find less satisfaction and decreased psychological well-being when husbands fail to share in housework and child care (Kessler & McRae, 1982; Krause & Markides, 1985; Lennon et al., 1991; Pleck, 1985; Ross & Mirowsky, 1988;

Ross et al., 1983; Yogev & Brett, 1985). Although an association between domestic arrangements involving the division of family work and psychological distress has been demonstrated, several unanswered questions remain. First, because studies to date have been based on cross-sectional data, the direction of association is ambiguous. Perhaps perceptions of housework and child care are colored by psychological distress, with depressed women reporting, for example, that they perform a larger share of work than they actually do. Before this question can be addressed, however, another basic question remains unanswered: What is it about family work that may be distressing?

Robinson and Spitze (1992) outline and investigate three mechanisms that may account for the association of domestic labor and psychological distress. First, as noted above, many employed women receive little help with household chores. As a result, they face a "second shift" of work. Compared with their husbands, they spend more time in paid and unpaid work and less time in leisure activities (Bielby & Bielby, 1988; Hochschild, 1989). The burden of this work overload may be psychologically distressing. Second, it has been proposed that many women who have primary responsibility for household chores may experience a sense of inequity when their husbands do not share in this work (Lennon & Rosenfield, 1994; Thompson, 1991). The sense of inequity or unfairness may contribute to increased marital dissatisfaction and greater psychological distress. Third, housework has been described as requiring little skill and being physically demanding, isolating, and routine. In this view, housework, like paid work, may be characterized by its structural imperatives (Schooler et al., 1983). It has been argued that engagement in tasks with such negative characteristics, whether on the job or in the home, may be depressing.

Although there is some evidence in the literature to support each of these explanations, much of the research done to date has focused on issues of overload or equity.

Studies find that depressive symptoms are higher for women in transitional marriages, where wives are employed and husbands do not share housework, than they are for employed women in marriages where husbands do share housework (Ross et al., 1983). Moreover, when the division of household labor is equal, employed women have levels of depressive symptoms equal to those of employed men (Rosenfield, 1989). However, these studies generally rely upon wives' reports about whether household chores are shared equally. As Hochschild (1989) has compellingly demonstrated in her qualitative study of dual-earner couples, wives may report that housework is shared equally even though they do a far greater share than husbands. Explanations for this discrepancy, although of interest in themselves, are not of direct concern here (see Thompson, 1991, for a review). What is of concern is that many studies that purport to examine the division of housework may rely on measures that may not assess adequately the division of work. Studies that used more objectively gathered data, such as those amassed from daily diaries or from reports of time spent on a range of specific activities, provide more accurate accounts of the amount and distribution of work. Results from these studies generally support the conclusion that time spent on housework is associated with psychological distress among employed wives, supporting the possibility that burden or overload may account for the distress associated with housework (Glass & Fujimodo, 1994).

With regard to equity, several studies find higher levels of depressive symptoms among women who believe they perform an unfair share of housework compared with women who see the distribution of housework as fair (Lennon & Rosenfield, 1994; Robinson & Spitze, 1992). These studies are limited, however, by the potential confounding of reports of fairness and symptoms of depression. Nevertheless, results from these studies are generally consistent with results from experimental studies on the association of fairness and satisfaction, which support the proposition that perceptions of unfairness give rise to feelings of dissatisfaction and distress (e.g., Austin & Walster, 1974; Markovsky, 1988). Thus perceptions of fairness are a plausible mechanism for the association between housework and symptoms.

With respect to the argument that housework in inherently stressful, few investigators measure the characteristics of housework directly. Rather, studies simply compare levels of psychological distress between housewives and employed wives. More symptoms among housewives, found in several studies, are then assumed to derive from the burdensome nature of housework, the positive features of employment, or both. Thus characteristics of housework and paid work are taken as constant across women. However, some research suggests that conditions of housework, like job conditions, vary among women and may include positive as well as negative dimensions (Bird & Ross, 1993; Schooler et al., 1983). This is especially apparent when the working conditions of homemakers are compared to the job conditions of employed women (Lennon, 1994).

Among the studies that use comparable measures of dimensions of paid work and housework (Bird & Ross, 1993; Grana et al., 1993; Kibria et al., 1990; Lennon, 1994; Schooler et al., 1983), only a few compare the conditions of work for full-time homemakers and employed women (e.g., Bird & Ross, 1993; Grana et al., 1993; Lennon, 1994). Results from one of these, a study I conducted comparing conditions of housework for homemakers with conditions of jobs for employed wives, indicate that homemakers experience more advantageous work conditions in terms of greater autonomy, fewer time pressures, and less responsibility for matters outside their control; they experience less advantageous conditions in terms of more routine, more physical demands, and more interruptions (Lennon, 1994; see also Bird & Ross, 1993; Grana et al., 1993).

In that study, I also found that differences in work activities between employed wives and homemakers have implications for depressive symptoms. Two of the dimensions examined—the extent to which the worker is responsible for things outside her control and the amount of routine the work involves—are associated with depressive symptoms among women, regardless of work status. Compared with employed wives, homemakers obtain a certain benefit from having less responsibility; compared with homemakers, employed wives appear to benefit from less routine on the job. On balance, as a result of these distinctive work configurations, employed wives and homemakers exhibit similar levels of depressive symptoms.

Although research to date has examined job conditions for employed wives, little is known about how their housework conditions compare with those of full-time homemakers. It is known that employed wives spend significantly fewer hours on housework than full-time homemakers (Baruch & Barnett, 1986; Pleck, 1985; Thompson & Walker, 1989); but it is unclear whether the nature of housework changes when wives are employed. Additionally, little is known about the relation of housework conditions to depressive symptoms for these two groups. The present study examines three factors that may account for the association of housework and depressive symptoms: overload, equity, and housework conditions. I first describe and compare the configuration of housework conditions for employed wives and full-time homemakers and then examine the relation of depressive symptoms to these conditions, overload, and equity.

METHODS

Sample

Data for this investigation come from telephone interviews conducted in 1991 with a stratified sample of employed women, employed men, and homemakers, selected to be representative of the U.S. population (Lennon, 1994). Using a sample of randomly generated telephone numbers, interviewers first determined whether a household member met criteria for inclusion. The sample was restricted to persons between the ages of 25 and 54 because these are the ages during which individuals are most actively involved in jobs and household tasks. The sample of employed women and men was restricted to those who worked 15 hours a week or more for pay, thus ensuring that a substantial share of their daily activities would be job related. The homemaker sample was restricted to women who were married or living with someone as if they were married, not in school full-time, and not working outside the home more than 5 hours a week. These restrictions were designed to produce a comparison group of women whose primary work-related activities were focused on homemaking. The subsample of full-time homemakers was all female; male homemakers are extremely rare in the general population.

In the screening of households for eligible members, priority was given to locating and interviewing full-time homemakers. When such a homemaker was identified, the probability of her being selected was 80%. In the remaining households, an employed individual was selected. Where more than one household member was eligible for the study, the person with the next birthday was included in the sample to ensure random selection (O'Rourke & Blair, 1983).

The final sample consisted of 300 employed women, 302 employed men, and 202 full-time homemakers. The response rate for the survey was 67%. My analysis focuses on comparisons of homemakers ($n = 202$) and employed women who were married or living with someone as if they were married ($n = 197$). Data on housework conditions are available from all homemakers but were not obtained from all employed wives. Questions about housework were restricted to employed individuals who spent at least 10 hours a week on household chores ($n = 167$). When missing data are taken into account, the final sample consists of 166 employed wives and 198 homemakers.[*]

Measures

Hours Worked

For homemakers, the number of hours spent on housework was assessed by asking respondents to report the number of hours they spent doing household chores during the week and on weekends. Employed women were asked to report the number of hours spent on housework during a working day and during a nonworking day. Answers to these questions were used to calculate the number of hours per week spent on housework. For homemakers, this is the measure of hours worked. For employed wives, the number of hours spent on housework was added to the number of hours spent on the job to derive a measure of hours worked.

There is a statistically significant difference ($t = -13.92$, $p < .001$) between the average number of hours spent by employed wives on their jobs and household tasks combined (64.7) and the hours spent by homemakers on housework (38.5). Employed wives report significantly fewer housework hours compared to homemakers, with a mean of 25 hours. When hours spent in paid work by employed wives are compared with hours spent in housework by homemakers, there is no significant difference. Thus the excess in total work hours among employed wives is due to time spent on housework.

Fairness

Perceptions of fairness of the division of housework were assessed by an item that in-

quired into wives' perceptions of their own involvement in housework as being "more than your share" (coded -1), "about your share" (coded 0), or "less than your share" (coded 1). Given the proposition in theories of social equity that unfairness, either to oneself or someone else, is more distressing than fairness, a multiplicative term, fairness squared, was also added to the equation.

Just over half of employed wives (50.9%) and homemakers (56.9%) think that their share of housework is fair, while 41.2% of employed wives and 40.6% of homemakers feel that they do more than their share. The remaining wives (7.9% employed and 2.5% homemakers) report that they do less than their share. These differences are of marginal statistical significance ($\chi^2_{2,262} = 5.75$, $p < .10$).

Working Conditions

Measures of housework conditions were developed specifically for this study. The conceptualization of many important dimensions of housework is based on the investigations of Kohn and colleagues (Kohn & Schooler, 1983; Schooler et al., 1983). Whenever feasible, questions focused on specific tasks or behaviors, rather than on subjective appraisals, to reduce the contamination between the measurement of housework conditions and psychological outcomes (see Frese & Zapf, 1989, for a discussion of the distinction between subjective and objective self-reports). Thus, instead of asking respondents whether they feel that their housework is time pressured, they were asked whether "there is more work than there is time to complete the work."

Seven dimensions of housework are considered in this investigation: autonomy, time pressure, responsibility, interruptions, physical effort, routine, and complexity. With the exception of questions about complexity, interviewees were asked to choose one of the following four responses to indicate how much each statement resembled their housework: very much (coded 4), somewhat (coded 3), only a little (coded 2), or not at

---

[*]When data were missing on sociodemographic variables, the mean level of the variables was substituted. Separate means were calculated for employed wives and homemakers. In addition, dummy variables indicating that the respondent had missing data were added to the equations, as recommended by Cohen and Cohen (1983). These dummy variables are not presented in the tables. Results presented here do not differ materially from those derived from analyses that excluded all cases missing data on any variable.

all (coded 1). The complexity items were phrased in terms of how often respondents performed particular household tasks. Response categories are *1* (never), *2* (occasionally), *3* (sometimes), and *4* (often).

Autonomy is assessed by averaging responses to four items: (*1*) you decide when to start and when to finish your household activities, (*2*) you can take breaks whenever you want, (*3*) you control the speed at which you do your household tasks, and (*4*) you decide on your own how to go about doing the work (alpha = .65 for employed wives and .56 for homemakers). *Time pressure* is measured by the average of three items: (*1*) you have to work under time pressure, (*2*) there is more work than there is time to complete the work, and (*3*) you have enough time to do the work you're supposed to do (reverse scoring). The alpha coefficient is .69 for each group. *Responsibility* is assessed by the average of three items: (*1*) you are held responsible for others' mistakes, (*2*) you are held responsible when things don't get done, and (*3*) you are held responsible when things happen even though you can't control them (alpha = .79 for employed wives and .76 for homemakers). *Interruptions* is measured by the average of three items: (*1*) you can complete your work without interruptions (reverse scoring), (*2*) there are distractions that interfere with your household activities, and (*3*) you are interrupted by other people or telephone calls while doing your tasks (alpha = .84 for employed wives and .72 for homemakers). *Physical effort* is measured by one item: your household activities require physical effort. *Routine* work is assessed by the average of four items: (*1*) household activities require doing the same thing over and over, (*2*) you usually know exactly what you'll be doing from one day to the next, (*3*) you follow the same routine day-in and day-out, and (*4*) your household activities involve repetition (alpha = .76 for employed wives and .71 for homemakers). *Complexity* is measured by averaging responses to seven items about the frequency with which the following tasks are performed: (*1*) prepare complete meals from scratch, (*2*) follow complicated recipes, (*3*) bake from scratch, (*4*) plan weekly menus, (*5*) repair or mend clothing, (*6*) sew or make whole garments, and (*7*) make curtains or other things for around the house. The alpha coefficients are .72 for employed wives and .69 for homemakers. Comparisons between employed wives and homemakers on housework conditions are presented below in the "Results" section.

Depressive symptoms are assessed by averaging 12 items from the Center for Epidemiologic Studies Depression Scale (Radloff, 1977). In separate factor analyses by gender, Ross and Mirowsky (1984) found that these items loaded on one factor for women and men. Examples of the items are: you felt lonely, you could not get going, and you felt depressed. The time frame for reports of symptoms was the preceding month. Reliability is .88 (coefficient alpha). Scale scores were log transformed to normalize the distribution of the residuals.

Control Variables

The analyses control for demographic and family variables that differentiate homemakers from employed wives or correlate with housework conditions or depressive symptoms. The demographic variables are age and education (measured in years), race (represented by a dummy variable contrasting whites with others), and family income, categorized by one of nine groupings, ranging from less than $5,000 to $100,000 or more. Income was recoded to the category midpoint and divided by 1000. The analysis also controls for the number of children living at home.

Table 22.1 presents the average values of these control variables separately for employed wives and housewives as well as *t*-tests assessing the statistical significance of differences between these two groups. Homemakers and employed wives do not differ materially on average age or race but do differ significantly on education, family income, number of children at home, and work hours. On average, employed wives re-

Table 22.1. Sociodemographic characteristics of samples of full-time homemakers and employed wives

Variable	Homemakers (n = 198) Mean (S.D.)	Employed wives (n = 166) Mean (S.D.)	t-Statistic
Age	37.9 (8.1)	38.7 (7.9)	−0.88
Years of education	13.1 (2.2)	13.7 (2.8)	−2.29°
Percent white	89	86	0.79
Family income	$41,883 ($23,237)	$47,451 ($22,073)	−2.34°
Number of children at home	1.8 (1.3)	1.5 (1.2)	2.88°°

°$p \leq .05$.

°° $p \leq .01$.

port more education, higher family income, and fewer children at home.

RESULTS

Conditions of Housework

Table 22.2 shows average levels of housework conditions separately for homemakers and employed wives. It presents two types of statistical tests: tests of the difference between the mean scores (t-statistics) and tests of the difference in the scores' variances (F-ratios). The t-tests are based on means statistically adjusted for age, education, race, income, and number of children at home.

The housework conditions of homemakers and employed wives differ significantly on just two dimensions: time pressure and complexity. Employed wives report greater time pressure than homemakers. Both groups score at or below the scale midpoint on this measure, with homemakers significantly below this point, indicating that, on

Table 22.2. Housework conditions of full-time homemakers and employed wives

Work conditions	Homemakers (n = 198) Mean (S.D.)	Employed wives (n = 166) Mean (S.D.)	t-Statistic[a]	F-ratio[b]
Autonomy	3.79 (0.35)	3.85 (0.29)	1.49	1.40°
Time pressure	2.31 (0.88)	2.53 (0.85)	−2.71°°	1.06
Responsibility	1.90 (0.90)	1.96 (0.90)	−1.25	1.01
Interruptions	3.22 (0.73)	3.12 (0.81)	0.78	1.22
Physical effort	3.36 (0.68)	3.36 (0.67)	−0.74	1.04
Routine	3.17 (0.70)	3.19 (0.72)	−0.71	1.07
Complexity	2.50 (0.59)	2.29 (0.60)	2.67°°	1.04

[a]t-Statistic for difference between mean scores, adjusted for age, education, race, income, and number of children at home.

[b]F-ratio for difference between variances.

°$p \leq .05$.

°°$p \leq .01$.

average, neither group experiences excessive time pressures from housework (although the standard deviation suggests a wide range of variability in the scores of both groups). In addition, the mean difference between the groups in not large (approximately one-quarter of a standard deviation). The difference between the groups on complexity is somewhat larger, about one-third of a standard deviation. Again, the average scores fall around the scale midpoint for both groups, with employed wives significantly below that point. There is a marginally significant difference in average housework autonomy scores, with employed wives reporting greater autonomy than full-time homemakers. The groups also differ in the variability in autonomy, with homemakers reporting greater variation in autonomy scores than employed wives. However, for both groups, the mean autonomy scores are quite high and the standard deviations are quite small. In fact, 62% of homemakers and 68% of employed wives achieve the highest possible score of "4" on this scale, indicating that housework provides a great amount of autonomy for the large majority of women.

Also of interest in Table 22.2 is that the relative rankings among the average housework conditions scores are quite similar for employed wives and homemakers. Because all scales have the same metric, scores may be compared across housework dimensions. Both groups describe housework as involving a high degree of autonomy, physical effort, routine, and interruptions (a score of 3 or greater). These results are consistent with descriptions of housework found in the literature (e.g., Berk, 1985; Berk & Berk, 1979; Ferree, 1984; Oakley, 1974).

The similarities in many of the housework conditions between employed wives and full-time homemakers stand in sharp contrast with differences I found in an earlier comparison of housework conditions of full-time homemakers and job conditions of employed wives (Lennon, 1994). To summarize these, relative to how employed wives describe their jobs, full-time homemakers see their housework as more subject to inter-

ruptions, more physically demanding, more routine, less time pressured, and involving less responsibility. In addition, for most work characteristics, homemakers describe a narrower range. Many of the conditions of housework, by contrast, are similar for employed wives and homemakers, with regard to both average scores and degree of variability. The primary exceptions are that, for employed wives, housework involves more time pressure and less complexity. These findings are consistent with the greater amount of time this group spends combining housework with paid work.

Housework Conditions and Depressive Symptoms

The next step of the analysis examines the associations of the conditions of housework and depressive symptoms. I conducted analyses using hierarchical regression procedures. As a first step, I tested whether the associations of housework conditions and depressive symptoms vary for employed wives and housewives by including a series of two-way interaction terms in the equation. Because these terms did not contribute significantly to the variance in symptoms, either singly or as a group, main effect models are presented.

The first step, shown in column *a* of Table 22.3, shows the results of regressing depressive symptoms on housework status and demographic variables. Homemakers and employed wives do not differ on average levels of symptoms. The demographic variables are related to depressive symptoms as expected, with fewer symptoms found among older women, more educated women, and white women. In addition, women with children at home have fewer symptoms than other women.

The second step, shown in column *b*, indicates the effect of work hours. The total weekly work hours are unrelated to symptoms. Given the hypothesis that housework is distressing because it constitutes a second shift of work for employed wives, I also tested for the interaction between hours and work status (not shown). This was not sig-

Table 22.3. Regression of depressive symptoms on work status, hours, fairness, work conditions, and control variables

Variable	(a) b s.e. (b)		(b) b s.e. (b)		(c) b s.e. (b)		(d) b s.e. (b)	
Work status (Homemaker = 1)	.027	(.020)	.049[†]	(.025)	.051°	(.025)	.062°	(.025)
Age	−.004°°	(.001)	−.004°°	(.001)	−.004°°	(.001)	−.004°°	(.001)
Years of education	−.011°	(.005)	−.012°	(.005)	−.010°	(.005)	−.012°°	(.005)
Race (White = 1)	−.076°	(.031)	−.074°	(.031)	−.060°	(.031)	−.076°°	(.031)
Family income	−.001°	(.001)	−.001[†]	(.001)	−.001[†]	(.001)	−.001	(.001)
Number of children at home	−.029°°	(.008)	−.031°°°	(.008)	−.030°°°	(.008)	−.032°°°	(.008)
Work hours			.001	(.001)	.001	(.001)	.000	(.001)
Fairness					.017	(.024)	.016	(.024)
Fairness squared					.070°	(0.28)	.048[†]	(.027)
Working Conditions								
Autonomy							−.013	(.032)
Time pressure							.036°°	(.013)
Responsibility							.033°°	(.011)
Interruptions							−.025[†]	(.014)
Physical effort							.008	(.015)
Routine							.023	(.014)
Complexity							−.024	(.017)
R^2	0.127		0.132		0.156		0.215	

[†]$p \leq .10.$
°$p \leq .05$
°°$p \leq .01.$
°°°$p \leq .001.$

nificant, indicating that hours of work are not associated with depressive symptoms for either employed wives or homemakers. This result suggests that the overload hypothesis is not supported in these data.

To examine the second mechanism, perceptions of equity, I added the linear and quadratic terms for perceived fairness to the equation. Results, shown in column c, are consistent with equity theory in that the lowest rates of symptoms are found among wives who feel that they perform their share of housework (see Lennon & Rosenfield, 1994). The positive sign of the quadratic term, coupled with the nonsignificance of the linear term, indicates that the lowest level of symptoms is found among women who see the division of housework as fair, while higher levels of symptoms are found

among women who believe that they do either more or less than their fair share.

The addition of the seven measures of housework conditions is shown in column d. Before examining these, note that the coefficient for work status has increased and is statistically significant (as it is in column c), a point to which I return later. The results for work hours and demographic variables are similar to those described earlier, with the exception that the effect of income is no longer significant. Because housework conditions are likely to associated with income, this result is not surprising.

Of the housework conditions in the equation, four are not related to symptoms: autonomy, physical effort, routine, and complexity. The coefficients for time pressure and responsibility for matters outside one's control are positive and significant, indicating that high scores on these dimensions of housework are associated with more symptoms. Surprisingly, the coefficient for interruptions is negative (but of marginal statistical significance) indicating that, all other housework conditions being equal, interruptions are marginally associated with lower symptoms.

Finally, the significant positive coefficient for work status suggests that, were employed wives and homemakers to experience similar housework conditions, depressive symptoms would be higher among homemakers. Thus it appears that homemakers may benefit because their housework is less time pressured than that of employed wives.

DISCUSSION

To summarize the results, women describe housework as characterized by a high degree of autonomy, routine, and physical effort, subject to frequent interruptions, and entailing a moderate degree of responsibility for things outside of their control. Employed wives and full-time homemakers are quite similar in these descriptions, with the tendency for employed wives to report somewhat more autonomy in their housework. Two differences, however, appear in their reports of housework conditions: homemakers describe their housework as more complex and less time pressured. Employed wives and homemakers differ as well on the number of hours that they spend on housework each week, with employed wives averaging fewer hours (25.0) than full-time homemakers (38.5). However, when hours on the job are added to the time spent on housework, employed wives average a total of 64.7 job and housework hours per week. Finally, and consistent with their fewer hours spent on housework, slightly more employed wives (7.9%) than full-time homemakers (2.5%) feel that they do less than their share of housework. The majority of women, however, report that they do their share (50.9% of employed wives; 56.9% of homemakers) of household chores, while a

large minority (41.2% of employed wives; 40.6% of homemakers) report doing more than their share.

These differences in specific work conditions, hours, and fairness have implications for levels of depressive symptoms among employed wives and homemakers. Before these variables are taken into account, employed wives and homemakers show little average difference on levels of depressive symptoms. However, when hours, work conditions, and fairness are added to equations predicting depressive symptoms, employed wives average significantly fewer depressive symptoms than nonemployed wives. In other words, the relationship between work status and symptoms appears to have been suppressed by the characteristics of housework that distinguish employed wives from homemakers. Both time pressure and unfairness are associated with greater levels of depressive symptoms. Were homemakers to share the high time pressure and sense of unfairness that employed wives express, they would exceed employed wives on symptoms.

These results suggest that combining paid work with housework reduces the benefits of employment for women. Although employed wives experience greater time pressure resulting from housework, they are no more disadvantaged than homemakers with respect to depressive symptoms. This suggests that they experience rewards from paid work that offset the difficulties they encounter with housework. Benefits of employment, such as earnings and access to networks of social support, may compensate for disadvantages of housework. Future research on these issues therefore should consider aspects of jobs as well as aspects of housework in understanding symptoms among employed wives.

In considering these results further, it is important to point out that this study is based on cross-sectional data. It is possible that women's choice of housework as a full- or part-time activity derives from certain of their distinctive characteristics. For example, some women may opt for full-time housework because they prefer work that involves less time pressure or more complexity. While the general issue of selection into employment merits further study, Gerson (1985) suggests that women's choice between employment and homemaking is not based simply on their personal characteristics or early socialization. Rather, the constraints and opportunities available in the labor market and in the family combine to shape the decisions and adaptations that women make.

The cross-sectional nature of these data also makes other inferences open to question. For example, measures of housework conditions and depressive symptoms may be confounded. Unfortunately, the strategy of using objective assessments of work conditions that has been adopted in the study of occupations (e.g., Eaton, 1990; Lennon, 1987; Link et al., 1993; see also Link et al., Chapter 21, this volume) cannot be applied to the study of housework. To accurately assess housework conditions in the home would require the use of outside observers, a task that would be difficult to manage on a large scale. Even were such data available, the issue of selection into work situations would remain unresolved.

However, I have argued that, it spite of their limitations, data from cross-sectional and self-report investigations are potentially useful for exploring the mechanisms that may account for the association between housework and depressive symptoms and thus for suggesting directions for future research efforts. Three mechanisms for the association between housework and depressive symptoms are considered here: overload, equity, and housework conditions. Both inequity and specific housework conditions contribute significantly to symptoms.

This investigation underscores the importance of specifying the ways in which social positions structure the content of daily life. It suggests the importance of specifying the nature of the day-to-day activities and tasks that constitute the daily work of domestic labor. In terms of domestic arrangements more generally, it suggests a strategy of investigation that focuses on the experiences encountered by individuals under various structural arrangements. By uncovering some of the complexity underlying social roles and positions, we will increase our understanding of the relation of these roles to psychological well-being.

REFERENCES

American Psychiatric Association. (1987). *Diagnostic and statistical manual of mental disorders* (3rd ed., rev). Washington, DC: American Psychiatric Press.

American Psychiatric Association. (1994). *Diagnostic and statistical manual of mental disorders* (4th ed.). Washington, DC: American Psychiatric Press.

Austin, W., & Walster, E. (1974). Reactions to confirmation and disconfirmation of equity and inequity. *Journal of Personality and Social Psychology, 30,* 208–216.

Baruch, G. K., & Barnett, R. C. (1986). Consequences of fathers' participation in family work: Parents' role strain and well-being. *Journal of Personality and Social Psychology, 51,* 983–992.

Barnett, R. C., & Baruch, G. K. (1987). Determinants of fathers' participation in family work. *Journal of Marriage and the Family, 9,* 9–40.

Berk, R. A., & Berk, S. F. (1979). *Labor and leisure at home: Content and organization of the household day.* Beverly Hills, CA: Sage.

Berk, S. F. (1985). *The gender factory: The apportionment of work in American households.* New York: Plenum.

Bielby, D. D., & Bielby, W. T. (1988). She works hard for the money: Household responsibilities and the allocation of work effort. *American Journal of Sociology, 93,* 1031–1059.

Bird, C. E., & Ross, C, E. (1993). Houseworkers and paid workers: Qualities of the work and effects on personal control. *Journal of Marriage and the Family, 55,* 913–925.

Cohen, J., & Cohen, P. (1983). *Applied multiple regression/correlation analysis for the behavioral sciences.* Hillsdale, NJ: Lawrence Erlbaum Associates.

Dohrenwend, B. P., & Dohrenwend, B. S. (1976). Sex differences and psychiatric disorders. *American Journal of Sociology, 81,* 1447–1454.

Dohrenwend, B. P., Shrout, P. E., Egri, G., et al. (1980). Measures of nonspecific psychological distress and other dimensions of psychopathology. *Archives of General Psychiatry, 37,* 1229–1236.

Ferree, M. M. (1984). Class, housework, and happiness: Women's work and life satisfaction. *Sex Roles, 11,* 1057–1074.

Frese, M., & Zapf, D. (1988). Methodological issues in the study of work stress: Objective vs. subjective measurement of work stress and the question of longitudinal studies. In C. L. Cooper & R. Payne (Eds.), *II. Causes, coping and consequences of stress at work* (pp. 375–441). Chichester: John Wiley & Sons.

Gerson, K. (1985). Hard choices: How women decide about work, career, and motherhood. Berkeley, CA: University of California Press.

Gibson, C. (1993). The four baby booms. *American Demographics, 15,* 36–40.

Glass, J., & Fujimodo, T. (1994). Housework, paid work, and depression among husbands and wives. *Journal of Health and Social Behavior, 35,* 179–191.

Gore, S., & Mangione, T. W. (1983). Social roles and psychological distress: Additive and interactive models of sex differences. *Journal of Health and Social Behavior, 24,* 300–312.

Gove, W. R., & Geerken, M. R. (1977). The effect of children and employment on the mental health of married men and women. *Social Forces, 56,* 66–79.

Grana, S. J., Moore, H. A., Wilson, J. K., et al. (1993). The contents of housework and the paid labor force: Women's perceptions of the demand levels of their work. *Sex Roles, 28,* 295–315.

Hochschild, A. (1989). *The second shift: Working parents and the revolution at home.* New York: Viking.

Horwitz, A. (1982). Sex role expectations, power, and psychological distress. *Sex Roles, 8,* 607–623.

Kessler, R. C., McGonagle, K. A., Zhao, S., et al. (1994). Lifetime and 12-month prevalence of DSM-III-R psychiatric disorders in the United States. *Archives of General Psychiatry, 51,* 8–19.

Kessler, R. C., & McRae, J. A. (1982). The effects of wives' employment on the mental health of married men and women. *American Sociological Review, 47,* 216–227.

Kibria, N., Barnett, R. C., Baruch, G. K., et al. (1990). Homemaking-role quality and the psychological well-being and distress of married women. *Sex Roles, 22,* 327–347.

Kohn, M. L., & Schooler, C. (1982). Job conditions and personality: A longitudinal assessment of their reciprocal effects. *American Journal of Sociology, 87,* 1257–1286.

Kohn, M. L., & Schooler, C. (Eds.). (1983). *Work and personality.* Norwood, NY: Ablex.

Krause, N., & Markides, K. A. (1985). Employment and well-being in Mexican American women. *Journal of Health and Social Behavior, 26,* 15–26.

Lennon, M. C. (1994). Women, work and well-being: The importance of work conditions. *Journal of Health and Social Behavior, 35,* 235–247.

Lennon, M. C., & Rosenfield, S. (1992). Women and distress: The contribution of job and family conditions. *Journal of Health and Social Behavior, 33,* 316–327.

Lennon, M. C., & Rosenfield, S. (1994). Relative fairness and the division of housework: The importance of options. *American Journal of Sociology, 100,* 506–531.

Lennon, M. C., Wasserman, G. A., & Allen, R. (1991). Husbands' involvement in child care and depressive symptoms among mothers of infants. *Women & Health, 17,* 1–23.

Lennon, M. C. (1987). Sex differences in distress: The impact of gender and work roles. *Journal of Health and Social Behavior, 28,* 290–305.

Link, B. G., Lennon, M. C., & Dohrenwend, B. P. (1993). Socioeconomic status and depression: The role of occupations involving direction, control and planning. *American Journal of Sociology, 98,* 1351–1387.

Markovsky, B. (1988). Injustice and arousal. *Social Justice Research, 2,* 223–233.

McGrath, E., Keita, G. P., Strictland, B. R., et al. (Eds.). (1990). *Women and depression: Risk factors and treatment issues.* Washington, DC: American Psychological Association.

McLanahan, S. S., & Adams, J. (1987). Parenthood and psychological well-being. *Annual Review of Sociology, 13,* 237–257.

Oakley, A. (1974). *The sociology of housework.* New York: Pantheon.

O'Rourke, D., & Blair, J. (1983). Improving random selection in telephone surveys. *Journal of Marketing Research, 20,* 428–432.

Paykel, E. S. (1991). Depression in women. *British Journal of Psychiatry, 158*(Suppl. 10), 22–29.

Pearlin, L. I. (1975). Sex roles and depression. In N. Datan & L. H. Ginsberg (Eds.), *Life-span developmental psychology: Normative life crises* (pp. 191–207). New York: Academic Press.

Pleck, J. H. (1985). *Working wives/working husbands.* Beverly Hills, CA: Sage.

Radloff, L. S. (1975). Sex differences in depression: The effects of occupation and marital status. *Sex Roles, 1,* 243–265.

Radloff, L. S. (1977). The CES-D scale: A self-report depression scale for research in the general population. *Applied Psychological Measurement, 1,* 385–401.

Radloff, L. S. (1980). Depression and the empty nest. *Sex Roles, 6,* 775–781.

Robins, L. N., & Regier, D. A. (1991). *Psychiatric disorders in America: The Epidemiologic Catchment Area study.* New York: The Free Press.

Robinson, J., & Spitze, G. (1992). Whistle while you work? The effect of household task performance on women's and men's well-being. *Social Science Quarterly, 73,* 844–861.

Rosenfield, S. L. (1980). Sex differences in depression: Do women always have higher rates? *Journal of Health and Social Behavior, 21,* 33–42.

Rosenfield, S. (1989). The effects of women's employment: Personal control and sex differences in mental health. *Journal of Health and Social Behavior, 30,* 77–91.

Rosenfield, S. (1992). The costs of sharing: Wives' employment and husbands' mental health. *Journal of Health and Social Behavior, 33,* 13–225.

Ross, C. E. (1984). The division of labor at home. *Social Forces, 65,* 816–833.

Ross, C. E., & Mirowsky, J. (1984). Components of depressed mood in married men and women: The Center for Epidemiological Studies Depression Scale. *American Journal of Epidemiology, 119,* 997–1004.

Ross, C. E., & Mirowsky, J. (1988). Child care and emotional adjustment to wives' employment. *Journal of Health and Social Behavior, 29,* 127–138.

Ross, C. E., Mirowsky, J., & Huber, J. (1983). Dividing work, sharing work, and in-between: Marriage patterns and depression. *American Sociological Review, 48,* 809–823.

Schooler, C., Kohn, M. C., Miller, K. A., et al. (1983). Housework as work. In M. C. Kohn & C. Schooler (Eds.), *Work and personality* (pp. 242–260). Norwood, NY: Ablex.

Thompson, L. (1991). Family work: Women's sense of fairness. *Journal of Family Issues, 12,* 181–196.

Thompson, L., & Walker, A. J. (1989). Gender in families: Women and men in marriage, work, and parenthood. *Journal of Marriage and the Family, 51,* 845–871.

Weissman, M. M., & Klerman, G. L. (1977). Sex differences in the epidemiology of depression. *Archives of General Psychiatry, 34,* 98–111.

Weissman, M. M., & Klerman, G. L. (1987). Gender and depression. In R. Formanek & A. Gurian (Eds.), *Women and depression: A lifespan perspective* (pp. 3–15). New York: Springer-Verlag.

Yogev, S., & Brett, J. (1985). Perceptions of the division of housework and child care and marital satisfaction. *Journal of Marriage and the Family, 47,* 609–619.

V

COMPLEMENTARY APPROACHES

Robert M. Rose

Previous sections have focused on observational research, especially psychosocially oriented studies using epidemiological methods. Although these studies can tell us a great deal about the role of adversity, they are not controlled experiments. They have not investigated genetic and physiological factors that are likely to be important in relations between adversity and psychopathology. In this section, therefore, we consider complementary approaches that help expose weaknesses and fill in gaps. More specifically, we look at an experimental simulation, some experimental research with animals, and an experimentally controlled trial of a preventive intervention. In addition, we learn about a behavioral genetic approach to the study of adversity and about an investigation of some physiological correlates of stress. Finally, we are invited to share a perspective on problems and possibilities of integrating different lines and levels of analysis of adversity, stress, and psychopathology.

Shrout and Link provide an intriguing computer simulation of Dohrenwend's quasi-experimental strategy for investigating inverse relations between socioeconomic status and psychopathology. In doing so, they make it possible to formalize our thinking about the assumptions underlying the

actual study reported earlier in this volume. They show where the logic of this quasi experimental test of the social causation–social selection issue with epidemiological methods holds up and where it is limited when examined in the light of results from a simulation experiment. The different findings for different disorders suggest the need for interventions with different emphases. For example, the social selection outcome for schizophrenia points to the need for tertiary prevention designed to diminish risk of chronicity, chronic disability, and further downward spiral. The social causation outcome for depression, by contrast, underlines the need for strategies designed to enhance adaptive abilities in the face of new adversity.

Kraemer and Bachevalier's work shows that we can develop a model of the effect of adversity during early development on future psychopathology through experimental studies of nonhuman primates. These investigators fault the field for continuing the "nature versus nurture" debate and emphasize, instead, that the environment causes biological changes in the brain. The studies point to the importance of interplay between physiological regulation and the evolution of behavioral repertoires. By way of illustration, Kraemer and Bachevalier examine the impact of altered rearing status of rhesus monkeys separated from their mothers and reared with only human contact or in peer groups. They have been able to document important differences in these non-mother-reared monkeys, such as inability to block irrelevant stimuli or excessive impulsiveness in making choices. They also have been able to tie alterations in cognitive processing to the profound social defects these monkeys show in group or dyadic behavior. In this work, they are articulating a much refined model of attachment theory, which attempts to link brain development and physiological regulation to the unfolding of behavioral propensities. Their work provides a basis for insights into the important interplay between genetic influences and developmental experiences.

Frank and Karp's chapter also argues for the need to integrate future studies of psychopathology with physiological measures that reflect the burden of exposure to adverse life events. As they point out, we need to investigate how chronic stress, or the accumulated effects of repeated attempts at adaptation to multiple stresses, leads to altered physiological states as well as psychological dysfunction. This has been called allostatic load; it involves changes in response to new challenges with resettings of homeostatic mechanisms. Although earlier research has focused on the potential effects of both acute and chronic stress on hormonal function, more recent work also has investigated effects on sleep and autonomic activity and, most recently, on immune function. Studying both psychological and physiological consequences broadens and deepens our understanding of vulnerability in relation to physical and mental health.

Kendler's report is a very important example of how to integrate perspectives from psychiatric genetics and epidemiology. He focuses on an area that is central to our concern with adversity— the risks for psychopathology associated with exposure to stressful life events. The first part of his argument relates to the nonrandom nature of exposure to life events. As pointed out in the past by the Dohrenwends and re-emphasized in this volume, it is important to differentiate between those life events whose occurrence is essentially beyond the control of the individual, such as deaths in the family, and those that are likely to be highly influenced by the person (e.g., being fired from work, getting divorced). We are aware that many life events seem to be products of our own behavior, personality, or temperamental attributes. If this is so, as it now appears to be from several different studies, one is led to ask if such exposure also can be a product of genetic influences. Using the Virginia Twin Study, Kendler finds that monozygotic twins were more similar than dizygotic twins in the frequency of occurrence of financial difficulties or being the victim of an assault or robbery; however, they were no different in experiencing a death of a family member or friend.

Kendler went on to investigate the question of whether individuals differ in their *sensitivity* to these events. In other words, even if one is exposed to the same event or same number of events, does the impact on psychological functioning differ? If so, what mechanism underlies the difference? Using the same Virginia Twin Study data, Kendler and his colleagues replicated the findings from other studies showing that stressful life events were strongly related to the onset of episodes of major depressive disorder. These investigators also found that individuals with strong family history and high genetic risk were about twice as likely to become depressed following exposure to stressful life events as those with lower genetic risk. This research illustrates the value of investigating *interactions* between genetic proclivity and environmental events. This need is often cited but rarely followed by such persuasive research.

The two preventive interventions introduced and evaluated by Kellam and associates are very compelling in helping us to understand the causal relationships between school and achievement and aggressive behavior. These studies are the more impressive in that they involved unusual interventions with an entire population of over 1000 first-grade students. There were two interventions, and students were randomly assigned to one or the other or to control groups. One (the Good Behavior Game) was designed to diminish inappropriate aggressive/disruptive behavior in the classrooms (i.e., verbal disruptions, physical disruptions, out-of-seat without permission, and noncompliance). Students were rewarded for maintaining good behavior, without disruptions, for increasing periods of time during the fall semester of their first year in school. The other intervention, also in the fall of the first year, involved learning (Mastery Learning). It consisted of a systematically enriched instructional strategy for the reading curriculum. Changes in the level of aggressive/disruptive behavior and learning achievement were assessed during the following spring of the first year.

Each intervention was effective in the same domain of behavior. That is, good behavior diminished future aggression/disruption, and mastery learning improved future schoolwork achievement. However, the authors are particularly concerned with the possible crossover effects. Did children who improved in their learning show diminished future aggressive behavior? Did those who showed a diminution of disruptive behavior have a greater enhancement of future learning?

Kellam and his colleagues report one very important crossover effect: improved learning associated with mastery curriculum led to diminished future aggression. This was most pronounced for boys who were unusually aggressive in the fall and also had higher gains in achievement while they participated the Mastery Learning curriculum.

By contrast, those students who showed improvement in aggressive behavior after participating in the Good Behavior Game did not show subsequent improvement in reading achievement. This was a universal, not a targeted, intervention, and the group-level effects are not large. More powerful changes might result from application of the mastery learning strategy to boys who show both problems in disruptive behavior as well as poor initial scholastic achievement. Nevertheless these are impressive findings. They strongly suggest that much aggressive behavior stems from the experience of failure and a sense of being blocked from acceptance and advancement.

These studies by Kellam and his colleagues are complex and require much work involving teachers, students, and parents. Skill, ingenuity, and persistence are required to carry them out. As this chapter shows, the results are worth the effort. The research is of crucial importance in providing us with insight into the complex interactions among learning, self-esteem or efficacy, and aggressive behavior.

In the last chapter in this section, Leighton describes, in historical context and from the vantage point of his functionalist theoretical orientation, something of the complexity of the challenge to integrate lines of research in biology, psychiatry, clinical psychology, and the social sciences. He brings depth as well as great breadth to his argument for the creation of "bridging structures" between differing levels of theory and research ranging "from molecules to organs of the body, to the whole person and beyond to social organizations of which the . . . [individual] is a part."

23

Mathematical Modeling and Simulation in Studies of Stress and Adversity

Patrick E. Shrout
Bruce G. Link

Randomized experiments are widely regarded as the best way to establish a causal link between a risk variable and an outcome, such as psychopathology (Holland, 1988). The logic is simple: Randomly assign subjects who do not have psychopathology into one of two groups, expose one group to the risk, and then follow them over time to see whether they exhibit signs and symptoms of mental disorder. The other group is left unexposed but is followed using the same procedures as the exposed group. The control group is included to inform us of what the exposed group would be like had they had not been exposed.

Although the logic of randomized studies may be simple, the ethical, logistic, and interpretive issues for studies of stress and adversity are not. Even with animals, one must think carefully about the benefits of inducing pain or stress in subjects who are otherwise not at risk. Ethical issues with human subjects are more troublesome and are not handled by routine informed consent procedures. Often the ethical issues are resolved by making the stress experience relatively innocuous, but then the generalizability of the experimental results to real-life

stress is called into question. Social experiments (Cook & Campbell, 1979) are conceivable[1] but seldom, if ever, carried out in practice. For these reasons, most of the research on adversity, stress, and psychopathology depends on nonexperimental data. This volume contains reports of many studies that have advanced our knowledge on the basis of such data.

The analysis and interpretation of nonexperimental data require vigilance against artifacts and spurious claims. Whether we use case–control designs or prospective risk designs, we must always be sure that sampling and measurement problems do not lead us to believe that there is a causal relation when no causality exists. Usually investigators guard against such artifacts using tools of sampling and statistical analysis. The most common method is *statistical adjustment*, through which we ask, "What if the exposed and unexposed groups were more similar than they really are?"[2] This hypothetical equating is achieved on the basis of mathematical models of the relations among the risk, outcome, and confounding variables. The logic of statistical adjustment requires that we have perfect measures of potential confounding variables, and that we can account for the mathematical relation among the variables.

In practice, we virtually never can be sure that we have perfect measures or that the specification of the statistical model is correct. Sometimes we can be sure of the opposite: that both our measures and model are flawed. We may want to control for previous psychopathology but only have available a retrospective symptom screening measure. We also may know that certain variables must be included in the model but have no measures of those variables. From statistical textbooks (Snedecor & Cochran, 1967), we know that measurement and model specification error will certainly bias the statistical analyses, but they will not necessarily invalidate the broad interpretation of findings. Statistical texts usually cannot help to determine the impact of bias in multivariate analyses, in large part because we often do not know exactly how the imperfect model differs from the ideal model.[3]

One way social scientists can learn about the validity of results from nonexperimental studies is through replications that vary the conditions and assumptions made in the nonexperimental test. When different studies produce the same pattern of results even though the samples, measures, statistical methods, and theoretical assumptions vary, we begin to be confident that the results hold. However, carrying out the additional empirical studies can be extremely costly and time consuming.

For some problems, we can learn about features of statistical models and measures without interviewing new subjects. If it is possible to formulate alternative statistical models, the impact of the different model specifications can be studied mathematically. Two approaches are used by quantitative scientists for such studies. One is the examination of sets of equations using formal mathematical logic. The other is a comparison of results obtained when the models are used to analyze simulated data. Although the former approach is preferred by mathematically inclined statisticians and social scientists, the latter approach is often

more accessible to empirical researchers and is hence the focus of this chapter.

To study model specification using simulation, we first specify a reference statistical model—one that we assume a priori in order to study it. As a simple example, we might assume that, on the average, symptoms of psychopathology increase linearly with increases in stressors. In algebraic terms, this reference model is $Y = B_0 + B_1X + e$, where Y stands for symptoms, X stands for stressors, B_0 is the expected symptoms for persons with no stressors, and B_1 is the expected symptom increase for a unit increase in stressors. The residual e represents a random error term, in recognition that most individual subjects' data will deviate somewhat from the linear trend.

Next we use statistical computer software to create hypothetical data that would result if the reference model were true. To do this, we first create a sample of X observations that has a realistic distribution. For example, if X were a count of stressors, the distribution would be positively skewed and would range from zero to some number such as 15. Ideally, this distribution would be constructed to resemble a real data set.

Next we would select realistic values for the parameters B_0 and B_1, and we would specify the variance of the random term e. These values determine the size of the multiple correlation (R^2) for the model. Ideally, we choose values that are consistent with the previous literature. Given X, B_0, B_1 and a set variance for e, it is possible to generate Y. Because part of Y comes from the random component e, Y itself is random. It is associated with but not completely determined by X.

Finally, we analyze the simulated data using alternative statistical models, several of which we know to be "wrong" (i.e., not the model used to generate the data). Through these analyses, we can observe if the alternative analyses produce misleading conclusions or merely produce biased effect-size estimates. For example, instead of analyzing symptom data as a linear function of the stressor data, we might ask how the results would change if the psychopathology out-

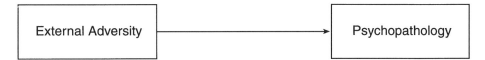

Figure 23.1. The victimization model.

come were redefined to be disorder present/absent, using some cut point on the symptom count. How would the stressor data relate to the binary outcome instead of the "correct" quantitative outcome? The simulation would provide clues, and a series of simulations would provide an answer.[4]

In the next section, we illustrate the simulation approach to investigate models of social selection and social stress. These models are substantially more complicated than the two-variable model used in the simple example discussed so far.

STATISTICAL MODELS OF STRESS, ADVERSITY, AND PSYCHOPATHOLOGY

The importance of model specification in the analysis of nonexperimental data can only be appreciated if we have explicit models of the stress process. Barbara Dohrenwend was a pioneer in formulating alternative explicit models, and a summary of five different models that she and Bruce Dohrenwend formulated in the early 1980s was previously presented at the American Psychopathic Association (APPA) meetings (Dohrenwend et al., 1986). Each of the models described how stressful life events, social situations, and personal dispositions

might relate in different ways to psychopathology as an outcome.

For example, one of the models is called the "victimization" model (Fig. 23.1). According to this model, psychopathology is caused solely by environmental adversity, such as that reflected in measures of stressful life events.[5] The victimization model provides one explanation for the often-observed *inverse relation* between psychopathology and social status—persons who are low on society's social hierarchy apparently have greater risk of psychopathology. According to the social causation explanation for the inverse relation, socioeconomic status (SES) disadvantage leads to increased risk of external adversity, which in turn leads to increased risk of psychopathology (Fig. 23.2). We can modify the victimization model to show this explicitly.[6]

Dohrenwend et al. (1992) examined this explanation and contrasted it to a social selection explanation; this posits that some people are selected into the lower rungs of the social hierarchy by psychopathology and that others are selected into the higher rungs by positive mental health. In contrast to the social causation model, the social selection explanation does not depend on a direct causal link between external adversity and psychopathology. Instead, it accounts for the inverse relation between SES and

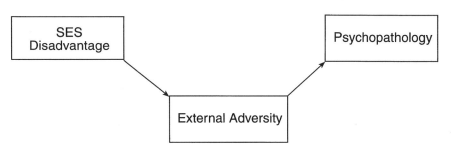

Figure 23.2. Social causation model.

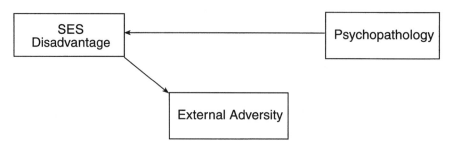

Figure 23.3. Social selection model.

psychopathology by hypothesizing that SES is directly affected by the mental health–psychopathology continuum (Fig. 23.3). This effect can occur within a lifetime or across several generations for psychopathology with a familial component. In the diagram of the model, we include the box for external adversity simply to make it comparable to the social causation model. External adversity could be eliminated from the diagram without doing an injustice to the central feature of the selection explanation.[7]

Although these models are explicit, they are difficult to study empirically. Experiments could establish which direction the arrow between SES and psychopathology should point, but the ethical issues we discussed earlier preclude their serious consideration. Instead, we must be content to survey persons with existing pathology, and whose adversity and SES disadvantage is not manipulated. However, both the social causation and social selection model make the same prediction regarding survey data, namely, that psychopathology will be correlated with both SES disadvantage and external adversity.

THE DOHRENWEND QUASI EXPERIMENT

In 1966, Bruce Dohrenwend suggested a quasi experimental strategy to break the impasse in the comparison of the social causation and social selection explanations of the inverse relation of SES and psychopathology. He identified a situation that could be examined with survey data for which the social causation and social selection explanations make different predictions. The situation is created by considering the impact of ethnic disadvantage at the same time that SES and psychopathology are examined.

According to the social causation explanation, ethnic disadvantage is another manifestation of adversity and should lead to psychopathology. If advantaged and disadvantaged ethnic groups are compared, the social causation hypothesis predicts that the disadvantaged ethnic group will show more psychopathology. This would be true even if SES is statistically controlled in the comparison because of ethnic discrimination and prejudice above and beyond their effects on SES.

According to the social selection explanation, ethnic disadvantage can be viewed as an additional factor in the sifting and sorting of selection. Prejudice and discrimination result in a larger proportion of the ethnic minority being restricted to the lower social strata. One of the many ways this general pattern occurs is less tolerance for psychopathology among the ethnic minority members relative to the ethnic majority. This means that ethnic minorities in the lower levels of SES will have trouble rising to the next social stratum if they exhibit even minor psychopathology, and that those in the higher levels of SES will lose social advantage unless they maintain exemplary mental health. In contrast, psychopathology will have less of an effect on the ethnic majority; social deviance in that group will be tolerated more through various social structures and supports.

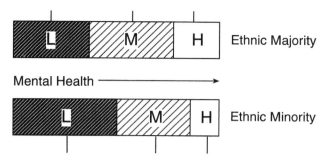

Figure 23.4. Schematic of social selection prediction.

Bruce Dohrenwend noted that the different selection thresholds for ethnically advantaged and disadvantaged persons will have an impact on the overall rates of psychopathology within the two groups, once SES is controlled. Under the selection process, the ethnic majority would have relatively higher rates of pathology than the ethnically disadvantaged in both the low and high ends of the SES continuum. In the upper SES levels, the ethnic *minority* will be highly selected and therefore will have less psychopathology than the ethnic majority. In the lower SES levels, the ethnic *majority* will experience the most extreme selection: only the most severe manifestations of psychopathology will push ethnic majority members into the lowest stratum.

Figure 23.4 illustrates in simplistic form the prediction of the social selection hypothesis. For the sake of clarity, the figure shows a perfect inverse relation between SES and psychopathology. The population of the ethnic majority is broken into low (L), middle (M), and high SES (H) on the basis of psychopathology/mental health. The bars above the breakdown indicate the median mental health level of each segment of the SES distribution. By comparing these to the corresponding bars for the ethnic minority, it can be seen that, although both populations span the same mental health continuum, the more stringently selected high-SES group in the ethnic minority has better mental health than the corresponding high-SES group in the ethnic majority. The same result is predicted for each of the SES strata.

The Dohrenwend quasi-experimental strategy calls for comparing rates of psychopathology in advantaged and disadvantaged ethnic groups while statistically adjusting for SES. To make these comparisons with adequate statistical power, the demographically unusual groups must be oversampled in the survey design: ethnically advantaged persons in the lowest SES levels and ethnically disadvantaged persons in the highest SES levels. The comparison must be made in a society where genuine social mobility exists, and with specific disorders that are known to be inversely related to SES. If rates of psychopathology are higher in the ethnic minority (SES held constant), then support for social causation obtains. If rates are higher in the ethnic majority (SES held constant), then support for social selection obtains.

Bruce Dohrenwend did not develop the quasi-experimental strategy through causal models such as those we presented previously, but it is of interest to see how ethnic disadvantage might be incorporated into the models. In Figures 23.5 and 23.6, we present plausible modifications of the earlier models. In the modifications, we characterize the external adversity construct as social adversity, by which we mean stressors associated with discrimination and prejudice.

Notice that the analysis proposed to test the quasi experiment, regressing measures of psychopathology on ethnic disadvantage and SES disadvantage, is quite different from the structural analyses of the models in Figures 23.5 and 23.6. The difference highlights the fact that the quasi experiment

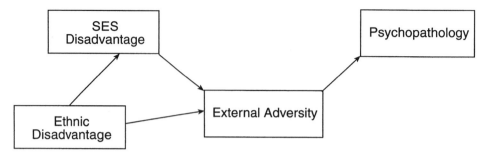

Figure 23.5. Social causation model with ethnic disadvantage.

is a heuristic device for testing the direction of the SES–pathology relation. Although it is designed for making a causal inference, it is not itself a causal model in the sense of Figures 23.5 and 23.6. Indeed, the analysis of the quasi experiment does not even require that adversity itself be directly measured. The impact of adversity is thought to become evident as one examines the multiple regression of psychopathology on ethnic group and SES.

TESTING THE QUASI-EXPERIMENTAL STRATEGY THROUGH SIMULATION

To understand the quasi-experimental strategy better, we examined it using simulation methods. We generated a data set using the causal model shown in Figure 23.5.[8] This is done by creating some random numbers that represent a hypothetical measure of ethnic disadvantage and then using this to create a hypothetical indicator of SES disadvantage. Both of these variables are used to create the social adversity measure, and

adversity is itself used to create the psychopathology measure. By creating each variable as a weighted sum of previous variables and random variation, the proper level of correlation between the variables can be created. Weights were chosen so that the observed correlation between SES disadvantage and psychopathology is .40.[9] The chapter appendix illustrates how the simulation may be carried out with the SAS statistical software system (SAS Institute, 1988).

When data created in accordance with the social causation model are analyzed using the quasi-experimental strategy, we find that psychopathology and ethnic disadvantage are positively related after SES disadvantage is statistically controlled. This is because ethnic disadvantage has a direct path to social adversity in addition to the indirect path through class disadvantage in Figure 23.5. Recall that this is precisely the prediction made by the quasi-experimental strategy: holding constant SES, ethnically disadvantaged persons are predicted to have higher rates of psychopathology.

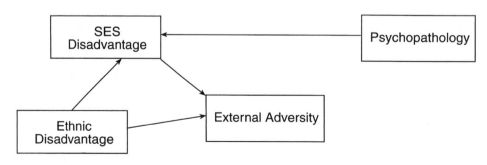

Figure 23.6. Social selection model with ethnic disadvantage.

Next, we generate some data using Figure 23.6. Again, weights are selected so that the overall correlation between social disadvantage and psychopathology is .40.[10] Note that according to this model, there is no reason to expect ethnic membership to be related to psychopathology when the two are considered separately. However, when SES is statistically controlled, then a negative relation between ethnic disadvantage and psychopathology emerges.[11] This corresponds precisely to the quasi-experimental prediction: when SES is held constant, the ethnically disadvantaged group will have better mental health than the advantaged group.

These analyses verify that the quasi-experimental strategy works well in differentiating the social selection from the social causation models when one or the other is operating. However, the models are not really mutually exclusive. It is possible that social selection may be the dominant mechanism, but that social causation contributes additional covariation between psychopathology and SES. Can the quasi-experimental strategy tell us which model dominates when both are operating to some extent?

This question can be addressed by merging two simulated data sets, one created using Figure 23.5 and another created using Figure 23.6. The weights in the models were selected so that the observed correlation between SES disadvantage and psychopathology is approximately .40 in both simulated sets, and the size of the two data sets were the same (1000 each). If the quasi-experimental test is valid in this case, it should show no association between ethnic group and psychopathology when SES is held constant. If the two effects are of equal size, they should cancel each other out in the quasi-experimental test.

The results of simulations carried out with mixed causal processes reveals a small bias in favor of the social causation hypothesis. However, the bias is so small that quite large sample sizes are needed to detect it statistically. For most purposes, we can expect the test to be indeterminate when the two processes are approximately equal.

To illustrate the utility of simulation studies to examine model specification variations, we examine an alternative social causation model to the one laid out in Figure 23.5. This variation suggests that psychopathology may be caused by SES disadvantage but through more than one causal pathway, not all of which are related to ethnic status. Instead of assuming that occupancy of lower SES positions simply exposes persons to adversity through prejudice, discrimination, and petty life stresses, we might also assume that lower SES persons experience environmental adversity that is largely unrelated to ethnic status. For example, low-SES persons (regardless of ethnic background) are more likely to be exposed to occupations involving noisome features such as excessive noise, hazardous conditions, fumes, or extreme heat, cold, or humidity (Link et al., 1986). Another example along these lines is the SES-related factor of low birth weight, which is associated with neurodevelopmental abnormalities that may cause subsequent psychopathology (McCormick et al., 1990). These additional sources of environmental adversity are the result of social causation, as illustrated in the modification of Figure 23.5 shown below in Figure 23.7.

Figure 23.7 is another plausible representation of the social causation model, but it does not produce exactly the same quasi-experimental results as the version in Figure 23.5. On one hand, if there is no social selection and the social causation follows Figure 23.7, then the quasi-experimental strategy produces the correct results. On the other hand, if both social selection and social causation as represented in Figure 23.7 operate equally, the quasi experiment produces biased results in favor of social selection. In this case, the ethnic variable does not fully represent the social causation processes, because only half of the causal effect of SES is shared with ethnic disadvantage. If the model in Figure 23.7 is correct and if both social causation and social selection mechanisms operate equally to produce the inverse relation between SES and a specific form of psychopathology, then the quasi-experimental test may lead to the biased

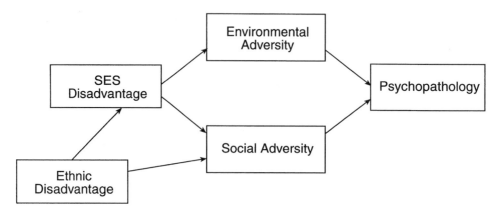

Figure 23.7. Modified social causation model.

CONCLUSIONS AND SUMMARY

Nonexperimental studies are not able to prove definitively which causal mechanisms operate in producing and maintaining psychopathology, but they can provide evidence about the plausibility of competing models. Inferences from nonexperimental studies depend heavily on the choice of statistical models used to represent the data. Although insights about the quality of the models are always gained when the models are used with real data, it is also sometimes possible to gain insights about the models with hypothetical data that are generated using alternative statistical models. We illustrated the utility of careful modeling with simulations in an examination of a quasi-experimental strategy for contrasting the social causation and social selection explanations of the inverse relation between SES and psychopathology. We found that the strategy was generally informative, but that it might produce misleading results if social causation involved paths through environmental adversity in addition to adversity attributable to discrimination and prejudice.[12]

Dohrenwend et al. (1992) applied the quasi-experimental strategy to survey data from Israel; they found that three of the four disorders they studied produced results

that were consistent with the social causation outcome. For schizophrenia, the results were consistent with the social selection outcome. Although the latter results are implausible without an important social selection component, our simulation analysis suggests that the relative importance of social causation in that analysis may have been underestimated. There is some evidence that the effects of social status on schizophrenia go through mechanisms that are not strictly social, and we found that the Dohrenwend quasi-experimental test is biased against the social causation hypothesis when the true mechanism involves nonsocial mechanisms.

REFERENCES

Cook, T. D., & Campbell, D. T. (1979). *Quasi experimentation: Design and analysis issues for field settings.* Chicago: Rand McNally.

Dohrenwend, B. P. (1966). Social status and psychological disorder: An issue of substance and an issue of method. *American Sociological Review, 31,* 14–35.

Dohrenwend, B. P., Levav, I., Shrout, P. E., Schwartz, S., Naveh, G., Link, B. G., Skodal, A. E., & Stueve, A. (1992). Socioeconomic status and psychiatric disorders: A test of the social causation–social selection issue, *Science, 255,* 946–952.

Dohrenwend, B. P., Shrout, P. E., Link, B. G., Martin, J. L., & Skodol, A. E. (1986). Overview and initial results from a risk-fact study of depression and schizophrenia. In J. E. Barrett (Ed.), *Mental disorders in the community* (pp. 184–215). New York: The Guilford Press.

Holland, P. (1988). Statistics and causal inference (with discussion). *Journal of the American Statistical Association, 81,* 945–970.

McCormick, M. C., Gormaker, S. L., & Sobol, A. M. (1990). Very low birthweight children: Behavior problems and school difficulty in a national sample. *Journal of Pediatrics, 117,* 687–693.

Link, B. G., Dohrenwend, B. P., & Skodol, A. E. (1986). Noisome occupations. *American Sociological Review, 51,* 242–254.

SAS Institute. (1988). *SAS/STAT user's guide.* Cary, NC: SAS Institute.

Snedecor, G. W., & Cochran, W. G. (1967). *Statistical methods* (6th ed.). Ames: Iowa State University Press.

NOTES

1. For example, a social scientist in the military might be able to convince authorities to randomly assign eligible soldiers to a stressful assignment and to randomly select a control group for follow-up.

2. Technically, we ask what effect the exposure would have had if the groups did not differ on a series of specific control (confounding) variables.

3. Although we often do not know the ideal mathematical model for describing the relations among variables, we can sometimes formulate competing models proposed by theorists working on a specific problem, such as stress and psychopathology. When competing explanations differ in their predictions about observable facts, we have the opportunity to use data to choose among them. In these cases, even imperfect statistical models can be used to evaluate the relative strengths of one theory over another.

4. A single simulation is like a single empirical study—it provides evidence, but the results must be replicated in order to be sure that they hold generally. The larger the size of the simulated sample, the more confident we can be that the simulated sample is not an unusual example of the hypothetical population.

5. Path models such as the victimization model in Figure 23.1 correspond to statistical models.

If psychopathology is measured by some variable Y, and external adversity is measured by some variable X, then Figure 23.1 says that Y is a linear function of X ($Y = B_0 + B_1X + e$, as in the previously discussed example.) As external adversity increases, psychopathology increases linearly.

6. Figure 23.2 corresponds to a system of statistical models (often called structural equation models). In the first equation, external adversity is modeled as a linear function of SES disadvantage, and in the second equation, psychopathology is a linear function of external adversity. Figure 23.2 explicitly hypothesizes that SES disadvantage will be correlated with psychopathology, but that the correlation will be completely accounted for by the external adversity that results from SES disadvantage.

7. Like Figure 23.2, Figure 23.3 corresponds to a pair of equations. In the first, SES disadvantage is expected to vary linearly with psychopathology level, and in the second, external adversity is expected to vary linearly with SES disadvantage.

8. Figure 23.5 corresponds to a system of three structural equations. SES disadvantage (CD) is represented as a linear function of ethnic disadvantage (ED) plus a random term; social adversity (SA) is a linear function of both ethnic disadvantage and SES disadvantage plus a random term; and psychopathology (PP) is a linear function just of social adversity and a random term:

$$CD = B_{01} + B_{11}ED + e_1$$

$$SA = B_{02} + B_{12}ED + B_{22}CD + e_2$$

$$PP = B_{03} + B_{33}SA + e_3$$

9. In terms of Figure 23.5, all three paths to the left were set to have weights of .4, and the path between social adversity and psychopathology was set to be .7143. In terms of note 8, $B_{11} = B_{12} = B_{22} = 0.4$, and $B_{33} = 0.7143$.

10. Figure 23.6 corresponds to a system of two equations. SES disadvantage (CD) is represented as a linear function of both ethnic disadvantage (ED) and psychopathology (PP) plus a random term; and social adversity (SA) is a linear function of ethnic disadvantage and SES disadvantage plus a random term.

$$CD = \beta_{01} + \beta_{11}ED + \beta_{31}PP + \varepsilon_1$$

$$SA = \beta_{02} + \beta_{12}ED + \beta_{22}CD + \varepsilon_2$$

For the simulation, all of the path coefficients were set to 0.4.

11. This fact may not be intuitively obvious, but consider the following. Suppose ethnic disadvantage and psychopathology have a bivariate correlation of zero, but both are positively related to SES advantage. When class is statistically partialled, its positive relation with both is subtracted from the zero correlation. This leaves a residual negative correlation among the statistically adjusted variables.

12. Technically, our simulation results hold only for the values of the parameters we chose when constructing the data. One should try a variety of plausible parameter values before making general statements. Our results did indeed hold for alternative parameter values representing weaker but nonzero relations among the variables.

APPENDIX

This program creates simulated data using the IML matrix programming language of the SAS software system. The example represents the following constructs with shorthand:

Psychopathology (PP)

Social Adversity (SA)

Environmental Adversity (EA)

Ethnic Disadvantage ED)

SES Disadvantage (CD)

PROC IML;
    *(A sample of size 1000 is constructed. First the ethnic disadvantage variable is constructed, with −1 representing advantaged and +1 representing disadvantaged. Since there are equal numbers of each group, this coding leads to an ED variable with mean zero and variance one.);
ED=J(500,1,−1); ED=ED/ /J(500,1,1);

*(SOCIAL SELECTION SIMULATION of Figure 23.3 (Part 1)—PP is exogenous predictor of CD. We create a distribution of PP that is standard normal.);
PP1=NORMAL(J(1000,1,0));
    *(PP and ED are used to create CD variable.);
DATA=ED| |PP1;
GAM1={.4 .4};
CD1=DATA°GAM1`;
    *(A random component is added to CD to make the correlation less than perfect. The random component is weighted so that the variance of the CD variable is about 1.);
EI1=SQRT(1-SSQ(CD1)/1000);
CD1=CD1+EI1#NORMAL(J(1000,1,0));
DATA=DATA| |CD1;

*(SOCIAL STRESS SIMULATION of Figure 23.5 (Part 2)—PP is caused by SA, which is caused by CD and ED. CD is a direct function of ED alone. A random component is again added.);
CD2=.4#ED;
EI2=SQRT(1-SSQ(CD2)/1000);
CD2=CD2+EI2#NORMAL(J(1000,1,0));
DATA=DATA| |CD2;
    *(Social adversity is a function of CD2 and ED.);
SA2=.4#ED+.4#CD2;
ESA2=SQRT(1−SSQ(SA2)/1000);
SA2=SA2+ESA2#NORMAL(J(1000,1,0));
DATA=DATA| |SA2;
    *(PP is a function of SA.);
PP2=.7143#SA2;
ED2=SQRT(1-SSQ(PP2)/1000);
PP2=PP2+ED2#NORMAL(J(1000,1,0));
DATA=DATA| |PP2;

*(SOCIAL STRESS SIMULATION of Figure 23.7 (Part 3)—PP is caused by SA and EA. The latter is caused by CD.);
EA3=−.4#CD2;
EPA3=SQRT(1−SSQ(EA3)/1000);
EA3=EA3+EPA3#NORMAL(J(1000,1,0));
DATA=DATA| |EA3;
PP3=.4167#SA2 +.4167#EA3;
ED3=SQRT(1−SSQ(PP3)/1000);
PP3=PP3+ED3#NORMAL(J(1000,1,0));
DATA=DATA| |PP3;

*(One data matrix with simulated PP variables under all three models has been simulated. Labels are assigned and a SAS system file is saved.);
LABS={"ED" "PP1" "CD1" "CD2" "SA2" "PP2" "EA3" "PP3"};
CREATE SIML.DAT FROM DATA [COLNAME=LABS];
APPEND FROM DATA ;

*(Descriptive statistics of the simulated data are examined.);
PROC CORR DATA=SIML.DAT COV;
VAR ED--PP3;
PROC MEANS DATA=SIML.DAT; VAR ED--PP3;
PROC MEANS DATA=SIML.DAT; VAR PP1--PP3; BY ED;

24

Cognitive Changes Associated with Persisting Behavioral Effects of Early Psychosocial Stress in Rhesus Monkeys: A View from Psychobiology

Gary W. Kraemer
Jocelyne Bachevalier

. . . all brains are, in essence, *anticipation machines.*
—Danial Dennett

Until the mid-1950s, it was commonly accepted that insults to the usual psychosocial or cognitive development of the child were causal factors in the later development of psychopathology. There was considerable diversity in proposed causal mechanisms. Psychoanalytic theory focused on challenges to the formation of the ego and defense mechanisms and on later inability to cope with ongoing stressors as a result of unresolved conflicts (Freud, 1969). Behaviorist theory focused on early conditioning and learning that leads to abnormal responses to stressors and deficient coping behavior later in life (Skinner, 1953). Psychological explanations of the cause of abnormal behavior became less prominent, however, following the discovery of pharmacological agents that were effective in treatment of depression and schizophrenia.

If any psychobiological reasoning could be awarded the status of theory in psychiatry by the late 1960s, it was that mental disorders might be caused by neurochemical changes that are the inverse of therapeutic drug effects. Examples of this reasoning would be that antidepressant agents increase availability of norepinephrine (NE) at the synapse by one mechanism or another;

therefore, the cause of major depression might be reduced NE system activity (Schildkraut, 1965; Schildkraut & Kety, 1967). In addition, most if not all neuroleptic agents block dopamine (DA) receptors, while drugs that increase dopaminergic transmission produce symptoms of schizophrenia, and therefore the cause of schizophrenia might be increased DA system activity (Garver et al., 1975; Snyder, 1973). What might cause the persisting changes in neurotransmitter system activity and what effects the neurotransmitters had on postsynaptic cells was not known. These psychobiological hypotheses also did not include any explicit propositions as to how stress might alter neurotransmitter system function or otherwise enter into the causal sequence of events leading to exhibition of psychopathology.

The brain mechanisms proposed to be responsible for psychiatric disorders have changed with advances in neuroscience research. In the 1970s to 1980s, reasoning about the causes of psychopathology moved from a "molecule without a mechanism" stage to a "mechanism without meaning" stage. One focus in neuroscience in the past two decades has been on receptor mechanisms and postsynaptic intracellular effects of neurotransmitters (Kraemer & McKinney, 1988). A plethora of publications have claimed that humans with psychiatric disorders exhibit changes in brain neurotransmitter and/or receptor systems. Few of these claims have withstood the test of time or, more correctly, been validated in further tests. As far as research on humans is concerned, we have yet to see a confirmed report substantiating the idea that changes in pre- or postsynaptic neurotransmitter mechanisms generally precede psychiatric disorders and play a causal role in their onset. Also, many more mechanisms must be considered than was the case two to three decades ago. For example, behavioral responses to stressors and exhibition of attachment behavior are now attributed by some researchers not to changes in neurotransmission, but to actions of neuromodulator, neurohormonal polypeptide regulatory mechanisms (e.g., corticotropin-releasing hormone and oxytocin, respectively) (Insel, 1992; Nemeroff, 1992).

What has tagged along with acceptance of a view that behavior is ultimately controlled by brain neurochemistry and structure are convictions that (*1*) variation in brain neurochemistry and structure from one individual to the next ultimately relates back to differences in genetic endowment, and (*2*) by implication, genetic endowment must play a major role in causing psychopathology because the latter is ultimately related to changes in brain neurochemistry and structure. In this framework, if stressors precipitate psychopathology, they must do this by challenging the function of brain neurotransmitter systems that were genetically "vulnerable" in the first place. There is societal acceptance of and even a fascination with this view [see works such as Franklin's (1987) *Molecules of the mind*, a Pulitzer Prize–winning work positively reviewed by the *New York Times Book Review* and endorsed by several prominent biological psychiatrists and neuroscientists]. An even more deterministic view is that stressors only increase the probability of onset of a psychiatric disorder (biological malfunction)

that has a reasonable probability of occurring in their absence (Cohen & Campbell, 1984). These views do not discount interactions with the environment as promoting factors for psychopathology (diathesis–stress), but they definitely put them in a second order of importance.

An important alternative to consider, however, is that one can hold a biological view of brain–behavior relations without necessarily accepting the idea that significant characteristics of brain neurochemistry and structure are genetically determined. Indeed, the crux of the problem in assigning more or less causal clout to the genes or the environment need not center on the issue of whether complex behaviors are attributable to actions of this or that brain mechanism. Instead, it is understanding what might cause changes in these mechanisms over time and produce variation in function from individual to individual that is critical.

RECONSIDERATION—BACK TO THE NATURE–NURTURE PROBLEM

The idea that the genetic program ultimately controls the expression of neurotransmitter systems and neural structures at some core or basic functional level has been traditionally accepted in some arenas (Fischer, 1987; Nowakowski, 1987). A further assumption—actually a leap of faith—is that, by controlling expression of brain mechanisms, genetic endowment also ultimately accounts for enduring social and functional characteristics of the individual. Among these might be personality, predispositions, intelligence, and vulnerability or immunity to the effects of stressors. Most would agree, though, that prevailing opinion about nature-versus-nurture causal relations favors interaction rather than dichotomy. Nevertheless, when "biological" changes associated with a persisting behavior pattern are found or even suspected, the hunt for the responsible molecule and genetic locus of control begins. For example, particular morphological characteristics of hypothalamic nuclei and the anterior commissure have been associated with male homosexuality (LeVay & Hamer, 1994). LeVay and Hamer suggested that it is unlikely that psychosocial factors leading to establishment of sexual preference and exhibition of a stable behavior pattern into adulthood could cause changes in brain morphology, and that a search for the genes responsible for the brain morphological characteristics of homosexual men is warranted.

Adventures of this sort have gained priority in research funding allocation despite the questionable validity of data and reasoning supporting the idea that genetic differences are responsible for either neurobiological or behavioral differences (Byne, 1994). Few studies claiming to demonstrate significant genetic control of complex behaviors or predispositions to pathology can stand up to a good debunking (Horgan, 1993). Indeed, behavioral geneticists have steadfastly maintained that *environmental factors* remain prominently associated with disorders that are constitutional in nature, and are at least as important as genetic factors (Plomin, 1989). Despite this, the idea that neurobiological variation is predominantly caused by genetic differences has been more compelling than the idea that neurobiological variation is caused by experience.

Nevertheless, there is substantial evidence that features of early psychosocial development and sustained patterns of social interaction produce enduring changes in brain neurotransmitter mechanisms and cytoarchitecture (Kraemer, 1992a, 1992b; Kraemer & Clarke, 1996). The major focus of debate here eventually returns to two clinical questions concerning psychopathology and stress that generally lead to an invocation of biological/genetic endowment as perhaps the only "reasonable" explanation:

1. Why is there an imperfect relationship between what most people accept as social causes of psychopathology (caregiver privation, deprivation, child abuse, poverty) and later exhibition of psychopathology by any given individual? Stated another way, why do some children growing up in terrible environments do well and others growing up in optimal environments do poorly? Do differences in biology account for these mismatches between environmental influences and behavioral outcomes?

2. Why is the expression of psychopathology so intractable and persistent in the face of salutary environmental change or psychotherapy? If clashes with the environment or rearing in a pernicious environment cause psychopathology, why cannot this be undone or reversed by subsequent experience in healthy and accepting environments? Do immutable pathological biological characteristics account for resistance to behavioral accommodation to the prevailing environment?

Scientists and theoreticians seem to have concluded that there is no nature-versus-nurture debate: nature and nurture interact. It seems that clinicians and patients (or parents and children) often conclude, however, that the abnormal behavior problem that they are grappling with cannot be attributed to the influence of the environment on genotype expression or laws of behavioral change or development. The problem must be biological! Levity aside, what is needed is a further understanding of the psychobiological mechanisms by which enduring characteristics of behavior are maintained. A second need is to understand whether the mechanisms that sustain normal behavior are different from those that sustain abnormal behavior. Finally, there is a need to provide a reintegration of the role that early stressors play in the promotion of later psychopathology that was acknowledged in the foundations of prior psychoanalytic and behaviorist theories. To address these needs, Post (1992) proposed a mechanism by which enduring changes in genetic regulation of neural plasticity and microstructure can be caused by exposure to psychosocial stressors. The effort herein is to propose a more global account of how psychosocial stress affects brain function and behavior at the system and organism level. The eventual view will be significantly different from prior diathesis–stress views of the interaction between stress and psychopathology that most readers might be expected to be familiar with.

PSYCHOBIOLOGICAL ATTACHMENT THEORY

Kraemer (1992b) proposed a psychobiological attachment theory (PAT) and then further expanded the theory to address causal mechanisms in psychopathology (Kraemer, 1992a). Grappling with attachment theory is an example of seeking ways to achieve a deeper understanding of how enduring (constitutional) characteristics of behavior develop and are maintained, and why they can be impervious to subsequent changes in the environment. PAT is based largely on research conducted in nonhuman primates and other animal species; it is a conceptual outgrowth of the ethological control systems theory (ECST) of attachment proposed by John Bowlby (1969, 1973, 1980).

People are often disconcerted when truly basic assumptions (premises) are challenged; perhaps they are surprised to find that logical premises are only assumptions that can be questioned. The following discussion may present such a challenge. Theories of attachment proposed around or after the turn of the century, including ECST, depend on the premise that the basic behavioral mechanisms of the neonate are heritable. These mechanisms exist as a result of prior Darwinian selection, and they surface in their preprogrammed form to greater or lesser degrees depending on the environment. In these views, the primary reason organisms initiate action (behave) is to survive. Psychoanalytical and behaviorist theory and ECST incorporate this premise in different mechanisms. In each theory, survival remains as the ultimate purpose for the behavior that is exhibited by living organisms, however.

One challenge is to see the tautology, that is, the circular and self-reifying reasoning.

For instance, is there anything that can be identified as living that does not move (behave), ever, and has no moving parts? Probably not. Life and movement are not the same thing, however. All things that move are not alive, but all things that are alive move at some point in their life history. Why do things that are alive move? Whatever answer we come up with will most likely complete the tautology. One example would be "living things move (behave) to be alive and survive." The only way out of this tautology is to assume, in truly Darwinian fashion, that the genome of a mammal, for example, produces a body that expresses movement (behavior). The behaviors expressed increase the chances of reproduction of the genome in a niche of the environment. This does not mean that behavior is goal directed toward the abstract concept of "survival," however. In fact, it is reasonable to suppose that many species, if not most, have no built-in concept of survival, nor is it a goal state for their nervous systems.

PAT differs from ECST in three major respects: (1) it does not depend on a "drive to survive" as an ultimate cause (motivator) of ongoing behavior, (2) it does not depend on energy or drive reduction as a proximal cause (motivator) of ongoing behavior, and (3) it does not depend on but does not discount behaviorist principles of conditioning to explain some of the causes of enduring behavioral change. Premises of PAT (Kraemer, 1992b) are as follows:

1. The genetic program does not express mechanisms with a mandate to survive. Human values, survival being one of them, are not encoded in the genome. Instead, the genetic program expresses mechanisms that are more or less adaptive.
2. The organization of brain function begins prenatally. Postnatal organization usually occurs within the context of caregiving. The emerging genetic program of the neonate is set to link with a caregiver.
3. Many of the primary cognitive and physiological characteristics of the ne-

onate are considerably more plastic than previously recognized. In particular, homeostatic systems emerge but they are not preset or tuned to the degree thought in the past.

4. The proximal cause of behavior has been referred to as "motivation" and described in terms of energy (psychoanalytic theory) or drive reduction (behaviorist theory). A premise of PAT is that behavior is caused by initially autonomous neural activity that is self-organizing in relation to experience. More specifically, action is initiated by neural working models of "what has happened," "what exists," "what should happen next," and "what should be." The basis of this view is grounded in American Pragmatism (James, 1890/1950; Peirce, 1878/1934), neuroscience and control systems theory (Craik, 1943; Hebb, 1949, 1982), and contemporary mind–brain philosophy (Dennett, 1991).

5. Brain functions traditionally discriminated as being regulatory, motivational, emotional, and cognitive are intertwined and organize postnatally. These functions are not attributable to actions of discrete and dedicated brain subsystems, however.

6. Attachment is a process by which neural systems in the neonate are usually "tuned" to those of an adult caregiver. Their eventual function depends on the environment that they develop in and the characteristics of the caregiver.

Given these premises, then, the next task is to examine what PAT implies about the causes of enduring characteristics of brain function (normal or abnormal).

Attachment (Formation of Brain Function) and Abnormal Behavior

Why do some children growing up in terrible environments do well, and others growing up in optimal environments do poorly? Does the explanation depend on invoking biological/genetic mechanisms? Despite common acceptance of the idea, it is not entirely clear that there are human children who grow up in optimal or terrible environments and do not conform to expectations of doing well or not well, respectively.

A number of longitudinal studies that illustrate the problem were conducted by Werner (1989a, 1989b) on the island of Kauai beginning in the 1950s. Of 698 infants born in 1955, 30% ($n = 201$) were identified as being "at risk" for mental illness or criminal delinquency on the basis of factors including perinatal stress, chronic poverty, low socioeconomic status and education of parents, parental discord, divorce, alcoholism, or parental mental illness. Of this population, 64% ($n = 129$) conformed to expectations and had mental health or delinquency records by age 18. The remainder, 36% ($n = 72$), "grew into competent young adults who loved well, worked well, and played well" (Werner, 1989a). Among these "survivors," constitutional factors including a fairly high activity level, a low degree of excitability and distress, and a high degree of sociability, combined with "the opportunity to establish a close bond with at least one caretaker from whom they received positive attention during the first years of life," were major protective factors that discriminated these children from those who did not do well. Beyond this, as resilient children developed, they demonstrated adequate ability to concentrate, as well as average or above-average problem-solving and reading skills, and seemed to find a great deal of emotional support outside their immediate family.

According to Werner (1989b) the "survivors" survived because they had both the wherewithal and opportunity to evade what she and most others would count as environmental risk. They found a social bolthole out of an ostensibly terrible environment. The major point regarding this research is that measuring the attributes of a risky environment in terms of socioeconomic status, family discord, and past history of the parent(s) may not reveal actual exposure to the real risk factor, which is disruption of early and continuing caregiver–child attachment. To dig down to this level however, we again need to examine what we should measure.

Attachment and Doing Well or Not Well

Ainsworth and Bowlby maintained that the infant is genetically primed to seek a secure base (Ainsworth et al., 1978; Bowlby, 1988). The bulk of developmental research conducted in the past two decades, however, does not support this proposition. Instead, the neonate is born with a sensory "shopping list" for multimodal stimuli that it requires initially to regulate its own behavior and physiology (Hofer, 1984, 1987). Cues associated with safety and sustenance are not at the top of the neonate's most preferred list of regulators. Instead, it appears that the neonate attends to surface perceptions that usually identify an adult caregiver (cuddly, nutritious, warm, and mobile, in order of preference) (Harlow et al., 1963, 1973). With persisting and predictable interaction with the caregiver, the neonate internalizes its own behavioral and physiological regulatory mechanisms (Kraemer, 1992b), which are modeled after those of the caregiver. Myron Hofer was among the first to propose that abnormal behaviors observed during or after maternal privation or deprivation were not specifically due to loss of a secure base or safety, but rather related to loss of regulation of the neonate's behavior and physiology (Hofer, 1987).

Abnormal Behavior Attributable to Interactions with the Environment

PAT suggests that the genome expresses a neurobiological structure that progressively incorporates aspects of the social environment at least at two levels and, in turn, acts upon the social environment correspondingly. At one level, persistent constitutional individual differences may be expressed in interaction styles, acquired habits, and possibly what may be referred to as variation in "temperament." The factors of extraversion versus neuroticism (Plomin, 1989), inhibited versus uninhibited (Kagan, 1992; Kagan

et al., 1990), and shy versus reckless (Jacobs & Raleigh, 1992) are examples of this idea. At another level, individuals appear to vary in their cognitive facility and capacity. The implication of this view is that the phenotype of the optimum social genome closely conforms to the social environment in which it develops. As individuals deviate from this optimum, they will be more or less "in tune," matched or mismatched, able to survive or not, and valued or devalued. Some individuals confront the environment with a less than optimal genetic endowment. This is one source of eventual mismatch between societal expectations and individual behavior. Beyond this, we can begin to determine how environmental factors usually contribute to or limit the expression of the genome regardless of its presumed optimal or deficient characteristics.

One cause of a mismatch between societally expected and expressed behavior could be privation of neonate–caregiver interaction. Another cause could be that the neonate attaches to or entrains itself to an inadequate or abusive caregiver. One major contribution of Harlow and colleagues was in demonstrating that sensory systems of the primate neonate that mediate attachment can be fooled. Rhesus monkey neonates will select attachment objects that have many characteristics of a caregiver but are in no way, shape, or form, secure bases or attentive and compassionate (Harlow et al., 1971). Neonates that attach to abusive or neglectful mothers display a more abiding and persistent attachment than monkeys reared with adequate mothers (Sackett, 1970). Such mistakes would not be possible if the neonate were preset to seek a secure base or adequate caregiver, or if its ultimate behavioral mandate were to survive. Through either privation of caregiving or abuse, the usual psychobiological trajectory of psychosocial development of the neonate is altered.

PAT also suggests that what constitutes an optimum versus deficient early social environment, or caregiver–infant interaction, is quite different from that portrayed in ECST. Bowlby, Ainsworth, and later proponents of ECST equate compassionate and attentive caregiving with secure base characteristics of the caregiver (Bretherton, 1985). That the caregiver acts as a secure base, in turn, is a prerequisite for optimum infant psychosocial development. The universal validity of this proposition has proved difficult to verify (Kagan, 1992; Lamb et al., 1984; Schneider Rosen & Rothbaum, 1993). PAT suggests instead that consistency, predictability, and availability of a caregiver who is functioning competently within the larger social group are optimal caregiver characteristics. Attentive and compassionate caregiving may be one style of caregiving that maximizes these critical factors in some societies. Nonetheless, the style of adequate caregiving can and demonstrably does vary widely across societies and cultures (Freedman, 1993; Hinde, 1982; Kagan, 1992). Rigidly structured and demanding caregiving may serve the neonate best in some environments.

Psychobiological explanations of what causes deflections from optimal trajectory also differ from classical psychoanalytical and learning theories and from ECST. For example, learning theory suggests that individual organisms necessarily incorporate different experiences, and different memories account for different behavior exhibited later. The foible here is that most learning theories assume that the basic mechanisms of learning remain constant regardless of experience. In contradistinction, PAT suggests that the rules for later incorporation of behavior patterns depend on first experiences of the neonate; that is, experiences change the rules for subsequent incorporation of experience. This view has implications for prevention of and intervention in psychopathology later in life.

Mechanisms Underlying Persisting Vulnerability to Social Stressors

Why is the expressed psychopathology, once it is established, so intractable and persistent in the face of salutary environmental change or psychotherapy? Is psychopathology ulti-

mately attributable to some immutable characteristic of the biological substrate that stressors reveal and that optimal development only glosses over most of the time?

One implication of PAT is that environmental stressors can produce biological changes in the organism that thereafter become an enduring but not immutable cause of abnormal behavior. Before continuing, however, it is important to place the body of research on nonhuman primates used to support further conclusions in its correct context. The external validity of the rhesus maternal privation/deprivation literature in extrapolations to the human condition has been questioned. Uppermost is the issue of whether there are any valid comparisons between laboratory-reared monkeys and humans reared in their "natural" environment. Critics cite the extreme or unnatural circumstance of being reared in a laboratory without caregiver contact as necessarily invalidating rhesus–human comparisons (Eiserer, 1992; Kagan, 1992; Kovach, 1992; Pérusse, 1992; Sigman & Siegel, 1992).

One basis of misapprehension disregards a mammalian mandate. Some critics are not familiar with how monkeys are reared in a laboratory. They maintain that the social experiential deprivation in the laboratory is so extreme that humans never experience it. One assumption, strange though it may be, is that laboratory-housed rhesus infants reared under "extreme" privation conditions somehow survive and mature with no caregiver. For instance, Kagan (1992) suggested that "if a monkey were fed and cleaned by a human for 30 minutes a day and, for the remaining hours, had only a variety of inanimate objects in the cage, it would not show the serious pathology characteristic of a completely isolated monkey." Mother Nature, however, dictates that all rhesus infants must have caregivers in order to survive. In the laboratory, some caregivers are humans and some are monkey mothers. Monkey mothers do better at rearing socially competent monkeys. Compassionate and attentive humans do better at rearing physiologically robust monkeys as assessed by survival rate and weight gain. Kagan's comment is one illustration of what seems to be a gulf in understanding across areas of endeavor.

Socially isolated monkey neonates are cared for by humans for much more than 30 minutes a day; they have diapers to roll up into and things to play with. Nevertheless, human-reared rhesus monkeys are social duds and regulatory wrecks as far as their behavior and neurobiology are concerned (Clarke, 1993; Clarke et al., 1996; Kraemer, 1995, 1997; Kraemer & Clarke, 1996). Even if they live socially with peers throughout early development, and are never socially isolated, human-reared rhesus monkeys never recover from the early insult of not having a monkey mother. One could still maintain that even institutionalized or orphaned humans are never reared by alien beings, and the case is still out of the bounds of human experience. It seems, however, that humans are reared in hospitals, in institutions, by siblings rather than parents, and by parents who are children (Carlson & Earls, 1996).

There is a spectrum of effects of nonhuman primate social privation. Cases more clearly analogous to the human condition produce biological changes consonant with those found in the extreme cases. For example, variation in foraging demands in bonnet macaques (*Macaca radiata*) affects the interaction between mother monkeys and infants (Rosenblum & Paully, 1984). Increased maternal foraging demand leads to decreased maternal attention and responsivity. Variation in maternal foraging demand alters the responsiveness of offspring to pharmacological agents affecting biogenic amine systems (Rosenblum et al., 1994). Hence, social environmental stress of mothers, well within the range accepted as occurring to humans, leads to longstanding biological differences in offspring. These changes are similar to those produced by more extreme manipulations. It is with increasing confidence that there are valid cross-species analogies, then, that the following litany of biological effects of disruption of early social development is rolled out.

ENVIRONMENTAL CAUSES OF BIOLOGICAL CHANGES

Figure 24.1 summarizes the proposed causal sequence by which deflection of usual psychosocial development leads to biological changes in the individual that could sustain abnormal behavior long after the early insult. In step 1, prenatal stress produces a number of changes in the neonate. These include impaired attention and neuromotor maturation, delay of cognitive acquisition of object permanence, altered behavioral and hypothalamic–pituitary–adrenal (HPA) axis responses to stressors, and changes in measures of biogenic amine system levels of activity (Clarke et al., 1994; Schneider, 1992a, 1992b, 1992c; Schneider & Clarke, 1993; Schneider and Coe, 1993; Schneider et al., in press). These effects leave the neonate less prepared to respond in the usual manner to common stressors. Responses are less likely to be adaptive. Prenatally stressed infants are more likely to challenge their caregivers, and the resulting interaction is less likely to be adaptive in the long run. The probability that the neonate will be exposed to subsequent stressors increases.

In step 2, disruption of the usual caregiver–infant "dance" leads to physiological dysregulation. Rhesus neonates reared with and without mothers differ in terms of behavior and either baseline levels or HPA and NE system responsiveness to stressors or pharmacological treatments affecting biogenic amine systems (Clarke, 1993; Higley et al., 1991b, 1992; Kraemer, 1985; Kraemer & McKinney, 1979; Kraemer et al., 1984, 1989, 1991). It is clear that some persisting organizational deficits are related to lack of early vestibular and temperature stimuli (Lubach et al., 1992; Schneider et al., 1991). Beyond this, it is evident that basic interactions between neurotransmitter systems thought to co-modulate each other fail to develop if the infant is deprived of maternal

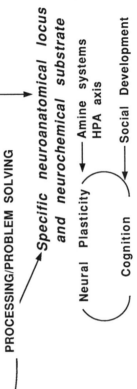

Figure 24.1. Proposed dynamic sequence of effects leading to persisting exhibition of abnormal behavior as a result of early psychosocial stress.

care (Clarke et al., 1996; Kraemer, 1997; Kraemer & Clarke, 1990, 1996).

Prior theories of neonatal development assume that physiological and cognitive capacities mature along a preset genetic plan. The view from PAT, however, is that the regulatory capacity of physiological systems and cognitive development of the neonate depend on interactions with an adequate caregiver. Early caregiver privation or abusive and inconstant caregiving produces alterations in the function of homeostatic mechanisms that the individual usually mobilizes to deal with stressors. This alters the ability to respond to future stressors. PAT further implies that caregiver privation produces changes in cognitive mechanisms used to solve problems and to avoid stressors in the future (step 3, Fig. 24.1). This is hypothesized to occur because the systems expressing both declarative and procedural knowledge initially develop in relation to the caregiver (Kraemer, 1992b).

Disorganization of cognitive mechanisms increases the probability that the neonate will be exposed to and fail to adequately cope with subsequent stressors (Kraemer, 1992b). Another implication is that subsequent interactions with the environment that could be viewed as restorative or therapeutic may not be so. The organism may not be able to perceive and process new experience in the usual way. If intervention does not occur at this point, the neonate will deflect further down this trajectory because it cannot be prepared for and is vulnerable to future stressors once it is disorganized by the initial insult. Empirical evidence supporting steps 1 and 2 has been cited. Next a computer systems analogy is used to explicate how the hypothesis associated with step 3, that early experience alters cognitive processing, is different from that which would be generated by prior theories. Then the rationale and results of initial studies are presented.

Effects of Experience on Cognition— Computer Systems Analogy

Psychoanalytical and behaviorist theories and ECST assume that mechanisms regulating behavior can be environmentally "programmed" in such a way that the behavior expressed is "abnormal," while the mechanisms that mediate the behavior remain inviolate, as genetically encoded. By analogy, I can take a computer and execute a program for action (software) that works well. I can also present the computer with instruction sets that are not compatible with its inner workings. In this case, I get errors in processing or the computer "crashes" altogether, and this aspect of computer behavior is entirely due to variation in the validity of the instruction set (program). Note that executing software that does not work as intended does not damage the hardware.

The view from biological psychiatry, conversely, is that abnormal behavior is due to a malfunction in mechanisms causing or regulating behavior. By analogy, I can run a valid program on machines that operate at different speeds, have different amounts of memory, are poorly designed or obsolete, or are malfunctioning. The program is always the same; therefore, variations in computer behavior are attributable to differences in the computer hardware.

From either viewpoint, and despite differences in machine/software behavior, in no case do I expect either the computers or the software to be enduringly modified in relation to what data they processed and what output they produced.

Suppose, however, that a computer must change its behavior over time in order to survive. A construct of memory is most often used to account for the changes in output (behavior) over time. Initially, the behavior of the system is determined entirely by input and the characteristics of the processor and its instruction set. However, the processor also accesses and uses memory. Once information has been stored in memory, subsequent input is processed in relation to memory. After first experience, output reflects input, memory, and processing. This view suggests that individuals behave differently as they mature because they have more experiences to access in processing new experience, and that individuals having different past experiences will behave differently because they are accessing different memories as part of processing input. The observable result is that behavior (output) varies across individuals in similar sensory environments (input) because they have different memories.

To give a human example, wandering around in public places as a 3-year-old is not the same as doing so as a 16-year-old or an adult. Individual differences in behavior in the same environment necessarily occur because memories differ from person to person and from age to age. From this perspective, most theories of social and/or cognitive development also imply that *processor function* (personality, temperament, predisposition, intelligence) is constant and peculiar to an individual; it is the experience and memories that differ. If one adds the idea that one can have malfunctioning or substandard machinery either by design (genetics) or by insult (environment), then these computer systems models are analogous in major respects to past psychological theories of psychosocial and cognitive development, and psychopathology as well.

The Computer Analogy Does Not Work: The View from Psychobiology

Neuroscience research suggests that memory and processing are only conceptually separable functions of the same mechanism (Kraemer, 1992b). In the brain, there is no functionally and structurally distinct instruction set controlling a functionally and structurally distinct processor that accesses memories stored in a functionally and structurally distinct memory bank. There is no gatekeeper to tell the processor what information to store and what to retrieve in order to process new information. Instead, it appears that what have been traditionally called memories and habits are no more or less than changes in brain processing mechanisms that are autonomously active. Perhaps the most difficult concept to cast away is that memories are static reflections of past experience. In PAT, memories and habits determine the course of brain information processing, and they are incorporated in

mechanisms that initiate action. Whereas the initial structure of the brain is genetically determined, memories are derived from interactions of the individual with the environment.

Hence, PAT depends on the idea that brain *processing* mechanisms change in relation to what they process and the consequences of actions that they initiate (feedback). That is, the functional capacities of brain systems and the way in which they regulate behavior adapt to environmental input and feedback. This does not mean that the molecular biology of the brain changes with experience. It does mean that the functional architecture of processing mechanisms can and does change in relation to experiences of the organism.

In order to test aspects of this hypothesis, it is necessary to show (1) that cognitive problem solving is affected by past experience, and (2) that differential memories and behavior patterns acquired as a result of experience are not responsible for the difference in performance. One test would be to show that monkeys having different experience (reared in one environment or another and subsequently stressed in one way or another) confront new cognitive problem solving differently on tasks in which past memories and established behavior patterns have no bearing. If differentially reared and differentially stressed monkeys approach new problem solving differently, this would help to sustain the hypothesis stated above; that is, that initial trajectory deflections in social development leading to enduring abnormal behavior can be sustained through persisting effects on cognitive processing.

COGNITIVE EXPERIMENT

It has already been established that monkeys reared in total social isolation differ from socially reared monkeys in their performance on cognitive problem-solving tasks. As reviewed earlier (Kraemer, 1992b), socially isolated monkeys exhibit deficits in inhibition of well-learned responses, blocking of redundant or irrelevant stimuli, and performance of oddity discrimination tasks by comparison with monkeys reared in relatively rich social environments (Beauchamp et al., 1991; Gluck & Sackett, 1976; Gluck et al., 1973; Harlow et al., 1971). While obviously not commenting on later findings, Harlow noted, however, that the cognitive deficits exhibited by socially isolated monkeys were surprisingly insignificant by comparison with the devastating behavioral disruption that social isolation produces in this species (Harlow et al., 1971). Hence the role of cognitive changes in producing the abnormal behavior associated with the isolation syndrome was deemed to be minimal.

One would also assume, then, that the probability that much less severe conditions of social privation and deprivation would produce alterations of cognitive function would be insignificant. Nevertheless, PAT suggests that first experiences with a caregiver and subsequent social rearing should alter the formation of cognitive mechanisms (the processor). It is well established that monkeys reared socially with peers but not having a monkey mother (peer reared) differ dramatically in their social competence from mother-reared monkeys. In particular, peer-reared monkeys are inordinately reclusive or impulsively aggressive (this varies unpredictably over time), and they are generally deficient in basic social skills common to mother-reared monkeys (Anderson & Mason, 1974, 1978; Harlow & Harlow, 1965; Harlow et al., 1971; Higley et al., 1991a). Motherless monkeys also display inordinate adverse responses to separation from peer group members later in life (Kraemer et al., 1991; Mason, 1979; Mason & Capitanio, 1988; Suomi et al., 1970). These deficits appear to endure throughout the life span despite long-term housing in relatively rich social environments. These behavioral changes are not due to social isolation. Rather, they are attributable to lack of early interaction with a maternal caregiver (Kraemer, 1995, 1997; Kraemer & Clarke, 1996).

Preliminary research leading up to the study reported herein suggested that Harlow and colleagues may have overlooked important variation in cognitive performance variables because (1) such variation does not always translate to significant deficits in correct performance of particular cognitive tasks (percentage of correct responses, however, is only one measure of cognitive performance); and (2) they did not use experimental groups that were large enough to allow detection of reliable rearing effects that may be subtle in the learning acquisition and performance environment but quite dramatic if exhibited in a social environment. Herein, we present only the results of a study that are critical to the present argument. A detailed report of the entire study will be presented elsewhere.

Cognitive Protocol

The monkeys in this study were exposed to two variations in early experience:

1. Rearing with or without a monkey mother. Twenty-four rhesus neonates were randomly assigned to one of two rearing conditions at birth: either mother reared ($n = 12$) or nursery reared ($n = 12$). Mother-reared neonates remained housed with their mothers after birth. Nursery-reared neonates were separated from their mothers 3–4 hours after birth and housed in individual cages. They were reared by humans for the first 6 weeks postpartum, during which time they were provided with daily peer socialization (30 minutes with two other peers) and were trained to self-feed. At 6 weeks of age, nursery-reared neonates were placed into peer groups of three monkeys each.

2. Repeated exposure to social deprivation. At approximately 8 months of age, mother-reared monkeys were separated from their mothers and housed in peer groups of three monkeys each. Nursery-reared monkeys were separated from their existing peer group and reorganized into new peer groups. Hence all subjects were separated

from pre-existing attachment objects at this time. Subsequently, half of the subjects in each natal rearing group were repeatedly separated from their peers for six 1 week separation–1 week reunion cycles. At the end of this treatment, the monkeys averaged 12 months of age. Subsequently, they remained undisturbed in their peer groups until they were approximately 16 months of age.

The monkeys in each group have different social memories. Half had mothers and half did not. Within these rearing groups, half experienced repeated separations from peers and half did not. These differences would account for and also confound measures of cognitive function in the social environment. Hence, the next step is to measure acquisition of problem-solving strategies in an environment in which social factors are canceled out and past social memories cannot be brought to bear.

Beginning at 16 months of age, and 4 months after the last separation stressor for half of the subjects, the monkeys were tested on three problems that challenge memory mechanisms that are broadly classified as nonlimbic, noncortical, and cortical. The monkeys were removed from their social group and tested individually in a Wisconsin General Test Apparatus using well-established procedures. In all cases, the monkey is presented with a flat surface with one or more objects on it. It must displace the "correct" object to receive a preferred food reward (raisin, sugar-coated cereal, chocolate) sequestered in a shallow well below the object. The monkeys were not food deprived for these tests. In all tests, the monkeys were trained to a criterion of 90% correct responding during the acquisition phase. The tests were:

1. *Concurrent Object Discrimination (COD) with a 24 hour intertrial interval.* For each test conducted on consecutive days, the monkey is presented with the same series of 20 pairs of objects. One object of each pair is always

rewarded, so the monkey must learn a list of 20 correct objects to gain all of the rewards. Monkeys learn to recognize and choose a series of familiar objects presented with unfamiliar distracter objects quite readily, and this is an easy task for monkeys beginning very early in life. This test measures visual habits and is not dependent on the integrity of either limbic or cortical mechanisms. Performance on this task was used as a control for global differences in affective responses to apparatus, objects, and test procedures that might alter performance on all tasks.

2. *Delayed Nonmatching to Sample (DNMS), with delays from 0 to 120 seconds.* This measures visual recognition and is dependent on the integrity of the limbic system (hippocampus – amygdala – diencephalon). The monkey is first shown one object. Then its vision is blocked by lowering a screen, and the first object and a new object are presented as a pair. When the screen is raised, the monkey must choose the new object in order to gain the reward. This task demands that the monkeys recognize and choose a new object over one they have seen before. A critical point is that this task requires memory of what has been presented but is biased toward rewarding "novelty preference." Most monkeys tend to choose novel over familiar objects without any other reward contingencies.

3. *Delayed Response Test (DRT), with delays of 0 to 120 seconds.* This measures spatial memory and is dependent on the integrity of the dorsolateral prefrontal cortex and striatum. The monkey observes while the reward is hidden in one of two places. Then the screen is lowered and raised immediately or after some delay. The monkey must retrieve the reward from where it observed the reward being hidden. This task demands that monkeys remember and seek a reward in a particular spatial location. There is no de-

mand on object recognition, nor is novelty seeking a significant factor.

In general, the difficulty of correctly responding to the latter two tasks increases with increasing delay. In all tasks, the monkey was given 120 seconds to respond to the problem. If the monkey did not respond, this was scored as a "balk."

These tasks do not involve social interactions, nor should variation in ongoing social behavior specifically interact with a test using only inanimate objects. There is a possibility that monkeys reared in different conditions could simply be more or less emotionally responsive to the test procedure, and this could affect performance (Harlow et al., 1971). Hence, the first assessment was to determine whether acquisition and performance of COD varied with rearing or prior separation. If monkeys varied on COD performance, then we would have to conclude that performance on cognitive testing was confounded with emotional responses to testing.

If there were no cognitive deficits on COD associated with rearing and/or separation, then a second objective was to determine whether such deficits could be localized in limbic or cortical cognitive problem-solving mechanisms. Based on prior work by Bachevalier and colleagues (Bachevalier, 1991; Bachevalier & Mishkin, 1986), it was hypothesized that (1) there would be no significant rearing differences in acquisition of tasks that do not depend on limbic or cortical mechanisms (COD), and (2) nursery-reared or socially deprived monkeys would display altered acquisition or performance on tasks that depend on prefrontal cortical association area or limbic functioning (i.e., DRT and DNMS).

Cognitive Testing Results

The results indicate that disruption of early social development (1) does not reliably affect acquisition or performance of COD, as anticipated, and (2) alters performance on cognitive tasks depending on limbic or cor-

tical mechanisms (DNMS, DRT). Repeated exposure to stressors also alters cognitive problem solving even when such stressors occurred months earlier. Two aspects of the data are presented to illustrate the nature of changes produced by differential rearing.

Delayed Nonmatching to Sample

Figure 24.2 shows the rate of acquisition of the DNMS task for individual mother-reared versus nursery-reared monkeys that were separated or not separated. Visual inspection of the data for monkeys that were not separated (Fig. 24.2A,B) suggests first of all, that mother-reared monkeys show a rather orderly progression to criterion (90% correct), whereas peer-reared monkeys start with a generally higher level of correct responses and on the whole achieve criterion somewhat sooner. By comparison, consideration of monkeys that were separated (Fig. 24.2C,D) suggests that separation tends to (1) increase trials required to reach criterion in some mother-reared monkeys but not others and (2) reduce initial correct responding but also the number of trials to reach criterion in some peer-reared monkeys.

Because one issue in acquisition is rate of increase in percent correct, group statistical comparisons were performed on data for the very first trial, and on the slopes and intercepts of least-squares regression lines over all trials required to reach criterion for each subject following the rationale and analysis of variance methods suggested by Kraemer and Thiemann (1989). On the first trial, there was a main effect of treatment groups ($F = 4.02$, df = 3/19; $p < 0.02$). Peer-reared monkeys that had been stressed previously by repeated separations had the lowest initial correct response rate. Their percent correct was significantly lower than mother- and peer-reared monkeys that were not separated ($p < 0.03$ and $p < 0.003$, respectively) but not significantly different from mother-reared monkeys that had been separated earlier. Analysis of the slopes of acquisition rate did not reveal any significant main effects; the interaction of rearing con-

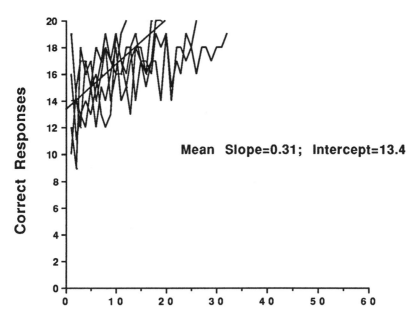

A. MOTHER-REARED NOT SEPARATED

Correct Responses

Mean Slope=0.31; Intercept=13.4

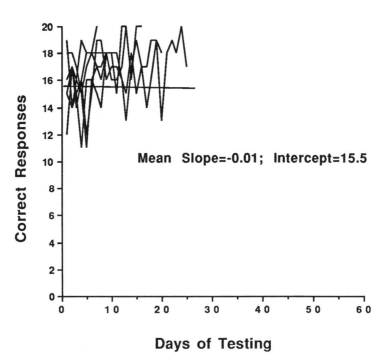

B. NURSERY REARED NOT SEPARATED

Correct Responses

Mean Slope=-0.01; Intercept=15.5

Days of Testing

Figure 24.2. Correct responses over days of delayed nonmatching to sample (DNMS) acquisition for subjects in four rearing groups described in text. Twenty trials were given each day until each subject correctly responded in 18 of 20 trials for 5 days in a row (90%). The last five trials for each subject (criterion) are not graphed. The mean slope and intercept of the regression line for correct responses versus days for all subjects in each group is presented for each group. *Illustration continued on next page.*

C. MOTHER REARED REPEATEDLY SEPARATED

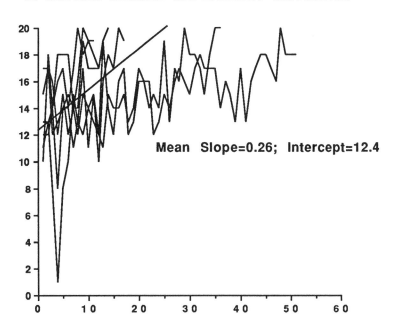

Mean Slope=0.26; Intercept=12.4

D. NURSERY REARED REPEATEDLY SEPARATED

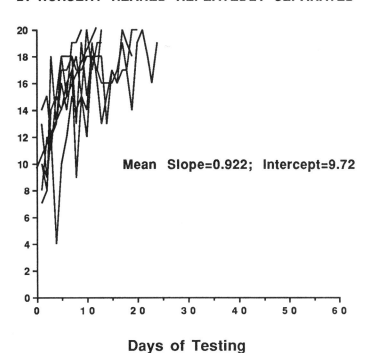

Mean Slope=0.922; Intercept=9.72

Days of Testing

Figure 24.2. *Continued*

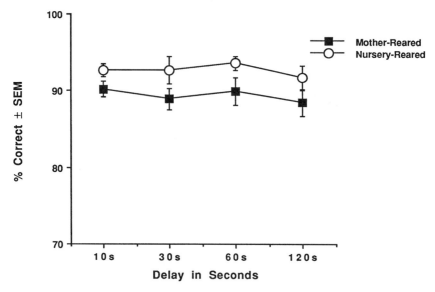

Figure 24.3. Percent correct responses over all delays in DNMS for mother-reared and nursery-reared monkeys (main effect of rearing, $p < .001$).

dition versus not being separated or being separated was of marginal significance ($p < 0.07$). Analysis of intercepts, however, showed that separated monkeys had significantly greater mean y-intercepts than non-separated monkeys ($F = 11.99$, df = 1/19; $p < 0.003$). There was a significant rearing condition versus separated versus not separated interaction. The interaction effect is attributable to nursery-reared monkeys that were not separated having the highest mean y-intercept and nursery-reared monkeys that were separated having the lowest y-intercept by comparison with all other groups (for the latter effect, $p < .033$ for all comparisons). These results indicate that, 4 months after the last social stressor (separations) and after training and performance on COD (approximately 6 months), monkeys performed differently on aspects of DNMS acquisition in relation to prior early rearing conditions and exposure to repeated separations.

Separation alters DNMS acquisition by increasing trials necessary to reach criterion in mother-reared monkeys and significantly and substantially reducing initial correct responding in peer-reared monkeys. Although not statistically significant, there was some

indication that peer rearing improves initial performance of DNMS (cf. Fig. 24.2A and 24.2B). This effect proved to be significant in subsequent testing with response delays imposed.

Figure 24.3 shows percent correct performance over all delays in mother-reared versus nursery-reared monkeys. Nursery-reared monkeys consistently displayed greater correct performance over all delays. Percent correct responding, however, does not tell the whole story about performance on this test.

Figure 24.4 shows the percentage of trials in which monkeys simply refused to perform the tasks (balk). Nursery-reared monkeys balked significantly more than mother-reared monkeys, and this effect was most prominent at short delays. The significance of these findings is discussed after considering aspects of performance on the DRT.

Delayed Response

In general, there were no differences in the final level of percent correct performance on the DRT attributable to rearing conditions or prior separations. This does not mean, however, that the monkeys in experi-

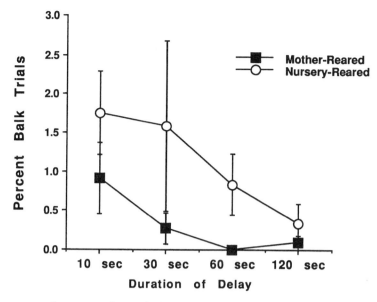

Figure 24.4. Percentage of DNMS trials on which mother-reared and nursery-reared monkeys failed to respond to the problem (balked).

mental and control groups responded equally to the task. The data to be presented concern percent error and time to respond to problem during the acquisition or "learning" phase. Differential rearing affects the time taken to respond to the problem in relation to the probability of making an error once a response was initiated.

On DRT, the baseline response occurs without obstruction of the monkey's vision of the location of reward. The monkey must simply retrieve the bait where it just saw the bait hidden. At 0 delay, the monkey's vision is obscured for as long as it takes to raise and lower a screen; in a third step, the monkey is titrated to perform with delays of 1–5 seconds between seeing the hiding spot and being allowed to displace the object. Figure 24.5 shows the correlation between percent error and time to respond for the nursery- and mother-reared monkeys at DRT of 1–5 seconds. These data illustrate findings characteristic of DRT acquisition across rearing groups. First, the data for nursery-reared monkeys are clustered with less variance than those for mother-reared monkeys. Second, percent error is correlated with time to respond for nursery-

reared monkeys but not for mother-reared monkeys.

Mother-reared monkeys eventually responded in significantly less time over delays of 10–120 seconds even though they took more time on average in responding when first acquiring the task at shorter delays. Nursery-reared monkeys balked more than mother-reared monkeys over all DRT conditions ($p < 0.001$).

DISCUSSION

These findings support the hypothesis that early rearing style and exposure to stressors significantly affect aspects of cognitive performance. The implications for theories about the relationship between stress and psychopathology are considered further here. A case can be made that the changes produced by peer rearing on DNMS and DRT would be counteradaptive in the social environment and may underlie some of the unusual social behavior exhibited by peer-reared monkeys.

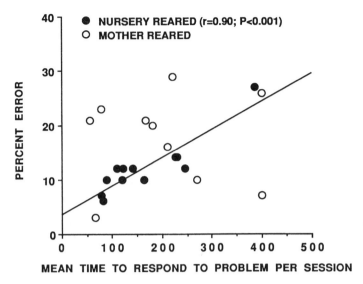

Figure 24.5. Relationship between error rate (% incorrect responses) and mean time per trial taken to respond to problem for mother- and nursery-reared monkeys.

Psychobiology of Cognition

Most theories of normal cognitive–emotional development either make no prediction about biological changes associated with abnormal behavior or imply that abnormal behavior is a normal response to an abnormal or at least unusual set of contingencies. In particular, Western behavioral cognitive–emotional theories do not suggest that mentally ill individuals should have unusual physiological responses to stressors, that they should have altered perceptions of stressors, or that the cognitive processes brought to bear to cope with stressors should be different. For example, organismic views, such as classical Piagetian cognitive developmental theory, suggest that developmental changes in cognitive processing per se occur independently of early experience (Piaget, 1963). Behavior that is affected by environmental influences is attributed to acquisition and retention of knowledge. The mechanisms by which the individual incorporates new knowledge (assimilation and accommodation) remain inviolate and constitutionally structured. Alternative dialectical views—Russian cognitive theory, for example—suggest that not

only are cognitive mechanisms affected by experience, but also that the structure of cognitive mechanisms is determined through interactions of the individual with the prevailing society and culture (Luria, 1976; Vygotsky, 1987).

PAT suggests that early exposure to stressors for which the organism is not prepared alters cognitive processing and the way in which future experience will be perceived and processed. This view does not deny that some individuals begin to behave differently from norm because they have unique experiences and stored memories. What this view adds is the idea that exposure to some circumstances entails that *new experience* will be processed differently. What the stressed neonate/juvenile perceives, incorporates, and uses to regulate behavior is different from what it would have been otherwise. PAT is more consistent with the views of Vygotsky and Luria, rather than Piaget.

Rhesus Cognitive Performance

Mother- and nursery-reared monkeys differ in cognitive problem solving in a number of respects. The data support the hypothesis that cognitive changes produced by prior rearing, and then further modified by subsequent stressors, underlie vulnerability to both exposure to and adverse responses to challenges in the future. A critical part of this perspective is the acceptance of mother-reared, not separated monkeys as the standard. These monkeys cope well with stressors. They are also resilient in the face of repeated stressors. It may seem puzzling, then, that on specific tasks (e.g., DNMS) nursery-reared monkeys appear to "do better" than mother-reared monkeys; they achieve a higher percent correct when they respond. As noted above, subtle but reliable increases in percent correct responses on some tasks, and altered timing of responses and correlations of this with correct responding, were not what previous investigators were looking for as a result of maternal privation. They were looking primarily for robust performance deficits. One can ask, though, whether the deficits we report are significant in any other than a statistical sense.

One interpretation of the DNMS data is that nursery-reared monkeys are more likely to attend to novel objects and to respond rapidly when these are presented. If they do not respond rapidly, they either balk or make significantly more errors in choosing among objects, especially at short delays. Capture of attention by novelty is suggested because the high rate of correct responding by nursery-reared monkeys on the first trial of DNMS acquisition suggests that an unlearned response tendency is responsible for the effect. Their cognitive processing appears to be rigidly locked to perceptual features of the test. Responding is "all or nothing," not modified by consideration of multiple cues that might be important in later problem solving and not flexible in timing and execution. Thus, peer-reared monkeys may not be learning the rules of the DNMS problem and may display increased correct responding on DNMS because they fail to inhibit reflexive responses to novelty. In the long run, this reflexlike responding

will lead to failure to extinguish old response patterns and perseverance of errors when the characteristics of the problem change. These effects are similar to effects found in totally isolated monkeys, suggesting a spectrum of privation effects.

Mother-reared monkeys, in contrast, do not appear to be stimulus or time locked. They respond at a particular level of percent correct regardless of how long they take to respond. They do not appear to be captured by novelty and make more errors as a result of selecting (shall we say preferring) familiar objects. They take longer to learn to seek hidden objects initially but with practice, they do it more rapidly and with virtually no balks. Mother-reared monkeys appear to attend to a broader array of stimulus and procedure cues. They are more successful in solving a variety of problems when the nature of the problem changes.

Rhesus Rearing and Cognition

The general picture produced by differential rearing is that of disorganization of cognitively mediated behavior with some abilities augmented at the expense of others. From a clinical standpoint, the social behavior of nursery-reared monkeys appears to be "impulsive" in many respects. Otherwise, they may be reclusive. These monkeys are highly distractible under some circumstances and oblivious to significant changes in the environment in others. The latter generally occurs while they are engaged in a well established behavior pattern, and aggression can be one of these. The results of cognitive testing reinforce the observation that peer-reared monkeys have difficulty in managing the flow of usual social interactions.

In many social encounters (a conversation between two people is a familiar and analogous example), a behavior pattern is initiated by one actor. This has a particular form and a usual beginning and end. A second individual is the audience while the first actor acts. Then the table turns. The actor pauses, the audience becomes the second actor, and the first actor, the audience. The second actor acts and pauses, and so it goes. A typical rhesus monkey vignette/conversation along these lines can be seen as they groom each other. The audience is always socially obligated to wait until the end of the act until an appropriate response can be made, even if what will be responded to was at the beginning of the act. If we translate the behavior of peer-reared monkeys on cognitive testing to these give-and-take social situations, then what we see is a tendency to be distracted by novelty, to respond rapidly to salient stimuli or balk or make an error in choice, and to be inflexible in timing of response. These are not endearing behaviors in rhesus society and do seem to be characteristic of the chaotic patterns of social behavior exhibited by peer-reared monkeys. Others have interpreted these behaviors as being indicative of increased anxiety and social tension (Higley et al., 1991a, 1991b).

The persistent exhibition of abnormal behavior exhibited by peer-reared monkeys might be labeled as psychopathology if exhibited by human juveniles. The closest analogies are to the commonalties shared among human childhood depression, anxiety, attention-deficit, attention-deficit/hyperactivity, and conduct disorders. The environmental etiology of such behavioral changes, particularly aspects concerned with early attachment and learning, is consonant with the premises of psychoanalytical and behaviorist theories and ECST. Hence, this new view reaffirms old views about the social and developmental risk factors for psychopathology. The probable mechanisms by which early disruption of social rearing produces enduring abnormal behavior, however, are different. Maternal privation or deprivation, or attachment to an inadequate or abusive caregiver, results in disruption of usual neonatal neurobiological organizational changes. Hence, exposing juveniles to repeated social and physiological stressors, and the challenge of ongoing attachments with peers, also affect physiological regulatory systems and cognitive processing.

Diathesis–Stress versus System Disorganization and Fractionation

One result of this difference in perspective is the conclusion that the individual is *different*, rather than fundamentally degraded or defective, following early maternal privation or social deprivation. Social privation–induced changes in cognitive processing (e.g., the enhanced speed at which novelty perception transfers to motor output) would provide a significant advantage in some situations (surviving in hostile environments) and appear to be maladaptive in others (the classroom). Most important, the cognitive abilities of motherless monkeys are not "weakened" or deficient as a result of privation. However, they may be maladaptive in most usual social environments. In the usual social environment, then, the individual may be repeatedly stressed because it cannot readily solve problems in the way others commonly do.

Thus the cognitive data do not fit within a diathesis–stress view in which the organism is vulnerable to subsequent challenges because it is less resilient or has fewer resources and wherewithal to bring to the situation. Instead, the data are consonant with the hypothesis that deflected developmental trajectories can be sustained because the organism confronts new problems differently than it would have otherwise. It is not likely that reversing changes in neurotransmitter systems through pharmacological treatment can affect this sustaining factor for altered behavior. Indeed, there is a wealth of evidence that pharmacological treatment of psychiatric disorder is often palliative but never remedial. Ultimately this means that psychotherapy must be tailored to what the individual can process.

Common sense and past theories about how individuals usually process information are not likely to be helpful in this endeavor. At present, the only mental health profession that specifically embraces the holistic view that sensorimotor integration is the critical substrate for health and well-being, and defines "health and well-being" in terms of purposeful activity, is occupational therapy. Understanding the relatively subtle cognitive deficits that, along with physiological changes, may be a core feature of stress-induced developmental psychopathology holds great promise in developing approaches to arrest or reverse the progression of these disorders.

Acknowledgments: Research and manuscript preparation supported by the John D. and Catherine T. MacArthur Foundation.

REFERENCES

Ainsworth, M. D. S., Blehar, M. C., Waters, E., et al. (1978). *Patterns of attachment: A psychological study of the strange situation*. Hillsdale, NJ: Lawrence Erlbaum Associates.

Anderson, C. O., & Mason, W. A. (1974). Early experience and complexity of social organization in groups of young rhesus monkeys (Macaca mulatta). *Journal of Comparative and Physiological Psychology*, 87, 681–690.

Anderson, C. O., and Mason, W. A. (1978). Competitive social strategies in groups of deprived and experienced rhesus monkeys. *Developmental Psychobiology*, 11, 289–299.

Bachevalier, J. (1991). Memory loss and socioemotional disturbances following neonatal damage of the limbic system in monkeys: An animal model of childhood autism. In C. A. Tamminga & S. C. Schulz (Eds.), *Advances in neuropsychiatry and psychopharmacology, Vol. 1: Schizophrenia* (pp. 129–140). New York: Raven Press.

Bachevalier, J., & Mishkin, M. (1986). An early and late developing system for learning and retention in infant monkeys. *Behavioural Brain Research*, 20, 249–261.

Beauchamp, A. J., Gluck, J. P., Fouty, H. E., et al. (1991). Associative processes in differentially reared rhesus monkeys (Macaca mulatta): Blocking. *Developmental Psychobiology*, 24, 175–189.

Bowlby, J. (1969). *Attachment and loss: Attachment*. New York: Basic Books.

Bowlby, J. (1973). *Attachment and loss: Separation, anxiety, and anger*. New York: Basic Books.

Bowlby, J. (1980). *Attachment and loss: Loss, sadness, and depression*. New York: Basic Books.

Bowlby, J. (1988). *A secure base*. New York: Basic Books.

Bretherton, I. (1985). The ontogenesis of attachment theory. In I. Bretherton & E. Waters (Eds.), *Growing points of attachment theory and research* (pp. 4–35). Chicago: University of Chicago Press.

Byne, W. (1994). The biological evidence challenged. *Scientific American*, 270, 50–55.

Carlson, M. & Earls, F. (1996). Psychological and neuroendocrinological sequelae of early social deprivation in institutionalized children in Romania. *Annals of the New York Academy of Science*, 807, 419–428.

Clarke, A. S. (1993). Social rearing effects on HPA axis activity over early development and in response to stress in young rhesus monkeys. *Developmental Psychobiology*, 26, 433–447.

Clarke, A. S., Hedeker, D., Ebert, M. H., et al. (1996). Rearing experience and biogenic amine activity in infant rhesus monkeys. *Biological Psychiatry*, 40, 338–352.

Clarke, A. S., Wittwer, D. J., Abbott, D. H., et al. (1994). Long-term effects of prenatal stress on HPA axis activity in juvenile rhesus monkeys. *Developmental Psychobiology*, 27, 257–270.

Cohen, R. M., & Campbell, I. C. (1984). Receptor adaptation in animal models of mood disorders: A state change approach to psychiatric illness. In R. Post (Ed.), *Neurobiology of mood disorders* (pp. 572–586). Baltimore: Williams & Willkins.

Craik, K. (1943). *The nature of explanation*. Cambridge, England: Cambridge University Press.

Dennett, D. C. (1991). *Consciousness explained*. Boston: Little, Brown.

Eiserer, L. A. (1992). Levels of explanation in theories of infant attachment. *Behavioral and Brain Sciences*, 15, 513–514.

Fischer, K. W. (1987). Relations between brain and cognitive development. *Child Development*, 58, 623–632.

Franklin, J. (1987). *Molecules of the mind*. New York: Dell.

Freedman, D. G. (1993). Attachment and the transmission of culture—an evolutionary perspective. *Journal of Social Evolution Systems*, 16, 297–329.

Freud, S. (1969). *An outline of psychoanalysis* (James Strachey, Transl.). New York: W. W. Norton.

Garver, D. L., Schlemmer, R. F., Maas, J. W., et al. (1975). A schizophreniform behavioral psychosis mediated by dopamine. *American Journal of Psychiatry, 132*, 33–38.

Gluck, J., & Sackett, G. E. (1976). Extinction deficits in socially isolated rhesus monkeys (Macaca mulatta). *Developmental Psychology, 12*, 173–174.

Gluck, J. P., Harlow, H. F., & Schlitz, K. A. (1973). Differential effect of early enrichment and deprivation on learning in the rhesus monkey (Macaca mulatta). *Journal of Comparative and Physiological Psychology, 84*, 598–604.

Harlow, H. F., & Harlow, M. K. (1965). The affectional systems. In B. M. Foss (Ed.), *Behavior of nonhuman primates* (Vol. 2, pp. 287–333). New York: Academic Press.

Harlow, H. F., Harlow, M. K., & Hansen, E. W. (1963). The maternal affectional system of rhesus monkeys. In H. L. Rheingold (Ed.), *Maternal behavior in mammals* (pp. 254–281). New York: John Wiley & Sons.

Harlow, H. F., Harlow, M. K., & Suomi, S. J. (1971). From thought to therapy: Lessons from a primate laboratory. *American Scientist, 59*, 538–549.

Harlow, H. F., Plubell, P. E., & Baysinger, C. M. (1973). Induction of psychological death in rhesus monkeys. *Journal of Autism and Childhood Schizophrenia, 3*, 299–307.

Hebb, D. O. (1949). *The organization of behavior.* New York: John Wiley & Sons.

Hebb, D. O. (1982). *The conceptual nervous system.* (Foundations in the Philosophy of Science & Technology Series, H. A. Buchtel, Ed.). New York: Pergamon.

Higley, J., Haseert, M., Suomi, S., et al. (1991a). Nonhuman primate model of alcohol abuse: Effects of early experience, personality, and stress on alcohol consumption. *Proceedings of the National Academy of Sciences USA, 88*, 7261–7265.

Higley, J. D., Suomi, S. J., & Linnoila, M. (1991b). CSF monoamine metabolite concentrations vary according to age, rearing, and sex, and are influenced by the stressor of social separation in rhesus monkeys. *Psychopharmacology, 103*, 551–556.

Higley, J. D., Suomi, S. J., & Linnoila, M. (1992). A longitudinal study of CSF monoamine metabolite and plasma cortisol concentrations in young rhesus monkeys: Effects of early experience, age, sex, and stress on continuity of individual differences. *Biological Psychiatry, 32*, 127–145.

Hinde, R. A. (1982). Attachment: Some conceptual and biological issues. In C. Parkes & J. Stevenson-Hinde (Eds.), *The place of attachment in human behavior* (pp. 60–76). New York: Basic Books.

Hofer, M. A. (1984). Relationships as regulators: A psychobiologic perspective on bereavement. *Psychosomatic Medicine, 46*, 183–197.

Hofer, M. A. (1987). Early social relationships: A psychobiologist's view. *Child Development, 58*, 633–647.

Horgan, J. (1993). Eugenics revisited. *Scientific American, 268*, 122–131.

Insel, T. R. (1992). Oxytocin and the neurobiology of attachment. *Behavioral Brain Science, 15*, 515–516.

Jacobs, B., & Raleigh, M. J. (1992). Attachment: How early, how far? *Behavioral Brain Science, 15*, 517.

James, W. (1950). *The Principles of Psychology,* (Vols. 1 and 2). New York: Dover (original work published 1890).

Kagan, J. (1992). The meanings of attachment. *Behavioral Brain Science, 15*, 517–518.

Kagan, J., Resnick, J. S., & Snidman, N. (1990). The temperamental qualities of inhibition and lack of inhibition. In M. Lewis & S. M. Miller (Eds.), *Handbook of developmental psychopathology* (pp. 219–226). New York: Plenum.

Kovach, J. K. (1992). Attachment and the sources of behavioral pathology. *Behavioral Brain Science, 15*, 518–519.

Kraemer, G. W. (1985). The primate social environment, brain neurochemical changes and psychopathology. *Trends in Neuroscience, 8*, 339–340.

Kraemer, G. W. (1992a). Psychobiological Attachment Theory (PAT) and psychopathology. *Behavioral Brain Science, 15*, 525–534.

Kraemer, G. W., (1992b). A psychobiological theory of attachment. *Behavioral Brain Science, 15*, 493–511.

Kraemer, G. W. (1995). The significance of social attachment in primate infants: The caregiver-infant relationship and volition. In C. R. Pryce, R. D. Martin, & D. Skuse (Eds.), *Motherhood in human and nonhuman primates: Biological and social determinants* (pp. 152–161). Basel: Karger.

Kraemer, G. W. (1997). Psychobiology of early social attachment in rhesus monkeys: Clinical implications. *Annals of the New York Academy of Science, 807*, 401–418.

Kraemer, G. W., & Clarke, A. S. (1990). The behavioral neurobiology of self-injurious behavior in rhesus monkeys. *Progress in Neuropsy-*

chopharmacology and Biological Psychiatry, 14(Suppl.), 141–168.

Kraemer, G. W., & Clarke, A. S. (1996). Social attachment, brain function, and aggression. *Annals of the New York Academy of Science*, 794, 121–135.

Kraemer, G. W., Ebert, M. H., Lake, C. R., et al. (1984). Hypersensitivity to d-amphetamine several years after early social deprivation in rhesus monkeys. *Psychopharmacology*, 82, 266–271.

Kraemer, G. W., Ebert, M. H., Schmidt, D. E., et al. (1989). A longitudinal study of the effects of different rearing environments on cerebrospinal fluid norepinephrine and biogenic amine metabolites in rhesus monkeys. *Neuropsychopharmacology*, 2, 175–189.

Kraemer, G. W., Ebert, M. H., Schmidt, D. E., et al. (1991). Strangers in a strange land: A psychobiological study of mother-infant separation in rhesus monkeys. *Child Development*, 62, 548–566.

Kraemer, G. W., & McKinney, W. T. (1979). Interactions of pharmacological agents which alter biogenic amine metabolism and depression: An analysis of contributing factors within a primate model of depression. *Journal of Affective Disorders*, 1, 33–54.

Kraemer, G. W., & McKinney, W. T. (1988). Animal models in psychiatry: Contributions of research on synaptic mechanisms. In A. K. Sen & T. Lee (Eds.), *Receptors and ligands in psychiatry and neurology* (pp. 459–483). Cambridge, England: Cambridge University Press.

Kraemer, H. C., & Thiemann, S. (1989). A strategy to use soft data effectively in randomized controlled clinical trials. *Journal of Consulting and Clinical Psychology*, 57, 148–154.

Lamb, M. E., Thompson, R. A., Gardner, W. P., et al. (1984).Security of infantile attachment as assessed in the "Strange Situation": Its study and biological interpretation. *Behavioral Brain Science*, 7, 127–171.

LeVay, S., & Hamer, D. H. (1994). Evidence for a biological influence in male homosexuality. *Scientific American*, 270, 44–49.

Lubach, G. R., Kittrell, E. M. W., & Coe, C. L. (1992). Maternal influences on body temperature in the primate infant. *Physiology and Behavior*, 51, 987–994.

Luria, A. R. (1976). *Cognitive development: Its cultural and social foundations*. Cambridge, MA: Harvard University Press.

Mason, W. A. (1979). Development of social interaction: Maternal attributes and primate cognitive development. In M. von Cranach, K. Foppa, W. Lepenies, & D. Ploog (Eds.), *Human ethology: Claims and limits of a new discipline* (pp. 437–455). Cambridge, England: Cambridge Universtiy Press.

Mason, W. A., & Capitanio, J. P. (1988). Formation and expression of filial attachment in rhesus monkeys raised with living and inanimate mother substitutes. *Developmental Psychobiology*, 21, 401–430.

Nemeroff, C. B. (1992). New vistas in neuropeptide research in neuropsychiatry: Focus on cortico-trophin releasing factor. *Neuropsychopharmacology*, 6, 69–75.

Nowakowski, R. S. (1987). Basic concepts of CNS development. *Child Development*, 58, 568–595.

Peirce, C. S. (1934). How to make our ideas clear. In C. Hartshorne & P. Weiss (Eds.), *The collected papers of Charles Sanders Peirce* (pp. 248–271). Cambridge, MA: Harvard University Press. (original work published 1878).

Pérusse, D. (1992). Attachment: A view from evolutionary biology and behavior genetics. *Behavioral Brain Science*, 15, 521–522.

Piaget, J. (1963). *The origins of intelligence in children*. New York: W. W. Norton.

Plomin, R. (1989). Environment and genes: Determinants of behavior. *American Psychologist*, 44, 105–111.

Post, R. M. (1992). Transduction of psychosocial stress into the neurobiology of recurrent affective disorder. *American Journal of Psychiatry*, 149, 999–1010.

Rosenblum, L. A., Coplan, J. D., Friedman, S., et al. (1994). Adverse early experiences affect noradrenergic and serotonergic functioning in adult primates. *Biological Psychiatry*, 35, 221–227.

Rosenblum, L. A., & Paully, G. S. (1984). The effects of varying environmental demands on maternal and infant behavior. *Child Develelopment*, 55, 305–314.

Sackett, G. P. (1970). Unlearned responses, differential rearing experiences, and the development of social attachments in rhesus monkeys. In *Primate behavior: Developments in field and laboratory research* (Vol. 1, pp. 111–140). New York: Academic Press.

Schildkraut, J. J. (1965). The catecholamine hypothesis of affective disorders: A review of supporting evidence. *American Journal of Psychiatry*, 122, 509–522.

Schildkraut, J. J., & Kety, S. S. (1967). Biogenic amines and emotion. *Science*, 156, 21–30.

Schneider, M. L. (1992a). Delayed object permanence development in prenatally stressed rhesus monkey infants (Macaca mulatta). *Occupational Therapy Journal of Research, 12*, 96–110.

Schneider, M. L. (1992b). The effect of mild stress during pregnancy on birthweight and neuromotor maturation in rhesus monkey infants (Macaca mulatta). *Infant Behavior and Development, 15*, 389–403.

Schneider, M. L. (1992). Prenatal stress exposure alters postnatal behavioral expression under conditions of novelty challenge in rhesus monkey infants. *Developmental Psychobiology, 25*, 529–540.

Schneider, M. L., & Clarke, A. S. (1993). Prenatal stress has long-term effects on behavioral responses to stress in juvenile rhesus monkeys. *Developmental Psychobiology, 26*, 293–304.

Schneider, M. L., Clarke, A. S., Kraemer, G. W., et al. (in press). Prenatal stress alters biogenic amine levels in rhesus monkeys. *Developmental Psychopathology*.

Schneider, M. L., & Coe, C. L. (1993). Repeated social stress during pregnancy impairs neuromotor development of the infant primate. *Development and Behavioral Pediatrics, 14*, 81–87.

Schneider, M. Kraemer, G. W., and Suomi, S. J. (1991). The effects of vestibular proprioceptive stimulation on motor maturation and response to challenge in rhesus monkeys. *Occupational Therapy Journal of Research, 11*, 135–154.

Schneider Rosen, K., & Rothbaum, F. (1993). Quality of parental caregiving and security of attachment. *Developmental Psychology, 29*, 358–367.

Sigman, M., & Siegel, D. J. (1992). The interface between the psychobiological and cognitive models of attachment. *Behavioral Brain Science, 15*, 523–524.

Skinner, B. F. (1953). *Science and human behavior*. New York: Macmillan.

Snyder, S. H. (1973). Amphetamine psychosis: A "model" schizophrenia mediated by catecholamines. *American Journal of Psychiatry, 130*, 61–67.

Suomi, S. J., Harlow, H. F., & Domek, C. J. (1970). Effect of repetitive infant-infant separation of young monkeys. *Journal of Abnormal Psychology, 76*, 161–172.

Vygotsky, L. S. (1987). Problems of general psychology: R. W. Rieber & A. S. Carton (Eds.), *The collected works of L. S. Vygotsky, Vol. 1*. New York, Plenum.

Werner, E. E. (1989a). Children of the garden island. *Scientific American, 260*, 106–111.

Werner, E. E. (1989b). High risk children in young adulthood: A longitudinal study from birth to 32 years. *American Journal of Orthopsychiatry, 59*, 72–81.

25

Physiological Correlates of Stress, Adversity, and Psychopathology

Ellen Frank
Jordan Karp

This chapter examines the available data on physiological correlates of stress, adversity, and psychopathology. It is in the development of depressive illness and posttraumatic stress disorder that life stress has been most strongly implicated. Thus it is not surprising that most of the literature we were able to locate relevant to the question of what the physiological correlates of stress and psychopathology might be focuses on these two disorders.

We would argue that examining both physiological and psychosocial parameters in the same subject over time is a most logical approach to the understanding of psychopathology, particularly to the understanding of etiopathogenesis. Indeed, three programs of research at the Western Psychiatric Institute and Clinic (WPIC) in Pittsburgh are currently focused on understanding such relationships. One focuses on depressed adolescents; a second, on midlife depressed patients; and a third, on depressed elderly. However, neither a review of the current literature nor our own data yield a particularly coherent story just yet. When one delves into this area by reading the extant literature or by trying to understand one's own data,

it becomes apparent that the picture is much more complicated than originally imagined. Nonetheless, we attempt to describe what is reported to date, review some of the results from our work at WPIC, suggest some reasons why a coherent picture fails to emerge, and finally suggest some future directions for research in this area. In doing so, we offer a reconceptualization of the possible psychophysiological correlates of stress, adversity, and psychopathology that takes into account what we believe are the true complexities of the parameters we are studying.

Our review of the complex interrelationships among stress, adversity, physiology, and psychopathology builds upon the elegant work of Zubin and Spring (1977), who developed the stress–diathesis/vulnerability model of mental disorders. Zubin and Spring suggested that, of the many theories of the etiology of mental disease (they were particularly interested in the etiology of schizophrenia), which included ecological, behavioral, and biological models, the vulnerability model succeeded in integrating these diverse and too-often independently researched schools of thought. They astutely acknowledged (*1*) the significance of the numerous components, including environmental, physiological, and genetic factors, that contributed to an individual's degree of vulnerability to mental disease; and (*2*) the importance of empirical measurement of those characteristics of vulnerability in individuals that might predict that an episode of illness will develop.

Zubin and Spring (1977) suggested that each individual differs in his or her response to stressors (both stressful life events and physiological stressors), and, as long as the level of stress remains below the personal vulnerability threshold, "the individual responds to the stressor in an elastic homeostatic way and remains well within the limits of normality" (p. 110). It is our goal to utilize this model to further elucidate how stressors such as life events or chronic psychosocial difficulties and presumed physiological reflections of stress, including sleep electroencephalogram (EEG) parameters and neuroendocrine responses, figure into the vulnerability model, and how this approach enhances our understanding of an integrated, longitudinally based hypothesis of the etiology of mental disorders and episodes of mental illness.

As a preview to this chapter, the authors acknowledge several biases. The first is that, in studying physiology, we view the cross-sectional approach as having serious limitations. We believe that investigators need to think about physiological parameters such as the sleep EEG in relationship to psychopathology from a longitudinal perspective, both within subjects and across subjects over the age span. Second, in studying stress, we believe it essential to distinguish between acute events and chronic difficulties that persist over time. Third, in integrating the two, we need to acknowledge that certain kinds of extreme stress, such as combat exposure or the experience of internment, may leave permanent physiological "scars" that, in their symptomatic expression, become themselves chronic stresses over time. Finally, we argue that any examination of how stress, adversity, and physiology fit together with psychopathology

must begin with a theory that leads to a testable hypothesis.

CURRENT RESEARCH FINDINGS

It appears there may be both a basic biological vulnerability to disorders such as depression and an influence of life stress on the expression of these disorders. Thus the physiological parameters investigated in the work described here tend to be those thought at one time or another to represent "biological markers" of psychopathological conditions [e.g., shortened rapid eye movement (REM) sleep latency as a "marker" of depression] or those thought to be the physiological parameters most responsive to psychological stress [e.g., the hypothalamic–pituitary–adrenal (HPA) axis].

Neuroendocrine Responses to Life Events

One of the earliest reports that attempted to integrate physiological parameters and stress was a study conducted by Dolan and colleagues (1985) that looked at the relationship between antecedent life events, clinical profile, and HPA axis function. The sample consisted of 72 depressed patients from psychiatric hospitals, general hospitals, and general practice in England. The investigators were interested specifically in the possible association between life events and the onset and clinical characteristics of depression, as well as the relationship between life events and neuroendocrine change, particularly patient status on the dexamethasone suppression test (DST).

The investigators used the Bedford College Life Events and Difficulties Schedule (LEDS; Brown & Harris, 1978) to assess the presence of both life events and ongoing difficulties. Ratings were made as to the independence, focus, and long-term contextual threat of both events and difficulties. On the basis of these ratings, only LEDS-defined provoking agents (i.e., *severe events* and *major difficulties*; Brown & Harris, 1978) were included in the analysis of clinical data. The investigators also noted the temporal relationship of the event to the onset of the disorder. Events were included if they occurred within 6 months of onset, and difficulties were included if they were present for at least 1 year before onset.

The study included a DST and two 24 hour urine collections to examine neuroendocrine status as a function of urinary free cortisol (UFC). Of the two 24 hour urine collections, the second occurred after the oral administration of 1 mg of dexamethasone before bedtime. Prior to the dexamethasone administration, a 4 P.M. blood sample was taken for plasma cortisol. The two 24 hour urine collections were assessed for pre- and postdexamethasone UFC, respectively.

Of the 72 patients who met entry criteria, 39% were inpatients, 60% were female, and the mean age was 41.6 years. Research Diagnostic Criteria (RDC; Spitzer et al., 1978) diagnoses of the patients were major depressive disorder ($n = 54$), probable major depressive disorder ($n = 9$), and minor depressive disorder ($n = 9$). In 39% of the patients, there was a severe life event before onset of their illness; in 21% of the sample, there was a major difficulty before onset. Fifty-four percent of the patients had either a severe event or major difficulty before onset.

At first glance, the investigators do not appear to articulate an explicit theory as to how they believed these variables might fit together; however, upon closer scrutiny of their report, it is apparent that they expected a stratification of the patients so that endogenous cases and dexamethasone nonsuppressors would have fewer life events. Dolan and colleagues (1985) found, however, that suppressor/nonsuppressor status on the DST was not associated with a greater or lesser likelihood of antecedent life events or difficulties. They report that 39% of both suppressors and nonsuppressors had a severe antecedent life event, and 21% of suppressors, compared with 20% of nonsuppressors, had a major difficulty before onset. The investigators also report that, within depressed subjects (who might be expected to have elevated values of UFC

to begin with), higher UFC values were associated with a greater number of stressful life events in both the 6 months before episode onset ($p < 0.05$) and the 6 months before entry into the study ($p < 0.05$). Of greater interest in this context was the fact that ongoing, chronic difficulties were even more strongly associated with elevated levels of UFC ($p < 0.005$) than were acute events.

Dolan et al. (1985) conclude that their findings cast a shadow of doubt on the value of the endogenous/nonendogenous distinction because of the failure of the DST to distinguish patients who had experienced life events and difficulties from those who had not. The investigators do not, however, specifically address the possible ways the parameters they studied might be related in terms of causality. Our own work (Frank et al., 1994) as well as that of Brown and coworkers (Brown et al., 1994) suggests that an important intervening variable in the relationship between endogenous/melancholic subtype and life stress is number of previous episodes of depressive illness. Our two research groups find a clear relationship between LEDS-defined (Brown & Harris, 1978) provoking agents and endogenous/melancholic subtype *except* in first-episode cases; these are equally likely to have had a provoking agent in the 6 months before onset whether the symptom picture is endogenous or nonendogenous. Dolan et al. (1985) apparently did not take number of previous episodes into account in this analysis, which may explain their failure to observe the expected relationships.

Another relatively early study that looked at the effects of life events on neuroendocrine levels was conducted by Roy and colleagues (1986). This study involved a homogeneous population of subjects as described in the *Diagnostic and Statistical Manual of Mutual Disorders (Third Edition)* (American Psychiatric Association, 1980), ($n = 23$) who met the criteria for major depression all of whom had sought treatment at the National Institute of Mental Health (NIMH) Clinical Center, a tertiary referral center. Of these 23 patients, 15 also met criteria for melancholia. Unlike the Dolan et al. (1985) report, Roy and colleagues (1986) explicitly stated that the "etiology of depression is considered to be multifactorial, with life events interacting with genetic and/ or other biological risk factors to produce a depressive episode" (p. 357). This hypothesis is congruent with the stress–diathesis model postulated by Zubin and Kietzman (1966), elaborated by Zubin and Spring (1977), and examined by Monroe and Simons (1991).

Roy and colleagues (1986) carried out lumbar punctures to obtain the cerebrospinal fluid (CSF) levels of seven monoamines and/or their metabolites thought to be biological markers of depressive illness. They also performed a DST with two subsequent blood draws. The results of the DST and the CSF levels were then analyzed with respect to the presence or absence of life events that had occurred during the 6 months prior to onset of the depressive episode. In addition to two separate clinical diagnoses, the Hamilton Rating Scale for Depression (HRSD; Hamilton, 1960) and the Bunney-Hamburg scale (Bunney & Hamburg, 1963) were completed for each patient to determine depression severity.

The Paykel Recent Life Events Interview was used to assess stressful life events within the 6 months before the onset of symptoms (Paykel et al., 1971). The Paykel 64 item interview includes details about changes in work, education, finances, health, bereavement, family and marital situation, and the like. Further probe questions were asked about the exact nature and timing of the event. The life events were also categorized by the interviewer as to whether they were desirable or undesirable. Additionally, a rating of the independence of the event (i.e., the extent to which the event might be considered a consequence of the depression) was determined by an independent psychiatric interviewer who did not know whether the subjects were patients or controls.

Fourteen of the 23 depressed patients and 9 of the 15 melancholic patients had experienced a life event prior to the onset of their depressive episodes. The mean time

between the onset of the depressive episode and the life event closest to it was 2.25 months (range, 3 weeks to 5 months). The mean time between experiencing an undesirable life event and the onset of depression was 1.7 months (range, 3 weeks to 3 months).

The results of the study revealed significantly lower CSF levels of dopamine ($p <$ .02), serotonin ($p <$ .004), and homovanillic acid ($p <$ .001) in those patients who had not experienced a severe event within the 6 months before the onset of illness. Similar findings were reported when the melancholic patients were analyzed separately. When only undesirable life events were examined, patients with major depressive episodes who had not experienced an undesirable life event (n = 12) had significantly lower CSF levels of homovanillic acid ($p <$ .05) than those patients (n = 8) who had experienced undesirable life events (e.g., death of a family member, demotion at work, imprisonment). Additionally, there was a trend for depressed patients without undesirable life events also to have lower CSF levels of serotonin ($p <$ .07). In the melancholic patients, there was no relationship between the presence (n = 4) or absence (n = 10) of undesirable life events and the level of any CSF metabolites.

Similar to the Dolan et al. study described earlier, there was no relationship between dexamethasone suppression/nonsuppression and the presence or absence of life events in general. However, there was a trend for the absence of an undesirable life event to be associated with a greater incidence of DST nonsuppression among the total group of patients with major depressive disorder (75% vs. 25%, $p <$ .06). This was not true for the melancholic patients.

Taking into account the severity and chronicity of illness of patients who typically enter the NIMH Clinical Center, it is reasonable to postulate that many of the subjects treated and studied by Roy et al. (1986) were ill for a very long time prior to hospitalization and evaluation for this study. Accounting for the fact that the investigators found no differences in the DST relating to the presence of life events, and a trend for those without undesirable life events to be more likely to be dexamethasone nonsuppressors, helps shape the stress–diathesis model toward that of a biologically marked form of illness present in those without events. However, one must also consider the effects of *chronic* stress (which were not distinguished from acute stressors in the Paykel scale) on the stress/biological vulnerability parameters. Additionally, one must consider those events that occur after episode onset; these were not included in the analysis and are probably relevant to any effort to interpret biological parameters in patients who have been ill for a long time at the point of evaluation.

Effects of Life Events on Sleep

Divorce

Another approach to the study of the biological implications of life events is to select a population that has experienced a particular life event and then examine the possible biological ramifications of that event. This approach was utilized by Cartwright (1983), who focused her attention on the effects of divorce on the sleep EEG. Cartwright first reported on a relatively small group of women (*n* = 56) between the ages of 30 and 55 years who were in the process of divorce. Follow-up evaluations were completed on 13 of the 56 subjects between 1 and 2 years later.

It should be noted that in most instances, divorce, an acute event that can be clearly marked in time, typically grows out of a chronic difficulty in the form of ongoing marital disputes. These domestic differences may stretch out over months or even years prior to a decision to divorce. The psychosocial and biological effects of such disputes are likely to be more similar to those created by an ongoing major difficulty than effects caused by a solitary severe event.

In the Cartwright study (1983), each subject was interviewed about her marital history and given a battery of psychological tests. These tests included the Adjective

Check List (Gough & Heilbrun, 1980), the Beck Depression Inventory (BDI; Beck, 1967), the Interpersonal Dependency Inventory (Hirschfeld et al., 1977), the Social Adjustment Scale (Weissman & Bothwell, 1976), the Social Role Inventory (Bem, 1974), and a role inventory developed by Cartwright. From the larger study population, 30 women were selected for the 6 night sleep laboratory evaluation. Although the investigator's primary interest was in the biological effects of a stressful event— divorce—on sleep EEG architecture and continuity, her hypothesis was quite different from the stress–diathesis model. Cartwright's hypothesis developed from her view of the adaptive significance of sleep and dreaming. She argued that sleep is used in the processing and accommodation of new or difficult affective information. Cartwright (1983) suggested that, in divorce, women who experience the most emotional distress would have a significant change in many REM sleep parameters; these include shortened REM latency, longer time spent in REM, greater density of eye movements within REM, and a longer REM period in the first half of the night compared with the second half of the night. The results of her study proved to be quite interesting. Cartwright reported the mean REM latency of all the subjects at baseline by dividing them into three levels of depression. Those ranked in the low range of depression (BDI = 5–14) had a mean REM latency of 84.8 minutes, while those in the middle (BDI = 15–19) and upper (BDI = 20–36) ranges of depression had mean REM latencies of 66.2 minutes and 59.7 minutes, respectively. Cartwright reported significantly shorter REM latencies (*p* < .01) in those subjects with more affective disturbance. Pooling the middle- and upper-range groups (those who were depressed) and comparing them with the subjects who had BDI scores of 5–14 (not clinically depressed) yielded a significant finding supporting her prediction of reduced REM latency in those subjects who are more distressed (*p* < .04).

Cartwright (1983) also noted that eye movement density and depression were significantly correlated (r = .39). Those subjects who were not depressed had a marked difference in eye movement density between the first and second half of the night (eye movement density mean = 0.74). Conversely, those who were more depressed had a flatter eye movement density distribution across the night (midrange depressed, mean eye movement density = 0.93; upper range depressed, eye movement density mean = 1.09) (p = 0.003). Thus, in one sense, her hypothesis of a greater change in REM variables for women who experience more stress from divorce was confirmed.

However, Cartwright (1983) presents a theoretical problem arising from her findings in the group of women studied at 1–2 years follow-up. She reports that REM latencies were longer in those women who were no longer depressed at follow-up (mean REM latency = 70.1 minutes) compared with those women who remained depressed at follow-up (mean REM latency = 60.1 minutes). Both averages, however, were still shorter than that of the group of women who were not depressed at initial testing or at follow-up (mean REM latency = 85.0 minutes). The finding of a shorter REM latency for the group of subjects still depressed at follow-up weakens Cartwright's argument that the shortened REM latencies observed at study entry were a result of affect processing. The findings at follow-up suggest that the REM latency sleep parameter actually may represent a biological marker of vulnerability to affective disorder. Women with this marker may be more predisposed to affective disorder in the face of adversity than those who do not express this trait (i.e., a stress–diathesis model). It should be noted that Cartwright's interesting findings at follow-up illustrate the limitations of cross-sectional studies and the benefits of longitudinal studies in this type of life stress research.

In 1991, Cartwright and colleagues further developed her original investigation of the biological implications of divorce as evidenced in EEG measures of sleep. In this later study, Cartwright et al. explicitly stated their research goals in terms of the stress–diathesis model, expecting those subjects who exhibited a particular REM sleep parameter to be predisposed to depression in the face of adversity. They again looked at their subjects both before (or rather during) the divorce and at 1 year follow-up. The investigators also included an inquiry into familial history of both depression and alcoholism to assess any genetic basis for an abnormal REM sleep parameter. In this particular study, the investigators were interested in whether the presence and persistence of early REM sleep was more characteristic of those experiencing depression than of their nondepressed counterparts. They also examined whether this trait was still present in those who were depressed at baseline but were remitted at follow-up, as well as whether those who exhibit this trait at both baseline and follow-up were more likely to have a positive familial history for affective disorders.

In this study, Cartwright et al. (1991) recruited a much larger population of subjects in the process of divorce (n = 214). The investigators included men (n = 110) as well as women. Seventy of these 214 subjects were selected for a standard 3 night EEG sleep study. Instruments similar to those used in the 1983 study were used to rate both the severity of depression and social and interpersonal adjustment. The Family History Research Diagnostic Criteria were administered to determine if an RDC diagnosis of major depressive disorder applied, whether there had been a previous episode of this disorder, and whether there was a family history of major affective illness. Sixty-one of the original 70 subjects returned for rediagnosis and to complete their 1 year follow-up sleep studies.

In this larger sample, Cartwright and colleagues (1991) found that, when seen close to the time of marital separation (baseline), approximately half of the subjects met RDC criteria for major depression, more than a third met Beck criteria (BDI $\geq$ 14), and about 30% met both criteria for major depressive disorder. However, only a few continued to meet both criteria after 1 year. At baseline, 30% of the 70 sleep subjects had

Table 25.1. Sleep EEG measures for three levels of depression

	Level of depression (BDI score)		
	5–14 (n = 10)	15–19 (n = 7)	20–36 (n = 12)
Sleep efficiency (percent)	92.2	89.1	90.4
Sleep latency (minutes)	20.1	24.6	19.1
REM latency (minutes)	84.8	66.2	59.7
Eye movement density (mean)	0.74	0.93	1.09

Adapted from Cartwright (1983).

a short REM latency (onset of REM sleep in less than 60 minutes). Seventy-one percent of the 21 subjects with short REM latency and 51% of the 49 subjects without short REM latency also met criteria for depression (positive RDC diagnosis and a BDI $\geq$ 14). Six (29%) of the subjects with and 24 (49%) of those without short REM latency were not currently depressed.

Cartwright et al. (1991) found that a short REM latency was not significantly related to a current affective disorder. However, when subjects who were currently depressed were combined with those who had recently recovered from an episode of depression according to the Schedule for Affective Disorders and Schizophrenia (SADS) interview, there was indeed a significant relationship between REM latency and depression (χ^2 = 9.8, p < .01). At follow-up, they found that, in general, REM latency tended to remain stable over 1 year. The authors note, however, that those subjects whose status changed from depressed to not depressed had less stable REM latency over the period of a year than those who remained depressed or who were not depressed on either occasion (Table 25.1). Interestingly, more subjects who were depressed and showed a normal REM latency continued to be depressed after 1 year compared to their counterparts who were depressed and had short REM latencies (χ^2 = 12.02, p < .05). In fact, none of the subjects with a stable short REM latency remained depressed at the follow-up point. Cartwright et al. (1991) note that the subjects who were depressed

but had a normal REM latency were slower to get over the divorce and make good postdivorce adjustment.

The rating of postdivorce adjustment was made by one of the authors and a blind rater (interrater reliability, r = .88) on the basis of an interview that assessed each subject's current functioning in the areas of work, children, friends, home, finances, relationship with ex-spouse, mood, and sleep. However, most of the subjects with a traitlike short REM latency on both occasions had scores indicating good adjustment, which is in contrast to those subjects whose initially short REM latency normalized a year later. The authors note that, although the population was small and the statistical power of the study minimal, it appears that, if one is depressed, having a stable, traitlike REM latency may predict recovery from depression and a more stable life adjustment at 1 year after the event.

These findings are interesting and, in many ways, call Cartwright's earlier notions regarding the use of sleep in the processing and assimilation of stressful events into question; if REM sleep were indeed used for processing difficult affect, she would not have found better adaptation and a higher recovery rate in those who exhibited a shortened REM latency trait. Cartwright and colleagues also note that those with stable short REM latencies were more likely to have a positive family history of affective disorder. Seventy-one percent of those who had shortened REM latencies, irrespective of clinical state, appeared to come from families with affective disorder. These findings are consistent with the family studies of REM latency by Giles et al. (1987).

Cartwright and colleagues (1991) conclude their paper by arguing that "a short REM latency may show not only a persistent, perhaps genetic, vulnerability to an affective response to a major stressful life event but also a greater capacity to recover from it" (p. 1534). They appear to move beyond describing the results of their study in terms of the stress–diathesis model and suggest that the presence of a consistently short REM latency may actually facilitate recovery and social adaptation from an adverse life event. They close with the suggestion that individuals who exhibit traitlike short REM latency should be followed at intervals and for longer periods of time to determine the true power of this sleep parameter as an indicator of *both* vulnerability to depression and capacity for recovery.

Single Severe Life Event

In a similar study, Hefez et al. (1987) examined the biological implications of a single severe life event on both sleep EEG and dreaming. Eleven patients participated in their study, five who were survivors of Nazi concentration camps, four who had been in active combat, and two who had survived a sea disaster. Three of the concentration camp survivors were clinically depressed, and all of the other subjects suffered from post-traumatic stress disorder (PTSD), some with a depressive tendency. The Holocaust survivors were studied as outpatients, and the postcombat and sea disaster survivors were studied as inpatients. All of the subjects underwent detailed physical and psychiatric examinations. Each of the patients slept in the laboratory for 2–5 nights and had basic EEG sleep studies. Respiration was monitored by a nostril thermistor and a respiratory belt, and leg movements were monitored by an accelerometer. Additionally, dream reports were documented by waking the subjects 10–15 minutes after the beginning of every REM period except the

first. Accounts of dreams also were collected after each spontaneous awakening.

In comparison with age-matched controls, all patients had low sleep efficiency indices, caused by a prolongation of sleep latency and larger amounts of "awake" plus "movement" time within sleep periods (Hefez et al., 1987). This was especially noticeable in the younger patients (sea disaster and postcombat survivors). Hefez et al. also report that REM sleep was significantly shorter in all patients than in controls. However, when the Holocaust survivors were compared with the postcombat and sea disaster survivors (these two groups were combined because of their closeness in age and similarity in sleep data), longer REM latency was seen only in the group of younger, more recently traumatized patients. Again, it should be noted that all of the younger patients were suffering from PTSD.

The researchers note that 4 of the 11 patients had laboratory-documented REM- and non-REM-related nightmares. None of the other patients reported any nightmares or night terrors during their laboratory nights. In fact, these seven patients had a surprisingly low rate of dream recall. Although the rate of dream recall was low, the overall REM density was significantly higher ($p < .05$) than that of the control subjects for the first three REM periods. Hefez et al. report that the average densities were 35.4% versus 21.6% for REM 1, 37.8% versus 24.4% for REM 2, and 40.1% versus 24.9% for REM 3. The small number of subjects in each group and the large differences in age and time since experiencing the trauma preclude meaningful interpretation of these results.

Psychosocial Stress and Depression

An interesting study begun by Monroe et al. (1992) at WPIC in Pittsburgh and analyzed at the University of Oregon also attempted to identify relationships between social factors, varying levels of depression severity, and REM sleep latency. Two specific questions guided the researchers in their investigation of an association between life stress and REM latency. First, they were interested in whether life stress predicts differences in REM latency. This question was suggested by their hypothesis that the greater the degree of life stress before the onset of depression, the lower the level of "biological vulnerability" to depressive illness and thus the longer the relative delay of onset of REM sleep. In contrast, lower levels of psychosocial stress would probably be accompanied by relatively reduced REM latency values. Second, the investigators also were interested in whether these markers (REM latency and life stress) from different levels of analysis suggest differences in the presenting picture of depression. Specifically, Monroe et al. predicted that increased stress would be associated with increased initial symptomatology and that reduced REM latency also would be related to greater severity.

The population included 61 outpatients with nonpsychotic, endogenous major depression. The average current age was 38 years, and 74% were women. Forty-eight percent of these patients were in their first episode of depression. Patients who met the entrance criteria—(1) RDC diagnosis of endogenous major depression, (2) HRSD ≥ 15, (3) duration of the index episode of less than 18 months, and (4) between 20 and 60 years of age—received the Psychiatric Epidemiology Research Interview (PERI) Life Events Scale (Dohrenwend et al., 1978). This scale asks patients to list all events that had occurred since 1 year before the onset of their symptoms. The modified version of the PERI that was utilized contains 110 life events and includes provisions for writing in events that are not listed. After completing the PERI, each patient underwent a semistructured interview to elicit details about each endorsed event.

Patients also were administered the SADS (Endicott & Spitzer, 1978) and the LEDS (Brown & Harris, 1978). The SADS was used to determine the duration of the current episode by establishing the date of onset. The LEDS utilized the information from the semistructured interview both in defining life events and difficulties and in rating the dimensions of the stressors. The LEDS investigators, who determined by consensus the significant events and difficulties of the patient's history, were unaware of the timing of onset, the subject's diagnosis, and any information about the patient's subjective response to the stressor. This allowed an objective and contextual analysis of each life event and difficulty.

Patients underwent three consecutive nights of EEG sleep studies. The analysis of each patient's EEG output yielded variables that covered different aspects of sleep maintenance, sleep architecture, and REM sleep. Additionally, patients were administered the 17-item HRSD and the 21-item BDI (Beck, 1967) to determine the severity of their illness at designated intervals.

Monroe et al. (1992) found that patients with acute severe events in the 6 weeks before onset had significantly longer REM latencies than their counterparts who did not experience such life events ($p < .05$). This was also significant at the trend level ($p < .08$) for those patients who experienced such an event in the 6 weeks before the interview. This finding was not significant for patients with severe difficulties (more chronic stressors) before onset versus those without difficulty. Similar nonsignificant associations with longer REM latency were found for patients who had experienced *either* a severe event or difficulty before the onset of depression versus patients who had experienced neither.

The investigators were also interested in the clinical implications of longer REM latency and life events on depression severity. Monroe and colleagues found that both severe events and REM latency were significantly and independently related to depression severity ($p < .05$). They state that, although both REM latency and stress independently predict severity, the association between REM latency and depression severity is especially pronounced for persons who have experienced a severe event prior to the onset of their episode.

STUDIES CONDUCTED AT WPIC

A study conducted at WPIC by Williamson et al. (1995) examined the effects of stressful life events on sleep EEG measures in depressed and normal adolescents. These investigators addressed the biological effects of life stress in the same manner as Cartwright et al. (1991) and Monroe et al. (1992), using the stress–diathesis model. Sixty-eight subjects were studied, 35 of whom were diagnosed as having major depressive disorder and 33 of whom were normal controls. All subjects were 12–18 years old.

Standard EEG sleep studies were conducted for three consecutive nights. Coinciding with the sleep studies, both the adolescents and their parent or guardian were interviewed about stressful life events that had occurred over the previous year. Life events were recorded with a modified version of the Life Event Record (LER; Coddington et al., 1972). The LER is a checklist, not an interview like the LEDS (Brown & Harris, 1978) or the PERI (Dohrenwend et al., 1978), and it clearly mixes acute life events with ongoing chronic stressors. After examining total life "events" occurring within the past year, subjects were classified as having had (1) no events, (2) one event, or (3) two or more events. In conducting their investigation, Williamson et al. pooled the events reported by both the parent and child for the year before the sleep study irrespective of date of illness onset.

Williamson and colleagues found a significant interaction between diagnostic group (major depressive disorder vs. normal control) and stressful life events for REM latency. They report that REM latency decreased as the number of events in the year preceding the sleep study increased among the normal controls, but remained constant for those adolescents with major depression ($p < .02$). Williamson et al. also found changes in delta sleep (stages 3 and 4) for both the control and depressed subjects, with delta sleep decreasing for both groups as the number of stressful life events increased. No differences between adoles-

cents with and without stressful life events were reported for sleep onset, total awake time after sleep onset, or total sleep.

In our own preliminary interpretation of the data presented by Williamson et al., we think it is important to stress two ideas. First, many family epidemiological studies (e.g., Weissman et al., 1987) suggest that such early onset of major depression (i.e., between ages 12 and 15) is strongly associated with a positive family history of depression. Thus we know that there is a high probability that these adolescents come from families with considerable loading for affective illness. The second consideration in interpreting these findings is that delta sleep generally is better preserved in adolescents than in adults; it may be especially insensitive to outside influence in this age-group irrespective of diagnosis, personal diagnostic history, or family history of depression.

In studies begun in 1989 at WPIC, Frank et al. (unpublished data) began an investigation of the relationship between a host of EEG sleep measures and severe life events, major difficulties, and all provoking agents as defined by the LEDS instrument (Brown & Harris, 1978) in the 6 months before the onset of major depression. The EEG sleep measures included parameters generated by computer analysis of the sleep EEG as well as traditional hand-scored variables. We began the study expecting results to support the stress–diathesis model; that is, those patients with abnormal sleep traits would be less likely to have experienced a stressful life event or chronic difficulty in the period before onset. We were unsure, however, which sleep parameters might prove to be statistically significant, and whether the relationship would be with a severe life event, ongoing major difficulty, or any provoking agent.

The 72 subjects studied were midlife patients with recurrent unipolar major depression. All patients were between the ages of 21 and 50. These patients were selected for having had at least two previous episodes. The average number of actual previous episodes, however, was six and the median was

Table 25.2. Effects of ongoing major difficulties on REM sleep measures from midlife recurrent depressed patients

Variable	Ongoing major difficulty		No ongoing major difficulty		F	p
	Mean	SD	Mean	SD		
Hand-scored REM measures						
Numer of REM periods	3.67	1.22	4.02	0.90	0.74	ns
REM latency (minutes)	87.67	63.42	69.80	27.20	1.18	ns
REM activity	88.67	34.86	167.66	77.28	10.97	0.002
REM percent	20.20	5.48	25.34	4.84	7.50	0.008
REM time	76.67	23.92	104.31	26.73	8.46	0.005
Computer-generated REM measures						
Total REM counts in first REM period	48.63	63.65	103.10	101.61	6.27	0.01
Average REM counts in first REM period	3.01	3.38	4.69	3.39	4.33	0.04
Total REM counts in second REM period	92.63	74.70	188.56	169.27	7.33	0.009
Average REM counts in second REM period	4.82	3.16	7.10	4.54	5.88	0.02
Total REM counts whole night	371.00	211.13	720.03	438.97	10.82	0.002
Average REM counts whole night	4.83	2.42	6.90	3.51	9.62	0.003

four, so it is obvious that the patients had a highly recurrent form of the disorder. This is significant to note because it makes the composition of this patient group quite different from that studied by Monroe et al. (1992), in which almost half of the patients were in their first episode of depression.

Despite the very clear histories of recurrent depression (presumably a more "biological" form of the illness) among these patients, they were far from free of either severe events or major difficulties according to LEDS criteria. Twenty-seven subjects had a severe event and nine subjects had a major difficulty in the 6 months before onset. When these two indices of life stress were combined, 31 of the 72 subjects were found to have experienced a provoking agent (either a severe event or a major difficulty) in the 6 months before onset. In other words, although conventional wisdom would suggest that such highly recurrent patients might appear to be suffering from exclusively "endogenous" depressions, a significant portion had experienced severe life stressors in the 6 months prior to the onset of the current episode.

What we found with respect to the relationship between sleep EEG and life stress was interesting but certainly not expected. No significant relationship was discovered between any of the 29 computer-generated or hand-scored measures and severe event status. We did find, however, that ongoing major difficulties were related to every REM sleep variable in this midlife population with the exception of REM latency and number of REM periods (Table 25.2). When all provoking agents (severe events and major difficulties) were examined, only percentage of time spent in delta sleep was significant in distinguishing patients who had experienced a provoking agent from those who had not ($F = 4.05$, $p < .05$); subjects who had *not* experienced a provoking agent showed decreased delta sleep.

The fact that no differences in EEG sleep were found for those patients experiencing an acute severe event compared with those who did not experience a severe event, whereas such differences were found for those patients who experienced an ongoing major difficulty, suggests possible physiological changes associated with chronic hardship. Cartwright's findings in her populations of divorcing subjects (if divorce is viewed as the end result of a chronic stressor involving ongoing marital tension and disputes) and Hefez's findings in a population who experienced traumatic events with longterm effects in terms of chronic depression and PTSD tend to support these preliminary findings. Two examples of the significant differences between those who had experienced an ongoing difficulty and those who had not in our study are the relative mean amounts of REM activity and the mean time spent in REM. Those with a chronic difficulty had REM activity values of 88.67 and spent 76.67 minutes in REM sleep, compared with activity values of 167.66 and 104.31 minutes of time spent in REM sleep in those without the difficulty. Thus, in this group of midlife subjects already heavily "scarred" by depression in terms of their physiology, it appears that REM is markedly diminished in the face of chronic adversity.

We also examined 58 late-life recurrent unipolar patients (ages 60–80) to determine if there were any differences on any of 29 EEG sleep variables between those with and without severe events, ongoing chronic difficulties, and all provoking agents. Similar to the midlife group of recurrent depressives, this older group was not free from stressors. Nineteen of the 58 subjects had experienced an acute severe event in the 6 months before onset, and 13 subjects had been living with a major difficulty during the same time frame. Close to half of the patients ($n = 26$) reported having experienced at least one provoking agent (either a severe event or a major difficulty) in the 6 months before they became ill.

There were no differences in EEG sleep between those patients who had experienced either a severe event or a major difficulty and their nonstressed counterparts. We did discover differences on two measures of delta sleep for those patients who had experienced any provoking agent ($n = 26$) versus those who had not ($n = 32$). Those with a provoking agent spent less time in stage 1 sleep (mean = 5.06%) than

with those without a provoking agent (mean = 7.14%) ($F = 4.24$, $p < .04$). There was also a difference between these two groups for total minutes spent in delta sleep. Patients who experienced a provoking agent had a mean of 43.04 minutes of delta sleep (standard deviation = 34.46) while their nonstressed counterparts had a mean delta sleep time of 24.82 (standard deviation = 25.05) minutes. No differences on any REM sleep measures were encountered in the analysis of provoking agents, severe events, or major difficulties.

COMMENT

How are we to understand the results reviewed here? The stress–diathesis model has been of great heuristic value in helping investigators to begin to think about the relationship among physiology, life stress, and psychopathology. In most cases, however, the model has been taken too literally. Interpreting Zubin's basic formula in a rather static way (which he almost certainly would have thought too simplistic), most of the investigations described above have approached the problem as a two-by-two contingency table, with stress/no stress on one axis and physiological perturbation/no perturbation on the other. The reality of the situation is undoubtedly much more complex. This does not mean we should abandon efforts to understand these relationships; rather, future efforts in this area must take into account the dynamic nature of the variables under investigation.

Physiology, by definition, does not remain static or show a single or immutable response to stress. Human physiology represents a constantly changing process, even in the absence of stress. In the face of challenge, the human body is prepared to respond and then re-equilibrate itself through a complex system of positive and negative feedback mechanisms. Even longitudinal studies can capture only small elements of this process. In addition, neither stress nor adversity is static. Sophisticated investigators in this area have long acknowledged that the threat associated with various kinds of adversity may wax and wane; some forms of adversity have little effect after a few hours or days, whereas other forms represent chronic challenges to the psyche and, almost certainly, to the body as well. Furthermore, some stressful experiences are relatively self-contained (e.g., temporarily losing one's child in a shopping center) with no long-term consequences or additional stress created by the event. Other kinds of events (e.g., the serious injury of one's child) can lead to multiple psychological, financial, and interpersonal stressors that follow from the event and extend forward in time. We would expect the physiological consequences of these two events to be quite different, particularly as time since the index event lengthens.

We still hold to the bias that the integrative approach is essential, yet more complex than many investigators, including ourselves, had acknowledged. In moving toward the future, it is clear that we need studies that take account of this complexity. It will be necessary to construct better articulated models through which we can explain how the internal workings of the body are affected by exogenous life stress, both in its acute form and when the stress itself or its internal representation in the form of traumatic memories or nightmares persists over time. A comprehensive model must take into account acute effects of stress, such as hypercortisolemia, sleep continuity disturbances, and increased REM activity, as well as the effects of persistent stressors such as elevated corticotropin-releasing factor levels and decreased REM activity. Whatever we do, very careful assessment of the acuteness versus the persistence of the stressors is required. A working model also must take into account the acuteness versus the chronicity of the psychopathology in question. This is necessary in order to be able to deal properly with both the physiological and psychological effects that prolonged periods of illness may have. In addition, as we look over the life course, we must think carefully about the natural age-related changes in the physiological parameters we examine, as well as changes in their perturbability as age increases. After understanding the aging process and its implications for a healthy individual, we can then proceed to examine the physiological correlates of adversity as they relate to psychopathology across the life span. A comprehensive, working model must encompass all of these changing aspects of stress and physiology, as well as the changing vulnerability to psychopathology over the life course even in the absence of life stress.

Acknowledgments: This work was supported in part by National Institutes of Mental Health grant MH30915 and by the John D. and Catherine C. MacArthur Foundation Networks on the Psychobiology of Depression and Psychopathology and Development.

REFERENCES

American Psychiatric Association. (1980). *Diagnostic and statistical manual of mental disorders* (3rd ed.). Washington, DC: American Psychiatric Press.

Beck, A. (1967). *Depression: Clinical, experimental, and theoretical aspects* (pp. 333–337). New York: Harper & Row.

Bem, S. (1974). The measurement of psychological androgyny. *Journal of Personality Assessment, 42*, 155–162.

Brown, G. W., & Harris, T. O. (1978). *The Bedford College Life-Events and Difficulty Schedule: Directory of contextual threat ratings of events.* London: Bedford College, University of London.

Brown, G. W., Harris, T. O., & Hepworth, C. (1994). Life Events and Endogenous Depression. *Archives of General Psychiatry, 51*, 525–534.

Bunney, W. E., & Hamburg, D. A. (1963). Methods for reliable observations of behavior. *Archives of General Psychiatry, 9*, 280–294

Cartwright, R. D. (1983). Rapid eye movement sleep characteristics during and after mood disturbing events. *Archives of General Psychiatry, 40* 197–201

Cartwright, R. D., Kravitz, H. M., Eastman, C. I., and Wood, E. (1991). REM latency and the recovery from depression: Getting over divorce. *American Journal of Psychiatry, 148*, 1530–1535

Coddington, R. D. (1972). The significance of life events as etiologic factors in the diseases of children—II. A study of a normal population. *Journal of Psychosomatic Research, 16,* 205–213.

Dohrenwend, B. S., Krasnoff, L., Askenasy, A. R., & Dohrenwend, B. P. (1978). Exemplification of a method for scaling life events: The PERI life events scale. *Journal of Health and Social Behavior, 19,* 205–229.

Dolan, R. J., Colloway, P. F., De Souza, F. V. A., & Wakeling, A. (1985). Life events, depression, and hypothalamic-pituitary-adrenal axis function. *British Journal of Psychiatry, 147,* 429–433.

Endicott, J., & Spitzer, R. L. (1978). A diagnostic interview: The schedule for affective disorders and schizophrenia. *Archives of General Psychiatry, 35,* 837–844.

Frank, E., Anderson, B., Reynolds, C. F., Ritenour, A., & Kupfer, D. J. (1994). Life events and the RDC endogenous subtype: A confirmation of the distinction using the Bedford College methods. *Archives of General Psychiatry, 51,* 519–524.

Giles, D., Roffwarg, H., & Rush, A. J. (1987). REM latency concordance in depressed family members. *Biological Psychiatry, 22,* 910–914.

Gough, H., & Heilbrun, A. (1980). *The adjective check list manual* (pp. 1–110). Palo Alto, CA: Consulting Psychologists Press.

Hamilton, M. (1960). A rating scale for depression. *Journal of Neurology, Neurosurgery, and Psychiatry, 23,* 56–62.

Hefez, A., Metz, L., & Lavie, P. (1987). Long-term effects of extreme situational stress on sleep and dreaming. *American Journal of Psychiatry, 144,* 344–347.

Hirschfeld, R., Klerman, G., Gough, H., et al. (1977). A measure of interpersonal dependency. *Journal of Personality Assessment, 41,* 610–618.

Monroe, S. M., & Simons, A. D. (1991). Diathesis-stress theories in the context of life stress research: Implications for the depressive disorders. *Psychological Bulletin, 110,* 406–425.

Monroe, S. M., Simons, A. D., & Thase, M. E. (1992). Social factors and the psychobiology of depression: Relations between life stress and rapid eye movement sleep latency. *Journal of Abnormal Psychology, 101,* 528–537.

Paykel, E., Prusoff, B., & Uhlenhuth, E. H. (1971). Scaling of life events. *Archives of General Psychiatry, 25,* 340–347.

Roy, A., Pickar, D., Linnoila, M., Doran, A. R., & Paul, S. M. (1986). Cerebrospinal fluid monoamine and monoamine metabolite levels and the dexamethasone suppression test in depression: Relationship to life events. *Archives of General Psychiatry, 43,* 356–360.

Spitzer, R. L., Endicott, J., & Robins, E. (1978). Research Diagnostic Criteria: Rationality and reliability. *Archives of General Psychiatry, 35,* 773–782.

Weissman, M., & Bothwell, S. (1976). Assessment of social adjustment by self-report. *Archives of General Psychiatry, 33,* 1111–1115.

Weissman, M., Gammon, D., John, K., Merikangas, K., Warner, V., Prusoff, B., & Sholomakas, D. (1987). Children of depressed parents. *Archives of General Psychiatry, 44,* 847–853.

Williamson, D. E., Duhl, R. E., Birmaher, B., Goetz, R. R., Nelson, B., & Ryan, N. D. (1995). Stressful life events and EEG sleep in depressed and normal control adolescents. *Biological Psychiatry, 37,* 859–865.

Zubin, J., & Kietzman, M. L. (1966). A cross-cultural approach to classification in schizophrenia and other mental disorders. In P. H. Hoch (Ed.), *Psychopathology of schizophrenia* (pp. 482–514). New York: Grune & Stratton.

Zubin, J., & Spring, B. (1977). Vulnerability—a new view of schizophrenia. *Journal of Abnormal Psychology, 86,* 103–126.

26

Adversity, Stress, and Psychopathology: A Psychiatric Genetic Perspective

Kenneth S. Kendler

How can the discipline of psychiatric genetics improve our understanding of the interrelationship between adversity, stress, and psychopathology? One logical way to begin addressing this question is to review possible mechanisms whereby genetic factors can interact with environmental factors to influence vulnerability to psychiatric illness (see Kendler & Eaves, 1986, for a more complete discussion of this topic).

MODELS FOR THE INTERACTION OF GENETIC AND ENVIRONMENTAL RISK FACTORS IN THE ETIOLOGY OF PSYCHIATRIC ILLNESS

When scientists consider how genes and environment impact on an individual's liability to psychopathology, they usually assume what might be termed the "additive model." This "commonsense" approach suggests that individuals inherit a certain level of genetic liability from their mothers and fathers, to which is added the liability created by their environmental experiences. Two important assumptions of this model are (1) that the impact of any given increase in environmental liability is the same for all individuals,

regardless of genotype and (2) that the probability of exposure to high-risk environments is likewise unaffected by genotype.

Two other models sometimes considered by geneticists can provide additional insights into the relationship between genetic factors and psychopathology. One of these models, best termed "genetic control of exposure to the environment," assumes that genetic factors influence liability to illness only indirectly, by altering the probability that an individual will be exposed to a high-risk environment. For example, there is ample evidence that familial factors, which are in part genetic, influence the risk for cigarette smoking (Eaves, 1980; Hughes, 1986). Researchers seeking a gene for adenocarcinoma of the lung might unknowingly come upon a gene that influenced the risk for smoking. Because at this time nothing would be known about the mode of action of this gene, and it would undoubtedly be noticed that people with the gene were at increased risk for developing lung cancer, the researchers might then conclude that they had found a "gene" for lung cancer. This would be true only in a special sense, however. In contrast to the oncogene, this "smoking" gene's action would be not physiological but environmental. By influencing the probability that an individual would expose his or her lungs to the carcinogenic components in cigarette smoke, this gene would create a high-risk environment. In one way, such a gene, like those that have a direct physiological effect, influences the risk for the end phenotype, but there are important differences. If cigarette smoking declined dramatically (e.g., as a result of increased taxation), then the impact of this gene on the risk for lung cancer would decrease. Such social action would have no impact on a more typical oncogene.

A second important model for the interaction of genes and environment in the etiology of psychiatric illness is often termed "genotype–environment interaction." It is usually easier to understand this kind of model if we call it "genetic control of sensitivity to the environment." This kind of gene action was first seen by animal and plant breeders. Some strains of plants could perform exceptionally well under ideal environmental circumstances (which might, for a plant, be soil type, fertilizer, sunlight, and rainfall). However, when these same strains were raised under poorer conditions, the yield was much worse. These "sensitive" strains (which were not very popular with farmers for obvious reasons) could be contrasted with "insensitive" strains, which might not do as well in the best environments but would do much better in the poorer environments.

One useful way to think about genetic control of sensitivity to the environment is that it is a result of endogenous homeostatic mechanisms. Insensitive strains have well-buffered physiological systems that can tolerate substantial deviations from ideal environmental conditions and still grow well. Sensitive strains, by contrast, are perfectly tuned to produce maximal output when the environment is "just right" but have little capacity to deal with environmental adversity. In tractable organisms (such as plants), we know that genes exist that influence the flexibility of these internal homeostatic processes (see Mather & Jinks, 1982, Chapter 5, for a more detailed discussion of this

topic). That is, genes exist that alter the *sensitivity* of the organism to the environment.

One example of this kind of gene action in humans is the hypertensive response to dietary sodium. Individuals differ widely in the degree of rise in blood pressure that accompanies an increase in sodium in their diet. This difference appears to be under at least partial genetic control (Kawasaki et al., 1978). That is, genes can make an individual relatively *insensitive* or *sensitive* to the hypertensive effects of dietary sodium.

GENETIC CONTROL OF EXPOSURE TO THE ENVIRONMENT

The subtler mechanisms of "gene action" in psychiatric illness are revealed in studies of possible genetic control of exposure to at least some forms of stressful life events (SLEs). Since their introduction over 25 years ago by Holmes and Rahe, SLEs have been a central concept in psychiatric epidemiology (Dohrenwend & Dohrenwend, 1984; Holmes & Rahe, 1967; Thoits, 1983). A model or hypothesis that is implicit in much of life event research is that individuals are passive recipients of their environments. This hypothesis predicts that the occurrence of SLEs should be largely random in a population because SLEs represent, in essence, bad luck (Fergusson & Horwood, 1987).

When stated this way, this hypothesis runs counter to common sense, clinical experience, and an accumulating research literature. The number of SLEs reported by individuals over time is significantly correlated (Andrews, 1981; Eaton, 1978; Fergusson & Horwood, 1984). That is, some individuals are more "event prone" than others. Research on specific events such as automobile accidents, industrial injuries, and criminal victimization has provided further evidence of consistent interindividual differences in "event proneness" (Gottfredson, 1981; McFarland, 1957; Tsuang et al., 1985). Other research has shown that the number of SLEs can be predicted by stable personal characteristics, including social class (Brown

& Harris, 1978, 1989; Kessler, 1979), self-esteem, social support, mood, and personality (Breslau et al., 1991, Brett et al., 1990; Brown & Harris, 1989; Cohen et al., 1988; Fergusson & Horwood, 1987; Lin et al., 1986; Newcomb et al., 1986; see also Kilpatrick et al., Chapter 10, this volume).

These results suggest that an etiological model for psychiatric illness in which individuals passively experience their environments is unlikely to be completely correct. An alternative hypothesis—that individuals actively help to create their environments—can be directly tested using genetic epidemiological designs, such as twin studies. One of the most powerful approaches to evaluating this genetic control of exposure to the environment is to analyze putative "environmental" variables like any other phenotype in a genetic analysis. This initially might seem counterintuitive. How can it make sense to submit an environmental measure to a genetic analysis?

Before answering this question, it will be helpful to clarify how genetic epidemiologists tend to think about the environment. When studying individuals reared in the same home environment, it is very useful to divide environmental risk factors into two categories. The first of these, alternatively called "common," "shared," or "familial" environment, reflects those environmental experiences that make members reared in the same family *similar*. Examples of such factors might be social class of rearing, dietary effects, cultural or religious influences, or parental rearing patterns that are consistently displayed to all members of a sibship. The second kind of environment, alternatively called "unique" or "individual specific," reflects those environmental experiences that make members reared in the same family *different*. Examples might include most stressful life events of adult life that are not shared with a sibling (e.g., being fired from a job, marital separation), childhood accidents, or aspects of the rearing environment that uniquely impact on one member of the family.

Returning now to the question of the genetic analysis of a putative environmental risk factor, if we performed a twin study (one could also get very similar information from an adoption study), it would be possible to understand how much of the individual difference in reports of this putative environmental risk factor is due to genetic differences between individuals, how much to differences in exposure to familial environmental factors, and how much to differences in exposure to individual-specific environmental factors. How would we interpret the results of such a study? If exposure to an environmental risk factor is *truly* random in a population, then relatives should be uncorrelated for exposure; a twin analysis should suggest that *all* the variance in liability to this environmental risk factor is individual specific. Many other risk factors might be correlated in families but for nongenetic reasons. In some cases, familial aggregation is a property of the event; a "network" event that occurs to a family member (e.g., death of parent) is, by definition, shared by other family members. Other risk factors might be related to the social class of the family or its place of residence.

In a twin study, such environmental factors should be correlated in twin pairs but, after accounting for sampling error, correlations should be equal in monozygotic (MZ) twins (who are genetically identical) and dizygotic (DZ) twins (who, like regular siblings, share on average half of their genes in common).

How would we expect these same twin study results to differ if it were true that individuals *actively* influenced their individual-specific environments? It could be that the traits that influence selection of environments are unrelated to genes, but the influence of genetic factors on human temperament and behavior is so pervasive (Eaves et al., 1989) that this is unlikely. What would we expect to find if genetically influenced traits such as extraversion or sensation seeking influenced the probability of experiencing putative environmental risk factors for psychiatric illness? We would expect that, in a genetically informative design such as twin studies, the "environmental" risk factor would be "heritable." In twin studies, the

Table 26.1. Twin correlations and the results of twin model fitting for selected categories of stressful life events

Life event/difficulty	Correlation[°] in		Parameter estimates of best-fit model[†]		
	MZ twins	DZ twins	a^2	c^2	e^2
Total	+0.43	+0.31	0.26	0.18	0.57
Network death	+0.47	+0.44	0	0.45	0.55
Network crises	+0.39	+0.33	0	0.35	0.65
Robbed/assaulted	+0.31	+0.19	0.33	0	0.67
Financial difficulties	+0.44	+0.12	0.39	0	0.61

[°]Polychoric correlation.

[†]Using Akaike's Information Criterion (Akaike, 1987) applied to results from LISREL analyses (Joreskog & Sorbom, 1989): a^2 = additive genetic effects; c^2 = common or familial environmental effects; e^2 = individual-specific environmental effects.

specific prediction would be that MZ twins would be more correlated for exposure to these "environmental" risk factors than would DZ twins.

Let us now turn to some data that can address these questions for SLEs. I am aware of five studies that have previously examined this question using a twin or family design. First, McGuffin and colleagues found that both depressed patients *and* their relatives had high levels of recent stressful life events (Bebbington et al., 1988; McGuffin et al., 1988). Second, Breslau et al. (1991), in a community sample, found that exposure to traumatic events was predicted by a family history of psychiatric illness. Third, in elderly Swedish twins reared together and apart, Plomin et al (1990) found that life events, reported over the entire life span, were significantly correlated in twin pairs, and the correlation in MZ twins substantially exceeded that found in DZ twins. Fourth, a similar finding was reported in the famous Minnesota study of MZ twins reared apart (Moster, 1991). Fifth, in an innovative use of the twin method, Lyons et al. (1993) found that exposure to combat stress in the Vietnam war was substantially more highly correlated in MZ than in DZ twin veterans.

In a sixth study examining this question, my colleagues and I examined stressful life events and difficulties (for convenience, both are here referred to as SLEs) reported

over the previous year in a large sample of twins from the population-based Virginia Twin Registry. The sample consisted of 2315 pairs of twins. SLEs were assessed by self-report questionnaire. Details of this study can be found elsewhere (Kendler et al., 1993); only the results of sex-independent models are reported here.

Illustrative results are seen in Table 26.1. For total life events, we found that the correlation in both MZ and DZ twins was highly statistically significant. SLEs were familial; they did not occur at random with respect to an individual's family membership. Equally important, however, the correlation of total SLEs was considerably higher in MZ twins (+0.43) than in DZ twins (+0.31).

When examined individually, most SLEs fell into one of two patterns. The first of these, illustrated by "network death" (i.e., death in a close relative or friend), was substantially correlated in twin pairs, but the correlation in MZ twins was very similar to that found in DZ twins. The second pattern was seen for most individual events (illustrated in Table 26.1 by "robbed/assaulted" or "financial difficulties"). Here, correlations in MZ twins were *much* greater than those seen in DZ twin pairs.

Model fitting further clarifies these results. For total life events, the best fit model suggested that genes, family environment, and individual-specific environment were all important, accounting for 26%, 18%, and 57%, respectively, of the population variance in total self-report life events. For network events, by contrast, the best fit model suggested that twin resemblance resulted solely from family environment. Sensibly, genes made no apparent contribution to the probability of experiencing death, illness, or a serious personal crisis in a close relative or friend. For most individual events, however, twin resemblance was due *solely* to genetic factors. In this sample, the "heritability" of being robbed/assaulted or having had a major financial crisis in the previous year was 33% and 39%, respectively.

What is the significance of these results? Clearly, genes do not "code" for life events as they do for cystic fibrosis or Huntington's disease. I would argue, however, that it is plausible that genetically influenced temperamental or personality factors, which are themselves moderately heritable (Eaves et al., 1989), influence the probability of experiencing life events. Our results are consistent with the hypothesis that some, or even most, life events are just "bad luck." For all the individual SLEs we studied, more than 60% of the variance was due to "individual-specific" environmental factors: events uncorrelated in twin pairs. However, these results argue strongly against a model in which the human organism is *entirely passive* with respect to its psychosocial environment. Rather, they suggest that, for psychiatric disorders, genetic control of exposure to the environment is probably important. In part because of differences in genetic constitution, individuals are more or less likely to select themselves into high-versus low-risk environments, exposure to which will influence their risk for psychiatric illness.

As summarized by Plomin (1994) in a thoughtful and provocative book, SLEs are not the only example of genetic control of exposure to the environment. Results from twin and adoption studies support a role, usually modest, for genetic factors in influencing social support, family environment, peer relations, and even television viewing.

Research has suggested that many measures traditionally used by psychiatric epidemiologists to reflect the "environment" are partially influenced by genetic factors.

These findings call for a rethinking of the concept of the "environment" in psychiatric epidemiology. Often in the past, epidemiologists have conceptualized the environment as something "out there" that impinges on the organism in a unidirectional manner. Our results support a more interactive concept of the environment in which the individual and the environment influence one another in a bidirectional fashion (Richman & Flaherty, 1985). Put in another way, these results argue for increased subtlety in considering gene action. For an organism as social as humans, our results are in accord with evolutionary theory (Dawkins, 1982) in suggesting that genetic effects mediated by behavior do not stop at the skin. Just as genetic factors in birds influence nest-building behavior, genetic factors in humans influence our social environment.

GENETIC CONTROL OF SENSITIVITY TO THE ENVIRONMENT

The other potential "subtle" model for the interaction of genetic and environmental risk factors for psychiatric illness noted above is genetic control of sensitivity to the environment. In this model, genes exert an indirect influence on the vulnerability to psychiatric illness by rendering the individual relatively sensitive or relatively insensitive to the pathogenetic effects of environmental stress. Previous studies of this question for psychiatric illness have been limited to adoption studies examining the possible interaction between genetic factors and early family experiences in the etiology of alcoholism (Cloninger et al., 1981), antisocial personality (Cadoret et al., 1983), and schizophrenia (Tienari, 1991). I here report results from analyses in the Virginia Twin Registry examining whether genetic factors influence the sensitivity of individuals to the depressogenic effects of SLEs. Details of this report are available elsewhere (Kendler et al., 1995). Briefly, we conducted logistic discrete time survival analyses [comprising 53,215 person-months of exposure and 492 onsets of major depression (MD)] in our on-going study of female–female adult twin pairs. Twins were divided into four categories of genetic risk as a function of zygosity and lifetime history of MD in the co-twin. In order of increasing risk, they are MZ twin/co-twin unaffected, DZ twin/co-twin unaffected, DZ twin/co-twin affected, and MZ twin/co-twin affected. SLEs and depressive onsets were assessed for the year prior to personal interview and dated to the nearest month. Our analyses examined nine personal events and three aggregate network events. We utilized criteria in the *Diagnostic and Statistical Manual of Mental Disorders (Third Edition, Revised)* (American Psychiatric Association, 1987) to diagnose MD except that episodes of "normal" grief meeting all other diagnostic criteria were not excluded.

As previously shown by many investigators (e.g., Bebbington et al., 1984; Brown & Harris, 1978; Costello, 1982; Paykel 1978), SLEs were strongly related to the onset of MD in our sample. Four events that had odds ratios of 10 or greater constituted a post hoc category of "severe" events: death of close relative, assault, serious marital problems and divorce/romantic breakup.

Because the dependent variable in these analyses—the onset of MD—was dichotomous, our discrete time survival analyses utilized logistic regression to test for the main effects of SLEs, the main effects of genetic risk, and their interaction in predicting onset of MD. Although logistic regression is a statistically convenient method of analysis, it is important to remember that, in these analyses, the dependent variable is *not* the probability of onset (p), but the natural logarithm of p [in the formula ln $p/(1 - p)$]. This use of a log scale dramatically changes the nature of what we mean by an interaction. *What is multiplicative on the scale of probabilities is additive on the scale of the log of probabilities.*

When both genetic factors and SLEs were entered as independent variables in our analysis, we obtained very strong statistical evidence for main effects of both variables in predicting depressive onsets. However, despite these massive main effects, we found no statistically significant interaction between genes and SLEs in predicting the onset of MD. This same pattern (strong main effects for both genes and environment but no significant interactions) was seen in nine of the ten individual SLEs. These results suggest that, on the scale of the log of probabilities, genes and SLEs act additively in predicting onset of MD. However, when viewed on the scale of probabilities, these results predict that their interaction should be multiplicative (as predicted by a model of genetic control of sensitivity to the environment, in which the absolute increased risk for MD would be greater in people with more sensitive genotypes). To test this on the scale of probabilities, we then performed, for any severe event, a laborious discrete time survival *linear* regression using an iterative method to reduce, but by no means eliminate, heteroscadasticity. As expected, we found very strong main effects for genetic factors and SLEs, but now the interaction term was statistically significant. On the scale of probabilities, genetic factors and SLEs do indeed interact to predict onset of MD.

This can be illustrated by examining the risk of onset of MD as a function of genetic risk and event exposure predicted by the best-fitting model. In those twins with the lowest genetic risk (MZ twin/co-twin with no lifetime history of MD), the probabilities of a depressive onset per month were estimated at 0.5% and 6.2% in those unexposed versus exposed to a severe SLE, respectively. In those at highest genetic risk (MZ twin/co-twin with a lifetime history of MD), the respective figures were 1.1% and 14.6%.

As predicted by the model of genetic control of sensitivity to the environment, the *absolute* increase in risk for MD, given a severe SLE, was about twice as high in those subjects at high genetic risk (14.6 − 1.1 = 13.5%) as in those at low genetic risk (6.2 − 0.5 = 5.7%). Although genetic factors do appear to increase the risk for MD in the absence of severe SLEs, they also increase the sensitivity of individuals to the depressogenic effects of stressful events.

psychiatric illness and that which has emphasized environmental causation will undoubtedly be to the benefit of both. (p. 288)

CONCLUSION

Genetic factors play an important etiological role in most, if not all, major psychiatric disorders. A thorough understanding of the interrelationship between adversity, stress, and psychopathology therefore will not be possible without considering gene action. My goal in this review was to suggest that genetic factors may influence vulnerability to psychiatric disorders in subtler (and more interesting) ways than are commonly considered. In particular, I have endeavored to show that psychiatric genetics and psychiatric epidemiology are natural allies in the endeavor to explicate the causes of psychiatric illness. Many (but not all) "environmental" effects on psychiatric illness can be fully understood only by considering the ways in which their etiology and impact on disease vulnerability are mediated by genetic factors. Many (but not all) genetic effects on the vulnerability to psychiatric illness cannot be fully understood without considering how, via genetic control of exposure to the environment or genetic control of sensitivity to the environment, they interact with environmental risk factors.

I close with a quotation from a paper I coauthored with Lindon Eaves (Kendler & Eaves, 1986):

It is our conviction that a complete understanding of the etiology of most psychiatric disorders will require an understanding of the relevant genetic risk factors, the relevant environmental risk factors, and the ways in which these two sets of risk factors interact. Such an understanding will only arise from research in which the important environmental variables are measured in a genetically informative design. Such research will require a synthesis of research traditions that have often been at odds with one another in the past. This interaction between the research tradition that has focused on the genetic etiology of

REFERENCES

Akaike, H. (1987). Factor analysis and AIC. *Psychometrika, 52,* 317–332.

American Psychiatric Association. (1987). *Diagnostic and statistical manual of mental disorders* (3rd ed., rev.). Washington, DC: American Psychiatric Press.

Andrews, G. (1981). A prospective study of life events and psychological symptoms. *Psychological Medicine, 11,* 795–801.

Bebbington, P. E., Brugha, T. S., MacCarthy, B., et al. (1988). The Camberwell Collaborative Depression Study: I. Depressed probands: Adversity and the form of depression. *British Journal of Psychiatry, 152,* 754–765.

Bebbington, P. E., Sturt, E., Tennant, C., et al. (1984). Misfortune and resilience: A community study of women. *Psychological Medicine, 14,* 347–363.

Breslau, N., Davis, G. C., Andreski, P., et al. (1991). Traumatic events and post-traumatic stress disorder in an urban population of young adults. *Archives of General Psychiatry, 48,* 216–222.

Brett, J. F., Brief, A. P., Burke, M. J., et al. (1990). Negative affectivity and the reporting of stressful life events. *Health Psychology, 9,* 57–68.

Brown, G. W., & Harris, T. O. (1978). *Social origins of depression: A study of psychiatric disorder in women.* London: Tavistock.

Brown, G. W., & Harris, T. O. (Eds.). (1989). *Life events and illness.* New York: Guilford Press.

Cadoret, R. J., Cain, C. A., & Crowe, R. R. (1983). Evidence for gene-environment interacton in the development of adolescent antisocial behavior. *Behavioral Genetics, 13,* 301–310.

Cloninger, C. R., Bohman, M., & Sigvardsson, S. (1981). Inheritance of alcohol abuse: Cross-fostering analysis of adopted men. *Archives of General Psychiatry, 38,* 861–868.

Cohen, L. H., Towbes, L. C., & Flocco, R. (1988). Effects of induced mood on self-reported life events and perceived and received social support. *Journal of Personality and Social Psychology, 55,* 669–674.

Costello, C. G. (1982). Social factors associated with depression: A retrospective community study. *Psychological Medicine, 12,* 329–339.

Dawkins, R. (1982). *The extended phenotype: The gene as the unit of selection.* London: Oxford University Press.

Dohrenwend, B. S., & Dohrenwend, B. P. (Eds.). (1984). *Stressful life events and their context.* New Brunswick, NJ: Rutgers University Press.

Eaton, W. (1978). Life events, social supports, and psychiatric symptoms: A re-analysis of the New Haven data. *Journal of Health and Social Behavior, 19,* 230–234.

Eaves, L. J., Eysenck, H. J., Martin, N. G., et al. (1989). *Genes, culture and personality: An empirical approach.* London: Oxford University Press.

Eysenck, H. J., & Eaves, L. J. (1980). The genetics of smoking. In H. J. Eysenck (Ed.), *The causes and effects of smoking* (pp. 140–314). Beverly Hills, CA: Sage.

Fergusson, D. M., & Horwood, L. J. (1984). Life events and depression in women: A structural equation model. *Psychological Medicine, 14,* 881–889.

Fergusson, D. M., & Horwood, L. J. (1987). Vulnerability to life event exposure. *Psychological Medicine, 17,* 739–749.

Gottfredson, M. R. (1981). On the etiology of criminal victimization. *Journal of Criminal Law and Criminology, 72,* 714–726.

Holmes, T. H., & Rahe, R. H. (1967). The Social Readjustment Rating Scale. *Journal of Psychosomatic Research, 11,* 213–218.

Hughes, J. R. (1986). Genetics of smoking: A brief review. *Behavioral Therapy, 17,* 335–345.

Joreskog, K. G., & Sorbom, D. (1989). *LISREL 7: A guide to the program and applications* (2nd ed.). Chicago, IL: SPSS, Inc.

Kawasaki, T., Delea, C. S., & Bartter, F. C. 1978). The effect of high-sodium and low-sodium intakes on blood pressure and other related variables in human subjects with idiopathic hypertension. *American Journal of Medicine, 64,* 193–198.

Kendler, K. S., Kessler, R. C., Walters, E. E., MacLean, C. J., Sham, P. C., Neale, M. C., Health, A. C., & Eaves, L. J. (1995). Stressful life events, genetic liability and onset of an episode of major depression in women. *American Journal of Psychiatry, 152,* 833–842.

Kendler, K. S., & Eaves, L. J. (1986). Models for the joint effect of genotype and environment on liability to psychiatric illness. *American Journal of Psychiatry, 143,* 279–289.

Kendler, K. S., Neale, M. C., Kessler, R. C., et al. (1993). A twin study of recent life events and difficulties. *Archives of General Psychiatry, 50,* 589–596.

Kessler, R. C. (1979). Stress, social status, and psychological distress. *Journal of Health and Social Behavior, 20,* 259–273.

Lin, N., Dean, A., & Ensel, W. (1986). *Social support, life events, and depression.* New York: Academic Press.

Lyons, M. J., Goldberg, J., Eisen, S. A., et al. (1993). Do genes influence exposure to trauma? A twin study of combat. *American Journal of Medical Genetics, 48,* 22–27.

Mather, K., & Jinks, J. L. (1982). *Biometrical genetics: The study of continuous variation* (3rd ed.). London: Chapman & Hall.

McFarland, R. A. (1957). The role of human factors in accidental trauma. *American Journal of Medical Science, 234,* 1–26.

McGuffin, P., Katz, R., & Bebbington, P. (1988). The Camberwell Collaborative Depression Study: III. Depression and adversity in the relatives of depressed probands. *British Journal of Psychiatry, 152,* 775–782.

Moster, M. (1991). *Stressful life events: Genetic and environmental components and their relationship to affective symptomatology.* Ph.D. thesis, University of Minnesota, St. Paul.

Newcomb, M. D., Huba, G. J., and Bentler, P. M. (1986). Life change events among adolescents: An empirical consideration of some methodologic issues. *Journal of Nervous and Mental Disease, 174,* 280–289.

Paykel, E. S. (1978). Contribution of life events to causation of psychiatric illness. *Psychological Medicine, 8,* 245–253.

Plomin, R. (1994). *Genetics and experience: The interplay between nature and nurture* (Sage Series on Individual Differences and Development, Vol. 6). Thousand Oaks, CA: Sage.

Plomin, R., Lichtenstein, P., Pedersen, N., et al. (1990). Genetic influences on life events during the last half of the life span. *Psychology and Aging, 5,* 25–30.

Richman, J. A., & Flaherty, J. A. (1985). Stress, coping resources, and psychiatric disorders: Alternative paradigms from a life cycle perspective. *Comprehensive Psychiatry, 26,* 456–465.

Thoits, P. A. (1983). Dimensions of life events that influence psychological distress: An evaluation and synthesis of the literature. In H. B. Kaplan (Ed.), *Psychosocial stress: Trends in theory and research* (pp. 33–102). New York: Academic Press.

Tienari, P. (1991). Interaction between genetic vulnerability and family environment: The Finnish adoptive family study of schizophrenia. *Acta Psychiatrica Scandinavica, 84,* 460–465.

Tsuang, M. T., Boor, M., & Fleming, J. A. (1985). Psychiatric aspects of traffic accidents. *American Journal of Psychiatry, 142,* 538–546.

27

Effects of Improving Achievement on Aggressive Behavior and of Improving Aggressive Behavior on Achievement Through Two Preventive Interventions: An Investigation of Causal Paths

Sheppard G. Kellam
Lawrence S. Mayer
George W. Rebok
Wesley E. Hawkins

Early learning problems and aggressive behavior have problematic consequences extending far into the life course, and they have been found to be correlated early in children's schooling (Jorm et al., 1986; Kellam et al., 1975; Maughn et al., 1985; Tremblay et al., 1992). However, the processes underlying the negative correlation between poor achievement and early aggressive behavior are not clear (Hinshaw, 1992). In this chapter, we report the results of experimentally testing whether improving one maladaptive response to classroom task demands produces change in the other in an effort to determine whether there is a functional and possibly etiological direction underlying their negative correlation.

Poor achievement has been shown to predict psychiatric distress, particularly depressed mood and possibly depressive disorder, among vulnerable children (Ialongo et al., 1993; Kellam et al., 1983; Kellam et al., 1991; Shaffer et al., 1979). Aggressive behavior in the form of breaking rules, truancy, and fighting at least as early as first grade has been found repeatedly to predict later antisocial behavior and criminality, as well as heavy substance abuse, including IV drug use, especially in boys (Block et al., 1988; Ensminger et al., 1983; Farrington et al., 1988; Kellam et al., 1983; Robins, 1978; Shedler & Block, 1990; Tomas et al., 1990; Tremblay et al., 1992). Some studies report common long-term outcomes from both poor achievement and early aggressive behavior (Farrington et al., 1988; Robins, 1978). Others reveal different specific outcomes of each maladaptive response (Ensminger et al., 1983; Kellam et al., 1983;

B. Maughn, personal communication, 1993; Maughn et al., 1985). In developmental epidemiological studies carried out in Woodlawn, a poor African-American neighborhood in Chicago, school dropout was predicted by a combination of early learning problems and aggressive behavior (Ensminger & Slusarcick, 1992), suggesting the possible developmental role of both poor achievement and early aggressive behavior in this outcome.

The etiological question is whether aggressive behavior is in part the vulnerable child's response to failure to master the teacher's demand to learn, or poor achievement is the consequence of aggressive behavior, or each leads to the other, or neither leads to the other but each stems from another source or sources shared with each other in a way that produces the correlation between them. The answers are important for understanding the etiological and developmental roles of aggressive behavior and poor achievement, and the prevention of later antisocial behavior, conduct disorder, and heavy drug use, as well as psychiatric symptoms, particularly depressive symptoms and possibly disorders, among vulnerable children. From a pragmatic perspective, the answers are important for determining whether developmentally based preventive intervention programs aimed at these target outcomes should be directed at poor achievement, aggressive behavior, both, or a third factor not yet identified.

The two preventive interventions were carried out in 19 elementary schools in eastern Baltimore. The first intervention, Mastery Learning (ML), was directed at improving reading achievement (Block & Burns, 1976; Dolan, 1986; Guskey, 1985). The second intervention, the Good Behavior Game (GBG), was directed at reducing aggressive behavior (Barrish et al., 1969; Robinson & Swanton, 1980). Each intervention resulted in measurable impact on its own target over the course of first grade (Dolan et al., 1993; Kellam et al., 1994b) and, at least in the case of GBG, as far later as the transition into middle school (Kellam et al., 1994a).

THE DEVELOPMENTAL EPIDEMIOLOGICAL FRAMEWORK

Our conceptual framework for this prevention research is centered on the integration of life course development, community epidemiology, and preventive intervention trials. Life course development calls attention to developmental paths leading to healthy or disordered outcomes, community epidemiology highlights the variation in developmental paths within a community and its ecological contexts, and preventive intervention trials focus on testing the malleability of antecedents along paths and the consequences for developmental outcomes of changing antecedents (Kellam & Rebok, 1992). This framework requires increasing specification and modeling of risk and resilience factors in the individual, in the environment, and in the interaction between the environment and the individual's behavioral, psychological, and physiological responses to social task demands [Kellam & Rebok, 1992; Kellam et al., 1975; National Institute of Mental Health (NIMH) Prevention Research Steering Committee, 1993; Sandler et al., 1991; Mrazek & Haggerty, 1994].

Specified risk factors from developmental models, such as aggressive behavior and poor achievement in the classroom, provide well-defined targets for preventive interventions aimed at determining whether an intervention can change the early risk condition, and whether the change produced can improve the risk of later problem outcomes. In this report, we are concerned with both the theoretical test of direction of effects and the practical issue of determining the effective strategy for preventing the distal consequences of each proximal target.

The interventions described here were developed out of this prevention research framework. The term *universal* was drawn from Gordon's (1983) schema and refers to the entire population (in this case entire classrooms) receiving an intervention, rather than only the high risk children. Our strategy involves directing universals at specific risk factors; determining those children who respond, and modeling the differences between those who do well compared with those who do not; and, in later stages of research, developing universals with integrated selected components for higher risk children. Behind the universal and the selected preventive interventions are the treatment levels of care which ultimately must be highly integrated with the levels of preventive interventions (Brown, 1993; Dolan et al., 1993; Kellam & Rebok, 1992; Mrazek & Haggerty, 1994; NIMH Prevention Research Steering Committee, 1993).

The theoretical framework focuses on the social task demands and the adequacy of responses of individuals in each social field relevant for each stage of life. At each stage of life, individuals are in a few major social fields where they are confronted with specific social task demands defined by a person or persons we have termed the *natural rater(s)*, who also rate the adequacy of performance of the individual. Parents function as natural raters in the family, and the teacher is the natural rater in the classroom. We have termed this demand–response process *social adaptation* and its measure by natural raters *social adaptational status* (SAS). Sometimes SAS is formal, as in grades in the classroom, and sometimes informal but having equally powerful consequences, as in parental responses to the child's behavior in the family. Chance, idiosyncrasy, and the actual performance of the individual play roles in the natural rater's rating (Kellam, 1990; Kellam & Ensminger, 1980; Kellam & Rebok, 1992; Kellam et al., 1975).

The framework distinguishes SAS from *psychological well-being* (PWB). By contrast to SAS, psychological well-being refers to the individual's affective status, self-esteem, psychiatric status, and neuropsychological and psychophysiological conditions, including the individual's cognitive processing. An example of the difference between SAS and PWB would be a child's poor grade on an arithmetic examination (SAS) versus the symptoms of depression (PWB) that might precede or succeed the test. Although SAS and PWB may be interrelated, they repre-

sent two distinct dimensions, and problems in each have very different long-term outcomes (Ensminger et al., 1983; Kellam, 1990; Kellam & Ensminger, 1980; Kellam et al., 1975, 1983).

At the center of this theoretical framework is the thesis that success or failure in each social field at each stage of life lays the foundation for subsequent social adaptation and psychological well-being. These relationships have been found to vary by gender and by the salience of a particular social field to the individual (see, e.g., Ensminger & Slusarcick, 1992; Ensminger et al., 1983; Kellam et al., 1983). The early antecedents targeted by the two interventions are socially maladaptive behavioral responses of first- and second-grade children to the specific, teacher-defined classroom tasks of learning the academic subjects and obeying rules and not fighting or disrupting classroom work (Kellam, 1990; Kellam & Ensminger, 1980; Kellam & Rebok, 1992; Kellam et al., 1975).

In this chapter we use data on standardized reading achievement scores from the California Achievement Test (CAT) and children's aggressive behavior ratings gathered from teachers during first grade. A major goal is to examine the mediating role that changes in each variable have on the other, or what we have termed *crossover effects*. Crossover effects concern the relationship between one intervention and the proximal target of another intervention in a set of parallel trials in which the proximal target of the first intervention is hypothesized to function in a mediational role in affecting the proximal target of the second intervention (Kellam & Rebok, 1992). In testing crossover hypotheses, we have been careful to distinguish analytically between mediated crossover effects and moderator effects involving interactions between the intervention and other independent variables (Baron & Kenny, 1986).

Results from previous intervention studies have produced only weak support for the existence of crossover effects. Although there is some evidence from the childhood hyperactivity literature suggesting that social learning–based interventions can lead to increases in on-task behavior and academic productivity, there is no evidence that such interventions can lead to normalization of academic achievement when deficits in basic academic skills are present (Gadow, 1985; Sprague, 1984). In such cases, as is discussed later, remedial academic instruction also is necessary (Gadow, 1985; Sprague, 1984). In a similar vein, Patterson (1986) points out that there is little evidence to suggest that crossover effects from academically oriented interventions to social behavior occur reliably in the absence of concurrent interventions targeting social behavior. For example, studies by Spence and Marzillier (1981) and Cohen (1980) showed that specific interventions for academic and peer-relational skills do not by themselves lead to reductions in antisocial behavior. However, in a study by Coie and Krehbiel (1984), academic skills training led to reductions in off-task behavior or, perhaps as a consequence, disruptive/aggressive behavior. Coie and Krehbiel also reported that social skills training resulted in improvements in reading comprehension, indicating the possibility of crossover effects.

There does appear to be some evidence for long-term crossover effects in the prevention of juvenile delinquency. In a review of early childhood interventions, Zigler et al. (1992) note:

Interestingly, longitudinal studies of some early childhood intervention programs are beginning to suggest that they may have an impact on future delinquency and criminality rates. These programs, although by no means standard in purpose and methodology, were never initiated to reduce delinquency but rather to prevent school failure among at-risk populations. (p. 997)

Zigler et al. (1992) cite as evidence several broad-based early intervention programs, such as the Perry Preschool Project and the Syracuse University Family Development Research Project, that have reported long-term impact on juvenile delinquency and predelinquent behavior. One interpretation of these results is that the programs produced greater school readiness, which in turn elicited more positive reactions from teachers, leading to a stronger commitment to school, followed by better academic achievement in later grades. This so-called snowball effect builds to more successful schooling, which eventually leads to reduced antisocial behavior and delinquency.

The major purpose of the present study was to test for crossover effects in an epidemiologically based sample of first-grade children through two parallel preventive trials. Consistent with a crossover model, we hypothesized that the achievement intervention (ML) would have a beneficial effect on aggressive behavior from fall to spring of first grade, and thus should reduce the risk of antisocial behavior and related problem behaviors in later childhood and adolescence. This effect results from improved school achievement leading to less aggressive behavior in the classroom; that is, achievement *mediates* the effect of ML on aggressive behavior. Alternatively, we recognized that there could be interactive effects among ML, fall achievement, achievement gain, and/or fall aggressive behavior on aggressive behavior in the spring. For example, children in ML who fail to make a sufficient gain in achievement might become more aggressive in the spring, in contrast to children who do make good gains. Or, the effect of achievement gain on spring aggressive behavior, for all children, could depend on the level of fall aggressive behavior. We have found examples of all these kinds of outcomes in related analyses of impact of the two interventions on their own proximal and distal targets (see Dolan et al., 1993; Kellam et al., 1994a, 1994b).

Our framework for understanding the etiology, course, and potential malleability of antisocial behavior relies heavily on the integration of our developmental epidemiological perspective with the developmental model of antisocial behavior described by Patterson et al. (1992), Patterson (1986), and Capaldi and Patterson (in press). In this view, children prove difficult for either teachers or peer groups to "teach" if their families have participated with the child in a coercive style of interaction regarding rules and compliance and have been unsuccessful in teaching children prosocial behavior. Deficits in academic achievement in these children are then a consequence of the rejection by teachers and peers that results from the child's noncompliant and aggressive responses. The GBG was directed at this rejection and the social integration of the child in the classroom, with the crossover hypothesis that, with better behavior by the child, teaching would improve and learning would then also improve. Based on this conceptualization, we hypothesized that the intervention for aggressive behavior (GBG) would have a beneficial effect on achievement. This effect was expected to occur as a result of the GBG reducing aggressive behavior. This reduction, in turn, would lead to improved achievement, that is, aggressive behavior would *mediate* the effect of GBG on achievement.

Once again, we recognized that there could be interactive effects among GBG, fall aggressive behavior, course of aggressive behavior, and fall achievement on spring achievement. For example, children in GBG who fail to improve in aggressive behavior may fail to increase, or even decline, in achievement. Alternatively, the effect of reduced aggressive behavior on spring achievement, for all children, could depend on the level of fall achievement. Because each intervention was specifically designed to affect its proximal target, no direct effects of ML on aggressive behavior, or GBG on achievement, were expected (Dolan et al., 1993).

METHOD

Design and Sample of the Two Preventive Interventions

This cohort of children began school during the 1985–1986 academic year. The interventions were implemented over 2 years; this study reports results at the end of first grade. The preventive trials are based upon a strong collaborative relationship between the Baltimore City Public Schools and the Johns Hopkins University Prevention Research Center, a necessary partnership for this kind of population- and community-based research (Jason, 1982; Kellam & Branch, 1971; Kellam & Hunter, 1990; Kellam et al., 1972; Rebok et al., 1991). The urban areas and schools were selected with the active involvement of the Baltimore City Public Schools and the Baltimore City Planning Department. Within five urban areas, three schools were selected and matched according to standardized reading achievement, percentage nonwhite, and percentage free lunch as described by Kellam et al. (1991). Within these matched triads, by random assignment, one school received ML, one received the GBG, and one served as an external control school. Four other schools were added as reserves to the 15 core schools. Two were randomly assigned one of the two interventions and the remaining two were assigned to the external control condition.

For each intervention school, teachers were randomly assigned to classrooms and intervention or internal control conditions; the children were assigned to classrooms in alphabetic rotation, thus holding constant school, family, and neighborhood differences. The internal controls provided for control over school, family, and community characteristics through randomly assigning children from the same community and school to classrooms and teachers within that school. Teachers were assigned to the intervention condition by a chance process, with the restriction that they intended to remain in the building at the same grade level for at least a 2 year period. The external control schools and children were an additional backup control group to safeguard against the possibility that teachers in the internal control classrooms might learn about and implement the intervention in their classroom, an issue that was constantly attended to by monitoring and training of intervention and control teachers. Teachers were representative of current elementary teachers in the 19 schools and were not selected because of specific interest in an intervention or because of positive evaluation by principals.

The Preventive Interventions

Both interventions were useful in the analyses reported in this chapter because of prior analyses showing success at improving their proximal targets (Dolan et al., 1993; Kellam et al., 1994a, 1994b). Although each was aimed as precisely as possible at its own proximal target, both addressed social adaptational processes in the classroom and classmate/peer group. The GBG was directed at integrating the behavioral expectations of teacher and classmates and, under the teacher's authority, reinforcing appropriate student behavior with collaboration of classmates and teacher, thus integrating the classmates and teacher in the classroom social system. ML also addressed the social integration of students in the classroom by assuring that the majority of children achieved a standardized level of mastery through group-based curriculum.

Details of the training are described in *The Good Behavior Game Training Manual* (Dolan et al., 1989b) and *The Mastery Learning Manual* (Dolan et al., 1989a). Teachers received approximately 40 hours of training in either ML or GBG before applying the intervention in the classroom. The training sessions continued throughout the intervention period. Great care was taken to provide equal time and incentives to all teachers, including control teachers.

Good Behavior Game

The GBG is a classroom team-based behavior management strategy that promotes good behavior by rewarding teams that do not exceed maladaptive behavior standards. The goal is to encourage students to manage their own behavior through group reinforcement and mutual self-interest.

After baseline measurement of precisely defined behaviors, the teacher assigned each child to one of three heterogeneous teams, ensuring that teams contained equally aggressive/disruptive children. While the GBG was in progress in the classroom, the teacher assigned a check mark on the blackboard next to the name of a team whenever one of its members displayed one of the specified disruptive behaviors. Disruptive behaviors included such items as *verbal disruption, physical disruption, out of seat without permission*, and *noncompliance*. A team could win if its total number of check marks did not exceed four at the end of the game period. Thus, all teams could win. Initially, children on the winning teams received tangible rewards (stickers, erasers), and later they engaged in a rewarding activity (extra recess, class privileges). In addition, all teams who won the most games during the week were termed the Weekly Winners and received a special reward on Friday.

During the first weeks of the intervention, the GBG was played three times each week for a period of 10 minutes. Duration increased approximately 10 minutes per game period every 3 weeks, up to a maximum of 3 hours, although the criterion for winning the game remained at four check marks. Initially, game periods were announced and the rewards were delivered immediately after the game. Later, the teacher initiated the game period without announcement and the rewards were deferred. Over time, the game was played at different times of the day, during different activities, and in different locations (such as in the hallway walking to the cafeteria). Thus, the GBG evolved from a highly predictable and visible procedure with a number of immediate reward props to a procedure with unpredictable occurrences and locations and deferred rewards.

Mastery Learning

This intervention consisted of an extensive and systematically applied enrichment of the ML instructional strategy in the reading curriculum. Key elements were clear statements of instructional goals and objectives; communication of high expectations for success; small, sequenced instructional units; use of formative and summative testing and use of corrective methods, with maintenance of teach–test–correct–test cycles; clear linkage between objectives, teaching, and testing; presentation of mastery standards for each instructional unit; immediate feedback to students; and clear and updated records of student progress.

Two critical aspects of ML were the development of a group-based approach to mastery and a flexible corrective process. With the group-based model, students did not proceed to the next learning unit until the majority (80%) of students fulfilled the learning objectives of the previous unit (achieving 80%–85% of objectives). The corrective process was tailored to the specific weaknesses of individual students and was flexible in terms of time, grouping strategy, and variety of correctives.

Study Population

The total population for the first phase of the intervention research consisted of 1196 children who entered the first grades of 19 Baltimore public schools during the 1985–1986 academic year, 1084 of whom were still present at first report card time when the first measures were done prior to intervention. By gender, the sample was 49% male, and by race/ethnic group, 65.6% African-American, 31.6% European-American, 1.6% other ethnic groups, and 1.2% unspecified. At the time of the first-grade assessments, the average age was 6.48 years (standard deviation ± 0.39). Among those not assessed, 27 either had transferred out of the participating schools prior to consent being requested or could not be reached for response to the consent request. About 5% of the parents of the 1196 children refused to allow their children to participate. Chi-square analyses revealed that refusal rates, although fairly low, varied as a function of geographic area, (χ^2_4 = 31.45, p < .0001). The highest rates of refusals were in Areas 1 and 4, which were made up primarily of middle-income, two-parent families living in well-maintained row or detached homes.

Assessments and Measures

Achievement Test Scores

Reading achievement was assessed by the total reading score (standard scores) from the CAT, Forms E and F (CTB/McGraw-Hill, 1985), administered in the classrooms during the fall and spring of the first grade by the Baltimore City Public Schools. The CAT scores were transferred to the Prevention Research Center as magnetic data files, with error and reliability checks.

Teacher Observation of Classroom Adaptation–Revised

Teacher Observation of Classroom Adaptation–Revised (TOCA-R) is a structured interview in which teachers rate the adequacy of performance of each child on the following social task demands: social contact, authority acceptance, and concentration. Teachers are interviewed for TOCA-R for about 2 hours during the school day in a private room by a trained member of the Prevention Research Center staff who follows a script precisely, responds in a sensitive and standardized way to issues the teacher raises, and records the teacher's ratings on each child. Teacher ratings in the fall and spring of one factor on the TOCA-R—Authority Acceptance (with the maladaptive behavioral response being aggressive behavior)—were used to analyze intervention crossover effects. The aggressive behavior scale includes items such as *breaks rules*, *harms property*, and *starts fights*. Two other factors—Social Contact (shy behavior) and Concentration (concentration problems)—also are included in the TOCA-R but are not included here because the focus was on aggressive behavior and achievement. The psychometric properties of the TOCA-R have been reported by Werthamer-Larsson et al. (1991). The alpha for the Authority Acceptance factor was .92. Test–retest reliability over a 2 week period was investigated in a subsample of 361 children from the sample of 1094. Spearman correlations and Pearson correlations between Time 1 and Time 2 behavioral factors were all significant, with coefficients ranging from .74 to .94. The behavioral factors were significantly associated with a set of concurrent measures, including spring standardized achievement scores, fourth quarter report card grades and work habits, and absenteeism during first grade. In addition, the behavioral factors were significantly associated with a set of antecedent variables, including gender, standardized achievement scores, kindergarten report card grades and work habits, whether the child repeats first grade, preschool experience, and changing schools between kindergarten and first grade.

In epidemiological terms, the TOCA-R and the CAT are first-stage assessment methods in that all children in the classroom are rated, thus providing an economical but ecologically valid method of simultaneously determining the social adaptational characteristics of the children and the social demand characteristics of their classroom environment.

RESULTS

Analyses of covariance were used to assess the direct effect of each intervention on the spring level of its proximal target, controlling for the fall level of the same target. Multiple regression was used to assess the direct and indirect effects of the first intervention on the spring level of the target of the other intervention. In these regressions, predictors of the spring level of this distal, or crossover, target include the fall level of this target, the change in the level of the proximal target of the first intervention, and a binary variable indicating membership in the intervention group or in one of the control groups (internal, external).

The control groups were pooled to decrease the standard error of the estimate and increase the power of the test of the relationship between the proximal target of the first intervention and the proximal target of the second. There was no indication that the relationship between the proximal and distal outcomes varied across the various

control groups, and thus no reason to avoid pooling. Separate analyses among the different internal and external control groups were examined, and results were essentially the same as with the combined controls. All analyses were conducted separately for males and females because of previous results showing marked gender differences (Dolan et al., 1993; Kellam et al., 1991). The statistical procedures and most of the statistics themselves are detailed in the tables rather than in the text to facilitate comprehension.

Effects of ML on Achievement and Aggressive Behavior

The first analysis of the crossover hypotheses examines the direct effects of ML on spring achievement and the direct and indirect effects of ML on spring aggressive behavior, with the indirect effect working 4 brendathrough achievement, the proximal target of ML. The results in Table 27.1 indicate that ML has a significant direct effect on spring achievement for both genders (p = .0006 for males; p = .001 for females). The second part of Table 27.1 indicates that, for males, there is a significant effect of gain in achievement on spring aggressive behavior controlling for fall aggressive behavior (t = −1.96, p = .05); there is no significant effect for females (t = −1.04, p = .30). The combination of the two results indicates a significant indirect relationship of ML to aggressive behavior in the spring for males but not for females. Table 27.1 also shows that there is no direct effect of ML on spring aggressive behavior controlling for fall aggressive behavior for either gender (t = .24, p = .81 for males; t = .91, p = .36 for females).

Effects of GBG on Aggressive Behavior and Achievement

The second analysis of the crossover hypotheses examines the direct effects of GBG on spring aggressive behavior and the direct and indirect effects of GBG on spring achievement, with the indirect effect work-

Table 27.1. Effects of mastery learning on achievement and aggressive behavior

Mastery Learning on Spring Achievement Adjusting for Fall Achievement (Analysis of Covariance)

Design group	N	Mean	Standard error
Males[*]			
Mastery learning	98	316	3.17
Controls	253	304	1.97
Females[†]			
Mastery learning	132	320	2.55
Controls	245	309	1.88

Mastery Learning and Achievement Gain on Spring Aggressive Behavior Adjusting for Fall Aggressive Behavior (Multiple Regression Analysis; Dependent Variable = Spring Aggressive Behavior)

Predictor	Coefficient	Standard error	t-value	Significance level
Males				
Constant	.72	.105	6.88	<.0001
Fall aggressive behavior	.74	.037	19.82	<.0001
Gain in achievement	−.002	.001	−1.96	.05
ML versus controls	.018	.077	.24	.81
Females				
Constant	.44	.08	5.44	<.0001
Fall aggressive behavior	.80	.034	23.01	<.0001
Gain in achievement	−.0009	.0008	−1.04	.30
ML versus controls	.04	.053	0.91	.36

[*]$t = 3.45$, $p = .0006$.

[†]$t = 3.16$, $p = .001$.

ing through the change in aggressive behavior, the proximal target of GBG. The results in Table 27.2 indicate that GBG, when compared with combined control groups, had marginally significant effects on spring aggressive behavior for both genders ($t = 1.54$, $p = .123$ for males; $t = 1.95$, $p = .056$ for females). These effects are less than those we found when we compared GBG with the randomized internal control children (Dolan et al., 1993). The second part of Table 27.2 indicates no significant effect of change in aggressive behavior on spring achievement controlling for fall achievement for either gender among either GBG or control groups ($t = −1.64$, $p = .101$ for males; $t = −1.52$, $p = .129$ for females). This analysis was then repeated, this time comparing GBG to the internal randomized control children to ensure that this null result was not due to GBG having a weaker effect when compared with combined controls. The comparison between the GBG group and the internal control group does produce significant effects of GBG on spring aggressive behavior controlling for fall aggressive behavior. The results were the same in regard to crossover effects; that is, no effect was found of improving aggressive behavior and thereby improving spring achievement.

Table 27.2. Effects of the good behavior game on aggressive behavior and achievement

Good behavior game on spring aggressive behavior adjusting for fall aggressive behavior (analysis of covariance)

Design group	N	Mean	Standard error
Males°			
Good behavior game	91	2.01	.072
Controls	235	2.14	.045
Females†			
Good behavior game	90	1.54	.052
Controls	244	1.66	.032

Good behavior game and change in aggressive behavior on spring achievement adjusting for fall achievement (multiple regression analysis; dependent variable = spring achievement)

Predictor	Coefficient	Standard error	*t*-value	Significance level
Males				
Constant	92.54	14.07	6.58	<.0001
Fall achievement	.83	.054	15.36	<.0001
Change in aggressive behavior	−3.83	2.31	−1.64	.101
GBG versus controls	.897	3.946	.23	.820
Females				
Constant	135.75	12.54	6.88	<.0001
Fall achievement	.682	.048	14.06	<.0001
Change in aggressive behavior	−5.27	3.45	−1.52	.129
GBG versus controls	1.42	3.88	.37	.714

°$t = 1.54$, $p = .1227$.

†$t = 1.95$, $p = .056$.

The combination of the two results indicates that there is not a significant indirect effect of GBG on spring achievement for either gender. Table 27.2 also shows that there is no direct effect of GBG on spring achievement controlling for fall achievement for either gender ($t = .23$, $p = .82$ for males; $t = .37$, $p = .71$ for females).

The above results indicate no indirect effect of GBG on spring achievement through aggressive behavior when any control group is compared with GBG. Also, there is no interactive effect on spring achievement between the intervention and fall achievement or between the intervention and change in aggression. Furthermore, the absence of a direct effect of either intervention on its distal target is demonstrated by the lack of significance of the direct effects in both tables.

Interaction Between Achievement Gain, Baseline Aggression, and Spring Aggression

Among males, rising achievement levels were associated with reduced aggressive behavior in the spring. There is evidence that ML produced a decrease in aggressive behavior by inducing higher achievement gain than occurred among control children. Turning to the issue of interactions, there is

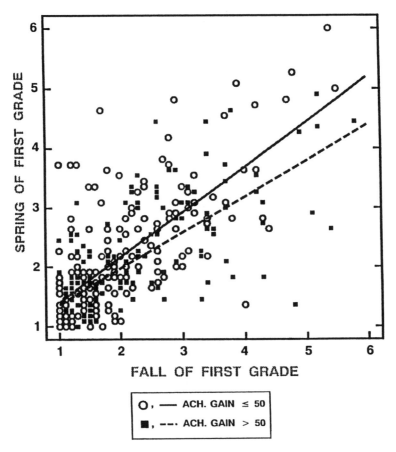

Figure 27.1. Teacher ratings of aggressive behavior in the fall and spring of first grade among males with lower and higher achievement gain.

no evidence that ML interacts with fall aggressive behavior or achievement gain to affect spring aggressive behavior. There is, however, a strong interaction that is consistent with the mediational model, namely, the interaction between gain in achievement and fall aggressive behavior. To demonstrate this interaction, we plotted spring aggressive behavior on fall aggressive behavior for males with higher gains in achievement and those with lower gains in achievement, regardless of intervention condition, cutting the children's scores at the median. These slopes and plots are presented in Figure 27.1. Examination of the plots indicates that the slope shifts because of a fairly uniform decrease in spring aggressive behavior among higher gainers and not because of a

small number of outliers. Males who were more aggressive in the fall and had a higher gain in achievement were less aggressive in the spring than those who were aggressive in the fall but had a smaller gain in achievement. The effect of the ML intervention among the males who were more aggressive in the fall was to produce higher gains in achievement (included among the high gainers in Figure 27.1) and, as a consequence of that, reduced aggressive behavior.

Crossover Effects of ML in Relation to Baseline Achievement

Next we tested the possibility that the crossover effects varied as a function of baseline levels of the proximal target. For the ML

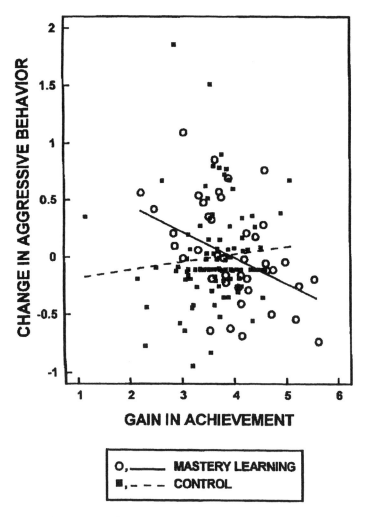

Figure 27.2. Change in teacher ratings of aggressive behavior from fall to spring of first grade among females with higher baseline achievement and higher gain in achievement in ML and control classrooms (multiple regression component plot).

intervention, we divided each gender into two groups based on their fall level of achievement, one group being below the median for that gender and the other being above. We repeated the previous analyses for these groups. For males, we found no significant effects, direct or indirect, and no significant interactions among intervention, fall aggression, and gain in achievement on spring aggression. For females who were above the median in fall achievement, we found a strong interaction between intervention status and changes in fall aggression

on changes in aggressive behavior from fall to spring (see Figure 27.2). Females who were higher achieving in the fall, were in ML classrooms, and had high achievement gain from fall to spring displayed significantly reduced aggressive behavior from fall to spring compared with females in control classrooms. Conversely, females who were higher achieving in the fall, were in ML classrooms, and had low achievement gain from fall to spring displayed significantly increased aggressive behavior from fall to spring over females in control classrooms.

Crossover Effects of GBG in Relation to Baseline Aggression

In assessing the variation in crossover effects of GBG, we divided each gender group into two groups based on their fall level of aggressive behavior, one group being below the median and the other above. We repeated the above analyses for each group. These analyses yielded no significant effects, direct or indirect, and no significant interactions among intervention, fall achievement, and change in aggressive behavior on spring achievement.

DISCUSSION

At least in first grade the direction underlying the correlation between reading achievement and aggressive behavior, based on these results, stems from reading achievement to aggressive behavior, not the reverse. If reading achievement is improved over the course of first grade, this leads to reduced aggressive behavior. This inference about directionality stems from the key crossover results and prior analyses of results of the two preventive trials. These show (1) achievement gains at appropriate levels over the course of first grade led to lower aggressive behavior among males, whether or not they were in ML classrooms, although the ML intervention contributed by inducing higher achievement gains; (2) females in ML classrooms had lower aggressive behavior in the spring if they were higher achievers in the fall and had higher achievement gains over the year; and (3) children who received the GBG intervention showed decreased aggressive behavior (see Brown, 1993; Dolan et al., 1993; Kellam et al., 1994a), but there was no increase in achievement.

Although at this stage of the analysis the correlation between achievement and aggressive behavior appears to stem from poor achievement to aggressive behavior, not the reverse, we need to be cautious in generalizing the results for several reasons. First, although the GBG intervention did not reveal evidence of changing achievement by reducing aggressive behavior, this finding is limited to this particular intervention and to the first-grade year. Furthermore, the relationship between changes in aggressive behavior and changes in achievement may be mediated by a third variable, with a likely candidate being concentration or attentional performance. In previous analyses, we found that concentration problems in first grade led to both aggressive and shy behavior as well as poor achievement in both genders (Kellam et al., 1991) and that concentration problems moderated the impact of the GBG intervention on aggressive behavior in males (Rebok et al., 1996). The role that concentration problems play as an antecedent to early aggressive behavior and poor achievement requires further exploration.

The absence of an effect of GBG on achievement through improving aggressive behavior could be due to a lesser effect of GBG on its own proximal target of aggressive behavior or due to other reasons. The amount of time teachers spent with children in the two interventions varied. The GBG was played initially for only 10 minutes a day 3 times a week during any subject, whereas the ML intervention was given every day for an entire reading period. However, each intervention had a highly specific effect on its own proximal target and not on the target of the opposite intervention. GBG, in particular, had measurable effects as late as the transition into middle school in these same children (Kellam et al., 1994a). The difficulty of interpreting a null result can only be resolved by replication with another possibly more intense intervention aimed at aggressive behavior.

The explanation of improving aggression not affecting improving achievement may lie in the nature of the skills each intervention induced. Aggression and achievement are not comparable with regard to individual skill components. Although GBG was effective at reducing aggression, learning to read requires new skills that may have to be deliberately taught through an improved curriculum. Unlike ML, which may have come closer to teaching new learning skills, GBG, in reinforcing reduced aggressive behavior, might require combination with a strengthened curriculum to link reduced aggressive behavior and increased achievement. It is possible that, over the course of the children's development and schooling, the impact of GBG on increasing achievement through reducing aggressive behavior will become apparent. We may find such results in later analyses, because longer term effects of GBG on aggressive behavior have been found (Kellam et al., 1994a).

Whereas the males generally showed an effect of improving aggressive behavior following improving achievement, only a subgroup of the females showed such an effect. The higher achieving females whose aggressive behavior was reduced in ML, but not in control classrooms, showed this effect. The reliability of this result requires replication and further modeling. These females entered first grade with a high level of achievement and continued to gain in achievement with a clear reduction in aggressive behavior. This result did not occur in control classrooms, suggesting that higher achieving children perceive the importance of reading and its rewards more clearly in ML classrooms than in control classrooms. Hypothetically, they learned through ML that their mastery of reading achievement was the key to greater acceptance by teachers and possibly classmates, and this provided them reinforcement for prosocial behavior. We inferred in an earlier paper that females are more attuned than males to how others, particularly the teacher, see them, at least in first grade (Kellam et al., 1991).

Why did the females mainly not respond in the same way as the males, with lowered aggressive behavior as a consequence of rising achievement? First we should recall that their level of aggressive behavior was far lower than that of males (see Kellam et al., 1994a). In addition, perhaps their sense of uncertainty regarding mastery affected them inwardly through depressive symptoms, rather than outwardly through aggressive behavior. We reported elsewhere that lower achievement in the fall of first grade

in females led to increased depressive symptoms by the spring, controlling on depressive symptoms in the fall (Kellam et al., 1991). This finding resulted from our earlier analyses of developmental modeling of social maladaptive and psychological responses to teacher's social task demands as baseline for the intervention trials. In another paper, we reported that increased achievement in females over first grade resulted in decreased depressive symptoms (Kellam et al., 1994b). Placing these last results about females with those about males reported in this chapter leads us to infer that males respond externally to uncertainty regarding their potential for mastery with aggressive behavior, whereas females respond internally with depressive symptoms.

Mastery of the core social task demand of learning to read appears to be central to developmental consequences that are specific to each gender. These results provide evidence for the role of mastery of reading achievement in aggressive behavior in males and in depression in females. The preventive trials provide evidence of the direction of effects and of the reversibility of the aggressive behavior and depressive symptoms by raising the level of reading achievement. The directionality of these results is consistent with other findings showing that cognitive problems lead to later aggressive behavior and conduct disorder (Schonfeld et al., 1988). However, other studies have shown that early conduct problems predict poor school achievement (Huesmann et al., 1987; McMichael, 1979) and future delinquency (Loeber et al., 1987). The lack of benefit on achievement of improving aggressive behavior reported here requires further testing, as we cautioned earlier. However, the results reported here provide a reasonably substantial basis for hypotheses as to the role of mastery in the antecedents of aggressive behavior in the classroom and the earlier stages of the gender differences in later delinquency, heavy drug use, and school dropout. Other reports cited above from these two preventive trials also provide hypotheses of the role of mastery in the early manifestation of depressive symptoms in the classroom and in later high rates of depressive symptoms and possibly disorder in vulnerable women as compared to men.

Why do males who enter school and succeed in appropriate achievement gain over the course of first grade have reduced aggressive behavior by spring? One hypothesis derives from the classic chapter by Robert Merton concerned with social structure and anomie (Merton, 1968). In this model, individuals who see themselves blocked from acceptance and advancement either become aggressive and lash out at others and the social system or withdraw or do both. Hypothetically, the males who are predisposed toward aggressive behavior respond to the uncertainty of acceptance by fighting others and the system as personified by the teacher and their classmates. If males can master reading and raise their achievement test scores by being assigned to an ML classroom, by having a gifted teacher, or by their own abilities, they may become more accepted within the social structure of the classroom. As a consequence of this reinforcement, they become less aggressive and more committed to school. Merton's model needs testing in greater depth to determine what cognitive processes are involved in the achievement link to aggression.

A child who fails to master a reading task and who feels blocked from the acceptance and status in class that mastery would bring might perceive the failure as leading to rejection by his or her teacher and respond aggressively in retaliation. Alternatively, the child might develop a pattern of interpreting such events in helpless and hopeless ways and respond by becoming withdrawn or depressed. This chapter is limited to the aggressive behavior–achievement correlation, but we note that the shy-behaving males may respond with social isolation to their failure to achieve and the teacher's and classmates' unacceptance, as suggested by Merton's model. Such socially maladaptive children will be the focus of another set of analyses. Our earlier Woodlawn developmental epidemiological studies in Chicago found strong predictive importance of aggressive behavior in first grade when cou-

pled with shy behavior (Ensminger et al., 1983; Kellam et al., 1975, 1983). Similar findings regarding the added risk to shy/aggressive individuals have been reported by Schwartzman et al. (1985), McCord (1988), Farrington et al. (1988), and Hans et al. (1992) in four very different populations.

In the next stage of research, we need to assess children regarding their own perceptions of how the teacher and classmates see them in regard to adequacy of performance, acceptance, and status in the classroom and classmate/peer group. The cogency of the Merton model rests on children's competence to compare their own status with that of others and to perceive the teacher's assessment of their social adaptation (Cicchetti & Schneider-Rosen, 1986).

A related explanation of the role of achievement gain in reduced aggression in males derives from the frustration–aggression hypothesis, originally advanced by Dollard et al. (1939). In this model, frustration leads to some form of aggression, and aggression stems from frustration. Thus the model would predict that a student whose achievement strivings are blocked or frustrated would respond by aggressing against others, and that this is the only factor leading to such reactions. However, it is clear that all aggression does not result from frustration per se, nor do frustrated individuals always aggress. As indicated above, they may react by withdrawing or becoming depressed. Subsequent revisions of the frustration–aggression model have attended to the mediating role of the affective experience (e.g., anger) evoked by the thwarting of goal-directed behavior (Berkowitz, 1969). Although the evidence that affective state gives rise to aggressive behavior has been inconsistent (Krebs & Miller, 1985), it does suggest some possibilities for prevention research. For example, if improving achievement improves children's affect, it may reduce the likelihood of later aggressive behavior. We presented in this chapter evidence that improving achievement reduces aggressive behavior. This may be mediated by improving the child's psychological well-being as reported in the paper on achievement and depression (Kellam et al., 1994b). The next analytical step will be to test whether the impact of raising achievement on aggressive behavior is mediated by the improvement of depressive symptoms that result from raising achievement.

We have reported evidence that achievement is strongly linked to depressive symptoms (Edelsohn et al., 1992); that lower achievement leads to depressive symptoms among females, and depressive symptoms lead to lower achievement among both genders (Kellam et al., 1991); that depressive symptoms have long-lasting importance from early in first grade (Ialongo et al., 1993); and that improving the experience of mastering reading results in reduction of symptoms of depression, particularly in females (Kellam et al., 1994b), and in less aggressive behavior, particularly in males. All of this demonstrated children's awareness of, and the importance they attach to, their SAS according to teacher and classmates. These findings are consistent with those of other research indicating that achievement plays a developmentally important role in children's social behavior with peers (Bursuck & Asher, 1986; Green et al., 1980).

We are already measuring the social adaptation of children in the classroom and the classmate/peer group, but we have not yet analyzed the child's own view of his or her social adaptation in these two social fields. Hypothetically, increased mastery of the social adaptational task of learning to read should lead to perception by the child of increased acceptance by the teacher and possibly also by at least some classmates. This increased acceptance should lead to reduced aggressive behavior as a result of seeing the classroom in a new light as a source of praise and acceptance. This acceptance also may provide higher achievers with greater amounts of practice and support in developing and refining their social adaptational skills (Coie & Kupersmidt, 1983; Green et al., 1980).

In studies such as this one, with multiple children in one classroom and one teacher doing the aggression ratings, the question of independence of the ratings is an important conceptual and analytical issue. One way to remove the nonindependence problem is to use the classroom as the unit of analysis. A major problem with this solution is that it ignores our overriding interest in the individual child in the context of classroom, peers, and family and the broader community. We have used peer ratings and independent observations in other reports (see Brown, 1993; Dolan et al., 1993), along with teacher ratings, but these are also not independent of each other from one child to the next in the same classroom. The problem is not merely one of nonindependence, but that the classroom is one of the set of hierarchically nested contexts that may influence ratings, development itself, and the impact of interventions. Other analyses we have reported include classroom, family, and peer characteristics in the models in the pursuit of mediators and moderators of development and its malleability (Kellam et al., in press). This is not a totally adequate solution, because the modeling of such complex sets of variables over time is certainly not a simple one. Multilevel modeling is an important concept addressing this issue, and we are applying and comparing analytical methods and results (Shinn & Rapkin, 1990).

As in our prior work on the impact of the two preventive interventions and the underlying developmental models, we found that impact differs for subgroups of children. Rarely do we find only general effects that fit all children in either of the two interventions. The predisposition or prior learning of the children may play a critical role in this variation. For example, all children may not respond according to the teacher's expectations; females may respond more than males at this age, some children may respond with shy/withdrawn behavior, others with aggressive behavior, and still others with both. Likewise, depressive symptoms play a major role in the children's achievement, and children may or may not be predisposed to depressive symptoms (Kellam et al., 1991, 1994a, 1994b).

Variation is usual in contextual influences and in children's responses to social task demands and the experience of failing the classroom tasks. This requires assessing variation among children in developmental modeling, not merely the means or central tendencies. These differences in the children and conditions also add to their variation in responding to preventive interventions. Indeed, the impact of the two interventions would be masked by diverse responses of children if we did not intentionally examine possible interactions of baseline severity and the interventions themselves with the effects on their proximal and distal targets.

The results presented in this chapter regarding crossover effects add improving reading as a key element to be further explored in preventing not only the consequences of poor achievement, such as depressive symptoms and possibly disorder, but also in reducing aggressive behavior and its consequences of delinquency, drug abuse, and school dropout. The vital importance of programs that enhance the mastery of reading and other academic tasks are supported by these data. If improving learning problems can reduce aggressive behavior with economical interventions such as ML, this kind of *universal* intervention can potentially help prevent the long-term negative consequences of both poor achievement and aggressive behavior. Children who need more than the universal intervention then become apparent by their poor responses to the universal intervention. A second (*selected*) level of preventive intervention can then be employed, with a third (*indicated*) level for those who need still more aid in socialization and development over the life course (Kellam & Rebok, 1992; Mrazek & Haggerty, 1994; NIMH Prevention Research Steering Committee, 1993).

Acknowledgments: We acknowledge the contributions of the City of Baltimore, its families and children, and the administration of the Baltimore City Public Schools. The Prevention Program is a collaboration between the Baltimore City Public Schools and the Prevention Research Center of the Department of Mental Hygiene, Johns Hopkins University School of Hygiene and Public Health. This work of the Prevention Program would not have been possible without the participation and support from the leadership, faculty, and staff of the School District. Our work has been based on the search of mutual shared interests in the assessments and interventions, and has been carried out under the aegis of the Board of Commissioners and the Superintendent. We also acknowledge the help of our dissemination coordinator, Ms. Natalie Keegan, who did her usual fine job. The studies on which this article is based have been supported by the following grants, with supplements from the National Institute on Drug Abuse: National Institute of Mental Health, NIMH Grant number P50 MH38725, Epidemiologic Prevention Center for Early Risk Behavior; NIMH Grant number 1RO1 MH42968, Periodic Outcome of Two Preventive Trials; and NIMH Grant number 1RO1 MH40859, Statistical Methods for Mental Health Preventive Trials; and for the follow-up NIDA Grant DA-00787.

REFERENCES

Baron, R. M., & Kenny, D. A. (1986). The moderator-mediator variable distinction in social psychological research: Conceptual, strategic, and statistical considerations. *Journal of Personality and Social Psychology*, 51, 1173–1182.

Barrish, H. H., Saunders, M., & Wolf, M. M. (1969). Good behavior game: Effects of individual contingencies for group consequences on disruptive behavior in a classroom. *Journal of Applied Behavior Analysis*, 2, 119–124.

Berkowitz, L. (1969). The frustration-aggression hypothesis revisited. In L. Berkowitz (Ed.), *Roots of aggression*. New York: Atherton Press.

Block, J., Block, J. H., & Keyes, S. (1988). Longitudinally foretelling drug usage in adolescence: Early childhood personality and environmental precursors. *Child Development*, 59, 336–355.

Block, J., & Burns, R. (1976). Mastery Learning. In F. N. Kerlinger (Ed.), *Review of research in education* (Vol. IV). Itasca, IL: F. E. Peacock Publishers.

Brown, C. H. (1993). Statistical methods for preventive trials in mental health. *Statistics in Medicine*, 12, 289–300.

Bursuck, W. D., & Asher, S. R. (1986). The relationship between social competence and achievement in elementary school children. *Journal of Clinical Child Psychology*, 15, 41–49.

Capaldi, D. M., & Patterson, G. R. (in press). Interrelated influences of contextual factors on antisocial behavior in childhood and adolescence for males. In D. Fowles, P. Sutker, & S. Goodman (Eds.), *Psychopathy and antisocial personality: A developmental perspective*. New York: Springer-Verlag.

Cicchetti, D., & Schneider-Rosen, K. (1986). An organizational approach to childhood depression. In M. Rutter, C. Izard, & P. Read (Eds.), *Depression in young people: Developmental and clinical perspectives* (pp. 71–134). New York: The Guilford Press.

Cohen, S. (1980). After effects of stress on human performance and social behavior: A review of research and theory. *Psychological Bulletin*, 88, 82–108.

Coie, J. D., & Krehbiel, G. (1984). Effects of academic tutoring on the social status of low-achieving, socially rejected children. *Child Development*, 55, 1465–1478.

Coie, J. D., & Kupersmidt, J. B. (1983). A behavioral analysis of emerging social status in boys' groups. *Child Development*, 54, 1400–1416.

CTB/McGraw-Hill. (1985). *California Achievement Test, Forms E and F*. Monterey, CA: Author.

Dolan, L. J. (1986). Mastery Learning as a preventative strategy. *Outcomes*, 5, 20–27.

Dolan, L. J., Ford, C., Newton, V., & Kellam, S. G. (1989a). *The Mastery Learning manual*. Baltimore: The Johns Hopkins Prevention Research Center.

Dolan, L. J., Kellam, S. G., Brown, C. H., Werthamer-Larsson, L., Rebok, G. W., Mayer, L. S., Laudolff, J., Turkkan, J. S., Ford, C., & Wheeler, L. (1993). The short-term impact of two classroom-based preventive interventions on aggressive and shy behaviors and poor achievement. *Journal of Applied Development Psychology*, 14, 317–345.

Dolan, L. J., Turkkan, J., Werthamer-Larsson, L., & Kellam, S. G. (1989b). *The Good Behavior Game training manual*. Baltimore: The Johns Hopkins Prevention Research Center.

Dollard, J., Doob, L. W., Miller, N. E., Mowrer, O. H., & Sears, R. H. (1939). *Frustration and aggression*. New Haven, CT: Yale University Press.

Edelsohn, G., Ialongo, N., Werthamer-Larsson, L., Crockett, L., & Kellam, S. (1992). Self-reported depressive symptoms in first grade children: Developmentally transient phenomena? *Journal of the American Academy of Child and Adolescent Psychiatry*, 31, 282–290.

Ensminger, M. E., Kellam, S. G., & Rubin, B. R. (1983). School and family origins of delinquency: Comparisons by sex. In K. T. Van Dusen & S. A. Mednick (Eds.), *Prospective studies of crime and delinquency* (pp. 73–97). Boston: Kluwer-Nijhoff.

Ensminger, M. E., & Slusarcick, A. L. (1992). Paths to high school graduation or dropout: A longitudinal study of a first grade cohort. *Sociology of Education*, 65, 95–113.

Farrington, D. P., Gallagher, B., Morley, L., St. Ledger, R. J., & West, D. J. (1988). Are there successful men from criminogenic backgrounds? *Psychiatry*, 51, 116–130.

Gadow, K. D. (1985). Relative efficacy of pharmacological, behavioral, and combination treatments for enhancing academic productivity. *Clinical Psychology Review*, 5, 513–533.

Gordon, R. S. (1983). An operational classification of disease prevention. *Public Health Reports*, 98, 107–109.

Green, K. D., Forehand, R., Beck, S. J., & Vosk, B. (1980). An assessment of the relationship among measures of children's social competence and children's academic achievement. *Child Development*, 51, 1149–1156.

Guskey, T. (1985). *Implementing Mastery Learning*. Belmont, CA: Wadsworth.

Hans, S. L., Marcus, J., Henson, L., Auerbach, J. G., & Mirsky, A. F. (1992). Interpersonal behavior of children at risk for schizophrenia. *Psychiatry: Interpersonal & Biological Processes*, 55, 314–335.

Hinshaw, S. P. (1992). Academic underachievement, attention deficits, and aggression: Comorbidity and implications for intervention. *Journal of Consulting and Clinical Psychology*, 60, 893–903.

Huesmann, L. R., Eron, L. D., & Yarmel, P. W. (1987). Intellectual functioning and aggression. *Journal of Personality and Social Psychology*, 52, 232–240.

Ialongo, N., Edelsohn, G., Werthamer-Larsson, L., Crockett, L., & Kellam, S. G. (1993). Are self-reported depressive symptoms in first grade developmentally transient phenomena? A further look. *Development and Psychopathology*, 5, 433–457.

Ialongo, N., Werthamer, L., & Kellam, S. G. (in press). Proximal impact of two first grade preventive interventions on the early risk behaviors for later substance abuse, depression and antisocial behavior. *American Journal of Community Psychology*.

Jason, L. A. (1982). Community-based approaches in preventing adolescent problems. *School Psychology Review, 11*, 417–424.

Jorm, A. F., Share, D. L., Matthews, R., & Maclean, R. (1986). Behavior problems in specific reading retarded and general reading backward children: A longitudinal study. *Journal of Child Psychology and Psychiatry, 27*, 33–43.

Kellam, S. G. (1990). Developmental epidemiologic framework for family research on depression and aggression. In G. R. Patterson (Ed.), *Depression and aggression in family interaction* (pp. 11–48). Hillsdale, NJ: Lawrence Erlbaum Associates.

Kellam, S. G., & Branch, J. D. (1971). An approach to community mental health: Analysis of basic problems. *Seminars in Psychiatry, 3*, 207–225.

Kellam, S. G., Branch, J. D., Agrawal, K. C., & Ensminger, M. E. (1975). *Mental health and going to school: The Woodlawn program of assessment, early intervention, and evaluation.* Chicago: University of Chicago Press.

Kellam, S. G., Branch, J. D., Agrawal, K. C., & Grabill, M. E. (1972). Woodlawn Mental Health Center: An evolving strategy for planning in community mental health. In S. E. Golann & E. Eisdorfer (Eds.), *Handbook of community mental health* (pp. 711–727). New York: Appleton-Century-Crofts.

Kellam, S. G., Brown, C. H., Rubin, B. R., & Ensminger, M. E. (1983). Paths leading to teenage psychiatric symptoms and substance use: Developmental epidemiological studies in Woodlawn. In S. B. Guze, F. J. Earls, & J. E. Barrett (Eds.), *Childhood psychopathology and development* (pp. 17–55). New York: Raven Press.

Kellam, S. G. & Ensminger, M. E. (1980). Theory and method in child psychiatric epidemiology. In F. Earls (Ed.), *Studies of children* (pp. 145–180). New York: Prodist.

Kellam, S. G., & Hunter, R. C. (1990). Prevention begins in first grade. *Principal, 70*, 17–19.

Kellam, S. G., Ling, X., Merisca, R., Brown, C. H., & Ialongo, N. (in press). The effect of the level of aggression in the first grade classroom on the course and malleability of aggressive behavior into middle school. *Development and Psychopathology.*

Kellam, S. G., & Rebok, G. W. (1992). Building developmental and etiological theory through epidemiologically based preventive intervention trials. In J. McCord & R. E. Tremblay (Eds.), *Preventing antisocial behavior: Inter-ventions from birth through adolescence* (pp. 162–195). New York: The Guilford Press.

Kellam, S. G., Rebok, G. W., Ialongo, N., & Mayer, L. S. (1994a). The course and malleability of aggressive behavior from early first grade into middle school: Results of a developmental epidemiologically-based preventive trial. *Journal of Child Psychology & Psychiatry & Allied Disciplines, 35*, 259–281.

Kellam, S. G., Rebok, G. W., Mayer, L. S., Ialongo, N., & Kalodner, C. R. (1994b). Depressive symptoms over first grade and their response to a developmental epidemiologically based prevention trial aimed at improving achievement. *Development and Psychopathology, 6*, 463–581.

Kellam, S. G., Werthamer-Larsson, L., Dolan, L., Brown, C. H., Mayer, L., Rebok, G., Anthony, J., Laudolff, J., Edelsohn, G., & Wheeler, L. (1991). Developmental epidemiologically-based preventive trials: Baseline modeling of early target behaviors and depressive symptoms. *American Journal of Community Psychology, 19*, 563–584.

Krebs, D. L., & Miller, D. T. (1985). Altruism and aggression. In G. Lindzey & E. Aronson (Eds.), *The handbook of social psychology* (Vol. 2, pp. 1–71). New York: Random House.

Loeber, R., & Stouthamer-Loeber, M. (1987). Prediction. In H. C. Quay (Ed.), *Handbook of juvenile delinquency* (pp. 325–382). Toronto: John Wiley & Sons.

Maughn, B., Gray, G., & Rutter, M. (1985). Reading retardation and antisocial behavior. A follow-up into employment. *Journal of Child Psychology and Psychiatry, 26*, 741–758.

McCord, J. (1988). Parental behavior in the cycle of aggression. *Psychiatry, 51*, 14–23.

McMichael, P. (1979). The hen or the egg? Which comes first: Antisocial emotional disorders or reading disability? *British Journal of Educational Psychology, 49*, 226–238.

Merton, R. K. (1968). Social structure and anomie. In R. K. Merton (Ed.), *Social theory and social structure.* New York: The Free Press.

Mrazek, P. G., & Haggerty, R. J. (Eds.). (1994). *Reducing risks for mental disorders: Frontiers for preventive intervention research.* Washington, DC: National Academy Press.

National Institute of Mental Health Prevention Research Steering Committee. (1993). *Prevention of mental disorders: A national research agenda.* Bethesda, MD.

Patterson, G. R. (1986). Performance models for antisocial boys. *American Psychologist, 41*, 432–444.

Patterson, G. R., Reid J., & Dishion, T. (1992). *A social learning approach: IV. Antisocial boys*. Eugene, OR: Castalia.

Rebok, G. W., Hawkins, W. E., Krener, P., Mayer, L. S., & Kellam, S. G. (1996). The effect of concentration problems on the malleability of aggressive and shy behaviors in an epidemiologically based prevent trial. *Journal of the American Academy of Child and Adolescent Psychiatry*, 35, 193–203.

Rebok, G. W., Kellam, S. G., Dolan, L. J., Werthamer-Larsson, L., Edwards, E. J., Mayer, L. S., Brown, C. H. (1991). Early risk behaviors: Process issues and problem areas in prevention research. *The Community Psychologist*, 24, 18–21.

Robins, L. N. (1978). Sturdy childhood predictors of adult antisocial behavior: Replications from longitudinal studies. *Psychological Medicine*, 8, 611–622.

Robinson, V., & Swanton, C. (1980). The generalization of behavioral teacher training. *Review of Educational Research*, 50, 486–498.

Sandler, I. N., Braver, S. L., Wolchik, S. A., & Pillow, D. R. (1991). Small theory and the strategic choices of prevention research. *American Journal of Community Psychology*, 19, 873–880.

Schonfeld, I. S., Shaffer, D., O'Connor, P., & Portnoy, S. (1988). Conduct disorder and cognitive functioning: Testing three causal hypotheses. *Child Development*, 59, 993–1007.

Schwartzman, A. E., Ledingham, J. E., & Serbin, L. A. (1985). Identification of children at-risk for adult schizophrenia: A longitudinal study. *International Review of Applied Psychology*, 34, 363–380.

Shaffer, D., Stokman, C., O'Connor, P. A., Shafer, S., Barmack, J. E., Hess, S., & Spaulten, D. (1979, November). *Early soft neurological signs and later psychopathological development*. Paper presented at the meeting of the Society for Life History Research in Psychopathology and Society for the Study of Social Biology, New York.

Shedler, J., & Block, J. (1990). Adolescent drug use and psychological health: A longitudinal inquiry. *American Psychologist*, 45, 612–630.

Shinn, M., & Rapkin, B. D. (1990). Cross-level research without cross-ups in community psychology. In P. Tolan, C. Keys, F. Chertok, & L. Jason (Eds.). *Researching community psychology: issues of theory and methods* (pp. 111–126). Washington, D.C.: American Psychological Association.

Spence, S. H., & Marzillier, J. S. (1981). Social skills training with adolescent male offenders. II. Short term, long term, and generalized effects. *Behavior, Research, and Therapy*, 19, 349–368.

Sprague, R. L. (1984). Hyperkinetic/attentional deficit syndrome: Behavior modification and educational techniques. In M. Rutter (Ed.), *Developmental neuropsychiatry* (pp. 404–421). New York: The Guilford Press.

Tomas, J. M., Vlahov, D., & Anthony, J. C. (1990). Association between intravenous drug use and early misbehavior. *Drug and Alcohol Dependence*, 25, 79–89.

Tremblay, R. E., Masse, B., Perron, D., LeBlanc, M., Schwartzman, A. E., & Ledingham, J. E. (1992). Early disruptive behavior, poor school achievement, delinquent behavior, and delinquent personality: Longitudinal analyses. *Journal of Consulting and Clinical Psychology*, 60, 64–72.

Werthamer-Larsson, L., Kellam, S. G., & Wheeler, L. (1991). Effect of first-grade classroom environment on child shy behavior, aggressive behavior, and concentration problems. *American Journal of Community Psychology*, 19, 585–602.

Zigler, E., Taussig, C., & Black, K. (1992). Early childhood intervention: A promising preventative for juvenile delinquency. *American Psychologist*, 47, 997–1006.

28

A Perspective on Adversity, Stress, and Psychopathology

Alexander H. Leighton

As an orientation regarding the meaning of the words, *adversity*, *stress*, and *psychopathology*, let me begin with some recollections of a case of Graves' disease that I encountered in the clinical literature while a medical student many years ago.

The patient was a young woman who set out one day to ride her bicycle through the Blackwall Tunnel under the Thames in London. When she was part way along, a team of horses, coming behind her pulling a brewer's wagon, escaped the control of their driver. The wagon was full of empty barrels, and the noise horrendous. The young woman peddled for dear life ahead of the plunging horses for the remainder of the distance through the tunnel, which was considerable. At length, she shot out the Greenwich end and leaped off her bike into the arms of a policeman. It was soon found that she had a full-blown case of Grave's disease—bulging eyes, tachycardia, fine tremor, inability to keep still and all the rest. Moreover, in subsequent months, as I recall, the disorder persisted until a portion of her thyroid had been removed.

Taking the word "stress" first, we may say that stress is that which happened to the lady—let us call her Miranda—in the tunnel, and we may note that in this case it was entirely psychological. Despite the fact that there had been a lot of noise, this was apparently never loud enough to do her physical harm.

Although her effort in peddling the bicycle was extraordinary and may have resulted in damage to her endocrine system, one can hardly call it pathological while she was in the tunnel because at that time it was part of an adaptation to the situation that functioned to preserve her life. In the aftermath, however, she was left badly handicapped as a result of one or more systems in her body having become overactive and unable to return to their ordinary relationships with other systems. The result was impairment of Miranda as an integrated unit —that is to say, as a person—and the chances are that without the surgery she would have died before long. An enduring element of danger had clearly emerged out of the complex of stress and adaptive responses.

Let us consider this in the light of a definition of pathology proposed by Rudolf Virchow, who is widely considered the founder of pathology as a scientific discipline (Ackerknecht, 1953; Virchow, 1860). Although

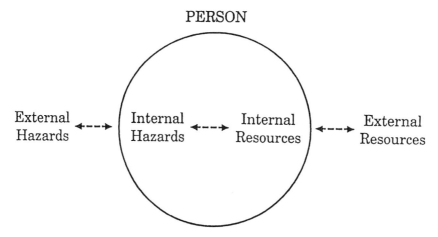

Figure 28.1. A person is a system of complex interactive and balancing variables. Stress is any influence that disturbs the balancing process. Pathology—including psychopathology—is an imbalance that places a person's survival at risk.

Virchow had organic pathology in mind, his notion is fundamental enough to include "psychopathology." Paraphrasing Virchow, one may say that pathology differs from normality by the obstruction of the functions on which life depends, or by their overstimulation, or by their occurrence in unusual locations or at unusual times. Such conditions involve risk to the survival of the person. Thus pathology differs from normality in *the character of danger* it poses for the continuance of life. Pathology, in other words, is not properly the presence of a lesion or a microbe and not a psychological condition of delusion or depression per se. These are happenings at the organically and/or psychologically emergent levels of integration that may play a role in the development of pathology. The pathology itself consists in the presence of a process that brings risk to the person's survival. It is not uncommon for it to consist of some normal process turned malfunctional.

One of the advantages of Virchow's perspective is that it makes it largely unnecessary to argue over whether a particular physiological or psychological pattern of reaction is "normal" or "abnormal." Any normal pattern that becomes life threatening is *ipso facto* pathological. Nothing is more normal than the clotting of blood, for example. It is

part of the mechanism that prevents us from bleeding to death in the event of minor cuts. However, if it occurs in a location such as the coronary arteries, under those conditions it is a pathological process. Virchow's definition of pathology, as you can see, is *functional* rather than structural or descriptive.

With respect to Miranda, her high level of metabolism in the tunnel was not in these terms pathological. However, its persistence after the restoration of ordinary circumstances *was* pathological because it was now itself a threat to her survival. The timing in relation to circumstances was clearly wrong.

Figure 28.1 may help in advancing our discussion. The person, represented by the circle, is here conceived as existing in an environment in which a heterogeneous mix of external hazards and external resources of varying degrees are of frequent occurrence on all sides. An important aspect of adaptation to life—the struggle to stay alive—consists in manipulating resources so as to neutralize the danger of hazards. In Miranda's case, the runaway horses were an external hazard, and her bike an external resource.

Comparable transactions occur inside the person between what may be called internal hazards and internal resources. Internal hazards consist in handicaps and vulnerabilities of various kinds among components of the person. Internal resources consist in the biological and psychological capabilities of the person.

So far as Miranda was concerned, it is reasonable to infer, because of the subsequent appearance of Graves' disease, that she had vulnerability somewhere among her systems that constituted an internal hazard. The burst of energy that got her out of the tunnel ahead of the horses suggests internal resources of considerable power in other parts of her physiological and psychological systems—at least for the short run.

It may now be seen that "adversity," "hazard," and "stress" have much commonality of meaning. The word *adversity* may have some greater suggestion of multiple components, prolonged duration, and bad luck. Having sketched certain main features of a frame of reference in which "adversity," "stress," and "psychopathology" can be understood, I must add some qualifications:

1. Had the clinical outcome for Miranda been more in the realm of psychological medicine—chronic anxiety, depression, or delusions, for instances—the relationships depicted in Figure 28.1 would be no less relevant but they would stand for different sets of particulars.

2. The fact that Miranda's case makes certain points vividly means that it is, as an ostensive definition, something of a caricature. The common run of cases in which stress plays a major role are much more gradual in onset and more multifaceted.

3. In previous publications I have used the terms *assets* and *liabilities* for what are here called "internal resources" and "internal hazards." The change implies no alteration in the frame of reference; rather, my desire in this paper is to emphasize connections among internal and external factors.

4. The word *hazard* as employed in the frame of reference signifies not only threatened injury but also actual affliction. In this it resembles the clinical term *insult*.

5. My presentation of stress is misleading because it fails to point out that low and absent stress conditions can be hazardous. Physiology, psychology, and clinical observation encourage interest in this other end of the stress dimension, especially during growth and development of the person. We also should have concern about conditions in the middle range between these extremes, where some degree of stress is often the optimal state for the maintenance of life.

Let us recognize also that we have bypassed the fact that the life of a person, as with many other organisms, goes according to a sort of "bauplan," a design plan that involves origination from a single cell, growth, development, maturity, reproduction, senescence, and death. As a consequence, the potentials for reaction to stress vary greatly depending on the part of this life arc a person is in.

Finally, we must note that the processes initiated by stresses in a person can spread laterally and vertically through *all levels of integration and their emergent properties* from molecules, to organs and systems of the body, to the whole person, and beyond to social organizations of which he or she is a part. Furthermore, this may be considered true whether the stress be run-away horses, experience of class or ethnic prejudice, destruction of culture, or loss of a confidant.

The "levels of integration," and the "emergent properties" of their phenomena at each level are empirical findings obtained according to the rules of hypothetico-deductive science. However, these have had much influence on forming the boundaries that separate academic disciplines, and with this has come strong melding with philosophical positions and traditional viewpoints. One consequence of this has sometimes been the formation of obstacles and false guidelines that mislead investigators who are trying to pursue questions across disciplinary boundaries.

AN ENVIRONMENTAL ETHOS

Some Origins

My impressions are in agreement with those of Dohrenwend (see Chapter 1, this volume), namely, that at midcentury there was widespread confidence in the etiological power of environmental factors. As Plomin and colleagues (1994) put it, "Environmentalism . . . peaked in the 1950s" (p. 1733). In terms of stress and the frame of reference just sketched, this can be described as a strong, even doctrinaire, belief in the determining power of external hazards.

If we think of a *zeitgeist* or ethos, however, there were a number of associated sentiments that also deserve mention. These included (1) a strong belief in science itself as a way to obtain greater knowledge about human motivation and behavior; (2) high confidence in the possibility of beneficial application of such knowledge; (3) a modest but definite inclination toward short-range hypotheses and empirical data, and skepticism regarding both the practical and the epistemological usefulness of monolithic theories at the present stages of knowledge; (4) willingness to work not only laterally within, but also up and down among levels of integration and their emergent properties; and (5) interest in collaboration among disciplines. Much of this latter interest was in conflict with traditional academic values, which tended to believe that each discipline should stay within the bounds of its own assigned parameters.

In the following discussion, I present some impressions regarding how such an ethos evolved. The topics chosen are only a small part of a much larger total, but I offer them as exemplifying the ambience in which the ethos arose and gained strength.

Between 1929 and 1945, two successive periods of history in North America and Europe did much to focus attention on external hazards and their potential for negative effects. The first was the great economic depression that spread across the 1930s, and the second was World War II.

Social scientists were among the first academics to be drawn into operational contact with problems posed by the depression. This was in large measure because the U.S. government recruited economists, and then sociologists and cultural anthropologists, as members of teams and task forces that were set up throughout the country to work first on measures regarding food, shelter, and bank closures, and later on how to promote recovery in socioeconomically deprived communities.

It was soon found that socioeconomic damage was enormously complex, with many streams of psychological, societal, and cultural domino effects leading to numerous unforeseen consequences. When sociocultural systems were thrown off balance in relation to each other by changes in economic circumstances, it seemed that they went through numerous swings and counterswings before an equilibrium of some kind again could be achieved. There were communities, for instance, that deteriorated in powers of adaptation to the point of becoming unable to utilize economic opportunities when they were again available—like a drowning person who cannot grasp a proffered rope. Remedial planners began to find it desirable to take such behavior into account. Aphorisms began to appear such as "If you destroy sociocultural structures of one kind, you destroy functional capabilities of many kinds."

Numbers of social scientists, together with many others who were trying to roll back the depression, came to think that socioeconomic malfunctioning constitutes a stress on individuals that in turn causes psychological reactions that seriously interfere with a return to a viable economy. Such reactions were seen as having numbers of different forms, one of which was "low morale," marked by copelessness and lack of initiative. Another consisted in paranoid ideation and violence, and this led to theorizing about "frustration" as a cause of "aggression." Again, it was anticipated that children growing up in malfunctioning families and communities would have their personalities malformed by their experiences and so become adults who were psychologically and socially impaired. It seemed that the effects of external hazards on adult individuals, together with their interference in the normal development of children, could lead to an array of malfunctioning individual patterns that would range from poor morale to psychopathy, criminality, and mental illness.

A sampling of the theoretical orientations being employed at this time would have to give prominence to sociological and cultural functionalism. Some of this took the form of updating Pareto and Durkheim and taking leads from the contemporary writings of Malinowski and Radcliffe-Brown—both of whom visited and taught in North America at this time. Cannon's (1932) "homeostasis" was also frequently mentioned, although it was on many occasions not clear whether the discussant regarded it as an analogy or as an ostensive definition. At any rate, the ground was prepared for the later popularity of Selye's (1956) concepts of stress, which were important to the North American studies in the psychiatric epidemiology of general populations (Murphy, 1986; Srole & Fischer, 1986).

The nature and location of many of the problems created by the depression inspired numerous studies of geographically defined communities. Of these, one of the most influential was the "Yankee City" work led by the anthropologist W. Lloyd Warner and his numerous colleagues from several different disciplines (Warner, 1937; Warner & Lunt, 1941). The act of choosing a community as a unit for investigation necessarily aroused interest in how the component systems interacted, and this created a favorable climate for cooperation among disciplines, for functional thinking, and for trying to synthesize theories that came from different levels of emergent properties, such as social structures, cultural values, and psychological notions of individual motivation.

I also should remark on the rise of problem-solving interests as contrasted to the more academic theory–oriented interests. Research often began with pragmatic questions and was expected to show results that could be used, and to do so as speedily as possible. Such a stance had its negative side, of course, in leading to haste, waste, and mistake, but it also helped foster an empirical orientation that gave rise to both practical results and, at times, contributions to basic knowledge. In this there was resemblance to how much of medical science works.

Psychiatry, unlike some of the social sciences, took little interest at first in the possibility of socioeconomic stresses playing a part in the etiology of mental illnesses. This fact may be traced to the net effect of two contrasting theoretical points of view within the discipline. One of these, "biological psychiatry," held strong convictions about the dominant role of inheritance and other biological processes as causes of mental illnesses. "Poor biological stuff" and "unmodifiable human material" were common expressions that summarized this perspective on causality.

The second point of view was equally rigid in holding that the answers to etiological questions were to be found in the psychosexual dynamics of early life. The distresses caused by economic losses were therefore regarded as mostly a matter of "normal human miseries" and consequently not of much relevance as causes of mental illnesses.

There was, however, a third point of view led by Adolf Meyer, the chief of psychiatry at Johns Hopkins. Meyer named his frame of reference "psychobiology," which today is confusable with "biological psychiatry" and the latter's concern with the organic causes of psychological phenomena. Meyer's meaning was different in that he focused on the functioning of the individual person as a whole—not on a part, a disease, or a lesion—as the object for psychiatric attention. In keeping with this, he put emphasis on multiple causes and the importance of the clinician's gathering and synthesizing all available "facts" about a patient's psychological, biological, social, and cultural experiences from infancy down to the present.

On the advent of World War II, the stresses in North America underwent change, but as a topic they continued to draw much attention. What was called "conduct in battle," for instance, grew to be a theme of major importance, and with this psychiatrists began taking an interest in external hazards. Two notable studies were Sargant and Slater's (1940) report on the retreat at Dunkirk and *Men Under Stress* by Grinker and Spiegel (1945). These and other works such as *Wartime Psychiatry* (Lewis & Engle, 1954) gave us new information about the great variety of patterns by which people react to severe external hazards, some of these patterns being clinically indistinguishable from mental illnesses. "Battle fatigue" became a commonly accepted model demonstrating how external hazards can produce psychopathology. Many such episodes had strong resemblances to Miranda's case.

Numerous discussions took place as to whether the main causes consisted in degree and kind of stress—in other words, hazards of the *environment*—or in degree and kind of individual vulnerability—such as *genotypic* structure, with environmental hazards playing a precipitating or unmasking rather than a causal role. Much less considered was the possibility that these ideas were too simple to be representations of the process, and that what most needed investigation was continuing *interaction* among the multiple factors and multiple reactions to these factors, which might then combine with each other to form networks composed of complex feedback loops.

In addition to clinically oriented studies, with an emphasis on how to prevent as well as treat "battle fatigue" and other psychiatric disorders, there were extensive investigations of the environmental factors that foster good and bad morale. With this went efforts to develop operations that could raise or (in the case of the enemy) lower morale

(Leighton, 1943, 1949; Stouffer et al., 1949a, 1949b). From these efforts came the need to reconcile psychological and sociological theories. Thus the word *anomie*, which originally represented a construct kept strictly at the sociological level, came to be widely accepted as a word also pertaining to the psychological level and to the interactive processes between these two levels. In the war context, morale was of course recognized by all as a matter of vital importance. The main question was whether psychiatrists, psychologists, and social scientists could discover things about it that made important sense. In the course of time, experience suggested that the answer should be a strong "yes."

When the period of economic depression followed by war was over, many of the scientists who had been working on human problems turned to the tasks of peace with a strong feeling that a new era was beginning. For numbers of us, this feeling of potential sprang from accomplishments observed during the war, and this gave it a sense of having a solid basis. No doubt it also was influenced by the public enthusiasm for science that followed the success of the atomic bomb, and from predictions by political leaders and popular writers that atomic energy would now "transform the way we live" (Udall, 1994). Depression and war had shown us how bad things could be but also gave visions of how to do better. From the perspective of social phenomena, this meant bringing about changes in some of the defective ways in which societies and cultures function. From an individual perspective, it meant alterations in the social environment such that external hazards would be reduced and external resources increased. As social scientists, psychologists, and psychiatrists of this period, we felt we had a start toward the necessary concepts and tools and were eager to get to work.

Expressions of the postwar ethos emerged on many fronts. A notable example by the Ford Foundation was the creation of both its Division of the Behavioral Sciences and its Center for Advanced Study in the Behavioral Sciences. However, perhaps the most influential event in North America was the formation of the National Institute of Mental Health (NIMH). It was largely crafted by Robert Felix, a U.S. Public Health officer and psychiatrist. Felix had had his psychiatric training in the Denver Psychopathic Hospital under Franklin Ebaugh, who in turn had been trained by Meyer and was a strong exponent of psychobiological psychiatry. Later, Felix had obtained an M.P.H. at the Johns Hopkins School of Hygiene and Public Health, where he came under the influence of Paul Lemkau, also a Meyer trainee. Felix was thus a third-generation psychobiologist, and, while at the School of Hygiene, he wrote a preliminary draft of what after the war became NIMH.

Thus we may note that, when the postwar ethos emerged, that portion of it most relevant to the study of stress and psychopathology had going for it two major and overlapping bodies of thought: *psychobiology* in psychiatry and a *functional orientation* in the social sciences.

Although *psychobiology* was mainly influential in psychiatry, it had extensions and recognition in general medicine and public health. It also was influential in the child guidance, mental hygiene, and mental health movements and stimulated bridging between such integrative levels as the person, the physiological levels below this, and the societal and cultural levels above. It is to this perspective that one may, at least in part, attribute the fact that the first three psychiatric studies in the epidemiology of general populations launched after World War II were initiated by former Meyer trainees: Paul Lemkau, Thomas A. C. Rennie, and myself.

In building his frame of reference, Meyer, whose own training was in neuropathology, utilized the ideas of the American pragmatic philosophers, especially John Dewey, C. S. Pierce, and William James, and "common sense" was a central part of his thinking (Winters, 1950). By these words, he meant to emphasize the relative dependability of concepts and methods that have been tested by much use in everyday problem solving,

as compared to the risks implicit in ideas that are novel and abstruse. One is reminded here of James Boyle and other founders of natural science in the 17th and 18th centuries who struggled hard to define "reasonableness," meaning a suitable basis for decision making in their scientific work as well as in religious thought. The upshot for them was the use of ostensive definitions drawn from the methods of problem solving in commerce practiced by successful merchants and in court decisions by distinguished jurists (Daston, 1988).

Although never himself a behaviorist—I suspect it put too great a strain on his attachment to common sense—Meyer was a strong believer in objectivity and gave appointments in his department to J. B. Watson, Curt P. Richter, and W. H. Gantt. Meyer also was close to the contemporary Chicago school of sociology and was an admirer of W. I. Thomas, George Herbert Mead, and the anthropologist Edward Sapir. He also was familiar with Ruth Benedict and the Columbia school of cultural anthropology; on the national scene, he was one of the directors of the Social Science Research Council.

It is from this array that one can understand how it came about that the psychobiological frame of reference required that diagnosis, treatment, research, and teaching in psychiatry give as much attention to the possibility of social and cultural etiologies as to intrapsychic and organic etiologies.

The *functional orientation* in the social sciences penetrated deeply among their main divisions and was implicit in such new developments as the scientific investigation of "human organizations," and "group dynamics." A list of major conceptualizers and practitioners would include such a diverse spread as Chester I. Bernard, Eric Trist, Kurt Lewin, Robert K. Merton, Talcott Parsons, and William F. Whyte.

Before turning to the next section on the decline of the environmental ethos, it is perhaps appropriate to remind the reader once more that I have been emphasizing selected temporal and contextual aspects of origins, not the whole story. The core ideas that were ushered into prominence by the ambience of the 1930s and 1940s were not newborn at that time. For example, the effort to apply scientific methods to understanding some aspects of human psychology occurred at least as early as 1650, when mathematicians began trying to discover a calculus that would capture the process by which consistently successful merchants and others were able to reach their patently useful decisions under conditions of incomplete and uncertain information (Daston, 1988).

The functional perspective must have begun much earlier when people first started making a distinction between what they thought of as natural phenomena and those they regarded as supernatural or magical. At any rate, it is already evident by the fourth century B.C. in the opposition of some Hippocratic writers to considering epilepsy a "sacred" disease rather than a natural disease. Functionalism began to take its modern form during the 18th and first half of the 19th centuries in consonance with the growth of observation and inductive reasoning in studies of natural history, society, and medicine. The notion of there being a natural order and natural causes came to permeate all three disciplines and their respective systems of explanation. Adam Smith, Thomas Malthus, Auguste Comte, Pierre Simon Laplace, Georges Leopold Cuvier, Charles Darwin, Louis Pasteur, Rudolph Virchow, and Claude Bernard are but a few of the many scientists who could be mentioned as exhibiting functional thinking in the sciences that deal with living things. Moreover, some mutuality existed in these influences, leading to functional thinking's most outstanding product, the theory of organic evolution.

Decline

The reasons for the weakening of the environmental ethos and its associated ideas after the middle of the 20th century may be divided in two parts: the general impact of historical changes on the human condition, which we all recognize; and the impact of changes more intimately related to the com-

position of the environmental ethos itself. In the discussion that follows, I make a few remarks intended for orientation only on the first part and then focus on those aspects of the second part that seem to me most relevant to our topic, to the immediate future, and to our tasks as researchers and teachers.

The dominant change in the societies of the world is sociocultural fragmentation and its concomitant psychological phenomena (Leighton, 1974). It is similar to the social disintegrative processes witnessed during the great economic depression of the 1930s, only it now seems more widespread and deadly. The driving forces include fast rates of technological change and accelerating increases in world population that seem to be exceeding the adaptive capacities of our species. Throughout the fabric of world society, systems of control that depend on fiducial relationships—governmental, familial, economic, religious, philosophic, ethical—are in serious states of malfunctioning, and so are the processes of education and knowledge discovery.

Sociocultural and psychological reintegrations are also in progress on a world scale, but they move at a rate that leaves outcome in doubt. The upshot is a flocculent—rather than either a coordinated or a completely chaotic—social and cultural environment in which external hazards are often many and severe, while external resources are often few and ineffectual. As a facet of sociocultural disintegration, the position of science in public esteem and support has undergone considerable deterioration. That this is different from the "euphoric expectations" of prevailing sentiments, even as little as 25 years ago, was much noted by the press during last year's commemoration of the first moon walk.

Turning now to factors more directly related to destruction from within the environmental ethos, I try to summarize most of my impressions in terms of four points. The first has to do with insufficient consensus regarding a frame of reference by which clinical psychiatry, psychology, and the social sciences could be aligned in such a way as to open doors to probing for etiological transactions. For one thing, the concepts employed were at different levels of integration and emergent properties—on the one hand individual in orientation, on the other social—and therefore in need of much attention to the development of epistemic, bridging structures. For another thing, a good deal of the theory within each level was so general that connections to specific phenomena of any kind were difficult to make. This constituted a serious obstacle to operationalizing investigations and to interpreting results.

In psychiatry, what I mean by these statements may be illustrated in the global and therefore vague way "mental health" and "mental illness" were used. More specific designations of disorder types such as "schizophrenia" and "psychoneurosis" were almost equally problematic because they served numbers of different purposes, such as indicating type of care needed, type of behavioral pattern exhibited, or type of theory attributed. The social scientists naturally found this bewildering and a hindrance to designating entities as targets for research. They were right to be critical up to a point, but they might have been able to make better use of psychiatric nosology had they taken the time necessary to understand the several different ways it was employed. They were also handicapped—as were the psychiatrists—by lack of training in the principles and methods of taxonomy and systematics.

In the social science field, the notion of culture may be taken as an example of a concept too global for the uses people tried to make of it. As Murphy (1994) has indicated, despite the importance attributed to culture as a determining environmental influence, the cultures of the world have never been described in systematic terms sufficient to facilitate the study of such an effect. One cannot, for instance, find generally accepted standards by which cultures and subcultures may be distinguished. Although there can be no doubt that "culture" has usefulness as a general orientation, it remains, like "mental health," too indefinite for operational procedures.

What has tended to happen, in lieu of work on systematics or on breaking global concepts down into components that frame more identifiable and therefore researchable topics, has been the reification of the global concept and then its treatment as if it were a thing instead of an idea about things. Such misidentification leads to searching for the reified concept as if it were an object in nature—a goal that can be satisfied only by the use of intuition. To accept this, however, means moving out of science into metaphysics.

To restate, it seems to be the case that at the time environmentalism was peaking in the 1950s, neither the clinical psychological disciplines nor the social sciences were far enough along toward developing the systematics called for in the examination of either environmental causes or mental illnesses. The boundaries in a number of the main variables were not identified and specified in nature with a sufficiently useful degree of consensus. We are beginning to get the systematics of psychiatric diagnosis in order now, but the systematics necessary to provide more adequate sociological and cultural variables—as pointed out by Zubin and Spring (1977)—has not yet emerged.

The second of the four points bearing on the weakening of the environmental ethos was the failure of environmentalists at this time to take advantage of opportunities created by the notable successes of the biological sciences in helping control the symptoms of psychiatric disorders, in advancing knowledge about genetics and other organic etiologies, and in techniques for the study of brain function. Many of the new increments to the comprehension of organic causality were steps toward clarifying the nature of environmental effects, or they could have been made so. This was especially true of genetics, where, for example, the concordance investigations of monozygotic twins showed that, in schizophrenia, no more than half the variance was attributable to inheritance. Somewhat similar opportunities were created by the adoption studies.

The reason for this indifference on the part of many of those interested in environmental influence was not just accidental oversight; it sprang from strong sentiments of hostility toward biological determinism in human affairs. The crux in this was dedication to the ideal of individual freedom—a current version of the ancient "free will" issue. However, it had been enhanced and made particularly poignant by the atrocities committed in the name of biological determinism by the Nazis and by the racism still evident in contemporary life. For many of the people appalled by these acts, biological determinism and all its works was the enemy. Although one must unite with demands for a just society and opposition to cruelty, it seems evident that the opposition to biology by many psychiatrists, psychologists, and social scientists was so indiscriminating and sweeping as to constitute a hindrance to scientific investigation.

Given that theories of environmental etiology also are deterministic, one may wonder why they did not meet with an opposition similar to that of biological determinism. It is my interpretation that environmental theories of cause appear much less rigid than biological theories. They seem to give the individual some room for making choices and for self-determined maneuvering. It was often said that, after all, a person can change to a different environment but cannot alter his or her inheritance.

The third point consists in the virtual disappearance after midcentury of psychobiology from psychiatry and neighboring fields and its replacement by psychoanalysis. This was accompanied by a great flowering of interest in psychodynamic theory and metaphysical psychology, with a concurrent diminution of concern about scientific methods of validation. On the heels of this came a rise of more and more effective medications that encouraged the scientific approach but narrowed its focus and its methods. In combination, these two trends served to reduce interest in possible causal factors in personality and in the sociocultural environment.

What disappeared with psychobiology was a frame of reference that proposed that an explanation of pathology in mental life must be sought simultaneously in at least three different levels of integration: the psychology of the person, his or her biological processes, and his or her sociocultural processes. This was a clinical frame of reference in that it was oriented by the practice of treatment and prevention of relapse among individuals, but it also offered a basis for constructing a research frame of reference oriented by the goal of uncovering valid generalizations about the interaction of causes of mental illnesses at all three levels, whatever their nature and however they might or might not combine. It did not thrust forward the notion that one of these levels must be primary in virtually every case; yet, at the same time, it did not reject the idea that one level might be primary in a particular case.

Psychobiology also took with it the emphasis on common sense. This not only encouraged spending a great deal of professional time and money in speculation about novel and abstruse ideas and on unresolvable arguments but also led to therapeutic practices that run the risk of severe damage to patients and their families, as recently reviewed by Paul McHugh (1994).

The fourth point concerns the downgrading of the functional orientation among the social sciences, a diminution that has many parallels to the fading of psychobiology. One such is the emergence of intense interest in the construction of theory with concomitant lack of emphasis on the use of objective evidence. Structuralism, ethnomethodology, semiology, phenomenology, neo-Nietzscheism, and numerous other theories are like psychodynamics in being metaphysical ideas that do not, for the most part, ask questions that require very much use of data aside from illustrative purposes. In the philosophical distinction that is made between *verstehen* and *erklären*, they belong in the *verstehen* division, and although dealing in great and important issues, these are not of a nature that can be answered by science. They also, as pointed out by Jaspers (1963), typically constitute questions for which different, and even opposite, answers are equally convincing (Slavney & McHugh, 1987).

A part of the reason for these tendencies may be the fact that psychology, sociology, and anthropology have only comparatively recently—about the middle third of the 19th century—laid claims to scientific competence and been recognized as disciplines that are distinct from philosophy. At any rate, they now tend to be gathering places for students and teachers who have very strong philosophical interests and activist positions, but who have comparatively little interest or experience in scientific processes.

It seems to me that what brews here are some of philosophy's most gripping questions that were left unsatisfied after the fairly consistent and tightly interwoven religious thought of the Middle Ages became broken up in the Renaissance and Reformation. These issues include the meaning of life and the existence of a unique *psyche* in each person, a psyche that possesses the previously mentioned free will and has rights and obligations to spiritual self-determination. The consequence is a mix of ideas in the social sciences in which the concepts and methods of science are often opposed by other ways of thinking. These include disbelief in the appropriateness of applying science to human motivation and behavior and distaste for all mechanistic interpretations that threaten to reduce the notion of person to Thomas Huxley's "automaton."

To many individuals, this dilution of science seemed all to the good, but what diminished with functionalism in the social sciences was a potential for bridges connecting these fields to psychiatry and medicine—and beyond that to all the other sciences that struggle to comprehend life scientifically at different levels of integration and emergent properties. One way of summarizing the diminution of the scientific component in the environmental ethos is to say that, first of all, there was absence of agreement that science was the way to go and then, second, there was little agreement among the advocates of science as to what their paradigm should be.

My remarks on the decline of the environmental ethos are, again, incomplete. For example, I have not mentioned the antimedical movement, the wars over the "medical model," and the influence these had on collaboration between social scientists and psychiatrists. My hope is that I nevertheless have said enough so that it will be reasonable to put forward some concluding points that seem to me fundamental.

CONCLUSION

Let me begin this final part with a quotation from a 1993 article by Vartan Gregorian, professor of history and president of Brown University.

The real challenge . . . calls for integrating and resynthesizing the compartmentalized knowledge of disparate fields: the ability to make connections among seemingly disparate disciplines, discoveries, events and trends and to integrate them in ways that benefit the commonwealth of learning (p. 609).

In the course of this chapter, I have drawn attention to three "nests" of problems that I suggest are of enduring importance if the scientific process is to be applied successfully to understanding relationships among stresses and psychopathologies and other phenomena of similar kind. The first nest concerns the levels of epistemological integration and their emergent properties and the need to recognize that their borderlands can serve as aids or hindrances to scientific research. The reason for this rests on the fact that a phenomenon seen at any one integrative level is not a summation of phenomenal properties at a lower level but has new, "emergent," properties. Thus the causal relationships between phenomena at any two levels are far from self-evident. As a result, there is considerable need for building conceptual bridges and testing them with empirical research. The academic tradition that scholars should work only at the level appropriate to their discipline may once have been a convenient one, and perhaps politically astute, but it is largely unworkable with the research questions we are considering.

The second nest of issues concerns dangers that lurk in two borderland areas: scientism on the one hand and failing to distinguish metaphysics from science on the other. This is really a subdivision within the first nest of problems, and its import is, again, that we must construct bridges and not simply ignore or be bound by the existence of the epistemic chasms between levels of integration.

By "scientism," I mean intemperate commitment to imitating the techniques of the physical sciences, especially classical physics, rather than following the thought processes that underlie the techniques. Commonly, the physical science techniques are the result of focusing on very different kinds of phenomena and very different kinds of questions from those encountered in problems of stress and psychopathology. There will be more about this presently.

Metaphysics is, of course, an important branch of philosophy and addresses a far greater range of questions than science is able to do. We cannot live our lives in such a way as to limit ourselves to decisions based only on scientific procedures. As Justice Holmes once said, "Every year if not every day we have to wager our salvation upon some prophecy based upon imperfect knowledge" (Trilling, 1949, p. 264). My point is only that, where science has been selected as the procedure of choice, it must not be confused with metaphysics, for otherwise there is danger of an error just as great as that of scientism. Metaphysics has common ground with science in the matter of theory construction, but the empirical connection to incremental data is missing. Instead, there is dependence on validation by intuitive conviction backed up by logical structures, illustrative analogies, and often rhetoric. Jaspers's (1963) discussion of *verstehen* and *erklären* are again helpful in this regard.

The third nest of problems involves the need for more attention to conceptual bridges across the borderland between biology on the one hand and psychiatry, psychology, and the social sciences on the other. It appears to me that strong prejudices in this region have put many barriers in the way of research advances regarding relationships among stresses and psychopathologies. I therefore focus in these final paragraphs on some of the ways in which biology has common ground with the psychological and social sciences and differs from the inorganic sciences.

Scientism is often justified by the statement that "there is but one science." If taken at face value, such a view ignores the profound differences that separate levels of integration and their emergent properties. Thus physics does not predict chemical phenomena, and scientific work with chemicals does not predict biological phenomena. What generally happens is that, following independent scientific work at adjacent levels of integration, connections are found whereby it becomes possible for physics to help explain a chemical phenomenon, or chemistry to help explain a physiological one, and so on. Thus the periodic table, which was in the beginning a chemical discovery, became illuminated by physics. A physiological phenomenon such as respiration can turn out to be in part explicable by the chemical reactions involved in metabolism. At the level of social behavior, a pattern such as the family can be partially explained as derived from person processes such as obtaining food, shelter, and sex, which are in turn partially explicable by physiological processes. Because of these differences in properties at different levels, the conceptualizations and methods of science must also differ according to level and to question being asked of nature.

Therefore, even though it is possible to conceive of science in terms so abstract that speaking of "one science" is permissible, for the purposes of conducting actual research, it works better to think of scientific methods as varying considerably—even if within limits—according to phenomena and research aim. It is my view that imitating physics is not a safe alternative to metaphysics.

The borderland between levels of integration that separates studies of physical phenomena from those of living phenomena is a particularly important one because the differences involved have profound effects on what kind of conceptualizations, what kinds of methods, and what kinds of questions can be usefully asked of nature. Pathology provides one example. It is at the center of our concerns in this book, but it does not exist in the world of inorganic phenomena. The reason for this is, as we have seen, that pathology is an outrider of the death process, and death occurs only where there is life. It is, in fact, part of the definition of life.

One may object to this and point out that stars, hurricanes, mountain ranges, and oceans all "die." My first response would be to suggest caution with regard to metaphors, but then I would have to make some concessions. While maintaining that the main foci of physical scientists are on processes whereby energy and matter undergo transformations and not extinctions, I would have to admit that these scientists do also deal in *patterns* of energy and matter, and that patterning—as distinct from energy and matter—can disappear. I would then further agree that at a very high level of abstraction, it would be reasonable to classify death as a kind of pattern discontinuation and therefore in a class that also has some physical phenomena in it.

I would still maintain, however, that in terms of emphasis and problem characteristics, significant differences exist between biologists and inorganic scientists. How fundamental this is can be seen in the fact that almost every living process we know anything about is oriented by death in the sense that the process operates directly or indirectly so as to promote survival by continuation and/or reproduction. All our theories and concepts in the life sciences are ingrained with this influence. Without it, we would not have concepts such as hazards, resources, stress, or pathology. Nor could we have the functionalist orientation or a theory of evolution. Because all such is based on patterned phenomena, ubiquitous among life forms, we must be prepared to find that biology has need for conceptual tools and technical methods that may differ considerably from those found useful in most of the inorganic sciences.

Another major difference between life processes and nonliving processes is the existence of very low-energy systems that are able to control the distribution and timing of very high-energy transactions. By this means, randomness in events is reduced and patterns are evolved that have a general tendency to perpetuate life. What I have in mind here can be illustrated by reference to the central nervous system and its neurobiochemical transactions. These are a main basis for the transmission of signals within and among organisms and thus central in the phenomenon termed *information* and the activities it encompasses. At the level of a vertebrate organism, this involves the perception of an item of information, its combining with other information, its analysis, its storage, and its function in releasing or inhibiting actions that involve comparatively huge transformations of energy, as in muscles or the total flight or fight of an entire organism. The sharing and storage of information in populations of individuals vastly increases the extent, duration, and complexity of information functioning in the rhythms of death and replacement of individuals while the survival of collective life continues with adaptations to changing conditions. A picture of the principles in the shaping of major energy patterns through low-energy signals can also be drawn from genetics and from immunology.

Readers interested in further discussion regarding the properties of biological phenomena may consult Ernst Mayr's *The Growth of Biological Thought* (1982). For my purposes, enough probably has been said in order to make two points. The first is that the advent of low-energy systems of information signaling—codes—that can determine whether greater energy events take place or not introduces a flood of contingencies that biologists must face at every turn but that do not confront students of the inorganic world. The "laws" of physics and chemistry, of course, still operate in living systems, and they set limits on what can happen, but they do not by themselves determine what does happen.

The second point is that the controlling power of information systems very often lies in differences of patterning. In other words, its power is configurational rather than dimensional. The difference between "yes" and "no" does not lie in how loudly one shouts but in difference of auditory pattern.

A caveat is relevant, however. What I am trying to say is not that configurations are more important in biology than dimensions, but rather that both are important and that the scientist needs both conceptualizations much the way a bird needs two wings. In scientism, one of the errors is to expect too much of dimensions and their quantitative treatment.

The gradual discovery of the importance of configurations in causal explanations influenced biology's early natural history phase and contributed toward its' branching out from the dimensional bent of other sciences and the invention of methods for pattern description, classification, and analysis, leading ultimately to taxonomy and systematics. These make up the infrastructure for some of biology's major contributions, such as organic evolution, the mechanisms of inheritance, and the etiologies of diseases. Some of the differences in outlook that have resulted may be summarized by saying that, whereas the physical sciences give emphasis to the measurement of dimensions, nomothetic generalizations, parsimony, and mathematical modeling, the biological sciences emphasize qualitative description as fundamental, followed by pattern classification, probabilistic reasoning, and functional analysis.

If this statement is approximately correct, then I would suggest that the biological sciences as systems of thought and programs of method have a great deal to offer the social and psychological sciences, and that the antipathies to biology mentioned in discussing the decline of the environmental ethos have seriously handicapped the advance of knowledge regarding human behavior and motivation. In saying this, I am not referring to biological discoveries and theories as such, but rather to biological modes of thought and ways of handling the myriad complexities, reactivities, and disappearances with which living systems confront the investigator.

Coming back to our concern with the relationship between environmental stress and psychological disorder, the work on psychiatric nosology and methods for describing and classifying different patterns of psychological disorder do seem to be moving in the right direction at the present time. This is in marked contrast to the time when the first *Diagnostic and Statistical Manual of Mental Disorders* was published (American Psychiatric Association, 1952) and documented the fact that mainstream clinical psychiatry in North America had great difficulty in distinguishing between science and metaphysics. There may now, however, be some new risk of a swing to scientism.

With regard to environmental stresses, the social sciences, which might have contributed to our needs in this regard, have been mostly off attending to other concerns such as symbols and the construction of meaning. Thus community studies are gone, social and cultural functionalisms are out of fashion, and cultural systematics has never developed. We are left, therefore, with mainly global orientations that continue to need reduction to more highly specified items of thought that can be compared with observable phenomena in nature.

If the interactions of stresses and psychological disorder are to be better understood and better controlled for the benefit of humankind, then there is need for a cognitive grasp that reaches without serious gaps from molecular phenomena, as in genetics and neurochemistry, to the behavior of whole persons such as Miranda, and then beyond them to the dynamic and configurational behavior of whole populations systems. This is far beyond what we can now do, of course, but perhaps what is important is that we can visualize it.

Acknowledgements: This chapter is based on a lecture presented on receipt of the Joseph Zubin Award at the 1994 Annual Meeting of the American Psychopathological Association in New York City.

REFERENCES

Ackerknecht, E. H. (1953). *Rudolf Virchow: Doctor, statesman, anthropologist* (p. 86). Madison: University of Wisconsin Press.

American Psychiatric Association. (1952). *Diagnostic and statistical manual of mental disorders*. Washington, DC: American Psychiatric Press.

Cannon, W. B. (1932). *The wisdom of the body*. New York: W. W. Norton.

Daston, L. (1988). *Classic probability in the enlightenment*. Princeton, NJ: Princeton University Press.

Gregorian, V. (1993). Education and our divided knowledge. *Proceedings of the American Philosophical Society, 137*, 605–611.

Grinker, R. R., & Spiegel, J. P. (1945). *Men under stress*. Philadelphia: Blakiston.

Jaspers, K. (1963). *General psychopathology: Verstehende Psychologie* (pp. 302–446); *Part III. Erklärende Psychologie* (pp. 451–551). (J. Hoenig & M. W. Hamilton, Trans.). Chicago: University of Chicago Press.

Leighton, A. H. (1943). A working concept of morale for flight surgeons. *Military Surgeon, 92*, 601–609.

Leighton, A. H. (1949). *Human relations in a changing world: Observations on the use of the social sciences* (pp. 43–95). New York: E. P. Dutton.

Leighton, A. H. (1974). The erosion of norms. *Australia and New Zealand Journal of Psychiatry, 8*, 223–227.

Lewis, D. C., & Engle, B. (Eds.). (1954). *Wartime psychiatry*. New York: Oxford University Press.

Mayr, E. (1982). *The growth of biological thought* (pp. 52–67). Cambridge, MA: Belknap Press (Harvard University Press).

McHugh, P. R. (1994). Psychotherapy awry. *American Scholar, 63*, 17–30.

Murphy, J. M. (1986). The Stirling County Study. In M. M. Weissman, J. K. Myers, & C. E. Ross (Eds.), *Community surveys of psychiatric disorders* (pp. 133–153). New Brunswick, NJ: Rutgers University Press.

Murphy, J. M. (1994). Anthropology and psychiatric epidemiology. *Acta Psychiatrica Scandinavica, (Supplementum. 385): 90*, 48–57.

Plomin, R., Owen, M. J., & McGuffin, P. (1994). The genetic basis of complex human behaviors. *Science, 264*, 1733–1739.

Sargant, W., & Slater, E. (1940). Acute war neuroses. *Lancet, 2*, 1–2.

Selye, H. (1956). *The stress of life*. New York: McGraw-Hill.

Slavney, P. R., & McHugh, P. R. (1987). *Psychiatric polarities: Methodology and practice* (pp. 31–41). Baltimore: The Johns Hopkins University Press.

Srole, L., & Fischer, A. K. (1986). The Midtown Manhattan Longitudinal Study: Aging, generations, and genders. In M. M. Weissman, J. K. Myers, & C. E. Ross (Eds.), *Community surveys of psychiatric disorders* (pp. 77–107). New Brunswick, NJ: Rutgers University Press.

Stouffer, S. A., Lumsdaine, A. A., Lumsdaine, M. H., et al. (1949a). *The American soldier: Vol. 2. Combat and its aftermath*. Princeton, NJ: Princeton University Press.

Stouffer, S. A., Suchman, E. A., DeVinney, L. C., et al. (1949b). *The American soldier: Vol. 1. Adjustment during army life*. Princeton, NJ: Princeton University Press.

Trilling, L. (1949). *Matthew Arnold* New York: Columbia University Press.

Udall, S. L. (1994). *The myths of August: A personal exploration of our tragic cold war affair with the atom* (A Cornelia and Michael Bessie Book). New York: Pantheon Books.

Virchow, R. (1860). *Cellular pathology as based upon physiological and pathological pathology* (F. Chase, trans.; pp. 88–92). New York: Robert N. DeWitt.

Warner, W. L. (1937). The society, the individual, and his mental disorder. *American Journal of Psychiatry, 94*, 275–284.

Warner, W. L., & Lunt, P. S. (1941). *The social life of a modern community*. New Haven, CT: Yale University Press.

Winters, E. E. (Ed.). (1950). *The collected papers of Adolph Meyer*. Baltimore: The Johns Hopkins University Press.

Zubin, J., & Spring, B. (1977). Vulnerability—a new view of schizophrenia. *Journal of Abnormal Psychology, 86*, 103–126.

VI

OVERVIEW AND INTEGRATION

Bruce P. Dohrenwend

In the introductory chapter, I stated that this book had two purposes: (*1*) to examine the evidence on the question of whether adverse environmental conditions are important in the etiology of psychiatric disorders; and (*2*) to develop a theoretical framework of concepts, ideas, and propositions that will stimulate further research. In this part of the volume, I attempt to provide an overview of the evidence and an integrative theoretical framework for future research.

With regard to the evidence, I focus especially on results from three sets of studies, all represented in this volume, of important types of disorders, including schizophrenia, major depression, antisocial personality, alcoholism, and substance use disorders. I argue that these three groups of studies provide an environmental analogue to the behavioral genetic family, adoption, and twin studies that have demonstrated a role for genetic factors in most of these same types of psychiatric disorders.

The three sets of studies are epidemiological investigations showing that overall rates of psychiatric disorders and the subtypes of schizophrenia, major depression (at least in women), antisocial personality, alcoholism, substance use disorders (at least in men), and post-traumatic stress disorder are inversely related to socioeconomic status (SES); quasi-experimental tests of the social causation–social selection issue posed by these relations between SES and various types of psychopathology; and research on the effects of exposure to events in extreme situations such as military combat and natural and humanmade disasters. Leads from this environmental analogue are integrated into a theoretical framework for investigating stress processes through which adversity contributes to the onset and course of the various types of psychiatric disorder that are inversely related to SES. Suggestions are made for future research.

29

Overview of Evidence for the Importance of Adverse Environmental Conditions in Causing Psychiatric Disorders

Bruce P. Dohrenwend

Guze (1989) and Heston (1988), quoted in my introduction to this volume, implied that, in the context of advances in behavioral genetic research, the burden of proof is on those who would provide a similar demonstration of the importance of environmental adversity in the development of psychiatric disorders. Is the evidence, especially the evidence presented in this volume, a basis for a positive response to this challenge? In this chapter, I argue that there are three sets of studies, all of which are represented in preceding chapters, whose results, taken together, provide compelling evidence that environmental adversity and stress are important in the development of major types of psychopathology.

These studies, I believe, are analogous to the three types of behavioral genetic studies—family, adoption, and twin studies—that have proved so persuasive in demonstrating a role for genetic inheritance. First, there are epidemiological studies of relations between both overall rates of disorder and the subtypes of schizophrenia, major de-

pression, antisocial personality, alcoholism and other substance use disorders, and posttraumatic stress disorder (PTSD) on the one hand and socioeconomic status (SES) on the other (see Breslau et al., Chapter 15, this volume; Kohn et al., Chapter 13, this volume). These correspond to the family studies, with similar strengths and weaknesses. The strengths are in the consistent relationships they have found; their weaknesses, in the problem that these relationships are open to plausible alternative environmental and genetic explanations.

Second, there are results from a quasi-experimental strategy for investigating the social causation–social selection issue posed by inverse relations between these types of disorder and SES (see Dohrenwend et al., 1992, Chapter 14, this volume). This strategy has provided indirect tests of the importance of environmental factors that are akin to the adoption studies that have been used to test the role of genetic factors.

Finally, there is research on the psychiatric consequences of life-threatening events in extreme situations, such as prolonged exposure to wartime combat and to natural and humanmade disasters that target whole communities or groups (see Giel, Chapter 4, this volume; Keane, Chapter 3, this volume; Levav, Chapter 1, this volume; Mollica et. al., Chapter 2, this volume). Such events, compared to events in more usual situations, vary environmental contrasts almost as strongly as do the genetic contrasts employed in twin studies; also, like twins, they are unusual experiments of nature.

As with each member of the behavioral genetic triad, each of these three groups of studies that focus on environmental adversity has different strengths and weaknesses. Taken collectively, what has this environmental triad demonstrated about the role of adversity in the development of major types of psychopathology? What has it failed to demonstrate?

EXTREME, LIFE-THREATENING EVENTS THAT TARGET WHOLE GROUPS OR COMMUNITIES

I begin, as does Part I of this volume, with the studies I nominated above as analogous to the twin studies by behavioral geneticists. These consist of investigations of events in extreme situations, especially the humanmade disaster of war. I believe they provide the most compelling evidence that adversity causes psychopathology, although this conclusion is not beyond controversy and requires qualification.

Events or combinations of events in extreme situations involve actual or threatened death or serious injury; other threat to the person's physical integrity; and an immediate response of intense fear, helplessness, or horror (American Psychiatric Association, 1994). Barbara Dohrenwend and I reviewed much of the early literature on war-related extreme situations, especially on the effects of the Holocaust on Jewish survivors (Dohrenwend & Dohrenwend, 1969) and of combat during World War II (Dohrenwend,

1975; Dohrenwend & Dohrenwend, 1969; Dohrenwend & Egri, 1981). This review led us to conclude, as others have done, that some of these events will produce a wide variety of symptoms and signs of psychopathology in previously normal persons.

The signs and symptoms caused by events in extreme situations are not limited to types included under such headings as traumatic war neurosis, combat fatigue, combat exhaustion, or, most recently, PTSD. There are reports, for example, of "three day" psychoses (Kolb, 1973, p. 438), "five-day schizophrenia" (Kormos, 1978, p. 4), and "twilight states" (Schneider, 1959, p. 58) that, in cross-sectional view, are indistinguishable from schizophrenia. Indeed, these reports suggested that a large portion of the signs and symptoms observed in psychiatric patients in civilian settings also have been observed in the form of reactions of nonpatients exposed to extreme situations. The chapters presented in Part I of this volume by Levav on the Holocaust, by Keane on exposure to combat during the Vietnam war, by Mollica et al. on Cambodian refugees, and by Giel on natural and humanmade disasters that are not war-related reinforce these conclusions. So does the growing evidence of co-morbidity of PTSD and other types of disorder (Kulka et al., 1990; Skodol et al., 1996; see also Breslau, et al., Chapter 15, this volume; Keane, Chapter 3, this volume).

Although ample evidence has been presented that the likelihood of developing severe psychopathology varies positively with the severity of adversity to which the individual is exposed, some individuals develop disorder under less extreme provocation than others. It also may be that some do not develop severe disorder even under extreme provocation (see, e.g., Beiser's introduction to Part I of this volume; Hendin & Haas, 1984; my later discussion of Yehuda & McFarlane, 1995). For many years, there have been two broad sets of ideas in the literature about individual differences in liability to PTSD (and related phenomena such as acute combat reactions, or older concepts such as shell shock, gross stress re-action, combat fatigue, or combat neurosis —see, e.g., Solomon, 1993). One set of ideas applies to individual differences in the likelihood that disorder will develop at all. The other set applies to individual differences in the course of disorder once it has occurred. Consider, first, the ideas about initial onset.

The terms *inoculation* and *vulnerability* (sometimes also called "stress sensitization") have been used with regard to individual differences in likelihood of initial onset (see, e.g., Bremner et al., 1995, pp. 159–160; Solomon, 1995, pp. 143–144). For example, the concepts of inoculation/vulnerability were used by Solomon (1995, p. 144) to describe the issue of whether prior experience with potentially traumatic events reduces (inoculates against) or increases vulnerability to subsequent traumatic events. It seems likely that experiences with severe fateful negative events such as being the object of child abuse early in life are far more likely to increase vulnerability than to inoculate (e.g., Solomon, 1995; see also Widom, Chapter 5, this volume). The question of whether inoculation effects do or do not occur may also turn not only on primacy (how young the person is when the experience occurs) but also on the severity of the event and the frequency of its occurrence (Solomon, 1995; Yehuda et al., 1995).

In general, however, the term, *inoculation/vulnerability* is not used in the literature on adverse psychological reactions to events in extreme situations to refer to precise processes underlying individual differences in onset of psychopathology. Rather it refers to sensitizing concepts to bracket an array of important questions about factors involved in individual differences in responses to similar events in extreme situations. I therefore include "inoculation factors," with its relatively specific connotations, under the broader heading of "protective factors," and I use "protective" and "vulnerability" to refer to the complex of factors that may decrease or increase risk of onset of severe psychopathology following events hypothe-sized to be "traumatic." In this formulation, "inoculation" is used to describe one variety of possible protective factors—for example, being "battle hardened" in previous milder combat and thereby being protected against the development of psychopathology in a future more severe exposure. Other possibly important protective factors, such as physical stamina and superior intelligence, are considered as well, although they do not fit closely the inoculation analogy.

Also broadly conceived, vulnerability factors include genetic predispositions to a particular disorder but are not limited to such risk factors; for example, the possibly damaging effects on adult personality of abuse and neglect in childhood would be included as well (see, e.g., Widom, Chapter 5, this volume). Moreover, protective factors/vulnerability factors are not limited to personal predispositions; factors in the ongoing situation, such as the presence or absence of supportive social networks, are included as important sources of protection and vulnerability as well.

With regard to course, questions have focused on the extent to which symptomatology and disturbance of functioning produced by events in extreme situations are transient and self-limiting. As Beiser (introduction to Part I of this volume) points out, ideas about the issue have changed over time. On the basis of clinical experience and psychiatric research during World War II, a consensus appears to have developed that, by contrast with so much of the symptomatology of clinical disorder observed in psychiatric patients, the symptoms that occurred in response to extreme situations tended to disappear unless exposed persons did not have "good adaptive capacity" to begin with. In this case, another diagnostic category was to be used [see, e.g., the sections on Gross Stress Reaction under Transient Situational Personality Disturbance in the *Diagnostic and Statistical Manual of Mental Disorders* (*DSM*; American Psychiatric Association, 1952) and Adjustment Reaction of Adult Life under Transient Situational Disturbance in the *DSM-II* (American Psychiatric Association, 1968); see also the account in Dohrenwend and Dohrenwend (1969, pp. 174–175)].

Barbara Dohrenwend and I called this phenomenon of the development of relatively transient symptoms "situational specificity," which we believed was the rule rather than the exception unless the symptoms were treated in ways that increased secondary gain (Dohrenwend & Dohrenwend, 1969, p. 171). Others have described what we were calling "situational specificity" as "stress evaporation" (e.g., Bremner et al., 1995, p. 160; Figley, 1978, pp. 59–69; Solomon, 1995, pp. 125–126). In our research on the nuclear accident at Three Mile Island (for the President's Commission that was formed to investigate the event), Barbara Dohrenwend, our colleagues, and I would have missed a sharp elevation of psychological distress if, among the several measures taken after the accident, we did not have one that was administered within a few weeks of the crisis (e.g., Dohrenwend, 1983). This seemed to us a vivid example of situational specificity or stress evaporation.

Yet it is unmistakably clear from research reported in this volume and elsewhere that, for some persons, the psychopathology is not situationally specific, and stress evaporation does not occur even with the lapse of many years following exposure to events in extreme situations. Others, for example, have found evidence of the persistence or recurrence of symptomatology among residents of Three Mile Island (Baum, 1990). Vivid illustrations of persistent psychopathology can be found in the reports in this volume covering the effects of the Holocaust on Jewish survivors (see Levav, Chapter 1) and of the Vietnam war on U.S. combat personnel (see Keane, Chapter 3). Another compelling example of persistent psychopathology has recently been provided by Engdahl and his colleagues (1997) who found that 29% of a nonpatient sample of United States prisoners of War met criteria for PTSD 40–50 years after their imprisonment in World War II. For those who were prisoners of the Japanese and faced the harshest conditions, the rate of current PTSD was 59%. Moreover, there have been findings of persistent or recurrent symptomatology in research on more usual and often life-threatening events such as rape and other individually targeted violence toward women (see Kilpatrick et al., Chapter 10, this volume) and in relations between histories of PTSD and co-morbid disorders and histories of a variety of "traumatic events" inventoried in civilian samples (see Breslau et al., Chapter 15, this volume).

Some have referred to this evidence of persistent psychopathology as indicating the presence of "residual stress" (e.g., Bremner et al., 1995, p. 160; Figley, 1978, pp. 59–69; Solomon, 1995, pp. 125–126). I use this term to refer to the complex of predispositional and situational factors and biological changes (e.g., Yehuda & McFarlane, 1995) that may increase or decrease risk of reoccurrence or persistence once PTSD or other severe psychopathology has developed.

One possibility, consistent with the *DSM-I* and *DSM-II* focus on the role of prior adaptive capacity, is that there is a continuum between protective/vulnerability factors in the personal predispositions of the individual and stress evaporation/residual stress factors. Some investigators have suggested that vulnerable predispositional factors may in fact be more important than exposure to events in extreme situations in the occurrence and persistence of PTSD. Taking this position, Yehuda and McFarlane (1995) have argued that it is time to reconsider the formulations of PTSD in the *DSM-III*, *DSM-III-R*, and *DSM-IV* (American Psychiatric Association, 1980, 1987, 1994) that emphasize the primacy of the stressor in the occurrence of the disorder. As they put it:

[F]indings from empirical studies of PTSD ... illustrate that contrary to what might have been predicted at the time the diagnosis of PTSD was established, many recent findings are inconsistent with the notion that traumatic events are the primary cause of symptoms and challenge the idea of PTSD as a typical stress response. (p. 1707).

To make this case, Yehuda and Mc-Farlane read the results of epidemiological research on PTSD as showing that "the occurrence of PTSD following a traumatic event is the exception rather than the rule" (1995, p. 1707). They point to reports of overall prevalence rates ranging from 3% to 58% in various studies to support this conclusion. They are aware that "In evaluating these results it is important to consider the nature and severity of the traumatic event, since a number of investigators have documented a relationship between severity of the trauma and the development of chronic PTSD" (p. 1708). However, in their analyses of the epidemiological evidence, they blur the distinction between factors in initial onset and factors in course, and they downplay the evidence of dose–response relationships (see, e.g., Keane, Chapter 3, this volume; Levav, Chapter 1, this volume; Mollica et al., Chapter 2, this volume).

For example, Yehuda and McFarlane (1995, p. 1707) refer to "one of the classical epidemiological studies" of Vietnam veterans that was conducted by Kulka et al. (1990). They correctly note that the investigators found that, 15–20 years after their war service, about 15% of theater veterans met criteria for PTSD within 6 months of the research interview; in addition to this current prevalence rate, these authors note that Kulka et al. (1990) found a lifetime rate of about 30%; Yehuda and McFarlane emphasize that both figures are well below 100%. These rates apply, however, to Vietnam theater veterans as a whole, a group that includes persons exposed to mild as well as to extreme stress.

The rate of current and hence, for the most part, chronic PTSD in male Vietnam theater veterans categorized as exposed to "High War Zone Stress" was estimated at 35.8%, a *fourfold increase* over the rate of current PTSD for those exposed to "Low/ Moderate War Zone Stress" (Kulka et al., 1990, pp. 60–61). Kulka and his colleagues do not give comparable dose–response figures for lifetime rate of PTSD, which is a mixture of chronic and more transient disorder, but it is possible to make an extrap-olation that is not unreasonable: The overall lifetime rate of 30.9% is slightly more than twice the overall current rate of 15.2% for male theater veterans; at the same ratio as for current, the lifetime rate of PTSD for those exposed to high war zone stress would increase to almost three-quarters (72.7%). Because the category "High War Zone Stress" is a large one, there is likely to be heterogeneity in severity of stress within it; if so, it is possible that the lifetime rates could approach 100% for those exposed to the highest stress levels within this category as the lifetime rates appear to have done in the sample of World War II prisoners of the Japanese mentioned earlier (Engdahl et al., 1977, p. 1578). When dose–response relations are considered, it is likely that the occurrence, although not necessarily the persistence, of PTSD is the rule rather than the exception.

There is some evidence that "a specific predisposition to PTSD or . . . general predisposition to mental illness that is triggered by adversity" (Yehuda & McFarlane, 1995, p. 1708) may not nudge aside the stressor as the primary factor in chronic (much less transient) PTSD. This comes from some remarkable research with samples of identical twins, one member of each pair exposed to combat and one not exposed (Goldberg et al., 1990). These investigators found that rates of current PTSD were 4.5 times higher in twins who served in Vietnam than in co-twins who did not serve in Vietnam. Among those twins exposed to heavy combat in Vietnam, current rate of PTSD was 9 times as high as in co-twins who were elsewhere at the time. These results indicate that genetic inheritance cannot account for the strong impact of exposure to combat on current (and hence largely chronic) PTSD.

With regard to this question about the primacy of the stressor, a particularly vivid case study was conducted by Sutker and her colleagues (1993) at the Veterans Administration (VA) Medical Center in New Orleans. The subjects of her study were a pair of identical twins who served in the Army Air Force during World War II. Here is my summary of some of the highlights of her account:

1. The twins enlisted together in the Army Air Force after completing college with majors in mechanical engineering and participation in the Reserve Officers Training Corp (ROTC). Neither had a prior history of psychiatric disorder nor, so far as could be learned, did either of their well-off, college-educated parents.

2. One twin, referred to as OR, opted for single-engine aircraft while the other, JR, chose multiengine aircraft. JR was stationed stateside and assigned to fly cargo planes. OR was trained as a Mustang pilot and was shot down after 22 missions and taken prisoner by the Germans. Possibly because he had a heart condition, he took the opportunity at age 67 to have a comprehensive physical exam offered to prisoner-of-war (POW) survivors as part of the former POW Benefits Act of 1981. He then helped to recruit his brother for the VA study.

3. Neither had had prior contact with the VA health services.

4. During the 11 months of his imprisonment, OR "was subject to interrogation, intimidation, personal death threats, solitary confinement, forced marches, transportation in box cars, exposure to extreme cold without adequate protection, and inadequate diet and medical care. He reported weight loss of 20 pounds which was 13% of his precapture body weight" (Sutker et al., 1993, p. 5).

5. Both OR and JR served in the Air Force until the war ended. After the war:
   - OR had three children; JR had four
   - Both were economically successful and provided comfortably for their families
   - At the time of the study, both were retired and active in community affairs
   - Neither ever sought help for mental health problems

6. However:
   - While the results of tests of cognitive abilities show longstanding strengths for both, the former POW's (OR) performance was less even. For example, OR showed poorer performance than his brother and his educational peers in general on arithmetic tests.
   - OR showed more elevated Minnesota Multiphasic Personality Inventory profiles than JR and met criteria for lifetime generalized anxiety disorder, panic attacks, and PTSD. The PTSD is described as "chronic" but episodic in nature, and waxed and waned depending on external factors such as exposure to external events.
   - When the twins were recalled to service during the Korean War, unlike JR, OR requested removal from flight status.
   - OR had bypass surgery in his middle 50s; JR had bypass surgery at age 65.
   - OR's postwar occupation was that of insurance salesman, despite his training as a mechanical engineer; JR was a college professor, presumably in his engineering field.

Sutker and her colleagues concluded that

[E]ven among the most advantaged and capable individuals who are inclined to minimize psychological suffering, there is a psychological and perhaps biological price to be paid for prolonged [exposure to] brutalization encompassing severe psychological degradation and physical handicap. (1993, p. 9)

It is hard to imagine a more compelling demonstration of the enduring nature of this price over the life span of even the healthiest among us than these investigators have provided.

It has been shown in research with veteran twins that prior vulnerabilities, including genetic predispositions (True et al., 1993), play a part along with dose–response relations that vary with the severity of the stress situation. A comprehensive account must therefore take both stressor severity and predisposing genetic factors into account. It seems reasonable on the basis of existing evidence of demonstrated dose–response relationships, however, to conclude that, at high dosage levels of exposure to life-threatening events such as those involved in combat, the development of at least transient disorder is virtually endemic. So far as the development of PTSD is concerned, the following proposition seems sensible as a point of departure for further research:

The more severe the event to which individuals are exposed, the less the role of individual differences in prior vulnerability/protection in the *onset* of PTSD and related psychopathology.

What seems considerably more at issue is the relation of antecedent vulnerability/protective factors and severity of the stressor to the stress evaporation/residual stress factors that determine the course of PTSD and related psychopathology following their initial occurrence.

Our future progress in assessing the role of exposure to events in extreme situations in *both* onset and course of PTSD and comorbid disorders will depend greatly on (*1*) the adequacy of our conceptualization and measurement of the severity of the stressor and (*2*) our ability to develop and test hypotheses about the similarities and differences between risk factors in onset and risk factors for persistence or recurrence, and about relations between the two sets of risk factors. These questions become even more compelling and more complex when we turn subsequently to consideration of the role of more usual types of adversity in the general population in times of peace.

EPIDEMIOLOGICAL STUDIES OF RELATIONS OF PSYCHIATRIC DISORDERS TO (SES)

The next of the three types of studies that constitute the environmental analogy with the behavioral genetic studies that I want to consider correspond to the family studies. These are the studies of psychiatric disorders in general populations that have given rise to one of the most persistent and challenging findings in psychiatric epidemiology—the finding that the highest overall prevalence rates of psychiatric disorders occur consistently in persons of the lowest SES (see Kohn et al., Chapter 13, this volume). Moreover, as a nationwide study in the United States found, the highest rates of persons with multiple psychiatric disorders (three or more) are found in the lowest SES groups (Kessler et al., 1994).

This finding of an inverse relation between overall rates of disorder and SES is evident in all three generations of epidemiological research reviewed, despite changes in concepts and methods of identifying psychiatric disorders and despite the fact that the more recent studies tended to sample households rather than study cohorts or whole community populations, as in first-generation research. Household surveys are more likely to miss low-SES individuals who are in jails or hospitals or die at earlier ages than persons of higher SES (see, e.g., the discussion of the biases likely to occur in household surveys in Robins, 1969 and my later comments).

As Kohn et al. (Chapter 13, this volume) show, nevertheless, our best evidence is that the inverse relationship between SES and overall rates holds for several of the important types of psychopathology: schizophrenia, antisocial personality, and alcoholism (at least in men). The evidence is less consistent for major depression, with the main exceptions being studies that used the Diagnostic Interview Schedule for diagnostic purposes. Our own research using the Schedule for Affective Disorders and Schizophrenia (see Dohrenwend et al., Chapter 14, this volume), and the research of others using the Present State Examination (e.g., Brown & Harris, 1978), suggests that major depression also varies inversely with SES, at least for women in urban settings. There is evidence that PTSD also varies inversely with SES (Kessler et al., 1995;

Kulka et al., 1990; see also Breslau et al., Chapter 15, this volume). The consistent behavioral genetic finding that most of these disorders tend to run in families raised questions about genetic versus environmental transmission. The epidemiological findings on the relation of these disorders to SES have done the same, in the form of the classical social causation–social selection issue that was the subject of the investigation reported by Dohrenwend et al. (Chapter 14, this volume).

In brief summary, the social causation explanation, proposed by environmentally oriented theorists, holds that disorder rates are higher in lower SES groups because of greater environmental adversity. The selection explanation, proposed by genetically oriented theorists, argues that rates of disorder are higher in lower SES groups because persons with the disorder or other personal characteristics predisposing to the disorder drift down into or fail to rise out of lower SES groups. It is highly likely that, even for schizophrenia, where the selection evidence is strongest, both processes are operating. What has been missing has been decisive indications of their relative importance. It is the recent conduct of just such a test that constitutes the third element of our environmental analogy to the behavioral genetic twin, family, and adoption studies.

A QUASI-EXPERIMENTAL TEST OF THE SOCIAL CAUSATION–SOCIAL SELECTION ISSUE POSED BY SES DIFFERENCES

Let me turn now to consideration of this test and the remaining analogy, that with the behavioral genetic adoption strategies. The analogous research on adversity consists of a quasi-experimental strategy for investigating the social causation–social selection issue posed by SES differences. It has been described, and some of the main results of its first systematic application have been summarized, by Dohrenwend et al. (1992); a more detailed report of the assumptions, theory, and some further findings have been

provided in this volume (Dohrenwend et al., Chapter 14). In addition, the theory and strategy involved have been investigated in a simulation study by Shrout and Link (see Chapter 23, this volume). The focus here is on the analogy between this strategy and the adoption strategy of the behavioral genetic triad, some relevant research by others, and the kinds of further tests of the strategy that would prove valuable.

The Argument

Both social causation and social selection hypotheses predict inverse relationships between SES and psychiatric disorders. The problem, as with the family and family history studies, has been to find a set of circumstances in which the two contrasting theoretical orientations lead to different predictions. The adoption strategies did just this, with genetic theory predicting higher rates in the biological families and the environmental theory predicting higher rates in the adoptive families. I have argued that the assimilation of ethnic groups into the SES structures of relatively open-class, urban societies like our own provides such an opportunity with regard to SES and psychiatric disorders (Dohrenwend, 1966; Dohrenwend & Dohrenwend, 1969, 1981; Dohrenwend et al., 1992; see also Dohrenwend et al., Chapter 14, this volume). In the adoption strategies, the strong comparison is on the genetic variable and is provided by the contrast between, for example, adoptive and natural parents; there is little environmental contrast among adoptive families, who are rarely very wealthy or very poor. The quasi-experimental strategy for testing the social causation–social selection issue, by contrast, emphasizes such environmental contrasts.

As noted by Dohrenwend et al. (Chapter 14, this volume), the logic of the quasi-experimental strategy suggests that resolution of the social causation–social selection issue could turn on simple questions of fact: Are the rates of disorders that vary inversely with SES higher or lower in advantaged or in disadvantaged ethnic/racial groups with SES controlled? The social causation hypothesis, assuming greater adversity from the pressures of ethnic/racial prejudice and discrimination, predicts higher rates in disadvantaged ethnic groups than in advantaged ethnic groups at the same level of SES; the social selection hypothesis, assuming that the greater pressure is holding down more healthy members of the disadvantaged ethnic/racial group, predicts the opposite.

The Results

We now have the results of such a study (for a detailed presentation, see Dohrenwend et al., Chapter 14, this volume). To summarize again briefly: For rates of all disorders combined, there was no statistically significant ethnic difference when SES was controlled. There were, however, striking findings for individual types of disorder. Although there was a social selection outcome for schizophrenia, there were strong social causation outcomes for major depression in women and for antisocial personality and substance use disorders, including alcoholism, in men. The results for schizophrenia and major depression were consistent with the results from the case–control study reported by Stueve et al. (Chapter 17, this volume), who found a stronger role for recent stressful events preceding episodes of depression. We concluded that the results of our quasi-experimental test offer a resolution of the longstanding social causation–social selection issue by strongly suggesting that the processes differ in relative importance by diagnostic type for one or both genders.

Alternative Interpretations

The validity of this conclusion is based in large part on the plausibility of the assumptions we have made in developing the theory and hypotheses for the quasi-experimental tests we have conducted. One of these assumptions is that there is no difference between the advantaged and disadvantaged ethnic groups in genetic vulnerability to the disorders of interest. For social causation outcomes in which the base rates are much higher for the disadvantaged ethnic group, this assumption is especially im-

portant. As mentioned by Dohrenwend et al. (Chapter 14, this volume), Goldman (1994) has shown with simulated data that social selection outcomes can be indistinguishable from social causation outcomes (as diagrammed in Figure 14.1, this volume) if, contrary to our assumption, the disadvantaged ethnic group is assumed to have a greater genetic predisposition to the disorder (see Goldman, 1994, p. 1254).

Goldman's alternative assumption is consistent with one made by many medical researchers that genetic factors are responsible when illness rates vary by ethnic/racial background. This assumption of genetic differences has been criticized by many writers (e.g., Cooper & David, 1986; Lillie-Blanton et al., 1996; Scribner, 1996; Williams & Collins, 1995). Although there is little direct evidence for this assumption for any but a small handful of relatively rare physical diseases such as sickle cell anemia, and no direct evidence for the psychiatric disorders with which we are concerned, the belief has tended to persist.

Moreover, the view is not specific to biomedical researchers concerned with physical illnesses. As noted above, Goldman (1994) made the assumption that there are specifically ethnic differences in genetic vulnerability in some of her simulations of social selection outcomes for SES differences. Some psychologists and social scientists have interpreted race differences in IQ as genetic, with Herrnstein and Murray (1994) the most recent. They argue that it is plausible to hypothesize that race differences in genetic predispositions are substantial contributors, along with environment, to the lower IQ scores of blacks when SES is controlled. Let us consider this position further.

Like the disorders with which we have been concerned, IQ is inversely related to SES and, also like some of these disorders, has been shown by behavioral genetic studies to have a substantial genetic as well as environmental component. The evidence that IQ scores around the world have been increasing over time indicates that this environmental component is substantial (Flynn, 1987). The SES differences in IQ therefore pose the social causation–social selection issue, although Herrnstein and Murray clearly favor the social selection alternative. Herrnstein and Murray (1994) review research showing that blacks and whites differ significantly in measured IQ *with indicators of SES controlled*. Unlike Herrnstein and Murray, I consider this a clear-cut social causation outcome.

The question of whether it is plausible to generalize from known genetic differences within groups to genetic differences between them turns on whether the environments of the two groups are similar or different. If they are substantially different, within-group differences in heritability are irrelevant to the issue of between-group differences in heritability (Neisser et al., 1996, p. 95). It seems to me that the 300 year history of blacks in the United States provides ample evidence of strong environmental differences (see Muntaner et al., 1996). Environmental contrasts between blacks and whites in the United States have been and still are great, probably greater than those between the advantaged European and disadvantaged North African Jews we have been studying in Israel. Moreover, whites and blacks in the United States are genetically more heterogeneous than either the Jews of European descent or the Jews of North African background in our research (Goodman, 1979). In addition, there is experimental evidence that such ethnic/racial differences are reflected in expectations associated with "stereotype threat" that adversely affect performance (Steel & Aronson, 1995).

In their review and analysis of issues and evidence about the meaning of intelligence test scores and the nature of intelligence in response to the work of Herrnstein and Murray (1994), Neisser et al. (1996) have concluded that there is little direct evidence for environmental factors in the racial difference in IQ and even less to support a genetic interpretation. In the absence of "direct" evidence on the matter, Neisser and his colleagues consider the question about the relative importance of environment and heredity in the racial differences an open one.

However, some direct evidence has recently been provided from ingenious analyses of National Longitudinal Survey of Youth (NLSY) data on cognitive ability in relation to education completed (Meyerson et al., 1998). The results show that, although black test scores improved much less than white test scores during high school, the scores of blacks improved much more than the scores of whites in college. The same blacks who showed dramatic improvement in college, like high school graduates who did not go on to college, showed little or no improvement in high school. The authors suggest that:

It is not surprising . . . that as black and white students complete more grades in high school environments that differ in quality, the gap in cognitive test scores widens. At the college level, however, where black and white students are exposed to educational environments of comparable quality . . . many blacks are able to make remarkable gains, closing the gap in test scores (Meyerson et al., 1998, p. 141).

I think, therefore, that Neisser et al. (1996) are wrong about even the qualified plausibility their above position seems to allow to Herrnstein and Murray's proposition about racial differences in genetic vulnerability with regard to low IQ, as is Goldman (1994) in her similar suggestion about the ethnic contrasts we found in rates of various types of psychiatric disorders. The evidence of contrast in environmental adversity between advantaged and disadvantaged ethnic/racial groups in modern urban societies is too great to allow much credence to a genetic alternative for which there is no evidence.

Nevertheless, the willingness of Neisser and his colleagues (1996) and Goldman (1994) to entertain hypotheses about genetic vulnerabilities that are racially or ethnically specific as causes of the outcomes at issue are reminders that our quasi-experimental strategy did not create the contrasting environments or randomly assign our respondents to the different status groups assumed to represent differential exposure to the contrasting conditions of advantage and disadvantage in these environments. Although implausible, as we argued in the case of the proposition above about ethnic/racial differences in genetic vulnerability, it is nevertheless possible to entertain this and other alternative explanations for our findings.

It is possible, for example, that some factor involving adversity that does not reduce opportunity to realize valued goals could put the members of the disadvantaged groups at risk of disorder. Goldman's (1994, p. 1254) simulations have shown that, if such a factor exists, SES-related social selection processes could yield results that closely resemble the diagram of the social causation hypothesis shown in Figure 14.1 (this volume). However, it is difficult to think of environmental adversities associated with disadvantaged ethnic status that do not limit opportunity to achieve valued goals, and Goldman does not provide examples of such adversities. Nor can I think of a parsimonious explanation for combining a process involving environmental adversity related to ethnic/racial disadvantage with a social selection process related to low SES in Figure 14.1 (this volume).

The Need for Replications and Extensions

Whether plausible and parsimonious or not, and I think those discussed above are implausible, these alternative explanations have not been excluded in our quasi-experimental tests. As was noted earlier (see Dohrenwend et al., Chapter 14, this volume), replication of this study with different sets of advantaged and disadvantaged ethnic groups in different assimilation settings would make it possible to rule out idiosyncratic cultural–historical and/or genetic factors that could affect the results in a particular setting.

It must be pointed out, however, that replications of these quasi-experimental tests will not be easy to conduct for a variety of reasons. For example, most members of disadvantaged ethnic groups are low in SES, whereas most members of assimilated advantaged ethnic groups are middle or high SES—with the result that the two variables are confounded in epidemiological studies that use random sampling designs; stratified sampling with optimal allocation according to ethnic status and SES is required to unconfound these status variables.

Second, there has been difficulty in securing unbiased estimates of the rates of the types of disorders that are inversely related to SES in contrasting ethnic/racial groups. The importance of this problem cannot be overemphasized. In a classical article published over a quarter of a century ago, Robins (1969) provided a comprehensive description of what is involved:

Recognizing the inadequacies of treated samples, we have turned to area samples of dwelling units in order to obtain untreated as well as treated cases. But the use of area samples creates errors in both our numerator and our denominator. One of the striking consequences of psychiatric disorder is that it affects one's chances of living at home and being located at home if one does live there, negatively for some groups, positively for others. For example, the rate of the criminally insane will be underestimated, since some of them will have been removed by the courts to hospitals and prisons. The estimate for the psychiatrically disturbed cannot be corrected simply by adding in hospital populations. Still missed will be the many psychiatrically disordered who are in jails, nursing homes, and flophouses and on the surgical and medical ward of general hospitals. Ringing doorbells for interviews, we will miss people with syndromes that are associated with marital conflict and break up, because they will have either no desire or no obligation to spend much of their time at home, and we will over-sample people with syndromes which result in reduced interaction with friends and relatives or reduced capacity to work and do errands. (p. 98)

The problem may be particularly large when the goal is to obtain accurate rates for disadvantaged ethnic/racial minorities. Even in the U.S. census, which is conducted with far more resources than are available for any sample survey of households and is completed with far fewer refusals, the undercount for black men has been estimated to be as high as 15% (Chodin, 1994). The problem is not limited to the United States. It has been encountered as well in studies of the treated incidence of schizophrenia in African-Caribbeans who migrated to or were born in the United Kingdom (Bhugra et al., 1997; Harrison et al., 1997).

It is one thing to recognize such problems and quite another to solve them (see Mortenson et al., 1997). For our purposes, the need to solve the problems has been compelling, because our tests require unbiased estimates of rates of the disorders of interest in contrasting gender, ethnic, and SES groups. Our solution was to conduct our first systematic test of the issue in Israel, which has the two things we needed: first, the presence of second-generation members of advantaged and disadvantaged ethnic groups in an urban assimilation situation; and second, a carefully maintained Population Register from which to sample birth cohorts from these advantaged and disadvantaged ethnic groups. These resources are not widely or readily available elsewhere.

Meanwhile, there are some relevant but fragmentary findings from two studies in the United States that were designed for other purposes. One is the VA study that was described by Keane (see Chapter 3, this volume). In this study, fortunately for the purposes of securing unbiased rate estimates, Vietnam era and theater veterans were sampled from military records rather than households. The results suggest that rates of PTSD and associated disorders are substantially higher in blacks and Hispanics than in non-Hispanic whites with indicators of SES controlled. However, the comparisons are for current PTSD 15–20 years after exposure to combat, so it is not clear to what extent factors in the persistence of PTSD rather than in its onset are involved.

In addition to the data from the VA study, Robins made available to me (Dohrenwend, 1975) a relevant comparison with data from the control groups in her studies of antisocial personality in cohorts of white and black schoolboys followed into adulthood many years later (Robins, 1966; Robins et al., 1971). The results are consistent with a so-

cial causation outcome for antisocial personality (Dohrenwend, 1975). However, there is a problem with this comparison for our purposes in that the whites were from an earlier generation than the blacks, a generation in which use of illegal drugs played less of a role in antisocial personality. These additional results help with questions of generalizability, but they do not obviate the need for further replication.

How might replications and extensions of the strategy be conducted? For example, how can the quasi experiment on the social causation–social selection issue be replicated with different ethnic groups in settings where there are no population registers? What extensions of the strategy are most important to undertake, perhaps involving certain physical disorders that are inversely related to SES (see Dew, Chapter 11, this volume)?

There is a clear need, on the basis of results so far, to focus explicitly on gender along with ethnic/racial status and SES in further theory and research on the social causation–social selection issue. It is tempting to consider, for example, whether designs can be developed in which gender, also an ascribed status that varies in advantage, may be substituted for ethnic status in the tests. A problem arises, however, about how such gender-focused tests would deal with the fact that there are gender differences in risk of developing particular types of disorders (such as alcoholism for men and major depression for women). Such gender-specific qualitative differences in the types of disorder likely to develop complicate, and may even undercut, predictions about the quantitative effects of greater versus lesser gender-related adversity.

Whether or not this problem can be solved, the role of gender in the quasi-experimental tests requires more attention. For example, the research to date raises a number of important questions about the circumstances under which major depression is inversely related to SES (see Kohn et al., Chapter 13, this volume). Does such a relationship occur only for women? Do gender ratios for depression change when rates of alcoholism and other substance use disorder in men are low, as may be the case in Israel (Levav et al., 1997; see also Kohn et al., Chapter 13, this volume)?

The replications called for and further work on gender would increase the value of this quasi-experimental strategy. The fact that important physical disorders also tend to be related to SES (see Dew, Chapter 11, this volume) suggests that it may be valuable to extend the tests to these disorders. Some analyses of research finding higher overall mortality especially in U.S. blacks compared to whites in various age groups under 65, with indicators of SES controlled, have been interpreted as evidence of social causation factors (Lillie-Blanton et al., 1996; Williams & Collins, 1995). The strong positive association between physical and psychiatric disorders (see Dew, Chapter 11, this volume) is further reason to consider including investigation of both broad types of disorder in the same research designs. The strongest need, however, is for direct examination of the processes and mechanisms by which adversity related to ethnic/racial status and SES contributes to the onset and course of various types of psychopathology.

CONCLUSIONS

As with the behavioral genetic trio, each of the three sets of studies—investigations of extreme situations, epidemiological findings on SES, and the quasi-experimental test of the social causation–social selection issue posed by SES differences—has weaknesses. Taken together, however, their results strongly suggest that adversity and stress play an important part in the etiology of some major types of psychiatric disorder.

Evidence of dose–response relationships from research on extreme situations makes it clear that environmental adversity, at high dosage levels, can produce at least transient PTSD and important types of related psychopathology in previously normal persons. It is less clear how important a role environmental adversity plays in the course of PTSD and co-morbid disorders.

There is also strong evidence that adversity associated with disadvantaged ethnic/ racial status and low SES contributes to the occurrence of major depression, antisocial personality, alcoholism, and substance use disorders in the general population. As with the adoption studies, however, the evidence is indirect. It does not test hypotheses about the mechanisms and processes involved.

It seems to me that questions about these processes are at the frontier of our understanding of the role of adversity and stress in the occurrence and distribution of psychiatric disorders in the general population. If we are to make progress on these fundamental questions, we must come to terms with some facts about the occurrence and distribution of psychopathology in more usual by contrast with more extreme situations:

1. In the aggregate, psychopathology and severe psychological distress are not rare in the general population. In the United States, for example, overall prevalence of diagnosable disorder for a period of a few months to about a year may be somewhere between 20% and 30% (Dohrenwend et al., 1980; Kessler et al., 1994). These rates do not appear to be unusually high compared to rates reported since World War II for communities in other countries (see Kohn et al., Chapter 13, this volume). Moreover, it has been estimated that an additional 25% or so of the general population may show severe nonspecific distress, although they do not meet criteria for the current prevalence of particular disorders (Link & Dohrenwend, 1980).

2. Extreme situations such as natural disasters and military combat that are most likely to contribute to current psychopathology are rare in general populations. Yet it is research on just such nonthreatened populations for whom the high rates of current psychopathology described above have been reported. It is by no means self-evident what events in the more usual situations of everyday life have in common with the events involved in extreme situations.

3. We have little systematic information about how gender, ethnic/racial status, and SES are related to the occurrence of stressful events over the life spans of persons in more normal times and places, although some evidence is beginning to be provided (e.g., Turner & Lloyd, 1995; see also Breslau et al., Chapter 15, this volume; Kilpatrick et al., Chapter 10, this volume).

The most challenging job, if we are to build systematically on what has been done, is to integrate the leads from the three lines of research that form the environmental triad. How this might be done is the subject of the next and final chapter.

REFERENCES

American Psychiatric Association. (1952). *Diagnostic and statistical manual of mental disorders.* Washington, DC: American Psychiatric Press.

American Psychiatric Association. (1968). *Diagnostic and statistical manual of mental disorders* (2nd ed.). Washington, DC: American Psychiatric Press.

American Psychiatric Association. (1980). *Diagnostic and statistical manual of mental disorders* (3rd ed.). Washington, DC: American Psychiatric Press.

American Psychiatric Association. (1987). *Diagnostic and statistical manual of mental disorders* (3rd ed., rev.). Washington, DC: American Psychiatric Press.

American Psychiatric Association. (1994). *Diagnostic and statistical manual of mental disorders* (4th ed.). Washington, DC: American Psychiatric Press.

Baum, A. (1990). Stress, intrusive imagery, and chronic distress. *Health Psychology, 9,* 653–675.

Bhugra, D., Leff, J., Mallett, R., et al. (1997). Incidence and outcome of schizophrenia in whites, African-Caribbeans and Asians in London. *Psychological Medicine, 27,* 791–798.

Bremner, J. D., Southwick, S. M., & Charney, D. S. (1995). Etiological factors in the development of posttraumatic stress disorder. In C. Mazure (Ed.), *Does stress cause psychiatric illness?* (pp. 149–185). Washington, DC: American Psychiatric Press.

Brown, G. W., & Harris, T. (1978). *Social origins of depression: A study of psychiatric disorder in women.* New York, The Free Press.

Chodin, H. M. (1994). *Looking for the last percent: The controversy over census undercounts.* New Brunswick, NJ: Rutgers University Press.

Cooper, R., & David, R. (1986). The biological concept of race and its application to public health and epidemiology. *Journal of Health Politics, Policy and Law, 11,* 97–116.

Dohrenwend, B. P. (1966). Social status and psychological disorder: An issue of substance and an issue of method. *American Sociological Review, 31,* 14–35.

Dohrenwend, B. P. (1975). Sociocultural and social-psychological factors in the genesis of mental disorders. *Journal of Health and Social Behavior, 16,* 365–392

Dohrenwend, B. P. (1983). Psychological implications of nuclear accidents: The case of Three Mile Island. *Bulletin of the New York Academy of Medicine, 59,* 1160–1176.

Dohrenwend, B. P., & Dohrenwend, B. S. (1969). *Social status and psychological disorder: A causal inquiry.* New York: John Wiley & Sons.

Dohrenwend, B. P., & Dohrenwend, B. S. (1981). Socioenvironmental factors, stress, and psychopathology: Part 1. Quasi-experimental evidence on the social causation-social selection issue posed by class differences. *American Journal of Community Psychology, 9,* 129–145.

Dohrenwend, B. P., Dohrenwend, B. S., Gould, M. S., et al. (1980). *Mental illness in the United States: Epidemiologic Estimates.* New York: Praeger.

Dohrenwend, B. P., & Egri, G. (1981). Recent stressful life events and episodes of schizophrenia. *Schizophrenia Bulletin, 7,* 12–23.

Dohrenwend, B. P., Levav, I., Shrout, P. E., et al. (1992). Socioeconomic status and psychiatric disorders: The causation-selection issue. *Science, 255,* 946–952.

Engdahl, B., Dikel, T. N., Eberly, R., et al. (1997). Posttraumatic stress disorder in a community group of former prisoners of war: A normative response to severe trauma. *American Journal of Psychiatry, 154,* 1576–1581.

Figley, C. R. (1978). Psychological adjustment among Vietnam veterans: An overview of the research. In C. R. Figley (Ed.), *Stress disorders among Vietnam veterans: Theory, research and treatment* (pp. 57–70). New York: Brunner/Mazel.

Flynn, J. R. (1987). Massive IQ gains in 14 nations: What IQ tests really measure. *Psychological Bulletin, 101*, 171–191.

Goldberg, J., True, W. R., Eisen, S. A., et al. (1990). A twin study of the effects of the Vietnam War on posttraumatic stress disorder. *JAMA, 263*, 1227–1232.

Goldman, N. (1994). Social factors and health: The causation-selection issue revisited. *Proceedings of the National Academy of Sciences of the United States of America, 91*, 1251–1255.

Goodman, R. M. (1979). *Genetic disorders among the Jewish people.* Baltimore: The Johns Hopkins University Press.

Guze, S. B. (1989). Biological psychiatry: Is there any other kind? *Psychological Medicine, 19*, 315–323.

Harrison, G., Glazebrook, C., Brewin, J., et al. (1997). Increased incidence of psychotic disorders in migrants from the Caribbean to the United Kingdom. *Psychological Medicine, 27*, 799–806.

Hendin, H., & Haas, A. P. (1984). Combat adaptations of Vietnam veterans without posttraumatic stress disorder. *American Journal of Psychiatry, 141*, 956–960.

Herrnstein, R. J., & Murray, C. (1994). *The bell curve: Intelligence and class structure in American life.* New York: The Free Press.

Heston, L. L. (1988). What about environment? In D. L. Dunner, S. Gershon, & J. E. Barrett (Eds.), *Relatives at risk for mental disorder* (pp. 205–213). New York: Raven Press.

Kessler, R. C., McGonagle, K. A., Zhao, S., et al. (1994). Lifetime and 12-month prevalence of DSM-III-R psychiatric disorders in the United States. *Arichives of General Psychiatry, 51*, 8–19.

Kessler, R. C., Sonnega, A., Bromet, E., et al. (1995). Posttraumatic stress disorder in the national comorbidity survey. *Archives of General Psychiatry, 52*, 1048–1060.

Kolb, L. C. (1973). *Modern clinical psychiatry.* Philadelphia: W. B. Saunders.

Kormos, H. R. (1978). The nature of combat stress. In C. R. Figley (Ed.), *Stress disorders among Vietnam veterans: Theory, research and treatment* (pp. 57–70). New York: Brunner/Mazel.

Kulka, R. A., Schlenger, W. E., Fairbank, J. A., et al. (1990). *Trauma and the Vietnam war generation.* New York: Brunner/Mazel.

Levav, I., Kohn, R., & Golding, J. M. (1997). Vulnerability of Jews to affective disorders. *American Journal of Psychiatry, 154*, 941–947.

Lillie-Blanton, M., Parsons, P. E., Gayle, H., et al. (1996). Racial differences in health: Not just black and white, but shades of gray. *Annual Review of Public Health, 17*, 411–448.

Link, B. G., & Dohrenwend, B. P. (1980). Formulation of hypotheses about the true prevalence of demoralization in the United States. In B. P. Dohrenwend, B. S. Dohrenwend, M. S. Gould, B. Link, R. Neugebauer, & R. Wunsch-Hitzig (Eds.), *Mental illness in the United States: Epidemiological estimates* (pp. 114–132). New York: Praeger.

Meyerson, J., Rank, M. R., Raines, F. Q., et al. (1998). Race and general cognitive ability: The myth of diminishing returns to education. *Psychological Science, 9*, 139–142.

Mortensen, P. B., Cantor-Graae, E., & McNeil, T. F. (1997). Increased rates of schizophrenia among immigrants: Some methodological concerns raised by Danish findings. *Psychological Medicine, 27*, 813–820.

Muntaner, C., Nieto, F. J., & O'Campo, P. (1996). The Bell Curve: On race, social class, and epidemiologic research. *American Journal of Epidemiology, 144*, 531–536.

Neisser, U., Boodoo, G., Bouchard, G., Jr., et al. (1996). Intelligence: Knowns and unknowns. *American Psychologist, 51*, 77–101.

Robins, L. N. (1966). *Deviant children grown up: A sociological and psychiatric study of sociopathic personality.* Baltimore: Williams & Wilkins.

Robins, L. N. (1969). Social correlates of psychiatric disorders: Can we tell causes from consequences? *Journal of Health and Social Behavior, 10*, 95–104.

Robins, L. N., Murphy, G. E., Woodruff, R. A., et al. (1971). Adult psychiatric status of black school boys: Social correlates of antisocial personality. *Archives of General Psychiatry, 24*, 338–345.

Schneider, K. (1959). *Clinical psychopathology.* New York: Grune & Stratton.

Scribner, R. (1996). Editorial: Paradox as paradigm—the health outcomes of Mexican Americans. *American Journal of Public Health, 86*, 303–304.

Skodol. A, E., Schwartz, S., Dohrenwend, B. P., et al. (1996). PTSD symptoms and comorbid mental disorders in Israeli war veterans. *British Journal of Psychiatry, 169*, 717–725.

Solomon, Z. (1993). *Combat stress reaction in the enduring toll of war.* New York: Plenum Press.

Solomon, Z. (1995). The effect of prior stressful experience on coping with war trauma and captivity. *Psychological Medicine, 25*, 1289–1294.

Steele, C. M., & Aronson, J. (1995). Stereotype threat and the intellectual test performance of African Americans. *Journal of Personality and Social Psychology, 69,* 797–811.

Sutker, B. P., Allain, A. N., & Johnson, J. L. (1993). Case study: Clinical assessment of long-term cognitive and emotional sequelae to World War II prisoner-of-war confinement: Comparison of pilot twins. *Psychological Assessment, 5,* 3–10.

True, W. R., Rice, J., Eisen, S. A., et al. (1993). A twin study of genetic and environmental contributions to liability for posttraumatic stress symptoms. *Archives of General Psychiatry, 50,* 257–264.

Turner, J. R., & Lloyd, D. A. (1995). Lifetime traumas and mental health: The significance of cumulative adversity. *Journal of Health and Social Behavior, 36,* 360–376.

Williams, D. R., & Collins, C. (1995). US socioeconomic and racial differences in health: Patterns and explanations. *Annual Review of Sociology, 21,* 349–386.

Yehuda, R., Kahana, B., Schmeidler, J., et al. (1995). Impact of cumulative lifetime trauma and recent stress on current posttraumatic stress disorder symptoms in Holocaust survivors. *American Journal of Psychiatry, 152,* 1815–1818.

Yehuda, R., & McFarlane, A. C. (1995). Conflict between current knowledge about posttraumatic stress disorder and its original conceptual basis. *American Journal of Psychiatry, 152,* 1705–1713.

30

Theoretical Integration

Bruce P. Dohrenwend

In the preceding chapter, I argued that there are three groups of studies that provide an environmental analogue to the behavioral genetic twin, family, and adoption studies that have proved so persuasive in demonstrating a role for genetic factors in most major types of psychiatric disorder. The environmental triad consists of studies of extreme situations such as exposure to combat and natural disasters; epidemiological research showing that overall prevalence of psychiatric disorders and, in men or women, the specific subtypes of schizophrenia, major depression, antisocial personality disorder, alcoholism, substance use disorders, and post-traumatic stress disorder (PTSD) are inversely related to socioeconomic status (SES); and a quasi-experimental investigation of the social causation–social selection issue posed by these SES differences.

Although this environmental triad shows that adversity is important, like the behavioral genetic triad, the three groups of studies it includes do not investigate directly the processes and mechanisms involved. My purpose in this concluding chapter is to develop a theoretical framework of integrative ideas, concepts, and propositions for investigating the processes by which adversity contributes to the occurrence and distribu-

tion of psychiatric disorders in the general population.

In seeking to explain how adversity is related to psychopathology in the general population, it is necessary to consider what kinds of stressful events are likely to be important and under what circumstances. I therefore begin by analyzing the nature of events in extreme situations such as exposure to combat, and then investigate how stressful events in more usual situations of everyday life in general populations compare with events in extreme situations.

CHARACTERISTICS OF EVENTS IN EXTREME SITUATIONS

Extreme situations involve events that are negative and involve loss rather than gain. All or most major events in extreme situations are "fateful," (Dohrenwend, 1979) in that the circumstances leading up to them and their immediate occurrence are beyond the control of the person and unaffected by his or her behavior. Their onset is often unpredictable; some of these major events in extreme situations are life-threatening and hence central to the needs and goals of the individual. They are large in objective magnitude in that they bring about great changes in the usual activities of the individual; all or some of these changes are beyond the control of the individual (e.g., the casualty rate in a soldier's company). Some of the events themselves or the uncontrollable changes that follow them tend to exhaust the individual physically. All of these characteristics are found, for example, in the experience of the Holocaust (see Levav, Chapter 1, this volume); they are present in the situations of Southeast Asian refugees (see Mollica et al., Chapter 2, this volume); all occur in severe, prolonged combat (see Keane, Chapter 3, this volume); and they are the lot of those most exposed to the kinds of disasters described by Giel (see Chapter 4, this volume).

SIMILARITIES AND CONTRASTS BETWEEN EVENTS IN EXTREME SITUATIONS AND EVENTS IN MORE USUAL SITUATIONS

The characteristics that define events in extreme situations occur to some degree in most of the major, individually targeted negative events investigated in the chapters in Part II of this volume. They are most evident in child abuse and neglect (see Widom, Chapter 5, this volume), where they are likely to have the added impact of primacy; that is, they strike at the most vulnerable stages of human development. Homelessness (see Herman et al., Chapter 8, this volume), when it occurs independently of the behavior of the person (as would sometimes be the case for adults and usually the case for the children in homeless families) and exposes the person to life-threatening events, also can share many of the characteristics of events in extreme situations. Some situations involving rape also have these characteristics (see Kilpatrick et al., Chapter 10, this volume).

Life-threatening physical illnesses and injuries (see Dew, Chapter 11, this volume) have much in common with events in extreme situations (which can, of course, include life-threatening injuries) but usually lack the wider threatening context of extreme situations and occur in contexts where social supports are more readily available. Infection with the human immunodeficiency virus (see Ouellette, Chapter 9, this volume) prior to the time that knowledge of its behavioral risk factors became available is one such illness. As Ouellette's analyses suggest, its occurrence in the context of the social supports organized by the gay community may have provided extraordinarily effective protection against what would otherwise be more traumatic psychological effects.

It is possible, however, for life-threatening events to be created by the behavior of the individual. Illnesses and injuries that result when persons engage in behaviors they know to be high risk are examples, as are some types of homelessness. There are also major events such as bereavement (see Clayton, Chapter 6, this volume) that are likely to be fateful but not life threatening. This is true of some types of unemployment such as layoffs that occur when an entire plant shuts down (see Kasl et al., Chapter 7, this volume). These contrasts and similarities are relatively clear cut.

Assessing the points of similarity and contrast between events in extreme situations and events in more usual situations of individuals in the general population becomes more complicated when we look at such events as a marital separation or divorce (see Bruce, Chapter 12, this volume), the full variety of events involving unemployment (see Kasl et al., Chapter 7, this volume), or some types of physical illness or injury that may not occur independently of the behavior of the individual (see Dew, Chapter 11, this volume). These types of events are clearly stressful, but their magnitudes vary greatly and their origins may as often be in the "stress generative" (Hammen, 1991) behavior of the individual as in the environmental conditions to which the individual is exposed. Still more frequently, such events are brought about by a complex mixture of the person's behavior and factors in his or her external environment. Moreover, how long the negative changes in usual activities that follow these events remain uncontrollable may depend more on the coping ability of the person (e.g., choosing a good lawyer prior to divorce; using a successful strategy of job search following unemployment) than on external factors in the wider environment (e.g., Allied forces liberating a concentration camp survivor).

Where life-threatening events in extreme situations are concerned, the *centrality* of the threat to the needs and goals of the individual is self-evident; all usual activities are disrupted and all of the individual's goals are in jeopardy. Some events in both unusual and usual situations may also have an extremely high degree of centrality even when they may not be life-threatening. One possible example consists in events that involve threats to physical "place" (Fullilove, 1996). The sources of such events differ greatly, ranging from war-created refugee situations that involve life threat to lesser dislocations resulting from slum clearance and job relocation.

Most events in more usual situations impact more selectively on particular activities of the individual and the goals related to these activities (e.g., marital separation impacts on family but not necessarily on work). These more specific goals vary with the type of event and the particular values and beliefs of the individuals who experience it: for example, the particular goods and services the individual needs or desires, or the particular sources of respect on which he or she relies. Often money is a convenient measure because it can be converted into many of these goods and services and serves as a proxy for goals consisting in the goods and services. A meaningful indicator of amount of negative change is thus often the proportion of income lost following an event. These varied and sometimes subtle threats (e.g., "keeping up with the Jones's") can involve relative deprivation as well as absolute deprivation as the individual compares his or her plight with the circumstances of more fortunate others (Merton & Kitt, 1950).

Major work must be done in developing taxonomies of goals and aspects of various kinds of life events that carry the potential to interfere with them. In the United States, these goals are embodied in broadest terms in the "American dream" of life, liberty, and the pursuit of happiness and, more particularly, in its group and individual variations. Barbara Dohrenwend and I (1969) took some initial steps in the direction of classification by distinguishing between "developmental versus nondevelopmental" stressors and "security versus achievement" stressors. However, the checklist measures of life events that we were using then were not adequate to the job of operationalizing these distinctions. Much more detailed information about the event and the changes in usual activities following it is required. Although we have developed a more satisfactory general approach to measuring life events (Dohrenwend et al., 1993), we have not yet constructed ratings—other than that of life threat—that would test congruence versus incongruence with valued goals of events and of changes in usual activities following them. Others have been working on the problem as well. In addition to Brown (see Chapter 18, this volume), for example, Thoits (1995) is developing ideas along these lines.

What I think is needed is an integration of knowledge gained from intensive case studies of individual events (e.g., bereavement, marital separation, unemployment) on the one hand and event inventory approaches that can be used in research on risk factors in unselected samples from the general population on the other. This would help us develop measures of the important dimensions of events that capture something of their richness and complexity (see Bromet and Dohrenwend's introduction to Part III of this volume) while retaining the ability to inventory them both retrospectively and prospectively in general population samples (see Eaton and Dohrenwend's introduction to Part II of this volume).

The threats that negative events pose to the important goals of the individual are translated into actualities when the events are followed by negative changes in the usual activities through which the individual pursues or maintains important goals, that is, negative changes in the person's ongoing situation. As noted above, when events involve threat to life, all of the usual activities in the individual's ongoing situation are at risk. Negative events in more usual situations as a rule threaten only some of these activities. In general, we can define the *objective magnitude* of any negative event as being indicated by the *hypothetical* amount of negative change the event is likely to bring about in the usual activities of most people who experience the event (Dohrenwend et al., 1993). For an event to be *major*, this hypothetical amount of change in usual activities must be substantial. It should affect goals that are widely thought to be important by most people in the society.

Actual amount of change, in turn, would be indicated by the centrality of disrupted usual activities for maintaining or achieving the most important goals of the individual and the proportion of these activities affected. These actual changes in a person's ongoing situation are determined by personal predispositions and resources in the ongoing situation as well as by the magnitude of proximal events, as is discussed in more detail later on.

RELATION OF CHARACTERISTICS OF EVENTS IN EXTREME SITUATIONS AND EVENTS IN MORE USUAL SITUATIONS TO TESTS OF THE SOCIAL CAUSATION–SOCIAL SELECTION ISSUE POSED BY SES DIFFERENCES IN RATES OF PSYCHIATRIC DISORDERS

The theory underlying the social causation hypothesis in the quasi-experimental test of the social causation–social selection issue is that encountering barriers to achieving highly valued goals produces stresses and strains toward deviant behavior (see Dohrenwend et al., Chapter 14, this volume). These barriers are assumed to vary with adversity stemming from differences in SES and ethnic/racial status. In the macro-level

tests that we reported (Dohrenwend et al., Chapter 14, this volume), these processes were not investigated directly. It is reasonable to assume, however, that the postulated processes can be investigated directly in research with persons of different gender, ethnic/racial background, and SES in the general population. The focus of such research would be on the events in extreme situations and events in other more usual situations that individuals in different social statuses encounter over their life spans while pursuing their goals.

As a step toward developing guidelines for this research, let me enlarge on the three main elements of life stress processes that I introduced in my general introduction to this volume. Figure 30.1 includes the original three components of proximal life events (i.e., events occurring within a few weeks to a year prior to the adaptive or maladaptive outcomes to be investigated); ongoing situation of usual activities that antedate the occurrence of proximal events; and personal antecedent predispositions. However, it links personal predispositions to biological background, and it links both personal predispositions and the ongoing situation to characteristics of the wider external environment in which and out of which they have developed. Moreover, it shows more connective lines among variables in the diagram to illustrate something of the complexity of the relationships we know to be involved.

A comprehensive assessment of the nature and strength of the contribution of adversity to the occurrence, persistence, or recurrence of disorder would determine (*1*) the importance of antecedent environmental factors compared to antecedent biological background, especially genetic inheritance, in the development of proximal life events, ongoing situation, and personal predispositions; (*2*) the relative importance of proximal life events, personal predispositions, and a priori liabilities in the ongoing situation (e.g., lack of social network that can provide material and emotional support) in bringing about the adverse health outcome; (*3*) how proximal life events, personal

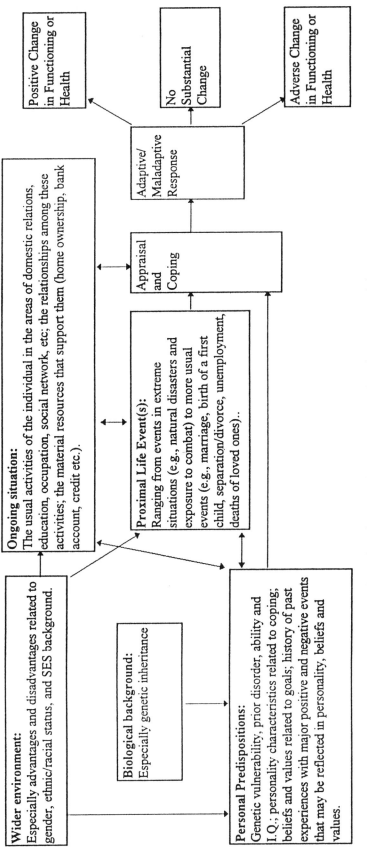

Figure 30.1. Relationship of proximal life events, personal predispositions, and the ongoing situation to wider environment, biological background, appraisal and coping processes, and health outcomes.

predispositions, and the a priori liabilities in the ongoing situation are related to each other in bringing about the negative outcome; and (4) similarities and differences in factors that contribute to onset of disorder on the one hand and to transient, by contrast with persistent or recurrent, course once disorder has occurred on the other hand. Next I consider what is involved in each of these determinations.

Importance of Antecedent Wider Environment

On the left-hand side of Figure 30.1 are two boxes portraying the impact of factors in the antecedent environment and personal predispositions as these may influence the occurrence of proximal life events; as was pointed out earlier, for example, when external environmental factors are far more important in the occurrence of a negative event than personal predispositions, the proximal event is fateful. Major fateful events are direct manifestations of adversity in close to one of the strongest dictionary definitions of adversity as quoted in my general introduction to this volume: "exposure to a set of unpropitious or calamitous circumstances implying previous well-being" (Webster, 1961, p. 14). When fateful events occur in the context of extreme situations such as combat, the fateful aspects of the event are likely to determine not only its occurrence but also uncontrollable changes in these ongoing situations. The experience described in the case study by Sutker and her colleagues (1993) of OR, the twin who was shot down during a World War II combat mission and taken prisoner, is a vivid example (see also Dohrenwend, Chapter 29, this volume).

We have developed procedures for measuring the extent to which events are fateful as well as other of their important objective characteristics, such as their magnitude (Dohrenwend et al., 1993). These involve obtaining a detailed narrative of what led up to the event and what happened at the time of its immediate occurrence. The distinction between fateful and nonfateful involves not just ascertaining whether the event is independent of prior disorder or of insidious onset of a new episode. The more comprehensive issue in assessing fatefulness is the extent to which individuals, by their own behavior, create the stressful events to which they are exposed (see Breslau et al., Chapter 15, this volume; Kendler, Chapter 26, this volume; Robins & Robertson, Chapter 16, this volume). When this occurs, it is possible that the personal predispositions (including but not limited to prior disorder) involved in the event-inducing behaviors have been influenced by genetic inheritance (Rutter, 1986). To the extent that this is the case, the occurrence of the events would be under genetic control (see Kendler, Chapter 26, this volume). The personal predispositions involved in the occurrence of such negative events may also contribute to maladaptive coping and prolonged uncontrollable negative changes in the individual's usual activities following the event.

Theory and stress research have focused less on positive events than on negative events; for example, positive events do not figure prominently in most life event inventories. The occurrence of most positive events is strongly influenced by the behavior of the person. Exceptions are rare examples of immense good fortune, such as winning a lottery, and some positive events that occur to significant others, such as a job promotion of one's spouse. Much of the significance of positive events whose occurrence is influenced by the behavior of the individual is that they indicate the presence of positive personal predispositions. It seems likely, moreover, that when they occur, self-generated positive events reinforce and strengthen these positive predispositions and coping behaviors related to the positive dispositions. Positive events can therefore be proxies for positive predispositions that contribute to the prevention of uncontrollable negative changes following negative events or, if uncontrollable changes do occur, to reducing their duration (e.g., Suh et al., 1996; Thoits, 1995; Zautra & Reich, 1983).

However, it is often the case that factors related to differences in gender, ethnic/racial status, and SES determine the types of both positive and negative events that it is possible for the individual to experience; these factors can thereby contribute an element of fatefulness even to events the occurrence of which also may be strongly influenced by the behavior of the individual. For example, women but not men directly experience gender-specific positive events such as a wanted pregnancy and negative events such as abortions, spontaneous or not; members of ethnic/racial minorities are more likely to be arrested whether for cause or not; persons of low SES are more likely to be in occupations with high turnover rates whether for cause or not. A major problem in assessing the nature of adversity represented by events in more usual situations is to isolate the fateful consequences of these status differences—that is, to assess the extent to which the status differences narrow the scope for individual differences in personal predispositions to come into play in bringing about the positive or negative events.

Let us turn now to variables in the other two components of life stress processes—personal predispositions and ongoing situation. Assessments of the relative importance of the effects of prior circumstances in the wider environment, on the one hand, and prior biological background, on the other, on the ongoing situation and personal predispositions are also necessary in evaluating the role of adversity. Consider, for example, occupational conditions in the ongoing situation of the individual, such as whether he or she is in the privileged position of owning the means of production (Wohlfarth, 1997); or of directing, controlling, and planning the work involved (see Link et al., Chapter 21, this volume); or rather is in much less advantaged circumstances. It would be necessary to examine whether such conditions of work vary with the ascribed characteristics of gender and ethnic/racial status or blue versus white collar parental SES, rather than with personal predispositions such as prior personal or family history of psychiat-

ric disorder (see, e.g., Link et al., Chapter 21, this volume). The same questions would need to be asked about differences in the ability of social networks to provide material resources such as financial aid, legal assistance, and physical health care to support the usual activities of individuals from different backgrounds (see Henderson, Chapter 20, this volume). For personality characteristics such as neuroticism, low attitudes of mastery, high external locus of control, or high sensation-seeking tendencies that are likely to contribute to maladaptive coping (see Skodol, Chapter 19, this volume), it would be necessary to investigate whether they are more strongly related to environmental factors such as adversity early in life (see Kraemer & Bachevalier, Chapter 24, this volume) or were more a function of genetic inheritance (see Kendler, Chapter 26, this volume).

Relative Importance of Life Events, Ongoing Situation, and Personal Predispositions

It is possible to conceive of circumstances in which the component of proximal stressful events is likely to be more important than either the strengths or weaknesses of personal predispositions or the assets or liabilities of the ongoing situation on which the events impact. When the overriding proximal negative events are fateful, we have referred to this as "victimization" (e.g., Dohrenwend & Dohrenwend, 1981). The most vivid examples are extreme situations such as prolonged exposure to combat during wartime in relation to the development of PTSD (see e.g., Keane, Chapter 3, this volume). These are clear "hazards" (see Leighton, Chapter 28, this volume) to psychological health.

By contrast with extreme situations of "victimization" are situations in which the role of personal predispositions is so strong that recent events and the factors in the ongoing situation are unimportant. An example would be genetic predisposition to a disorder such as Huntington's disease. This is an illustration of what we have referred to as a "proneness" model (Dohrenwend & Dohrenwend, 1981). In still further contrast with "victimization" by an extreme proximal event are circumstances in which the adverse conditions of the person's ongoing situation are paramount; for example, exposure to loud sounds, extreme heat or cold, or arduous physical tasks as part of one's job (see Link et al., Chapter 21, this volume) or inequitable domestic arrangements (see Lennon, Chapter 22, this volume). These are some of the types of conditions in ongoing situations that we have described as involving "chronic burden" (Dohrenwend & Dohrenwend, 1981). As Wheaton (1990) has pointed out, the impact of some events (e.g., divorce) may actually alleviate the burden of difficult components of ongoing situations (e.g., a longstanding problematic marriage).

Structural Relations among Life Events, Ongoing Situation, and Personal Predispositions

I gave examples above of "victimization," in which proximal life events are likely to carry greatest risk; "proneness," where personal predispositions dominate; and "chronic burden," in which the ongoing situation is most important. Usually, the three components are more nearly equal in importance. A variety of formulations of how they are related to each other in bringing about adverse health changes has centered on the idea of "vulnerability" (e.g., Dohrenwend & Dohrenwend, 1981; Zubin & Spring, 1977; Dohrenwend, 1981; see also Brown, Chapter 18, this volume). Here strengths and weaknesses in personal predispositions and assets or liabilities associated with the individual's usual activities in the ongoing situation amplify or reduce the impact of proximal life events on the ongoing situation, as discussed in Part IV of this volume (see Mechanic's introduction to Part IV; Henderson, Chapter 20; Lennon, Chapter 22; Link et al., Chapter 21; Skodol, Chapter 19).

An alternative to vulnerability models involves the hypothesis that strengths and weaknesses of personal predispositions and

assets and liabilities of the ongoing situation make independent causal contributions rather than modifying the impact of life events. We have termed this the "additive burden" model (e.g., Dohrenwend & Dohrenwend, 1981).

Psychological Integration of Relations between Proximal Events, the Ongoing Situation, and Personal Predispositions in Relation to Personal Goals: Appraisal, Threat, and Coping

For any particular event in the context of any particular ongoing situation, personal predispositions—especially the presence of prior psychopathology, differences in normal personality characteristics related to coping, and the relevance of the event to important personal goals—will determine how the event is perceived and reacted to (e.g., Dohrenwend & Martin, 1979). These appraisal and coping processes, in turn, often can increase or decrease the amount of negative change in the usual activities of the ongoing situation of the individual and increase or decrease the duration of these changes. To the extent that the coping efforts increase the amount or duration of the negative changes, they contribute to the uncontrollability of these changes.

Given the same event, we can estimate whether coping is *adaptive* or *maladaptive* by assessing whether the negative change in the usual activities of a particular individual who experienced the event is less or greater than the negative change that most normal individuals facing such an event would be likely to show. For example, in a study of patients suffering from chronic pain compared with controls free of this disorder, Lennon et al. (1990) found that the pain patients reported more negative changes in their lives following recent negative events (other than episodes of pain), than did controls who experienced negative events of similar objective magnitude.

The social statuses of gender, ethnicity, and SES are likely to be related to appraisal and coping processes through their relation to personal predispositions, perhaps especially personal values and beliefs. A particularly compelling example of how disadvantaged ethnic/racial status may be involved was mentioned in Chapter 29 (this volume). It is contained in research by Steele and Aronson (1995) on "stereotype threat." These investigators demonstrated experimentally the impact on aptitude test scores of increments of threat related to prejudice and discrimination in the wider environment of ethnic/racial minorities.

Gender, ethnic/racial status, and SES are also likely to be related to appraisal and coping processes through the relation of these statuses to the individual's assets or resources in the ongoing situation. When these resources provide inadequate means to sustain or achieve valued goals, there is likely to be an increase in feelings of relative deprivation, reactions of anger or pessimism or helplessness, and behavior that contributes to an increase in uncontrollable negative changes in usual activities. Just how the occurrence of different types of major fateful and nonfateful negative events affect these appraisals of relations between valued goals and the adequacy of available means to achieve them, feelings of relative deprivation, and different types of subsequent adaptive and maladaptive coping efforts are major questions (Merton & Kitt, 1950).

Although studies show that adverse health outcomes such as depressive episodes are likely to follow closely (within a few weeks to a few months) the occurrence of major negative events (see, e.g., Stueve et al., Chapter 17, this volume), are there nevertheless "incubation" effects for some events and for some people (e.g., Bebbington et al., 1993)? Under what circumstances do individuals habituate by reordering the importance of goals, abandoning them altogether, or developing alternative legal or illegal means for pursuing them? Is the new ongoing situation more or less viable (Thoits, 1995; see also Bromet and Dohrenwend's introduction to Part III of this volume; Eaton and Dohrenwend's introduction to Part II of this volume)? If the ongoing situation becomes increasingly less viable, at what point does the individual come to feel powerless to achieve or maintain his or her goals—find himself or herself in an "intractable predicament" (Frank, 1973, pp. 312–318), and develop behavior that shows the pointlessness and purposelessness that is characteristic of psychopathology (Horwitz, 1982, p. 28)?

Initial Onset and Course of Disorder

In Figure 30.1 and the theoretical considerations set forth above about the relationships it portrays, I have not confronted directly the important matter of distinguishing between factors in the initial onset of disorders by contrast with factors in their course following such onset. I have anticipated the question, however, with my discussions of the idea that proximal events can be followed by uncontrollable negative changes in the ongoing situation that themselves have lasting impact. I want to take up now in more detail the question of whether and, if so, to what extent risk factors in onset are the same as or different from risk factors in course. To address this question, I return to the concepts of protection/vulnerability with regard to onset and stress evaporation/residual stress with regard to course that I introduced in Chapter 29 (this volume) in relation to discussion of the development of PTSD following exposure to negative events in extreme situations. I attempt to develop these concepts as they link amplification or reduction of uncontrollable changes in the ongoing situation to health outcomes.

As emphasized earlier, negative events in extreme situations have in common with negative events in more usual situations the fact that both can lead, albeit usually by different routes, to uncontrollable negative changes in the ongoing situation. It seems reasonable to assume, therefore, that it is the uncontrollable negative changes that precipitate the onset of disorder: *The more central the uncontrollable changes and the greater the proportion of usual activities they involve, the greater the likelihood of onset of disorder.*

This proposition about the pathogenic role of exposure to uncontrollable negative changes is strongly supported by the parallels between research on PTSD in extreme situations such as combat and animal experiments on the effects of controllable and uncontrollable shock (Foa et al., 1992). It has, however, much wider applicability. This is illustrated in experiments with humans on the psychological and biological effects of much milder uncontrollable stressors (e.g., Boyd, 1982; Brier et al., 1987) and in experiments with animals involving the effects of exposure to uncontrollable shock on a variety of adverse physical and psychological outcomes (e.g., Jackson et al., 1979; Laudenslager et al., 1983; MacLennan & Maier, 1983; Visintainer et al., 1982).

Even in extreme situations, however, major fateful events are not the only determinants of the magnitude of uncontrollable negative changes in the ongoing situation. (Being placed in a concentration camp or being taken prisoner of war probably approach being exceptions.) Foa and her colleagues (1992) concluded on the basis of their review of the animal experiments, for example, that unpredictability of onset in addition to uncontrollability of onset make contributions to various types of adverse outcomes that seem congruent with some of the dimensions of PTSD in humans.

In the animal research reviewed, the investigators had experimental control over onsets and offsets of negative events (e.g., electric shock). Separation of unpredictability from uncontrollability is far more difficult to achieve in nonexperimental research with humans. As Foa et al. (1992, p. 222) note, there is considerable overlap between the two constructs. Some investigators, ourselves included, have used unpredictability as one of the criteria for uncontrollability of onset in our work on measuring fatefulness. We considered, for example, such things as whether a person had been previously divorced in evaluating narrative material for the likely contribution of the individual's behavior to the occurrence of the divorce.

Despite their close relationship, however, uncontrollability and unpredictability are not the same thing (e.g., sudden death of a loved one in an accident in contrast with death of a loved one after a long illness known to be fatal; an unexpected natural disaster in contrast with one for which there is advance warning). Predictability offers an opportunity to take action that may reduce uncontrollable negative changes and can therefore modify the impact and hence the adverse psychological consequences of a negative event. Whether such action is taken, of course, depends on a number of other factors such as whether the individual has the relevant information about the likelihood of the event occurring, his or her coping ability, material resources, and social supports.

As this discussion of the role of unpredictability suggests, vulnerability factors and protective factors contained in the personal predispositions and ongoing situation, components of Figure 30.1, are likely to play major parts, along with proximal negative events, in determining the magnitude of uncontrollable negative changes. Because both personal predispositions (e.g., personality characteristics) and elements in the ongoing situation (e.g., the person's social network) are likely to persist over time, the vulnerability/protective factors they contain affect not only the magnitude of uncontrollable negative changes following exposure to negative events, but also the duration of these changes and the occurrence of new, nonfateful negative events. For these reasons, vulnerability and protective factors affect not only the likelihood of initial onset of disorder but also the likelihood that disorder, once it occurs, will be transient, persistent, or recurrent.

The processes underlying these characteristics of course of disorder were described with the terms *stress evaporation* with regard to transience and *residual stress* with regard to persistence or recurrence—used as sensitizing concepts as in our earlier discussion of PTSD (Chapter 29, this volume). Although they reflect the continuing influence of vulnerability and protective factors, stress evaporation/residual stress factors also consist in new variables that do not apply prior to the initial onset of disorder; for example, psychiatric treatment and the possibility of both symptom control (see Frank & Karp, Chapter 25, this volume; Keane, Chapter 3, this volume) and labeling associated with such treatment (e.g., Link et al., 1989). There is increasing evidence that residual stress is also increased by biological changes (see Frank & Karp, Chapter 25, this volume; Keane, Chapter 3, this volume; Kraemer & Bachevalier, Chapter 24, this volume; Rose's introduction to Part V of this volume); by psychological "scarring" (Rohde et al., 1994); and by deficits in social functioning (Häfner et al., 1995) following the onset of disorder. Unless reduced by therapeutic interventions, such changes would be expected to increase the duration of the disorder or the likelihood that it will recur even when habituation to the negative changes in the ongoing situation has occurred.

The fact, as mentioned above and shown in Figure 30.1, that personal predispositions can contribute to the occurrence of events has implications for understanding the complex processes through which some types of events contribute to onset and course. To the extent that personal predispositions involve actions by the individual that bring about the occurrence of negative events, these events are nonfateful. A nonfateful negative event may therefore reflect vulnerability factors in these personal predispositions. Because such predispositions tend to be persistent over time, the negative, nonfateful events are likely to contribute not only to the initial onset of disorder but also to persistence or recurrence.

The occurrence of positive events usually also is affected by the behavior of the individual. Positive events therefore can reflect protective factors related to positive personal predispositions. Because positive predispositions, like negative predispositions, are likely to be persistent, positive events related to these predispositions are likely to reflect not only protection, by contributing to adaptive coping that minimizes the number of negative changes in the ongoing situation following negative events, but also

stress evaporation, by reducing the duration of their uncontrollable effects. The first, protective role decreases the likelihood that disorder will develop; the second, stress-evaporating role decreases the likelihood that it will persist if it does develop. In sum, nonfateful negative events and many positive events can be, in varying degrees depending on the magnitude of the role of personal predispositions in their occurrence, proxies for personal predispositions. As such, these events themselves have vulnerability/protective and residual stress/stress evaporation functions. Figure 30.2 builds on Figure 30.1 by incorporating these added distinctions about protection/vulnerability in relation to onset and stress evaporation/residual stress in relation to course.

Type of Disorder

The term *disorder* in Figure 30.2 applies to the types of psychopathology that are inversely related to SES among women or men, especially those that showed social causation outcomes in the macro-level quasi-experimental test. These include PTSD (on the basis of the study of Vietnam veterans referred to by Keane, Chapter 3, this volume), major depression, antisocial personality, alcoholism, other substance use disorders, and nonspecific psychological distress or demoralization (on the basis of Dohrenwend et al., Chapter 14, this volume). Which of these types of disorder develops will be influenced by personal predispositions (especially family history, type of prior Axis I and Axis II disorders, and normal personality characteristics); type and severity of threat posed by proximal life events or uncontrollable negative aspects of the ongoing situation (e.g., threat to life and PTSD; loss of loved ones and depression); and gender (a risk factor for depression in women and for antisocial personality, alcoholism, and substance use disorders in men). By extension, co-morbid disorders will occur when the risk factors for more than one disorder are present.

Some of the symptoms of each type of disorder that we have been considering

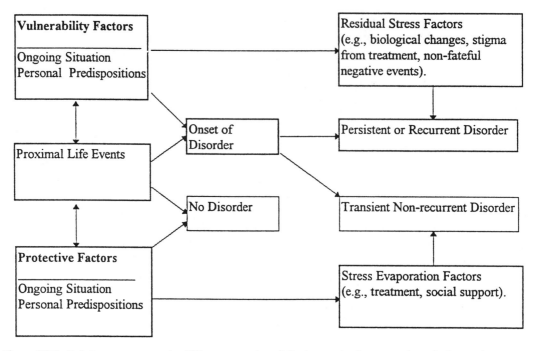

Figure 30.2. Relations among proximal life events, vulnerability/protective factors, and residual stress/stress evaporation factors to the onset and course of disorder.

show striking congruencies with uncontrollable negative changes in the ongoing situation. The intrusiveness/avoidance symptoms of PTSD are continuing reflections of the impact of life-threatening events even when the extreme situation in which they occurred may be over (Baum, 1990). The feelings of helplessness, hopelessness, and low self-esteem that help define "demoralization" seem compatible with an uncontrollable change of diverse origins that Frank (1973) refers to as an "intractable predicament" (pp. 312–318). The sadness and loss of pleasure and interest integral to major depression seem to correspond to abandoning goals under the impact of uncontrollable changes in the ongoing situation. The anesthetizing qualities of alcoholism and drugs may allow the individual to temporarily and unrealistically resurrect these goals. The adoption of illegal or violent actions as alternatives to disrupted or never-available conventional activities also can be understood as seizing on alternative means of achieved valued goals.

Some General Propositions

Based on the assumptions, definitions and distinctions set forth in relation to the variables in Figures 30.1 and 30.2, it is possible to set forth a few general propositions about how adversity and stress contribute to the onset and course of various types of psychopathology that are inversely related to SES in men or women. I begin with onset and then continue with course.

Initial Onset of Disorder

- The greater and more central the uncontrollable negative changes in usual activities in the ongoing situation following exposure to a negative event, the greater the likelihood that disorder will develop.
- The more unpredictable the negative changes, the greater the likelihood that they will be uncontrollable.
- Uncontrollable negative changes in the ongoing situation will increase with the

objective magnitude of proximal fateful and nonfateful negative events, the centrality of these events, the unpredictability of their onset, the amount of vulnerability in personal predispositions leading to maladaptive coping, and the lack of material and psychological supports in the ongoing situation, as well as combinations of these.

- The amount of environmental adversity represented by proximal negative events will increase with the events' fatefulness, objective magnitude, and centrality.
- The type of disorder that develops will vary with personal predispositions, characteristics of the proximal negative event, age, and gender.

Course of Disorder Once It Occurs— Transience, Persistence, or Recurrence

- The greater the contribution of personal predispositions, compared to proximal fateful events, to uncontrollable negative changes in the ongoing situation, the greater the likelihood that the changes will persist.
- The fewer the resources of material and psychological support in the ongoing situation, the greater the likelihood that uncontrollable negative changes will persist.
- The duration of disorder will vary directly with the duration or recurrence of uncontrollable negative changes in the ongoing situation.
- The longer the disorder persists once it has occurred, the fewer the new uncontrollable changes in the ongoing situation required to precipitate reoccurrence.

Social Status and Adversity

- The primacy, frequency, and recency of life-threatening and other major fateful negative events over the life course vary with ethnic/racial status (greater in disadvantaged ethnic/racial groups in

assimilation situations) and SES (greater in lower SES groups).
- Material resources in the ongoing situation that stem from the wider environment vary over the life course with ethnic/racial status (fewer in disadvantaged ethnic/racial groups) and SES (fewer in lower SES groups).

IMPLICATIONS FOR RESEARCH

The purpose of research designed to investigate these propositions would be to understand the role of adversity in the occurrence and course of psychopathology in general populations. The enterprise, therefore, would be epidemiological at its core.

As was evident in the quasi-experimental research on the social causation–social selection issue, however, the required contrasts are not likely to be provided by individuals drawn from representative samples of households with "survey methods better suited to predicting votes than to identifying psychiatric cases" (Robins, 1969, p. 103). Moreover, not all of the most important variables we have been considering lend themselves to investigation with cross-sectional designs and retrospective methods that, for practical reasons, are characteristic of most research in psychiatric epidemiology.

Fortunately, many of the important variables are relatively well suited to retrospective designs such as case–control studies (see, e.g., Stueve et al., Chapter 17, this volume). These variables include—along with measures of gender, ethnic/racial status, and SES—major negative and positive life events and some indicators of change in the ongoing situation following these events (e.g., changes in network characteristics and proportion of income lost). However, care must be taken with the measurement to avoid serious recall biases that can inflate relations between even such relatively objective risk factors and psychiatric outcomes. Such biases may be especially severe with self-report, checklist measures of stressful life events (Southwick et al., 1997). Intensive interviews and use of multiple methods and expert raters for measuring both life events and psychopathology offer more assurance (Dohrenwend, 1990; Dohrenwend et al., 1993).

As much of the research in this volume shows, substantial advances can be made by using prospective and longitudinal designs as well (see, e.g., Bruce, Chapter 12, this volume; Kilpatrick et al., Chapter 10, this volume; Widom, Chapter 5, this volume); there is a call for more prospective and longitudinal studies by the authors who introduced the various parts of this volume. Innovative designs with prospective and longitudinal components are mandatory for investigation of personality characteristics that could be state dependent appraisal processes, coping behaviors, and many details of the ongoing situation. Many of these more subjective variables resist accurate and unbiased recall (see Mechanic's introduction to Part IV of this volume). For example, the investigation of subjective appraisals of events that are direct indicators of the threat they embody for the individual must be conducted in the context of prospective research designs if interest is in antecedent risk factors rather than post hoc distortions and rationalizations.

Ideally, multiple measures at closely spaced intervals would be employed. When this use of frequent measurement over time is impractical, the type of procedure used by Brown (see Chapter 18, this volume) in one of the investigations he reports seems very promising. It involves, first, assessing the likely importance of goals by measuring the individual's prior commitment in various domains of life, such as marriage, motherhood, and work, in a baseline assessment. Once this is done, the second step is to monitor major events over the following year. The significance of these events can be assessed in terms of their centrality—that is, how relevant they are to the goals to which the individual is highly committed before the event occurred.

Like me, most of the researchers who have contributed to this volume work with epidemiological and other nonexperimental methods and develop their research within largely psychosocial orientations to etiology. To fully respond to the challenge of investigating the role of adversity in the development of psychopathology in further research, help would be needed from five sets of colleagues who use different methods or employ different theoretical frameworks: those in the field of behavior genetics (see, e.g., Kendler, Chapter 26, this volume); investigators of biological correlates of vulnerability, stress, and various types of psychopathology (see, e.g., Frank & Karp, Chapter 25, this volume; Keane, Chapter 3, this volume; Kraemer & Bachevlier, Chapter 24, this volume); animal researchers (see, e.g., Kraemer & Bachevelier, Chapter 24, this volume); people who do simulation studies (see, e.g., Shrout & Link, Chapter 23, this volume); and those who do preventive trials (see, e.g., Kellam et al., Chapter 27, this volume).

The twin strategies of behavior geneticists may be especially important for the information they can provide about the extent to which even fateful negative events are under genetic control (see Kendler, Chapter 26, this volume). Biological researchers could help investigate the important possibility that "certain kinds of extreme stress, such as combat exposure or the experience of internment, may leave permanent physiological 'scars' that, in their symptomatic expression, become themselves chronic stresses over time" (see Frank & Karp, Chapter 25, this volume). Animal experiments allow the manipulation of important environmental conditions (e.g., early rearing environments) that are analogous to important environmental conditions among humans that cannot be examined under conditions of experimental control (see Kraemer & Bachevlier, Chapter 24, this volume); computer simulations can test the logic of key theoretical assumptions based on nonexperimental observations (see Shrout & Link, Chapter 23, this volume). All of the authors who introduced the preceding sections of the volume point to the promise of preventive trials that are designed to reduce risk factors that are both potentially important and malleable. Work such as that of Kellam and his colleagues (see Chapter 27, this volume) may help us not only to modify the negative effects of adversity but also to establish the direction of relationships among the possible risk factors and the outcomes of interest (see also Eaton & Dohrenwend's introduction to Part II of this volume).

IN CONCLUSION

The three lines of research in the environmental triad that were examined—studies of extreme situations, epidemiological studies of relations between SES and psychiatric disorders, and quasi-experimental tests of the social causation–social selection issue posed by the SES differences—strongly suggest that environmentally induced adversity is a source of important risk factors for most major disorders, excepting schizophrenia, that are inversely related to SES. To return to Heston's (1988) question, "What about environment?", described in my introductory chapter to this volume, the collective results of the three lines of research provide strong evidence that the environment has been there all along and figures importantly not only in PTSD but also in the development of major depression in women and of antisocial personality and substance use disorders (including alcoholism) in men.

There are also clues to the specific risk factors and causal processes involved. Prolonged exposure to adversity in the form of fateful, unpredictable, and life-threatening events in extreme situations is probably sufficient for the occurrence of PTSD. The evidence is less clear about the importance of exposure to such extreme adversity in the course of PTSD and in its tendency to be accompanied or followed by other comorbid disorders, especially major depression and alcoholism. Questions about these matters are of fundamental importance to the whole idea of what is meant by the term *disorder*. They are even harder to answer about the role of adversity in other disorders that develop in more usual situations. Some leads are contained in Figures 30.1 and 30.2

and the definitions, distinctions, and propositions related to them.

The central integrating proposition is that the greater the uncontrollable negative changes in the ongoing situation (in terms of the centrality and proportion of usual activities affected) following the occurrence of a negative event, the greater the likelihood that disorder will develop. Ongoing situations become uncontrollable by different routes in which adversity is involved to greater or lesser extents. The uncontrollable negative changes in the ongoing situation are thus a final common pathway by which the different environmental and predispositional sources lead to adverse health outcomes. It is in the different environmental and predispositional sources of uncontrollability in extreme and more usual situations that adversity plays its part. These sources vary with gender, ethnic/racial status, and SES in modern, urban societies.

EPILOGUE

This theoretical formulation grew out of my attempt to integrate leads from the three lines of research mentioned above. They focus on adversity that is initiated or exacerbated by inequalities of gender, ethnic/racial status, and SES. Research on such adversity must deal with facts that are inconsistent with the most hallowed ideals of our society about equality and the right to life, liberty, and the pursuit of happiness. These propositions therefore have a subtext that is hard to put into words. I found help in expressing it when I came across a poem by Robert Frost (1979) about equality and The Declaration of Independence:

That all men are created free and equal . . .
That's a hard mystery of Jefferson's.
What did he mean? Of course the easy way
Is to decide it simply isn't true.
It may not be. I heard a fellow say no.
But never mind, the Welshman got it planted
Where it will trouble us a thousand years.

That Thomas Jefferson, the author of the position on equality, owned slaves and spoke of men but not women are historical manifestations of the continuing contradiction between the ideal and the harsh reality. It is through research on the nature and consequences of this potent anomaly that we may come to understand how adversity contributes to the development of psychopathology in our society.

Acknowledgements: This work has been supported by National Institute of Mental Health (NIMH) Research Scientist Award K05MH14663 and NIMH Research Grant MH30710. I would like to express my appreciation to Patrick E. Shrout for his very helpful comments and criticisms.

REFERENCES

Baum, A. (1990). Stress, intrusive imagery, and chronic distress. *Health Psychology*, 9, 653–675.

Bebbington, P., Geoff-Der, B. M., Wykes, T., et al. (1993). Stress incubation and the onset of affective disorders. *British Journal of Psychiatry*, 162, 358–362.

Boyd, T. L. (1982). Learned helplessness in humans: A frustration-produced response pattern. *Journal of Personality and Social Psychology*, 42, 738–752.

Breier, A., Albus, M., Pickar, D., et al. (1987). Controllable and uncontrollable stress in humans: Alterations in mood and neuroendocrine and psychophysiological function. *American Journal of Psychiatry*, 144, 1419–1425.

Dohrenwend, B. P. (1979). Stressful life events and psychopathology: Some issues of theory and method. In J. F. Barrett, R. M. Rose, & G. L. Klerman (Eds.), *Stress and mental disorder* (pp. 1–15). New York: Raven Press.

Dohrenwend, B. P. (1990). The problem of validity in field studies of psychological disorders revisited. *Psychological Medicine*, 20, 195–208.

Dohrenwend, B. P., & Dohrenwend, B. S. (1969). *Social status and psychological disorder: A causal inquiry*. New York: John Wiley & Sons.

Dohrenwend, B. P., Raphael, K. G., Schwartz, S., et al. (1993). The structured event probe and narrative rating method (SEPRATE) for measuring stressful life events. In L. Goldberger & S. Bresnitz (Eds.), *Handbook of*

stress: Theoretical and clinical aspects (2nd ed., pp. 174–199). New York: The Free Press.

Dohrenwend, B. S., & Dohrenwend, B. P. (1981). Socioenvironmental factors, stress, and psychopathology—Part 2: Hypotheses about stress processes linking social class to various types of psychopathology. *American Journal of Community Psychology*, 9, 146–159.

Dohrenwend, B. S., & Martin, J. L. (1979). Personal versus situational determination of anticipation and control of the occurrence of stressful life events. *American Journal of Community Psychology*, 7, 453–468.

Foa, E. B., Zinbarg, R., & Rothbaum, B. O. (1992). Uncontrollability and unpredictability in post-traumatic stress disorder: An animal model. *Psychological Bulletin*, 2, 218–238.

Frank, J. D. (1973). *Persuasion and healing*. Baltimore: The Johns Hopkins University Press.

Frost, R. (1979). "The Black Cottage." In E. C. Latham (Ed.), *The poetry of Robert Frost* (pp. 55–59). New York: Henry Holt.

Fullilove, M. T. (1996). The psychiatric implications of displacement: Contributions from the psychology of place. *American Journal of Psychiatry*, 153, 1516–1523.

Häfner, H., Nowotny, B., Loffler, W., et al. (1995). When and how does schizophrenia produce social deficits? *European Archives of Psychiatry and Clinical Neuroscience*, 246, 17–28.

Hammen, C. (1991). The generation of stress in the course of unipolar depression. *Journal of Abnormal Psychology*, 100, 555–561.

Heston, L. L. (1988). What about environment? In D. L. Dunner, S. Gershon, & J. B. Barret (Eds.), *Relatives at risk for mental disorder* (pp. 205–213). New York: Raven Press.

Horwitz, A. V. (1982). *The social control of mental illness*. New York: Academic Press.

Jackson, R. L., Maier, S. F., & Coon, D. J. (1979). Long-term analgesic effects of inescapable shock and learned helplessness. *Science*, 206, 91–93.

Laudenslager, M. L., Ryan, S. M., Drugan, R. C., et al. (1983). Coping and immunosuppression: Inescapable but not escapable shock suppresses lymphocyte proliferation. *Science*, 221, 568–570.

Lennon, M. C., Dohrenwend, B. P., Zautra, A. J., et al. (1990). Coping and adaptation to facial pain in contrast to other stressful life events. *Journal of Personality and Social Psychology*, 59, 1040–1050.

Link, B. G., Cullen, F. T., Struening, E., et al. (1989). A modified labeling theory approach to mental disorders: An empirical assessment. *American Sociological Review, 54,* 400–423.

MacLennan, A. J., & Maier, S. F. (1983). Coping and the stress-induced potentiation of stimulant stereotypy in the rat. *Science, 219,* 1091–1093.

Merton, R. K., & Kitt, A. S. (1950). Contributions to the theory of reference group behavior. In R. K. Merton & P. F. Lasarsfeld (Eds.), *Continuities in social research: Studies in the scope and method of "The American Soldier"* (pp. 40–105). Glencoe, IL: The Free Press.

Robins, L. N. (1969). Social correlates of psychiatric disorders: Can we tell causes from consequences? *Journal of Health and Social Behavior, 10,* 95–104.

Rohde, P., Lewinsohn, P. M., & Seeley, J. R. (1994). Are adolescents changed by an episode of major depression? *Journal of American Academy of Child and Adolescent Psychiatry, 9,* 1289–1298.

Rutter, M. (1986). Meyerian psychobiology, personality development, and the role of life experiences. *American Journal of Psychiatry, 143,* 1077–1087.

Southwick, S.M., Morgan, C. A., III, Nicolaou, A. L., et al. Consistency of memory for combat-related traumatic events in veterans of Operation Desert Storm. *American Journal of Psychiatry, 154,* 173–177.

Steele, C. M., & Aronson, J. (1995). Stereotype threat and the intellectual test performance of African Americans. *Journal of Personality and Social Psychology, 69,* 797–811.

Suh, E., Diener, E., & Fujita, F. (1996). Events and subjective well-being: Only recent events matter. *Journal of Personality and Social Psychology, 5,* 1091–1102.

Sutker, B. P., Allain, A. N., & Johnson, J. L. (1993). Case study: Clinical assessment of long-term cognitive and emotional sequelae to World War II prisoner-of-war confinement: Comparison of pilot twins. *Psychological Assessment, 5,* 3–10.

Thoits, P. A. (1995). Stress, coping, and social support processes: Where are we? What next? *Journal of Health and Social Behavior,* 53–79.

Visintainer, M. A., Volpicelli, J. R., & Seligman, M. E. P. (1982). Tumor rejection in rats after inescapable or escapable shock. *Science, 216,* 437–439.

Webster, M. (1961). *Webster's New Collegiate Dictionary.* Springfield, MA: C. & C. Merriam.

Wheaton, B. (1990). Life transitions, role histories, and mental health. *American Sociological Review, 55,* 209–223.

Wohlfarth, T. (1997). Socioeconomic inequality and psychopathology: Are socioeconomic status and social class interchangeable? *Social Science and Medicine, 45,* 399–410.

Zautra, A. J., & Reich, J. W. (1983). Life events and perceptions of life quality: Developments in a two-factor approach. *Journal of Community Psychology, 11,* 121–132.

Zubin, J., & Spring, B. (1977). Vulnerability: A new view of schizophrenia. *Journal of Abnormal Psychology, 86,* 103–126.

Index